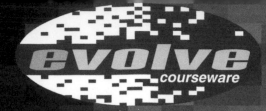

The Latest *Evolution* in Learning.

Evolve provides online access to free learning resources and activities designed specifically for the textbook you are using in your class. The resources will provide you with information that enhances the material covered in the book and much more.

Visit the Web address listed below to start your learning evolution today!

▶▶ **LOGIN:** *http://evolve.elsevier.com/Gerdin/*

Evolve Online Courseware for Gerdin, *Health Careers Today*, 3rd Edition offers the following features:

- **Web Links**
  Students and instructors can check out these sites to find out more information about health care and health care careers in the United States.

- **Image Collection**
  This collection of figures from the third edition allows instructors to provide visual tools for their students.

- **Teaching Tips and Content Updates**
  Check this feature for teaching tips from the author as well as any new and important health care career information.

Think outside the book...*evolve.*

Health Careers Today

Third Edition

Judith Gerdin, BSN, MS

Paradise Valley High School
Phoenix, Arizona

With 384 illustrations

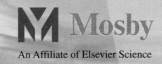

Mosby

An Affiliate of Elsevier Science

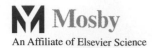

An Affiliate of Elsevier Science

11830 Westline Industrial Drive
St. Louis, Missouri 63146

HEALTH CAREERS TODAY   0-323-01867-X
Copyright © 2003, Mosby, Inc. All rights reserved.

Previous editions copyrighted 1991, 1997.

Library of Congress Cataloging in Publication Data

Gerdin, Judith A.
    Health careers today/Judith Gerdin.—3rd ed.
        p. cm.
    Includes index.
    ISBN 0-323-01867-X
      1. Medicine—Vocational guidance. 2. Allied health personnel—Vocational guidance. I. Title.

R690 .G47 2003
610.69—dc21   2002040976

Acquisitions Editor: Shirley Kuhn
Developmental Editor: Amy Holmes
Publishing Services Manager: Deborah L. Vogel
Senior Project Manager: Ann E. Rogers
Design Manager: Bill Drone

GW/QWK

Printed in The United States of America.

Last digit is the print number: 9 8 7 6 5 4 3 2 1

Dedication

To my father, Harold Gerdin, who has tirelessly researched, reviewed, and edited pages for this textbook. I would not have been able to do it without his help.

Instructor Preface

During the writing of this edition of Health Careers Today, the world, as we knew it in America, changed. The terrorism of September 11, 2001 brought a new commitment by and respect for the people who provide care for the sick and injured. We have tried to incorporate the new developments in health care that have been taken in response to that event.

Health care is evolving daily to respond to new knowledge as it is gathered. Research is finding new information that may be the cure or successful treatment for many of our health concerns. Technological innovations are announced in the news each day. Health care workers of the future will need to be able to find, evaluate, and learn to use new information and treatment techniques.

This book is divided into three units: Core Knowledge, Anatomy and Physiology, and Career Clusters. The Core Knowledge chapters provide the foundation from which all health care workers must operate. The Anatomy and Physiology chapters provide background information in health as they relate to the human body. The Career Clusters provide a sampling of information about the jobs, knowledge, and skills in each cluster area. With this book, we hope that an educated decision may be made about a career path in the health care field.

We are pleased to be partners with you in this adventure. Enjoy it.

Acknowledgments

I am always overwhelmed by the number of people to whom I owe gratitude when I finish a project. I am especially indebted to my family, for all they do for me which allows me time to work. My sisters, Karen Ellis and Susan Fathauer, my brother, Doug Gerdin, and their families provided me with emotional support and help with the daily tasks of living during the year and a half this project lasted. My aunt, Doris Cordonnier, was always available to lend an ear. My friends, Sandy Harness and Becky Laidig, kept me informed of happenings in the world of education and the health care field.

I would like to thank the staff and editors of Elsevier Science who provided the style for the book, editing, artwork, and all other parts of production. I would also like to thank my fellow workers at Paradise Valley High School, especially Cara Herkamp, who came to my rescue at the last minute to create the test bank for this work.

I must always thank my students who daily challenge me to learn something new and thereby renew my enthusiasm for and commitment to education.

Judith Gerdin, BSN, MS

Contents

Tables

Boxes

Skills

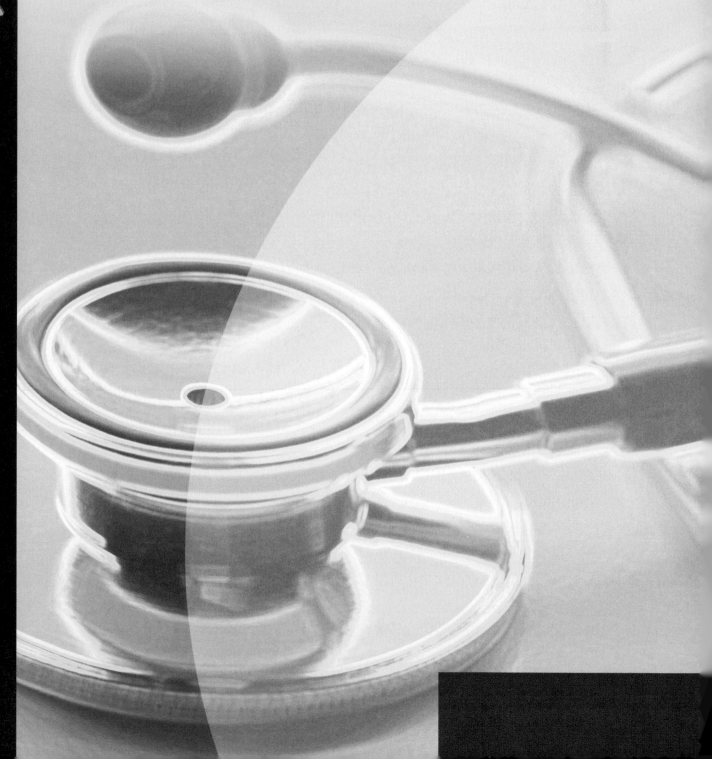

Core Knowledge

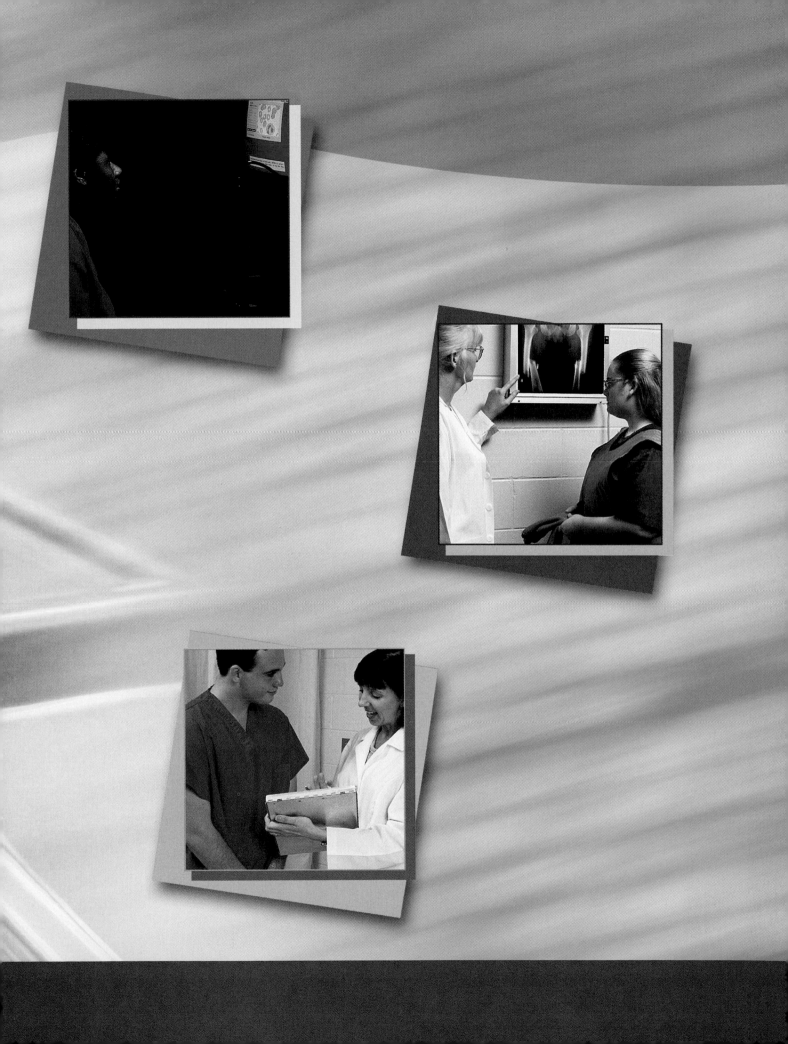

1

Health Care of the Past, Present, and Future

Learning Objectives

Define at least 10 words relating to health care of the past, present, and future.

Identify three socioeconomic factors that influence the health care industry.

Describe at least three advantages to following a career in the health care field.

Describe a career ladder for at least one health care occupation.

List at least five factors to be considered when choosing an occupation.

Identify at least five milestones in the advancement of health care.

Describe at least two factors that have contributed to the rising cost of health care.

Describe at least two methods being used to reduce health care costs.

Describe at least three types of health care services.

Key Terms

Accreditation
(uh-kred-uh-TAY-shun) Official authorization or approval

Career
(kuh-REER) Occupation or profession

Certification
(sert-uh-fuh-KAY-shen) Documentation of having met certain standards

Diagnosis-Related Grouping
(die-ug-NO-sis ree-lay-ted GROOP-ing) Predetermined payment structure for health care services established by the federal government

Health
(helth) State of optimal well-being, achieved through prevention of illness and injury

Insurance
(in-SHER-ens) Payment for health care expenses, which may or may not occur, in return for a specified payment in advance

Licensure
(LISE-en-sher) Legal authority to perform an activity

Litigation
(lit-uh-GAY-shen) Legal dispute; lawsuit

Occupation
(ahk-yoo-PAY-shen) Vocation, activity in which one participates

Paraprofessional
(par-uh-pruh-FESH-uh-nel) Worker who assists a professional in the performance of duties

Profession
(pruh-FESH-un) Occupation that requires specialized knowledge and often long and intensive academic training

Quackery
(KWAK-uh-ree) Treatment that pretends to cure disease

Registration
(rej-is-TRAY-shun) Official record of individuals qualified to perform certain services

Health Care of the Past

In the earliest civilizations, health needs were met by a specific person or group. Ancient treatments were harmful in some cases and helpful in others (Box 1-1). Some of the most helpful were the use of herbs and plants for medication. Some of these remedies, such as quinine for malaria and digitalis for heart conditions, are still in use today.

Hippocrates (460-377 BC) is considered the father of modern medicine. He initiated the oath of practice that, in adapted form, most physicians still adopt (Box 1-2).

In early times plagues or epidemics caused millions of deaths. Many of these diseases are now preventable through vaccination and improved methods of cleanliness and sanitation. Although communicable diseases still cause many deaths in less-developed countries, new technological advances are being used to provide better health care throughout the world.

Box 1-1   Medical Milestones

1518	College of Physicians is established in London.
1543	First anatomy textbook is published by Vesalius.
1590	Zacharis Janassen invents the compound microscope.
1628	William Harvey describes the circulation of blood.
1666	Anton van Leeuwenhoek uses the microscope to view microorganisms.
1670	Thomas Willis makes a connection between sugar in the urine and diabetes.
1796	Edwin Jenner develops the smallpox vaccine.
1816	Rene Laennec invents the stethoscope.
1818	James Blundel performs the first successful blood transfusion in humans.
1839	First dental school is founded in Baltimore.
1842	Crawford Long develops ether anesthesia.
1854	Florence Nightingale begins nursing soldiers and reforming the nursing profession.
1863	International Red Cross is established.
1865	Sir Joseph Lister uses asepsis in surgery.
1868	Thermometer is introduced to take body temperature.
1869	Gregor Mendel develops the laws of heredity.
1882	Robert Koch discovers that pathogens cause disease.
1887	Anne Sullivan helps Helen Keller communicate for the first time.
1893	Aspirin is developed.
1895	Wilhelm Roentgen discovers x-rays.
1898	Ronald Ross discovers that malaria is carried by mosquitoes.
1900	Blood groups are discovered.
1901	Jyokichi Takamine isolates the first hormone, adrenaline.
1910	Marie Curie isolates radium, later used to treat cancer.

1912	Sir F. Gowland Hopkins determines that some diseases are caused by lack of "accessory substances," later named vitamins.
1914	John B. Watson establishes the behaviorist theory of psychology.
1918	Francis Benedict develops a procedure to test basal metabolic rate.
1922	Frederick G. Banting treats diabetes with insulin.
1928	Sir Alexander Fleming discovers penicillin.
1937	First blood bank is established in Chicago.
1937	Alton Ochsner and Michael De Bakey link lung cancer to cigarette smoking.
1944	First kidney dialysis machine is developed.
1944	DNA is proved to be hereditary plan.
1948	Philip Hench and Edward Kendall synthesize cortisone.
1952	Jonas Salk develops a vaccine to prevent poliomyelitis.
1953	First heart-lung machine is used for successful open-heart surgery.
1953	First successful kidney transplantation is performed.
1957	Alick Isaacs and Jean Lindermann discover interferon.
1961	First continuously operating laser is developed for surgical use.
1962	Rachel Carson, in Silent Spring, describes the poisoning of the environment by pesticides.
1963	Thomas Starzl performs the first human liver transplantation.
1964	James Hardy performs the first human lung transplantation.
1966	First hormone, insulin, is synthesized.
1967	Christian Barnard performs the first successful heart transplantation.
1967	First hospice is founded in England.

Box 1-1   Medical Milestones—cont'd

1967   First penicillin-resistant pneumococcal strain is reported.

1969   Denton Cooley implants the first temporary artificial heart.

1972   Computerized axial tomography (CAT scan) is introduced.

1975   Lyme disease is reported for the first time.

1976   Legionnaire's disease outbreak occurs in Pennsylvania.

1977   Human growth hormone is produced by bacteria using recombinant DNA technology.

1978   The first "test tube" baby is born in England.

1981   AIDS is identified as a disease.

1981   First successful surgery on a fetus is performed in California.

1984   First baby is conceived from a frozen embryo in Australia.

1984   Virus that causes AIDS is identified.

1990   Genetically engineered blood cells are used to treat immune disorders, first gene therapy.

1992   Method for detection of cystic fibrosis gene is developed in England.

1993   Embryos are screened for genetic abnormalities before implantation.

1993   Human embryo is cloned.

1993   Genes that cause glaucoma, amyotropic lateral sclerosis, Mende's syndrome, colorectal cancer, xeroderma pigmentosum, Hirschsprung's disease, Canavan's disease, and Wilms' tumor are identified.

1994   Breast cancer gene (BRCA 2) and 22 mutations are identified.

1994   Test is developed for detection of colon cancer caused by mutant gene.

1994   Gene therapy is used to treat inherited form of high cholesterol.

1994   Normal gene is transferred into lungs of individual with cystic fibrosis.

1994   Scientists in Boston devise eye examination to detect Alzheimer's disease.

1997   Dolly, a sheep, is introduced as first mammal to be cloned from somatic cells.

1998   Stem cells are isolated from fetal tissues.

2000   Human genome mapping project is completed.

2001   Human embryo is created through cloning.

Box 1-2   The Hippocratic Oath

I swear by Apollo Physician, by Asclepias, by Health, by Heal All, and by all the gods and goddesses, that, according to my ability and judgment, I will keep this oath and stipulation; to reckon him who taught me this art equally dear to me as my parents, and share my substance with him and relieve his necessities if required. To regard his offspring as on the same footing with my own brothers and to teach them this art if they should wish to learn it, without fee or stipulation; and that by precept, lecture, and every other mode of instruction I will impart a knowledge of my art to my own sons and to those of my teachers and to disciples bound by a stipulation and oath according to the law of medicine, but to none others.

I will follow that method of treatment which, according to my ability and judgment, I consider for the benefit of my patients, and abstain from whatever is deleterious and mischievous. I will give no deadly medicine to anyone if asked, nor suggest any counsel.

Furthermore, I will not give to a woman an instrument to produce an abortion.

With Purity and with Holiness, I will pass my life and practice my art. I will not cut a person who is suffering with a stone, but will leave this to the practitioners of this work. Into whatever houses I enter I will go into them for the benefit of the sick and will abstain from every voluntary act of mischief and corruption; and further from the seduction of females or males, bond or free.

Whatever, in connection with my professional practice, or not in connection with it, I may see or hear in the lives of men which ought not to be spoken abroad, I will not divulge, as reckoning that all such should be kept secret.

While I continue to keep this oath inviolated, may it be granted to me to enjoy life and practice the art, respected by all men, at all times, but should I trespass and violate this oath, may the reverse be my lot.

Florence Nightingale may be credited with raising nursing to the level of a profession. Nurses were trained before her time, but not with the strong educational background that increased the respect for nurses.

When Nightingale asked to attend nursing training, her parents refused to allow it. She continued to learn on her own by visiting hospitals and finally obtained 3 months of training. She became superintendent of a small hospital and was quickly offered a position in a larger institution because of her strong views on social welfare.

In 1854, Florence Nightingale led a group of 38 nurses to travel to Turkey to care for soldiers injured in the war in which England was involved. Although the nurses were not welcomed by doctors because they were women, they improved the terrible conditions and organized and restructured the care greatly.

In 1860, the Nightingale School of Nurses opened with funding that was provided by the English government in appreciation for the service of these nurses. Nightingale believed that nursing was an art that must be founded on organized, practical, and scientific training. She taught that the person, not the disease, should be treated. Although in poor health, Nightingale lived to be 90 years of age.

In the past, the "patient" of the health care industry was a passive recipient of the treatment recommended by the health care professional. The relationship was a dependent one, with the health care provider as the guiding force. The patient often accepted without question the treatment suggested by health care providers.

Society has traditionally accorded respect to health care providers. The ancient Egyptians, Greeks, and Chinese who practiced the art of surgery or were witch doctors or neighborly herbalists all enjoyed stature in their communities. The arts of the past have become the **professions** of today (Box 1-3). These health care professions have many educational and training requirements.

Health Care of the Present

In the United States, the focus of health care has shifted from prevention of contagious diseases to those, such as cancer, drug abuse, and heart disease, that are the result of lifestyles. However, some communicable diseases are still a primary focus, including acquired immune deficiency syndrome and tuberculosis. As of December 31, 2000, the Centers for Disease Control and Prevention (CDC) report that 774,467 persons have been reported with AIDS in the United States. Of those, 448,060 have died and the status of 3,542 is unknown.

Institutional health care is provided by general hospitals, convalescent care centers, health maintenance organizations, home health agencies, and public health agencies (Table 1-1). Voluntary organizations provide education and support to individuals with specific concerns. The organizational structure of the facility defines the role of the health care worker (Figure 1-1).

The federal agency that oversees the nation's health care is the Public Health Services, which is part of the Department of Health and Human Services (HHS). It was established in 1798 to provide care for the American merchant seamen but has expanded to cover many other facets of health care (Box 1-4). The Department of Labor also regulates some health concerns through the Occupational Safety and Health Administration (OSHA).

Health care is one of the largest industries in the United States. Currently, the supply of workers is less than the demand, creating many opportunities and job security in many areas of health care. The cost of health care in the United States continues to increase much faster than other factors in the cost of living. Currently, the cost of health care is more than 14.3% of the gross national product. Two of the main reasons for rising health care costs are the advanced technological developments and the increase in malpractice **litigation.**

The United States is the only industrialized nation in the world that does not guarantee health care to all of its citizens. A third-party payer or **insurance** company assumes most health care costs. The federal government and states provide some insurance benefits for groups of the population with special needs and the elderly.

Since 1984 the federal health program for people over 65 years of age, Medicare, has reimbursed for services based on the diagnosis instead of the actual cost. **Diagnosis-related groupings** (DRGs) have greatly affected the health care industry by shortening the time allowed for treatment.

Table 1-1 Agency Health Care Providers

Agency	Service
General hospital	Provides short-term care, acute care, and diagnostic and rehabilitation services; may be for profit or nonprofit, teaching or nonteaching
Specialty hospital	Provides treatment for a specific condition such as tuberculosis, mental health disorders, or rehabilitation services
Practitioner office	Provides diagnosis, simple testing, treatments, and counseling services; may be independent or group practice
Long-term care center	Provides personal care for elderly and extended convalescent care
Outpatient care facility	Provides surgical, diagnostic, and ambulatory care
Clinic	Provides combination of practices, which may or may not be supported by public health care funding
Health maintenance	Provides health services at group rates
Home health care	Provides care in the home of the patient; may be publicly or privately owned
Hospice care	Provides medical and psychological care for the terminally ill, either in the home or at a hospice facility; may be private or part of another facility
Day care	Provides care for the elderly or children and may include care for illness
Public health care	Provides care through federal, state, and local agencies for those who cannot afford to pay for health care, and provides preventive services for the entire population
Voluntary organization	Provides research, education, and support for specific concerns; funded by donations and grants

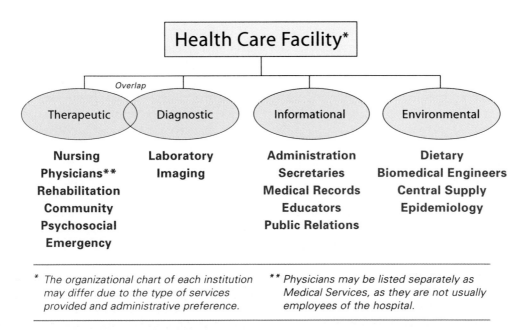

Figure 1-1 The organization structure of a health care facility.

Box 1-4 Department of Health and Human Services (HHS) Divisions and Functions

Administration for Children and Families (ACF): Responsible for programs that assist needy children and families including administration of the state-federal welfare programs such as Head Start

Administration on Aging (AOA): Provides services for elderly, including "meals on wheels"

Agency for Healthcare Research and Quality (AHRQ): Provides information through research to help people make better decisions about health care in the areas of safety, medical error, and effective service

Agency for Toxic Substances and Disease Registry (ATSDR): Conducts health studies, assessments, and education training to prevent exposure to hazardous substances in waste sites

Centers for Disease Control and Prevention (CDC): Monitors and prevents outbreaks of disease including maintaining statistics and providing immunizations

Centers for Medicare and Medicaid Services (CMS): Provides Medicare and Medicaid services for aged and indigent populations, which includes about one in every four Americans

Food and Drug Administration (FDA): Regulates safety of food, cosmetics, pharmaceutical, biological products, and medical devices

Health Resources and Services Administration (HRSA): Provides services for underserved populations such as the migrant, homeless, public housing residents. This division is also responsible for the organ transplantation system, infant mortality and services to people with AIDS.

Indian Health Service (IHS): Supports the hospitals and health centers that provide care to 557 federally recognized tribes of American Indians and Alaska Natives

National Institutes of Health (NIH): Supports more than 35,000 research projects in diseases such as cancer, diabetes, and AIDS

Program Support Center (PSC): Provides service-for-fee support services such as training and grant administration throughout the federal government

Substance Abuse and Mental Health Services Administration (SAMHSA): Works to improve substance abuse and mental health prevention and services

---

Insurance companies have established options designed to lower cost coverage, including health maintenance organizations (HMOs), preferred provider organizations (PPOs), and larger deductibles for individuals paying for insurance independently. Employers have reduced benefits and shifted the cost of health care to the employee. Others offer a "cafeteria-style" selection from which employees may choose various types of coverage up to a specified cost limit (Figure 1-2).

Hospitals are meeting the challenge of increased cost by becoming large corporate facilities and by forming partnerships with physicians for services such as extended care. Many smaller hospitals have been forced to close or sell to larger corporations, which, because of their size, have better buying power. Some hospitals have refused care for patients who have conditions or diagnoses for which treatment is not financially profitable.

The rise in professional malpractice insurance has contributed greatly to the increase in health care costs. To prevent the risk of liability, some physicians practice defensive medicine, such as ordering many tests and avoiding care for high-risk patients. In the field of obstetrics, the cost has led some physicians to stop delivering babies. In many states the obstetrician has been held financially responsible for children up to 18 or 21 years of age for damage that may have occurred at birth. Studies indicate that, in most of the court cases, the abnormalities were not related to medical care.

Pharmaceutical companies are also using defensive economic strategies by reducing the manufacture of valuable drugs that have a high risk of adverse affects. Only one company is now manufacturing vaccines because of the actual and potential litigation resulting from adverse reactions to these drugs. The Federal Drug Administration (FDA) requires extensive testing of drugs before allowing their use. The Orphan Drug Act allows the FDA to release some drugs early to meet needs of the ill when other medications have not been developed for the disease.

Health care in the United States is influenced by the state of the economy, the values of society, the law of supply and demand, and technological developments. The industry, patients, and workers are currently adapting to the new technologies and challenges of an advanced society. Health is no longer considered to be just the absence of ill-

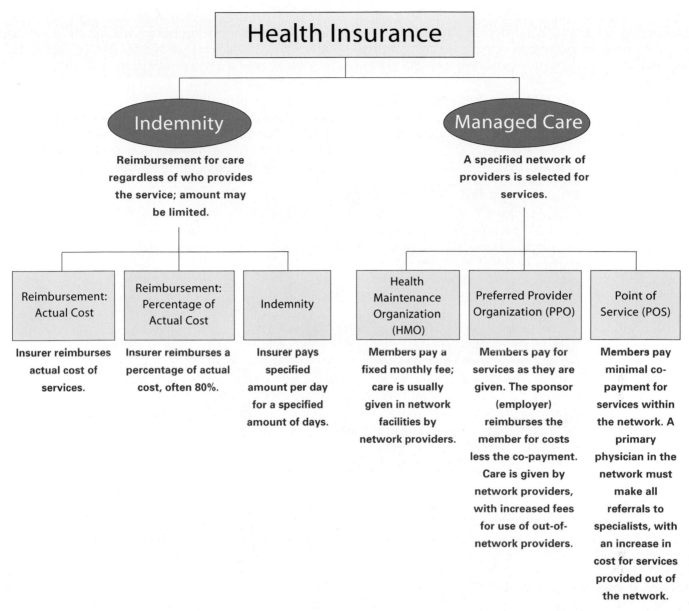

Figure 1-2   Health care insurance model.

ness or injury. **Health** is a state of optimal well-being, achieved through prevention of illness and injury. The health care workers of today are concerned with the physical, emotional, and social needs of their patients.

Those who choose a **career** in the health field seek more than economic security. Other factors to consider include the nature of the duties, the working conditions, and the opportunities for advancement in health care **occupations.** It is also important to know the number and location of jobs, methods and qualifications for employment, and the psychosocial factors involved in the work. Health care provides an opportunity to work with people, data, or things

to complement the interests and abilities of the worker (Figure 1-3).

Most health care careers provide the worker with an opportunity to meet new challenges, enjoy a stable salary and employment, and to move to new locations. Jobs in health care offer a good working environment, and the workers are respected by others. Many people have reached top-level positions in health care through a series of occupations or a career ladder, both of which provide experience and support during the process. Advancement is based usually on additional experience, education, and training (Table 1-2).

With the advances in technology, the need for a strong academic background and continuing education is even more critical for the health care worker. Those in **paraprofessional** careers help provide care to more people. For example, the physician assistant, nurse practitioner, and midwife provide more care than in the past, especially in rural areas. Prehospital emergency care has become a new area of practice. The knowledge and technology that make it possible to save many trauma victims have created many new career opportunities.

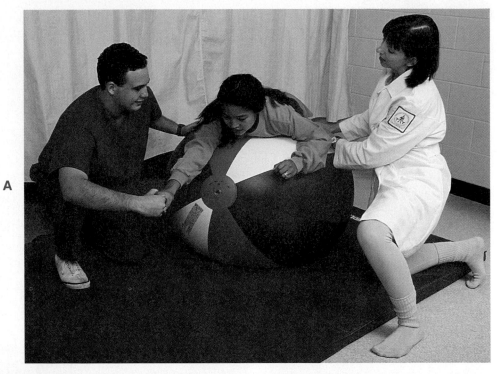

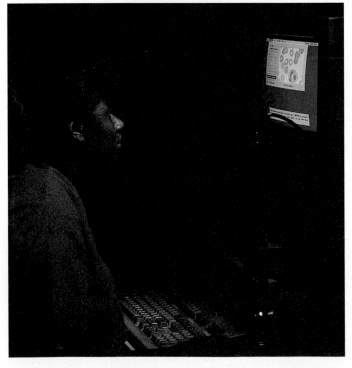

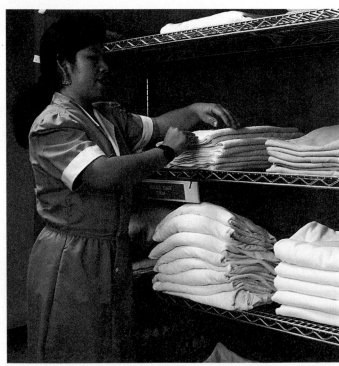

Figure 1-3   Health care today provides a variety of working conditions for employees who want to work with **A,** people; **B,** data; or **C,** things.

The "patient" of today has become a "client" or consumer of health care services. A shift in responsibilities has resulted in the client's taking more responsibility for his or her own care. In 1972 the American Hospital Association adopted the "Patient's Bill of Rights," which describes the rights of the client to participate in the system of care (Box 1-5). Obtaining second opinions, shopping for the lowest health care costs, and seeking alternative and complementary providers have become common practice.

Clients of health care of today are consumers with a greater awareness of the effect of their lifestyle on related health conditions. To avoid confusion, the term *patient* will be used throughout this text.

As those seeking care have more critical needs, advanced skills are required of workers. Professional associations and government agencies set standards to ensure the quality of education and training. Agencies of **accreditation** have been established to determine if a training pro-

Table 1-2   Career Ladder in Health Care

Title	Educational Requirement	Example
Aide	On-the-job training	Laboratory aide
Assistant	Up to 1 year of classroom and clinical preparation	Laboratory assistant
Technician	A 2-year community college or vocational training program	Laboratory technician
Technologist	A 3- to 4-year college program	Laboratory technologist
Professional	A 4-year degree, advanced degree, and clinical training	Pathologist (medical doctor)

Box 1-5   Patient's Bill of Rights

The American Hospital Association presents a Patient's Bill of Rights with the expectation that it will contribute to more effective patient care and be supported by the hospital on behalf of the institution, its medical staff, employees, and patients. The American Hospital Association encourages health care institutions to tailor this bill of rights to their community by translating and/or simplifying the language of this bill of rights as may be necessary to ensure that patients and their families understand their rights and responsibilities.

1. The patient has the right to considerate and respectful care.
2. The patient has the right to and is encouraged to obtain from physicians and other direct care givers relevant, current, and understandable information concerning diagnosis, treatment, and prognosis.

Except in emergencies when the patient lacks decision-making capacity and the need for treatment is urgent, the patient is entitled to the opportunity to discuss and request information related to the specific procedures and/or treatments, the risks involved, the possible length of recuperation, and the medically reasonable alternatives and their risks and benefits.

Patients have the right to know the identity of physicians, nurses, and others involved in their care, as well as when those involved are students, residents, or other trainees. The patient also has the right to know the immediate and long-term financial implications of treatment choices insofar as they are known.

3. The patient has the right to make decisions about the plan of care prior to and during the course of

Continued

Box 1-5   Patient's Bill of Rights—cont'd

treatment and to refuse a recommended treatment or plan of care to the extent permitted by law and hospital policy and to be informed of the medical consequences of this action. In case of such refusal, the patient is entitled to other appropriate care and services that the hospital provides or transfer to another hospital. The hospital should notify patients of any policy that might affect patient choice within the institution.

4. The patient has the right to have an advance directive (such as a living will, health care proxy, or durable power of attorney for health care) concerning treatment or designating a surrogate decision maker with the expectation that the hospital will honor the intent of that directive to the extent permitted by law and hospital policy.

   Health care institutions must advise patients of their rights under state law and hospital policy to make informed medical choices, ask if the patient has an advance directive, and include that information in the patient records. The patient has a right to timely information about hospital policy that may limit its ability to implement fully a legally valid advance directive.

5. The patient has a right to every consideration of privacy. Case discussion, consultation, examination, and treatment should be conducted so as to protect each patient's privacy.

6. The patient has the right to expect that all communications and records pertaining to his or her care will be treated as confidential by the hospital, except in cases such as suspected abuse and public health hazards when reporting is permitted or required by law. The patient has the right to expect that the hospital will emphasize the confidentiality of this information when it releases to other parties entitled to review information in these records.

7. The patient has the right to review records pertaining to his or her medical care and to have the information explained or interpreted as necessary, except when restricted by law.

8. The patient has the right to expect that, within its capacity and policies, a hospital will make reasonable response to the request of a patient for ap-

propriate and medically indicated care and services. The hospital must provide evaluation, service, and/or referral as indicated by the urgency of the case. When medically appropriate and legally permissible, or when a patient has so requested, a patient may be transferred to another facility. The institution to which the patient is transferred must first have accepted the patient for transfer. The patient must also have the benefit of complete information and explanation concerning the need for, risks, benefits, and alternatives to such a transfer.

9. The patient has the right to ask and be informed of the existence of business relationships among the hospital, educational institution, other health care providers, and payers that may influence the patient's care and treatment.

10. The patient has the right to consent or decline to participate in proposed research studies or human experimentation affecting care and treatment or requiring direct patient involvement, and to have those studies fully explained prior to consent. A patient who declines to participate in research or experimentation is entitled to the most effective care that the hospital can otherwise provide.

11. The patient has the right to expect reasonable continuity of care when appropriate and to be informed by physicians and other care givers of available and realistic patient care options when hospital care is no longer appropriate.

12. The patient has the right to be informed of hospital policies and practices that relate to patient care, treatment, and responsibilities. The patient has the right to be informed of available resources for resolving disputes, grievances, and conflicts, such as ethics committees, patients' representatives, or other mechanisms available in the institution. The patient has the right to be informed of the hospital's charges for services and available payment methods.

gram meets acceptable standards. The professional associations of the health care occupation provide most agencies of accreditation. Recently, the federal government has required specific training for nursing assistants working in extended care facilities.

Many occupational areas are regulated by law to ensure that the quality of care is acceptable. Health workers may need **licensure, certification,** or **registration** to practice. Licensure is controlled by the state and is usually based on successful completion of an examination. Certification, which may be given by an agency or a training program, indicates successful completion of a particular course. Individuals who have met a criterion of excellence or legal responsibility may be registered in some fields. Registration may be earned through the state or an agency. It is illegal to practice without holding the proper credentials in the professions that are regulated.

Health Care of the Future

All people in the United States use the health care system during their lifetime. Health care of the future will continue to emphasize wellness and prevention instead of cure. Wellness services will include nutritional advice, stress reduction counseling, habit cessation management, and exercise instruction (Box 1-6). Technology will continue to drive the type and pace of changes in the industry.

One main area of service in the future will be care of the elderly. The population of the United States continues to age and live longer. With fewer children being born each year, the average age of an American has risen to 34 and will continue to increase. It has been predicted that 20% of the US population will be over 65 years of age by 2030. The elderly require three times the amount of health care as those in younger groups. Many older people experience at least one chronic disease, and about half the elderly are limited in movement in some manner. Health care of the future will provide rehabilitative services for the elderly population.

More small hospitals will close their doors, and the number of large urban institutions and state-of-the-art intensive care units will increase. Hospitals will continue to provide care for only the severely ill and injured and will reduce the number of beds for other patients who will be treated in other settings, especially home care.

Alternative providers and treatments will continue to develop. One alternative that has gained increased popularity and acceptance is holistic health. In this type of care, patients are seen as being responsible for their own care and as unique people. Holistic health care uses many methods of diagnosis and treatment, of which traditional

---

Box 1-6   The Leading Health Indicators*

- Physical activity
- Overweight and obesity
- Tobacco use
- Substance abuse
- Responsible sexual behavior
- Mental health
- Injury and violence
- Environmental quality
- Immunization
- Access to health care

*The leading health indicators were selected to reflect the major health concerns in the United States at the beginning of the twenty-first century by the Healthy People 2010 project.

---

medical practice is just one. The National Institutes of Health (NIH) is currently providing research money for unconventional therapies through the Office of Alternative Medicine. These therapies include the use of bee pollen to control asthma, acupuncture for depression, hypnosis to speed bone healing, yoga to control addiction, and shark cartilage to reduce tumors. Development of alternative provisions may lead to an increase in the incidence of **quackery** as patients look for alternative treatments (Box 1-7).

In 1994 the Congress considered and rejected a comprehensive health care proposal. Some of the problems in the current methods of coverage addressed by the plan included health care for everyone and for every condition (universal coverage). The primary debate centered on whether health care is a "public good," such as schooling or a commodity to be purchased by those who can afford it. In 2001 Congress considered a Patient Bill of Rights that would allow the consumer to hold HMOs legally responsible for treatment choices and practices. Other provisions of the law would have allowed health care patients to seek care at the nearest emergency room, obtain perinatal care without a referral, and use a pediatrician as the primary physician for children.

The impact of technology can only be imagined for the future. Some innovations that may become common include the inventions of nanotechnology and telemedicine. It is now possible for a physician to view the intestines from the inside after the patient swallows a small camera.

Box 1-7   Twenty-Five Ways to Spot Quacks and Vitamin Pushers*

How can food quacks and other vitamin pushers be recognized? Here are 25 signs that should arouse suspicion:

1. When talking about nutrients, they tell only part of the story.
2. They claim that most Americans are poorly nourished.
3. They recommend "Nutrition Insurance" for everyone.
4. They say that most diseases are due to faulty diet and can be treated with "nutritional" methods.
5. They allege that modern processing methods and storage remove all nutritive value from our food.
6. They claim that diet is a major factor in behavior.
7. They claim that fluoridation is dangerous.
8. They claim that soil depletion and the use of pesticides and "chemical" fertilizers result in food that is less safe and less nourishing.
9. They claim you are in danger of being "poisoned" by ordinary food additives and preservatives.
10. They charge that the Recommended Dietary Allowances (RDAs) have been set too low.
11. They claim that under everyday stress, and in certain diseases, your need for nutrients is increased.
12. They recommend "supplements" and "health foods" for everyone.
13. They claim that "natural" vitamins are better than "synthetic" ones.
14. They suggest that a questionnaire can be used to indicate whether you need dietary supplements.
15. They say it is easy to lose weight.
16. They promise quick, dramatic, miraculous results.
17. They routinely sell vitamins and other "dietary supplements" as part of their practice.
18. They use disclaimers couched in pseudomedical jargon.
19. They use anecdotes and testimonials to support their claims.
20. They claim that sugar is a deadly poison.
21. They display credentials not recognized by responsible scientists or educators.
22. They offer to determine your body's nutritional state with a laboratory test or a questionnaire.
23. They claim they are being persecuted by orthodox medicine and that their work is being suppressed because it's controversial.
24. They warn you not to trust your doctor.
25. They encourage patients to lend political support to their treatment methods.

Courtesy Stephen Barrett, MD, Allentown, Penn.
*Written by Stephen Barrett, MD, and Victor Herbert, MD, JD.

Some forms of blindness will be cured with a microchip within 10 years. Some patients are receiving daily monitoring of health care conditions through remote data collection and consultations using computers. Distance surgery has been performed using similar technology. Recombinant DNA techniques will allow new types of gene therapy and fetal stem cell research. Technology will stimulate controversy such as that over the use of cloning of humans and their organs.

The Internet provides the patient with a wealth of information about a condition or disease. The information may or may not come from a reputable health care practitioner. It gives the consumer access to clinical trials and research results. It also provides a way to buy pharmaceuticals, which may or may not be effective. With the increase use of computers and technology in health care, the issue of privacy of information will become a central concern of the future.

The health care team will become more responsible for relieving some of the ills of society, such as the "border babies" and other abandoned children. Border babies are well infants who are left in hospitals because their mothers are unable to care for them because of drug addiction or poverty. Some states have passed laws that allow a mother to abandon a baby at a site designated a "safe haven" without fear of legal repercussions.

The worker of the future must be trained for a broad range of skills and know about many areas of care (Figure 1-4). Additionally, the worker must be flexible, know how to solve problems as they arise, and use independent judgment. The worker must be willing to continue to learn and to adapt to new technologies. The health care workers of the future will be highly regulated to ensure the quality of care that is provided. Technicians will continue to be trained to become multicompetent and thus able to offer more than one kind of service. Expanded skills for health

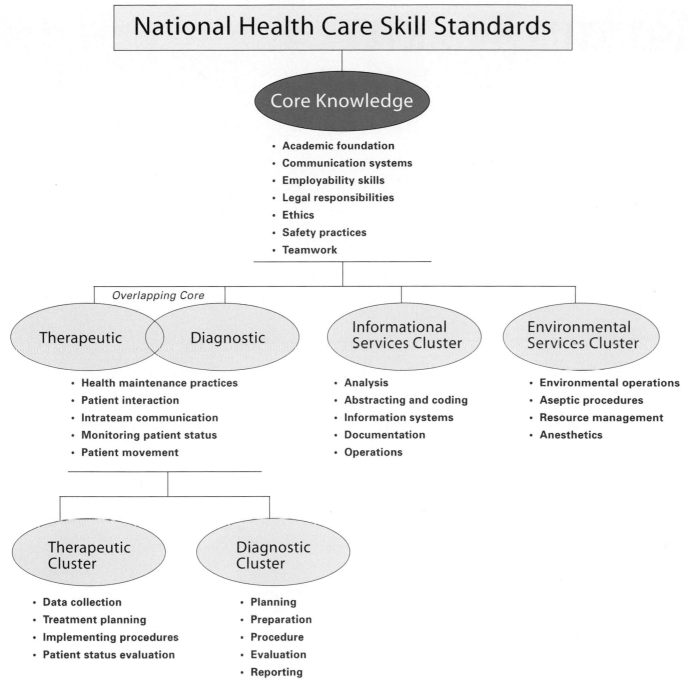

National Health Care Skill Standards

Core Knowledge

- **Academic foundation**
- **Communication systems**
- **Employability skills**
- **Legal responsibilities**
- **Ethics**
- **Safety practices**
- **Teamwork**

Overlapping Core

Therapeutic   Diagnostic

- **Health maintenance practices**
- **Patient interaction**
- **Intrateam communication**
- **Monitoring patient status**
- **Patient movement**

Informational Services Cluster

- **Analysis**
- **Abstracting and coding**
- **Information systems**
- **Documentation**
- **Operations**

Environmental Services Cluster

- **Environmental operations**
- **Aseptic procedures**
- **Resource management**
- **Anesthetics**

Therapeutic Cluster

- **Data collection**
- **Treatment planning**
- **Implementing procedures**
- **Patient status evaluation**

Diagnostic Cluster

- **Planning**
- **Preparation**
- **Procedure**
- **Evaluation**
- **Reporting**

Figure 1-4   National health care skill standard model. *(Courtesy WestEd, San Francisco, Calif.)*

practitioners will be used in many facilities, especially in small hospitals as less professional and more technical staff are employed.

On September 11, 2001, the World Trade Center and Pentagon suffered attack by terrorists, killing more than 3,000 people. After that date, several cases of anthrax occurred in various parts of the country. The health care team will need to make adjustments with the rest of society to deal with this new phase of American history. Emergency care providers and procedures will grow in number and specialization to deal with the reality of bioterrorism. Additionally, security measures for research in addition to health care facilities will be a concern along with all other public facilities.

Review Questions

1. The term that best describes the worker who assists the professional would be the _____.

2. The term that describes an occupation that requires specialized education and training is _____.

3. Research does not support the claim that static magnets are effective in relieving pain. What term best describes the use and sale of such magnets?

4. Compare the meaning of the terms *certification* and *licensure.*

5. List three factors of society that influence the health care industry.

6. Describe five advantages to pursuing a career in the health field.

7. Describe the factors that should be considered in choosing an occupation.

8. Describe the influence of advanced technology, malpractice coverage, and expanded roles of the health care industry on increased health care costs.

9. Compare the educational preparation and level of responsibility of the assistant, technician, technologist, and professional.

10. Identify at least three occupations in each area of the hospital organization.

Critical Thinking

1. Defend or deny the idea that the microscope is the most important milestone in health care.

2. Investigate the cost of malpractice insurance for five health care professionals. Hypothesize reasons why the rates for some professions such as neurosurgery and gynecology are higher than others.

3. Use medical milestones (Box 1-1) to trace the development of a treatment modality in health care. For example, trace the development of transplantation of organs or gene therapy. Synthesize the information gained to predict the future of this type of health care treatment.

4. Investigate a person famous for a health care discovery. Using information gathered about the person's life, form a hypothesis as to the events that led the person to that discovery.

5. Investigate the use of advanced technologies such as cloning or stem cell research. Develop guidelines for the safe use of this technology.

6. Investigate a form of alternative or complementary treatment to determine its use and effectiveness. Design an experiment or research project that would prove or disprove the usefulness of the treatment.

2

Interpersonal Dynamics and Communication

Learning Objectives

Define at least 10 words relating to the health care worker's characteristics and abilities.

Describe the relationship among values, attitudes, and behavior.

Describe the hierarchy of needs established by Abraham Maslow.

Identify at least five methods of maintaining good personal health and professional appearance.

Use a problem-solving system to make a decision that involves identification of alternatives, risks, and evaluation of the outcome.

Identify the elements of effective communication and at least three factors that might interfere with it.

Describe at least one example of assertive communication that requests a change in behavior.

Key Terms

Attitude
(AT-ih-tood) Mental position or feeling with regard to a fact or situation

Behavior
(be-HAY-vyer) Manner of conducting oneself

Character
(KARE-ik-ter) Distinctive qualities that make up an individual

Communication
(kuh-myoo-ni-KAY-shun) Exchange of information

Habit
(HA-bit) Act performed voluntarily without conscious thought

Hierarchy
(HI-er-ark-ee) Graded or ranked series

Nonverbal
(non-VER-bul) Communicating without using language

Personality
(per-sun-AL-it-ee) Set of traits, characteristics, and behaviors that make each person unique

Value
(VAL-yoo) Rate of usefulness, importance, or general worth

Verbal
(VER-bul) Relating to or consisting of words or sounds

Interpersonal Dynamics

To provide adequate care, the health care worker must be able to recognize and accept the values, attitudes, and beliefs unique to each person. The health care worker must be able to communicate effectively, provide leadership when needed, and use technological equipment. The health care worker also must maintain the ethical code of the profession and be aware of the legal considerations of health care. More than any other single characteristic, the health care professional of the future must be flexible to adapt to the changing industry. The industry is changing daily because of new medical discoveries, technological advances, and evolving health concerns.

Interpersonal skills allow an individual to relate with friends, family, co-workers, and patients. Some skills helpful in interpersonal relationships include the ability to communicate well, act independently by making decisions, and demonstrate sincere compassion for others.

Self-Awareness

Understanding and accepting the differences that exist between people of different backgrounds relies on an understanding of one's own values and motives. Understanding and accepting the self leads to development of high self-esteem. Psychologists believe that how a person thinks about an experience determines the feelings and behaviors that result because of the event. Each mentally healthy person can choose the feelings that result from events that occur in life.

Personality is the sum of the traits, characteristics, and behaviors that make each individual unique. **Behavior** is the action of an individual that can be seen by others. Society prefers some behaviors to others. **Habits** are acts that are performed voluntarily but without conscious thought. Habits can be changed by repetitive behavior changes. Many behaviors result from habit and can be changed by the individual.

The behavior that an individual displays in a situation is seen as a reflection of an **attitude**. Attitudes are the mental views or feelings formed by an individual or group. With new information and experience, individuals can change their attitudes.

Attitudes are formed from personal **values.** Values make up the system each individual uses to measure or evaluate the worth of ideas, people, and things in the world. They are formed early in life as a result of the environment and experience. Values are difficult to change. An undesirable value such as prejudice may not even be recognized by the individual who holds it (Figure 2-1). The sum of the behavior, attitudes, and values that a person exhibits to others is called **character.**

The patient and other caregivers expect certain characteristics, attitudes, and behaviors in the health care worker (Box 2-1). Undesirable behavior can be changed if it is recognized and if the desired behavior is practiced.

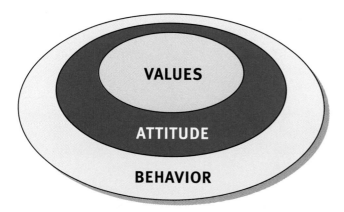

Figure 2-1   Values form the basis on which attitudes are molded. Attitudes are reflected by behavior. Behavior is made up of the actions seen by others.

Box 2-1   Characteristics of the Health Care Worker

- Communicates concisely and accurately in a clear, well-modulated voice
- Dresses neatly and appropriately
- Maintains controlled and upright posture
- Promotes good health through lifestyle
- Shows patience and poise when under pressure
- Remains tactful and courteous at all times
- Has sincere interest in and tries to understand others
- Takes responsibility for own actions
- Exhibits reliability, perseveres to accomplish tasks
- Is able and willing to follow directions
- Is flexible when changes in routine are necessary
- Displays humor but not at the expense of others
- Accepts criticism and makes an effort to improve
- Maintains ethical conduct including promptness, honesty, care of equipment, and respect for the organization's policies
- Shows initiative in tasks but knows limits of practice and does not exceed them

Hierarchy of Needs

Psychologist Abraham Maslow established a **hierarchy** of human needs that is still widely used to understand behavior (Figure 2-2). Maslow stated that people strive to meet their most basic needs first. Once these needs are met, the higher levels of needs can be attempted. Unless the more basic needs of physical security and social concerns are met, the individual cannot establish a feeling of self-respect and worth. Unless self-respect and an inner worth are felt, the individual will neither take the risks necessary for personal growth nor set goals to reach self-fulfillment or self-actualization.

Personal Health

Good personal health is basic for an individual to establish high self-esteem. The World Health Organization defines health as a state of physical, mental, and social well-being. It is not just the absence of illness or injury. The foundation of good personal health, cleanliness, is maintained by a daily routine that includes bathing, using a deodorant, shampooing the hair, and cleaning the teeth (Table 2-1). Nutrition, exercise, sleep, posture, eye care, and good personal habits are also needed to maintain good health. Some specific daily behaviors that indicate good personal grooming include the use of mouthwash, shaving, nail care, change of undergarments, and clean clothing that fits properly. Health care workers wear min-imal jewelry to prevent both its loss and the spread of microorganisms.

People form first impressions based on personal appearance. This impression is then modified by the behavior that is observed. Patients notice the personal appearance of the health care worker's face, hair, nails, dress, odor, skin, posture, and teeth. Appearance reflects self-esteem and how workers view themselves. The appearance of the health care worker is doubly important because it represents the employer and the worker.

Stress and Time Management

Health care is one of the most stressful occupations. The work affects the most fundamental part of the client's and health care worker's lives. One of the first psychologists who studied stress related disease was Claude Bernard. He proposed that the body has an "internal milieu" or need to maintain a consistent internal environment. Canon used the term *homeostasis* to describe the body's self-regulating processes including the "fight or flight" reaction to stress. Hans Seyle noted that many diseases share similar signs and symptoms such as fatigue, weight loss, aches, and gastrointestinal problems. He stated that these result from a general stress reaction that results from increased adrenal gland secretions, shrinkage of lymphatic tissues, and increased secretion of hydrochloric acid in the stomach. Seyle proposed that illness results from too small or too

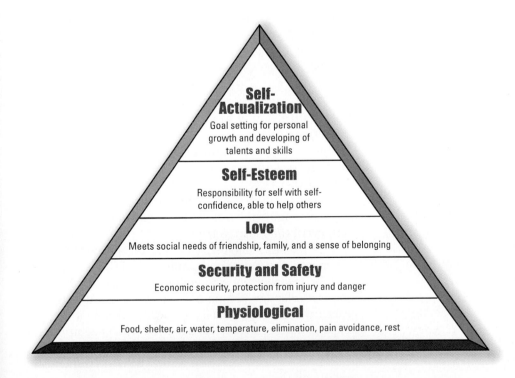

Figure 2-2 Maslow's Hierarchy of Needs.

Table 2-1 Good Grooming Habits for Health Care Workers

Habit	Action
Oral hygiene	Brush at least twice daily, and use mouthwash once daily
Hair care	Shampoo regularly, style hair away from the face and off the collar
Skin care	Cleanse regularly; treat rashes, blemishes
	Wear nylons or socks to prevent skin shedding (exfoliation)
	Use lotion to prevent drying
	Use antiperspirant, no perfume
Nail care	Clean nails, trim close to fingertips
	Use minimal or no polish color
Clothing	Appropriate, modest
	Clean, pressed, well fitting
	Mended, comfortable, allowing movement
	Undergarments changed daily, well fitted, not visible through clothing
	Minimal or no jewelry
	Name pin and watch in place
Foot care	Socks or stockings clean daily
	Toenails trimmed regularly
	Shoes cleaned and polished
	Shoes sturdy, nonskid, low heeled with closed toes

Box 2-2 Stress Management Techniques

- Plan and organize your workload. Use time management techniques.
- When possible, do things one at a time until they are completed.
- Occasionally, plan to escape and have fun.
- Be positive about things, and avoid criticizing others.
- Avoid unnecessary competition. Learn to negotiate.
- Get regular exercise.
- Tolerate, forgive, and learn to accept others.
- Talk to someone about things that are troubling you.
- Use relaxation methods such as biofeedback or deep breathing.

large of a reaction by the body's stress adaptation mechanism (Table 2-2).

Some methods used to manage stress include proper nutrition, exercise, relaxation techniques, and personal behavior changes (Box 2-2). Stress is not the result of events that occur but rather the attitudes that are formed about the events. Another stress management technique includes methods of time management.

Time management uses organization of a schedule to maximize effectiveness and productivity. The key to effective time management is planning. The basic tool for planning is a calendar. Setting both short-term and long-term goals increases the probability of accomplishment of them. Keeping focused on the goal helps the person complete the action steps needed to reach it. Learning and meeting the behavioral expectations of the setting help the worker concentrate on the task at hand.

Table 2-2 Stress-Related Illness

Body Process	Effect of Stress
Cardiovascular system	Heart attack (myocardial infarction)
	High blood pressure (hypertension)
	Heart pain (angina)
	Migraine headache
	Stroke (cerebrovascular accident)
Digestive system	Ulcer
	Colitis
	Constipation, diarrhea
Skeletal system	Arthritis
Muscular system	Headache
	Backache
Respiratory system	Asthma
Endocrine system	Diabetes (non–insulin dependent)
Nervous system	Accident proneness (decreased attention)
Immune process	Increased rate of infection
	Allergies
	Autoimmune disorders
Psychosocial process	Fighting and conflicts
	Alcoholism and drug abuse

Box 2-3 Model for Problem Solving and Decision Making

1. Recognize that a problem exists. Recognition may result from a feeling, observation, or conversation with others.
2. Describe the problem and clarify *what* the basic issue or question is and the factors that affect it. Identify *who* is involved, *where* the problem exists, and *when* and *how* it occurs.
3. Identify alternative methods of resolving the problem. Any alternative can be considered even if it is not immediately seen as practical.
4. Choose the best method for resolving the problem and implement it.
5. As the plan is being implemented, evaluate the results and adjust the method if necessary.

Box 2-4 Elements of Critical Thinking

- Ask questions
- Define a problem
- Examine evidence
- Avoid emotional reasoning
- Analyze assumptions and bias
- Avoid oversimplification
- Consider other interpretations
- Tolerate ambiguity
- Think about one's own thinking

Problem Solving

Problem solving is one method that can be used to make decisions (Box 2-3). It is based on evaluation of the factors involved in the decision, the risks, and possible solutions. The problem must first be well understood and clarified. Once the problem is identified, brainstorming is one way to seek possible solutions. Brainstorming generates but does not evaluate the practicality of ideas. The ideas can then be considered and possible solutions evaluated, based on the risks and consequences of each. When chosen, the solution can then be implemented and the results can be evaluated for use in making future decisions. Most problems and decisions have more than one solution. The merit of each decision can be evaluated only by its results.

Critical Thinking

Critical thinking has been identified as a necessary competency for workers in health care. It includes the ability to think creatively, make decisions, solve problems, visualize situational descriptions, learn new information, and reason (Box 2-4). Most formal definitions of critical thinking characterize it as the intentional application of rational, higher-order thinking skills. Critical thinking focuses on the application of logical concepts to everyday reasoning and problem-solving. Critical thinking skills allow the health care worker to apply concrete information, such as facts of anatomy and physiology, and draw conclusions to determine the kind of care that would be best for a patient.

Leadership

In an organization, a group of individuals joins together to reach a goal by cooperation and division of tasks among themselves. Groups can accomplish goals faster and more easily than individuals. An organizational chart shows the relationships among, and the roles of, the members.

Organizational frameworks may be planned using management practices and theories. This is usually called *organizational development*. The goal of organizational development is to increase productivity, quality, and worker satisfaction. The health care worker plays an important part in the health care organization by setting goals, meeting challenges, and implementing ideas.

The Team

Health care workers participate as a team to provide care for the patient. Members of the team have differing responsibilities. Some members provide direct care, working in contact with the patient, whereas others may not ever see the individual. Nevertheless, all members of the team are important in providing the best care possible for the patient.

The National Health Care Standards describe four clusters for careers in health occupations. The diagnostic careers provide a picture of the patient's health status and include technicians in radiology, medical, dental laboratory, and cardiography. The therapeutic careers provide treatment over time and include such providers as physicians, dentists, veterinarians, nurses, pharmacologists, and emergency personnel. Information careers process data and provide documents; these include administration, secretaries, and medical records personnel. Environmental careers provide a supportive environment for the patient and include nutrition services, central supply, and facility management personnel.

Communication

Communication is the sharing of an idea or information that results in understanding. Reading, writing, hearing, touching, and seeing are various forms of communication. If it involves language, communication is said to be **verbal,** and if it does not, then it is called **nonverbal.** Communication can take place on a one-to-one basis, in small groups, or with a large audience. Mass communication reaches large groups of people through television, radio, film, and newspapers.

In health care, communication between workers is completed in a professional and precise manner. The health

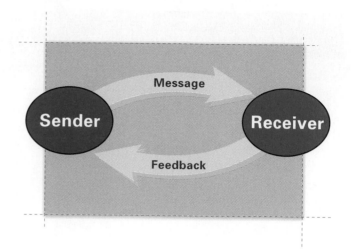

Figure 2-3   Feedback helps the receiver make certain that the message was understood.

care worker must determine to whom a message is being given before choosing the correct words to use. For example, the patient might not understand the medical term *hypertension,* but a colleague would immediately know that this word means high blood pressure. The goal of the health care worker's communication to other members of the team is to convey information concisely and accurately. In the health care team, there is usually a "chain of command" or hierarchy of practitioners. The assistant, for example, may not report directly to the department head but through a team leader. This chain of command is structured to provide the department head with concise information and provide the assistant-level workers with immediate supervisory guidance as needed. Each organization has its own structure for communication and leadership that must be learned by every new health care employee.

Verbal Communication

Effective communication may be defined as a shared understanding of a message. Effective communication consists of three parts. These are the sender, the message, and the receiver (Figure 2-3). The English language is made up of approximately 100,000 words, of which most people use 30,000 to 60,000. Of these, 5000 have a double meaning. It is estimated that 7% of a message is conveyed by words, 38% by the tone of voice, and 55% by nonverbal behavior. The message also may be distorted because of interference from the sender, receiver, or the environment. The quality of care given to a patient is often perceived on the basis of effective communication.

Feedback is a method to determine if the message was received accurately. Feedback is a response by the receiver to indicate how the information was understood. One factor that may influence the communication process is the attitude of each person. Communication attitudes are based

---

Box 2-5   Attitudes and Behaviors That Act as Barriers to Effective Communication

- Advising
- Closed-mindedness
- Commanding
- Distracting
- Judging
- Lecturing
- Moralizing
- Name calling

- Offering solutions
- Off-on listening (tuning out)
- Ordering
- Preaching
- Prejudging
- Red-flag listening (reacting automatically to certain words)

- Speaker-centeredness instead of subject-centeredness
- Stereotyping
- Teaching
- Threatening
- Warning

Box 2-6   Guidelines to Avoid Defensive Communication

- Be descriptive rather than critical of observed behaviors.
- Speak in terms of beliefs in viewpoints rather than certainties of rightness.
- Be spontaneous rather than manipulative. Don't have a preconceived outcome of the conversation.
- Communicate on an equal basis rather than as a superior.
- Approach the discussion with a goal of mutual problem solving rather than controlling the other person.
- Speak with empathy, showing concern for the other person.

Box 2-7   Good Listening Guidelines

- Allow the other person to talk more than half of the time.
- Listen thoughtfully. Try to see the other person's point of view.
- Speak your mind freely. Say what you mean. If you disagree, say so in a friendly manner.
- If you don't understand what is being discussed, ask for clarification. Use examples and paraphrasing as needed.
- Be prepared for the discussion. Bring notes if necessary to remember all points.
- Keep an open, friendly posture even when in disagreement.
- Don't argue if the dispute is over a fact or record. Have someone look it up.
- Evaluate the discussion for accomplishments and feelings.
- Be patient in allowing the other person time to form his or her thoughts.
- Do not display anger during communication.
- Find a quiet location to talk or remove distractions.
- Speak slowly, softly, and clearly.
- Look for the humor in negative situations if appropriate.

---

on previous knowledge, culture, and the communication skills of the sender and receiver. The complexity of the message is also a factor as is interference such as noise from the environment. Some attitudes may block effective communication (Box 2-5). Methods of communication that may lead to defensive responses from others include avoidance, unresolved anxiety, and poor self-esteem. Tone of voice, manner of speech, or the words may be perceived as criticism or an attempt to control the other. Lack of interest or dogmatism (certainty of rightness) also can result in a defensive response. There are methods of communication to help avoid a defensive pattern of communication (Box 2-6).

One technique that can improve communication is called *assertiveness* (Skill 2-1). Assertiveness is a learned skill that develops self-confidence and maintains individuality in stressful situations. The goal of assertiveness is to reduce the inner stress caused by inaccurate communication or lack of communication. The basis of assertiveness is that

every person has a right to express feelings, opinions, and beliefs in a respectful and appropriate manner without feeling guilt. Aggressiveness results if the rights of others are violated during the communication. If either person's rights are overlooked, respect is lost and resentment results.

Good listening skills can be learned (Box 2-7). Listening may be done on several levels. Social listening is for enter-

Skill 2-1

Assertive Behavior

1. Take a few long, deep breaths. Allow time to gain composure so the message can be delivered in matter-of-fact, unemotional tones.

2. Describe the behavior that you would like the other person to change. Be specific about one incident or action.

3. State the effect or how you feel when the behavior occurs.

4. State the positive behavior you would like to see rather than the one you do not like.

5. State the consequences that will occur if the behavior is not changed. These consequences must be timely, reasonable, enforceable, and clearly understood by the other person.

6. Follow through with the consequences if the behavior does not change.

7. Evaluate the success of the confrontation with the other person. Demonstrate appreciation for the change in the behavior.

Box 2-8 Active Listening Guidelines

1. Stop all other activities.
2. Look at the person speaking for nonverbal as well as verbal messages.
3. Focus attention on what is being said.
4. Confirm understanding with paraphrasing, clarifying, reflecting, validating, or encouraging.
5. Give own opinion only after listening.

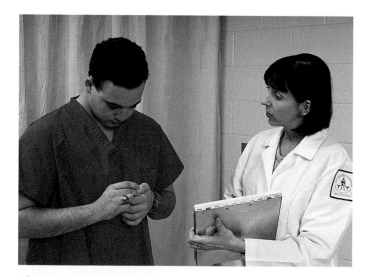

Figure 2-4 Body language may lead to varied interpretations of the message.

tainment. It does not need to be completely attentive. Discriminating or critical listening helps analyze the information to form a judgment or to take notes. Faking attention to the message, having prejudice against the sender, and listening to only part of the information (selective listening) may distort the meaning. Other actions that may interfere with communication include showing boredom, criticizing, and distracting behavior.

Good listeners are usually people with good self-concepts. They are able to pay better attention to the speaker because they are not worried about what the speaker will think of them or what their response will be. Active listening is an important part of effective com-

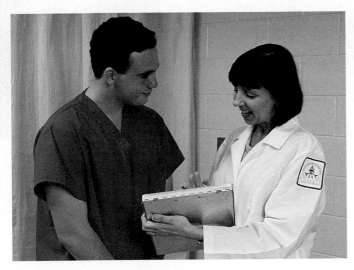

Figure 2-5   The nonverbal message should be the same as the verbal message.

munication (Box 2-8). The receiver interacts with the sender and provides feedback to indicate understanding of the message. The health care worker must listen for feelings in addition to facts by observing nonverbal behavior (Figure 2-4).

Nonverbal Communication

Messages are conveyed by appearance, facial expression, body motions (gestures), tone of voice, and the distance kept between the sender and receiver. These nonverbal methods of communication may be called *body language*. Body language includes the eye and facial movement (oculesics), personal appearance, gestures (kinesics), the spacing (proxemics), and time allowed for and pace of speech (chronemics). Use of touch (haptics), reaction to smells (olfactics), and pitch, inflection, tone, and volume of the voice also communicate a message. For effective communication, nonverbal and verbal messages to the patient should convey the same meaning (Figure 2-5).

Reading and writing skills are used in the health care field to convey information such as the instructions for

Box 2-9   Guidelines for Charting Health Care Records

- Records are kept on all patients receiving care or treatment. The chart is considered the property of the facility.
- Written consent of the patient, or a legal representative, is needed to release any information contained in the chart.
- The agency policy determines who can write in the chart or enter information in the computer.
- The professional status of the person charting (e.g., RN, MD, NA) is clearly shown with all entries.
- All entries in the chart must be legible and written in ink (black ink is preferred).
- All entries must be dated, timed, and signed by the writer.
- No part of the record may be erased, altered, destroyed, or obliterated. Do not chart before an event occurs.
- Never leave a blank space in the chart and never chart for another person.
- Charting should be a concise, accurate report of the care given.
- Chart only the facts. This includes things that can be seen, felt, heard, or smelled.
- Use only appropriate symbols and abbreviations. The agency determines which symbols are approved.
- Remember that the chart is the legal record of the care given. If care given is not charted, legally it may be considered to have not been provided.

medication, treatment, and care. Records of health care (charting) must be precise, clear, and concise to record the activities of care. The chart is the written documentation that serves as the legal record of the care given to the patient (Box 2-9).

Review Questions

1. The type of communication that best describes the use of body language is _____.

2. The sum of a person's values, attitudes, and behavior is called _____.

3. Define and describe the interrelationship of values, attitudes, and behavior. Which is most easily changed? Which is the most difficult to change?

4. Explain the hierarchy of needs as described by Abraham Maslow.

5. Draw a figure that represents a well-groomed health care worker.

6. Describe an example of the decision-making process using a problem-solving method.

7. List the three elements necessary for effective communication.

8. Describe an example of assertive communication.

Critical Thinking

1. Explain the statement made by psychologists that how a person thinks about an experience determines the feelings that result from it.

2. Describe some student behaviors that teachers prefer. Describe some that teachers find less desirable. How would these behaviors relate to patients in the health care setting?

3. Choose one aspect of personal appearance on which to improve. For 20 days keep a daily log recording the activities used to improve appearance.

4. Develop a plan to change an undesirable habit. Keep a log for 20 days documenting the amount of repetition of the habit.

3

Safety Practices

Learning Objectives

Define at least 10 terms relating to safety practices in health care.

Describe the methods of Standard and Transmission-Based Isolation Precautions that prevent the spread of microorganisms.

Describe three levels of medical asepsis.

List at least three principles of surgical asepsis.

Identify the functions of OBRA and OSHA.

Describe the guidelines for using good body mechanics.

Describe the signs and symptoms of general and localized infection.

Key Terms

Anthrax
(AN-thraks) An infectious disease of warm-blooded animals (such as cattle and sheep) caused by a spore-forming bacterium *(Bacillus anthracis),* characterized by external ulcerating nodules or by lesions in the lungs

Antiseptic
(ant-uh-SEP-tik) Substance that deters the growth of microorganisms

Asepsis
(a-SEP-sis) Freedom from infection; the methods used to prevent the spread of microorganisms

Autoclave
(AW-toe-klaev) Unit that uses steam under pressure to sterilize materials

Contaminated
(kon-TAM-in-ayt-ed) Soiled, made unclean, or infected with pathogens

Disinfectant
(dis-in-FEK-tent) Substance that kills microorganisms except viruses and spores

Pathogen
(PATH-uh-jen) Disease-causing microorganism

Standard Precautions
(STAND-erd pre-CAW-shuns) CDC guidelines for infection control that are applied to all body fluids of all patients all of the time

Sterile
(STARE-uhl) Free from living microorganisms

Transmission-Based Precautions
(trans-MISH-un baest pre-CAW-shuns) CDC guidelines for infection control applied to patients with known or suspected infections

Disease Transmission

The Infectious Process

Infection requires three elements: a source of microorganisms, a susceptible host, and a means of transmission to the host. The source may be the patient, other humans, or inanimate objects. The host must be lacking sufficient resistance or be susceptible to the infecting agent. Five main methods of transmission include contact, droplet, airborne, common vehicle, and vectors. Contact transmission may be direct or indirect, through an inanimate object. Common vehicle transmission includes items such as water, food, or **contaminated** equipment. Vectors include mosquitoes, flies, rats, and other such vermin.

Infection is a reaction caused by a microorganism. Infection may be symptomatic or asymptomatic (with or without expression of health). A local infection is an infection limited to a small area of the body. A systemic infection is an infection located throughout the body. Infection may occur in a general or local manner. General signs and symptoms of a general infection include a fever, chills, pain, an ache or tenderness, general feeling of tiredness, and night sweats. A local infection in a wound or incision may have redness, heat, swelling, pain, or fluid that is white, yellowish, or greenish coming from it.

Infection Control

Isolation Precautions

In the past, isolation procedures and precautions were based on the patient's diagnosis (Box 3-1). Someone with an infection was separated from others to prevent the spread of the microorganisms. In 1996 the Hospital Infection Control Practices Advisory Committee (HICPAC) of the Centers for Disease Control (CDC) established a two-level set of guidelines for isolation precautions designed for acute care hospitals. The two levels are Standard Precautions that are applied to all patients and Transmission-Based Precautions, which are applied to patients with known or suspected infections. These guidelines also may be applied to other health care delivery systems (Table 3-1).

Standard Precautions combine features of the previously used Universal Precautions (UP) and Body Substance Isolation (BSI) guidelines. They are applied at all times to all patients and all body fluids except perspiration. They are designed to reduce transmission of microorganisms from both diagnosed and undiagnosed infection sources (Box 3-2).

Transmission-Based Precautions are used for patients with known or suspected infections. They are used in ad-

Box 3-1 Evolution of Infection Control Procedures

1877: Hospital handbooks recommended patients with infectious conditions be placed in separate facilities.

1910: Cubicle system introduced in multiple bed wards, also known as "barrier nursing," required washing of hands and disinfecting contaminating materials between patient contacts.

1950-1960: Infections disease hospitals, except those for tuberculosis, were closed.

1960-1970: Tuberculosis hospitals closed.

1970: Manual published by CDC introducing a seven category system of isolation procedure including strict, respiratory protective, enteric, wound and skin, discharge and blood precautions.

1983: CDC manual for disease-specific isolation was revised to include strict contact, respiratory, tuberculosis, enteric drainage/secretions, and blood/body fluid precautions.

1985: Universal Precautions (UP) were instituted to combat the spread of HIV through needle sticks and skin contamination with patient blood. Emphasis was placed on applying infection precautions to every patient regardless of diagnosis. Hepatitis B vaccination of health care workers became a requirement.

1987: Body Substance Isolation (BSI) was introduced to focus on all moist and potentially infectious body fluids regardless of diagnosis.

1989: OSHA published a ruling regarding blood-borne pathogens.

1990: CDC published Standard Isolation guidelines for all patients that combine UP and BSI principles. It also combined the disease-specific categories into three sets of Transmission-Based Precautions.

dition to Standard Precautions. There are three categories of Transmission-Based Precautions guidelines including airborne, droplet, and contact precautions. Additionally, special precautions may be used for antibiotic resistant microorganisms and patients with immunosuppressed conditions. Isolation guidelines also include procedures in the event of the use of bioterrorism agents such as **anthrax** (Box 3-3).

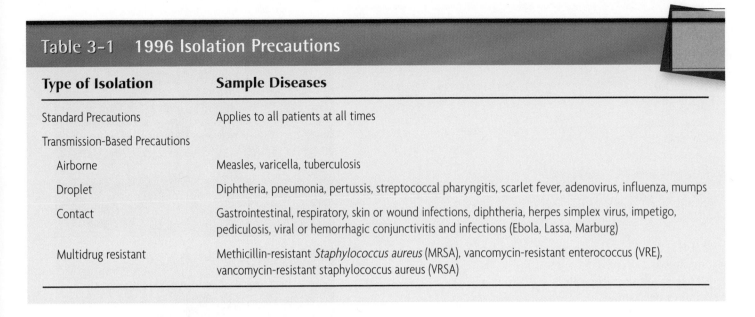

Table 3-1   1996 Isolation Precautions

Type of Isolation	Sample Diseases
Standard Precautions	Applies to all patients at all times
Transmission-Based Precautions	
Airborne	Measles, varicella, tuberculosis
Droplet	Diphtheria, pneumonia, pertussis, streptococcal pharyngitis, scarlet fever, adenovirus, influenza, mumps
Contact	Gastrointestinal, respiratory, skin or wound infections, diphtheria, herpes simplex virus, impetigo, pediculosis, viral or hemorrhagic conjunctivitis and infections (Ebola, Lassa, Marburg)
Multidrug resistant	Methicillin-resistant *Staphylococcus aureus* (MRSA), vancomycin-resistant enterococcus (VRE), vancomycin-resistant staphylococcus aureus (VRSA)

Box 3-2   Requirements of Standard Precautions

Handwashing

Whenever visibly soiled
Before and after patient contact
After contact with body fluids or moist surfaces
After removing gloves

Personal Protective Equipment and Attire (PPE)

Gloves
Gowns
Eye protection
Head cover
Footwear

Engineering and Work Practice Controls

Leakproof sharps disposal
No recapping of needles

Education

Training records to be kept for 3 years

Housekeeping, Waste Disposal, and Laundry

Surfaces cleaned and decontaminated
Regulated or biowaste disposal
Sharps disposal boxes
Soiled laundry—minimum contact and agitation

Hepatitis B Vaccine

Offered at no cost

Employee Exposure Protocol

Injured employee seen and treated within 2 hours of
   incident
Written exposure control plan

Records and Written Plans

Employee medical records confidential and maintained
   for 30 years

The primary method of protection from infection is good handwashing technique (Figure 3-1; Skill 3-1). The hands are washed thoroughly at the beginning of the work period, between each patient contact, before and after eating, before and after using the restroom, and before leaving the work environment. Gloves are worn when contact is made with body fluids, mucous membranes, or wet secretions (Figure 3-2; Skill 3-2). Wet secretions include urine, blood,

saliva, feces, wound drainage, and sputum. Disposable aprons, goggles, and masks are worn with a chance of the secretions splattering. Infections acquired by the patient as a result of the care or as a result of **pathogens** in the facility are called *nosocomial*. Epidemiology is a science devoted to studying health-related events in the human population. Principles of epidemiology are used to trace the source and minimize the risk of nosocomial infection.

Box 3-3 Bioterrorism Agents*

Bacterial

Anthrax
Brucellosis
Cholera
Glenders (rare)
Bubonic plague
Pneumumonic plague
Tularemia
Q Fever

Viral

Smallpox
Venez, Equine encephalitis
Viral encephalitis
Viral hemorrhagic fever

Toxins

Botulism
Ricin
T-2 Mycotoxins
Staphylococcus, Enterotoxin B

*Plans for containment of bioterrorism agents include strategies for isolation, placement, transport of patients, cleaning and disinfection of equipment, discharge management, and post-mortem care.

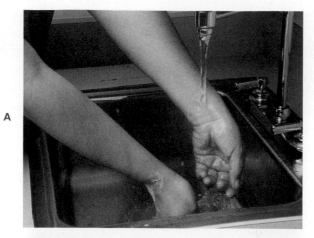

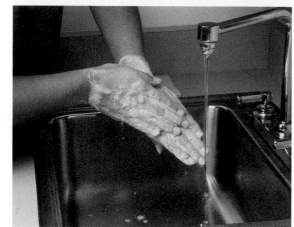

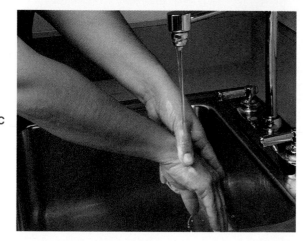

Figure 3-1 Handwashing technique. **A,** Keep the hands lower than the arms during the procedure. **B,** In addition to soap and water, friction or rubbing also cleans the skin. **C,** Rinsing hands thoroughly prevents skin irritation from soap. *(From Kinn ME, Woods M: The medical assistant, ed 8, Philadelphia, 1999, WB Saunders.)*

The most common method of transfer of pathogenic organisms that cause serious illness in the health care worker is contact with a contaminated needle or sharp instrument. To prevent contamination, needles should not be recapped but should be disposed of in a container specifically designed for the purpose. Other environmental risk factors are minimized with the use of hepatitis B vaccination and devices for cardiopulmonary resuscitation that eliminate mouth-to-mouth contact with mucous membranes during the procedure. Methods that are not considered effective include disposable eating utensils, "protective" isolation, **disinfectant** fogging, and double bagging for the removal of waste and linens. Waste and linen should all be disposed of according to individual agency specifications designed to prevent contact with secretions.

Principles of Asepsis

Asepsis is the absence of disease-causing microorganisms (pathogens). Asepsis also includes the methods used to prevent the spread of microorganisms. Medical asepsis is a state of cleanliness or the use of clean technique. An area or object that becomes unclean is considered contaminated. Medical asepsis can be evaluated on three levels:

1. **Antiseptic:** Antiseptics inhibit the growth of bacteria. They can be used on the skin.

Skill 3-1

Handwashing

1. Maintain medical asepsis by using good handwashing technique and wearing gloves according to Standard and Transmission-Based Isolation Precautions.

2. Hands should be washed at the beginning of the workday, between each contact with a patient, and at the end of the day. They should also be washed before and after eating and using the restroom.

3. Wet the hands completely with water before applying the soap. Keep the hands lower than the arms during the procedure. The hands are washed and rinsed from the least contaminated area to the most (clean to dirty).

4. Rinse the soap bar before using it and replacing it in the dish. Soap can carry microorganisms to another person. In addition to the soap and water, friction or rubbing actually cleans the skin.

5. Using a circular motion, rub the surface of each wrist at least 2 inches above the hand. Friction helps to remove the dirt from the skin surface.

6. Wash the palms and back of the hands after both wrists are cleaned. After they are cleaned, the wrists are not retouched to prevent contamination by microorganisms from the less clean areas of the hands.

7. Clean each finger and thumb of each hand. Do not retouch the less clean areas (backs of the palms). The fingers are considered to have four sides. Special attention is needed to the area underneath the nails and between the fingers.

8. Rinse each hand from the wrist to the fingers, keeping the hands below the level of the arms.

9. Using a circular motion, dry each hand thoroughly from the wrist to the fingertips. Use a separate towel or dry portion of the towel for each hand. Most skin irritations result from soap or moisture that remains on the skin after washing.

10. Use a dry towel to turn off the faucet handle and clean the sink area. Faucets and other metal fixtures (fomites) can also transmit microorganisms.

2. **Disinfectant:** Disinfectants are agents that destroy most bacteria and viruses. They can be caustic or harmful to the skin. Disinfection can be accomplished by boiling as well as by using chemical agents.

3. **Sterile:** Surgical asepsis is a state of sterility or the use of sterile technique. Sterilization is the removal of all microorganisms including viruses and endospores. Sterilization can be accomplished using an **autoclave.** One type of autoclave is a pressure cooker that uses steam and pressure to destroy microorganisms. Other autoclaves use dry heat or chemical vapor to kill all microorganisms. Sterile technique also includes special methods of handling sterile equipment, maintaining sterile fields, changing dressings, and disposing of contaminated materials.

Gloving

1. Maintain medical asepsis by using good handwashing technique and wearing gloves according to Standard and Transmission-Based Isolation Precautions.

2. The hands can never be sterile. If any part of the hand touches the sterile outside of the gloves, the gloves are contaminated.

3. Touching only outside and edges of the wrapper, open the sterile glove wrapper on a clean, dry surface. The inside of the wrapper creates a sterile field.

4. Remove one glove from the wrapper by grasping only the inside surface of the glove. Avoid touching the glove on the edges of the sterile field. Edges are considered contaminated. If the bare skin passes over the sterile part of the gloves, the gloves are contaminated.

5. With a smooth, upward motion, pull on the glove.

6. Using the gloved (sterile) hand, remove the remaining glove from the package, touching only the outside (sterile) surface.

7. Pull the remaining glove onto the ungloved hand in an upward motion without touching the outside (sterile) surface of either glove to the skin. Keep the hands above the level of the waist. Items below the waist and behind the back are considered contaminated.

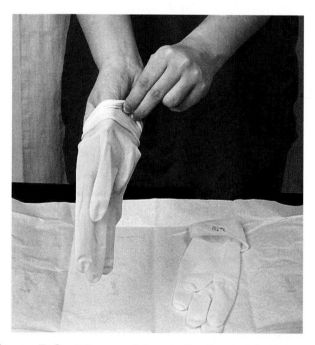

Figure 3-2 When applying sterile gloves, it is important not to allow the unsterile hand to cross over the sterile part of either glove.

OBRA and OSHA Regulatons

OBRA

In 1987 the Congress passed a law that requires training for nursing assistants that includes competency testing of skill performance. In addition to completing a written examination, the nurse assistant must demonstrate the ability to perform skills correctly. OBRA (Omnibus Budget Reconciliation Act) applies to all states and facilities in which nursing assistants are employed. Other requirements of OBRA include continuing education, periodic evaluation of performance, and retraining if the nursing assistant does not work in the field for 2 years or more at one time. In addition to training for nursing assistants, the Act also requires long-term care and home health facilities to provide specific care for the residents. For example, it requires the provision of a doctor for each resident and limits the use of restraints.

OSHA

The Occupational Safety and Health Administration was established in 1970 as one of the agencies of the Department of Labor. OSHA has two functions. They are to establish standards of safety for the workplace and to enforce those standards. In 1971 the National Institutes of Health established the branch called the *National Institute of Occupational Safety and Health* (NIOSH) to research and provide documentation to OSHA regarding the safe level of exposure to hazards in the workplace. OSHA must prove to the Office of Management and Budget (OMB) that the health standards set are economically feasible for the industries to which they apply.

In 1985 regulations established by the federal government began requiring employers to tell employees of potential hazards in the workplace. This "right-to-know" information includes details of any health and safety hazards related to working with hazardous or toxic materials. The information is often described in the Material Safety Data Sheet (Box 3-4). In 2001 OSHA revised the bloodborne pathogen standard to reduce the incidence of needlesticks to include broader and more specific definitions of "sharps" and reporting requirements.

Safe Movement

Body Mechanics

Body mechanics is the way the body is moved to prevent injury to oneself and to others. It is accomplished by using knowledge of proper body alignment, balance, and movement. Posture is the position of body parts in relation to each other. Balance is the ability to maintain a steady position that does not tip. Six principles of movement can be used to maintain good body mechanics (Figure 3-3; Skill 3-3).

When the ability to move (mobility) or feel (sensation) is lost, many complications can occur in the human body. Determining proper body alignment or positioning may be necessary if the patient is unable to move independently. Body positioning may be ordered by the physician or may be determined by the judgment of the health care worker (Figure 3-4). Additionally, side rails or restraints may be ordered by the physician to ensure safety of the patient (Skill 3-4).

The international symbol of access in more than 60 countries indicates that a person with a disability can enter

---

Box 3-4   Material Safety Data Sheet

Section I: Product Identification
Section II: Hazardous Ingredients
Section III: Physical Data
Section IV: Fire and Explosion Hazard
Section V: Health Hazards
Section VI: Reactivity
Section VII: Spill and Disposal
Section VIII: Protective Measures
Section IX: Special Precautions

MSDSs are often prepared by the product's manufacturer and provide only basic information.

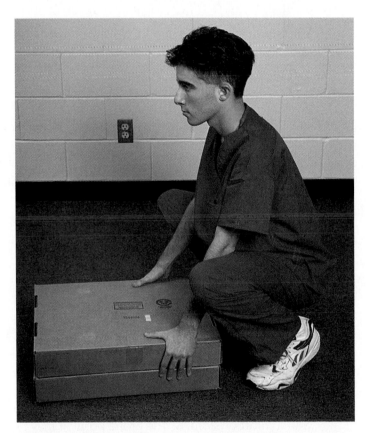

Figure 3-3 Principles of good body mechanics include keeping the back straight.

---

and use a building without being blocked by architectural design (Figure 3-5). The symbol indicates, for example, that wheelchair ramps are available, doors are wide enough to accommodate a wheelchair, the elevators have Braille indicators, and telephones and drinking fountains are placed

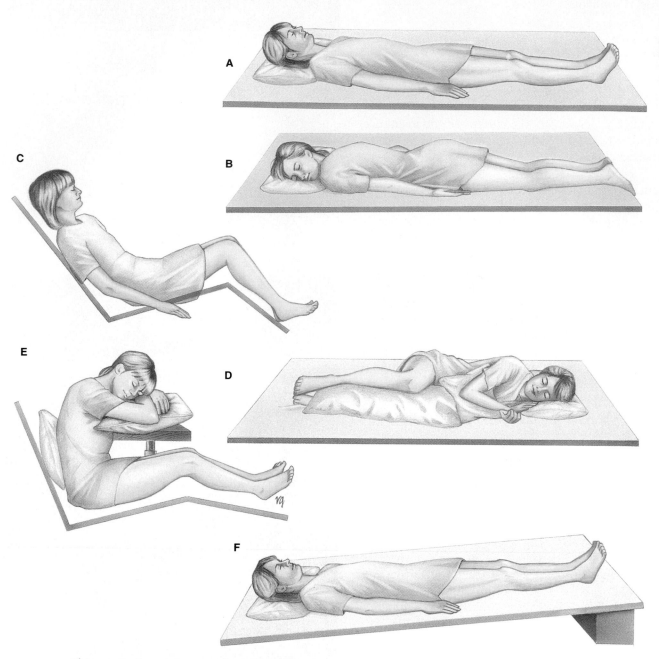

Figure 3-4 Body positions. **A,** The horizontal or supine position may be used for comfort or sleep. **B,** The prone position may be used for comfort or treatments to the back. **C,** Semi-Fowler's position may be used for comfort or to decrease pressure on the abdominal organs. **D,** The left Sims' position is used for taking a rectal temperature and for administering enemas. **E,** The orthopneic position may be assumed to ease respiratory distress. **F,** The Trendelenburg position, or a modified version that raises only the legs, may be used to treat conditions of lowered blood pressure such as shock.

Skill 3-3

Good Body Mechanics

1. Maintain medical asepsis by using good handwashing technique and wearing gloves according to Standard and Transmission-Based Isolation Precautions.

2. Identify the patient and explain the procedure.

3. Size up the load to be moved. Get help if needed.

4. Keep a broad base of stance, with feet 12 to 18 inches apart.

5. Bring the object or patient close before attempting the move.

6. Squat by bending at the knees, and keep the back straight.

7. Do not lift anything that can be pushed or pulled.

8. Turn the body as a unit by pivoting the feet, not turning at the waist.

at a lower height. Physical devices that are used to provide better access by disabled individuals include the walker, cane, wheelchair, and crutches. Hydraulic mechanical lifts may be used so a small force can lift a heavy object or person. With environmental adjustments and devices, the disabled individual may be able to perform activities of daily living such as eating, bathing, dressing, and moving about independently.

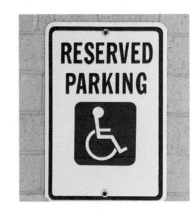

Figure 3-5 Parking sign designating parking space for persons with disabilities.

Skill 3-4

Positioning the Patient

1. Maintain medical asepsis by using good handwashing technique and wearing gloves according to Standard and Transmission-Based Isolation Precautions.

2. Identify the patient and explain the procedure.

3. Determine the position to be assumed. The appropriate position is determined by the health care worker or ordered by the physician.

4. Keep all unattended side rails in the upright position for safety.

5. Move cranks or electrical adjustments to achieve desired position. Replace adjusting devices to their original position. Injury may occur to the patient or health care worker if devices protrude from the bed.

6. Cushion points of pressure with pillows or linens. Points of pressure include areas where bones are close to the surface of the skin, such as the elbows, heels, tail bone (coccygeal) area, and knees. Impaired circulation on pressure points may lead to formation of bedsores (decubitus ulcers).

7. Assess the body alignment of the patient. The body should be aligned as naturally and comfortably as possible to prevent points of pressure and contracting of limbs.

Identifying and Reporting Hazards

Fire and Electrical Hazards

Fire may occur in the home or health care facility as a result of equipment that is damaged or circuits that are overloaded. Smoking may also cause fires. For a fire to burn, it must have oxygen, fuel, and heat. A fire may be controlled or extinguished by removing any one of these elements. Health care workers are responsible for preventing and reacting to fires to protect their patients.

Although each facility has a procedure to follow in the case of fire, it is common practice to sound the alarm, notify the switchboard, and move any patient who is in danger first. If the fire is small, a fire extinguisher may then be used to extinguish it. All windows and doors may be closed to decrease the amount of air to the fire. Oxygen and electrical equipment may be turned off. Exits are kept clear at all times to allow patients and workers to leave if needed. If smoke is present, the worker and patients should crawl or move close to the floor toward the exit because the smoke will rise. A damp towel or similar cloth may be used to cover the mouth and nose for breathing.

Portable chemical fire extinguishers are useful in extinguishing small fires. Four classes of chemical fire extinguishers include the following:

Class A: for use on paper, wood, trash, cloth, upholstery, rubber, and similar materials

Class B: for use on fuel oil, gas, paint, solvents, and other flammable liquids

Class C: for use on electrical equipment, fuse boxes, wiring and appliances

Class D: for use on metals

Some extinguishers may be designed for multiple purposes. For example, an ABC extinguisher may be used for the home. Fire extinguishers are also rated by the size of fire that can be extinguished. When extinguishing a fire, a person should aim the stream from the extinguisher at the base of the fire.

Hazardous Waste

In health care, waste is divided into two categories including biomedical and general. Infectious and hazardous waste produced in health care facilities may sometimes be poured into the sewage system or disposed of by incineration. One concern that has been raised because of local incineration of wastes is the production of toxic gases containing dioxin, acid gases, and heavy metals. According to the federal Office of Technology Assessment, hospitals release 10 to 100 times more of these elements into the air than other incinerators found in a city.

In health care facilities, hazardous and infectious waste is usually placed in sealed bags before removing it from the area of use. The bag is labeled and sealed to indicate the kind of

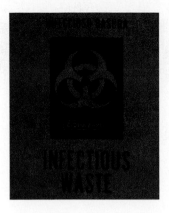

Figure 3-6   A biohazard symbol.

waste hazard that may exist and alert other workers in the facility (Figure 3-6). Some general guidelines for bagging waste for disposal includes separating items into categories such as linens, plastics, glass, and wet or dry. If the bag is contaminated during loading, it may be double bagged.

Emergency Disaster Procedures

A disaster may be caused by nature or by man and is considered to be any catastrophic event that injures or kills many people at one time. Some examples include tornadoes, explosions, plane crashes, earthquakes, and similar events. Policies and procedures for actions to be followed in a health care facility during a disaster depend on the type of facility. Some personnel may be asked to work in another area such as the emergency department or at an unscheduled time. In hospitals, some patients may be asked to go home or are moved to another facility.

Review Questions

1. Use the following terms in one or more sentences that correctly relate their meaning.
   Antiseptic
   Asepsis
   Contaminate
   Disinfect
   Sterile

2. Compare the signs and symptoms of localized and general infections.

3. Compare standard and transmission-based isolation precautions.

4. List and describe three levels of asepsis.

5. Describe the functions of OBRA and OSHA.

6. List the six guidelines for maintaining good body mechanics.

Critical Thinking

1. Describe the precautions that might be used to isolate a person with an infection of a surgical wound. Include the principles of isolation including patient placement, transport, cleaning and disinfection of equipment, discharge management, and post-mortem care.

2. Describe the precautions that might be used to isolate a person with an infectious cough. Include the principles of isolation including patient placement, transport, cleaning and disinfection of equipment, discharge management, and post-mortem care.

3. Describe the precautions that might be used to isolate a person with leukemia. Include the principles of isolation including patient placement, transport, cleaning and disinfection of equipment, discharge management, and post-mortem care.

4. Investigate the local emergency disaster procedures.

4
Legal and Ethical Principles

Learning Objectives

Define at least 10 terms relating to legal and ethical principles.

Describe at least five examples of ethical behavior for the health care worker.

Identify at least five situations that show improper ethical or legal behavior.

Explain the importance of confidentiality in health care including privacy issues resulting from advanced technology.

Describe at least two examples of rights of the health care patient.

Describe the role of the health care worker regarding current legal issues including advance directives and telemedicine.

Key Terms

Confidential
(kahn-fuh-DEN-chel) Private or secret

Ethics
(ETH-iks) Dealing with what is good or bad, determining moral duty and obligation

Jurisprudent
(jur-is-PROOD-ent) Understanding the science or philosophy of law

Legal
(LEE-gul) Deriving authority from or founded on law

Liable
(LIE-uh-bul) Legally responsible

Libel
(LIE-bul) Communicating something untruthful and harmful about another person in writing

Malpractice
(mal-PRAK-tiss) Failure of professional skill or learning that results in injury, loss, or damage

Moral
(MORE-ul) Relating to principles of right and wrong

Negligence
(NEG-li-jens) Failure to execute the care that a reasonable (prudent) person exercises

Slander
(SLAN-der) Verbally communicating something untruthful and harmful about another person

Legal and Ethical Terminology

TERM	DEFINITION
Assault	A threat or an attempt to injure another person in an illegal manner
Battery	Unlawful touching of another person without consent, with or without injury
Breach	Breaking the law, an obligation, or the terms of a contract
Civil law	Defines the legal relationships between individuals
Common law	Unwritten law; customs that may have authority or have been established by prior court decisions
Conduct	Behavior or a person's actions
Consent	Permission granted by a person voluntarily and in sound mind; written consent is most easily proved
Crime	Performing an act that is forbidden or omitting a duty required by public law, making the offender liable for the action
Criminal law	Defines the legal obligation between an individual and the state or society
Custom	An accepted behavior or common practice
Duty of care	By law, health care workers must perform services in a manner that meets common standards of practice
Ethics	Standards of behavior and practice that are established by a professional organization for its members
Felony	A serious crime for which the penalty is imprisonment for more than 1 year
Ideal	Standard of perfection or excellence
Illegal restraint	Holding or detaining a person against his or her will
Invasion of privacy	Unlawfully making known to the public any private or personal information without the consent of the wronged person
Liable	Legally responsible for own actions
Libel	Communicating something untruthful and harmful about another person in writing
Licensure	Authorization by the state to perform the functions of an occupation for which educational and examination standards are specified
Litigation	A lawsuit or legal action
Malpractice	Bad or harmful practice that injures another person
Misdemeanors	Crimes that are less serious than felonies and result in imprisonment for less than 1 year
Negligence	Failure to perform duties in a reasonable and customary way
Privileged communication	Personal or private information relating to the care given by health care personnel
Reasonable care	Services given in a manner appropriate to the level of education and experience of the health care worker
Slander	Verbally communicating something untruthful and harmful about another person
Statutory law	Law established by the legislative branch of government that determines what is legal
Tort	Civil wrong
Unethical	Action that does not represent ideal behavior but may not be illegal
Value system	Ideals and thoughts that determine what is considered worthwhile or meaningful, right or wrong
Will	Written document that allows a person to distribute property after death

Professional Codes of Conduct

Ethical and legal responsibilities are a central part of all health care occupations. The worker must understand and follow ethical practices including respect for cultural, social, and ethnic differences of the patients and other workers. **Legal** responsibilities include practicing within the guidelines of laws, policies, and regulations established for each type of employment.

Health care has become an industry that involves many complex professions and technologies. Every day the health care worker must make legal and ethical decisions.

Box 4-1   Code of Ethics

- The primary goals of the health care worker are to promote an optimal level of wellness, preserve life, and provide for a peaceful death when necessary.
- The health care worker respects the religious beliefs and cultural values of all patients.
- The health care worker provides adequate and continuous care for all patients regardless of age, gender, race, or nature of the illness or injury.
- The health care worker knows the limits of practice for which he or she is competent and stays within those limits.
- The health care worker maintains competence and current knowledge by pursuing continuing education.
- The health care worker practices jurisprudent behavior at all times by avoiding unethical or illegal practices.
- The health care worker respects the dignity and rights of each patient by maintaining confidentiality and a professional attitude regarding all information relating to the patient.
- The health care worker asks for clarification and assistance when unsure of any aspect of care.
- The health care worker participates in professional activities and organizations to provide better health care.
- The health care worker maintains a high standard of ethical and legal behavior in his or her private and professional life.

Ethics are the principles and values that determine appropriate behavior. An individual, community, or society adopts moral standards that distinguish right from wrong. **Morals** are based on the experience, religion, and philosophy of the individual and the society. The basis of ethical behavior in the health care field is the respect for the needs and rights of others.

Ethical codes are guidelines for the actions of people in a profession. They are established by the professionals to whom they apply, and they may not be legally binding. What is ethical in one society or profession may not apply to another and may change over time. In most health care professions, the rules of ethics are preserved in an oath or code of standards. Physicians established the first code of ethics for a profession. The lawyers followed them. The third and fourth professions to establish a code were the pharmacists and veterinarians.

Ethical standards apply to relationships with fellow workers, patients, and the community. These are based on individual morals and society's expectations. Some ethical standards are the same for all health occupations (Box 4-1). Each profession may have an oath or pledge that states the basic beliefs and goals of the group (Box 4-2).

The health care worker must be **jurisprudent** or aware of the laws that influence the industry. Workers in every health occupation are legally responsible **(liable)** for their behavior and the care given. The employer also may be liable for the actions of the worker that are not reasonably prudent **(negligent)** or that reflect bad practice **(malpractice)**. It is **slander** to verbally communicate something that is untrue and harmful about another person, and **libel** to put it in writing. Some of the most common incidences of

Box 4-2   Nightingale Pledge

I solemnly pledge myself before God, and in the presence of this assembly, to pass my life in purity and to practice my profession faithfully.

I will abstain from whatever is deleterious and mischievous and will not take or knowingly administer any harmful drug.

I will do all in my power to maintain and elevate the standard of my profession, and will hold in confidence all personal matters committed to my keeping and all family affairs coming to my knowledge in the practice of my profession.

With loyalty I will endeavor to aid the physician in his work and devote myself to the welfare of those committed to my care.

liability for the health care worker result from inadequate charting. Another concern is the violation of a patient's trust that may result in invasion of privacy or illegal restraint.

Hospitals and other health care facilities may have an institutional or internal review board that meets to oversee the agency's guidelines for ethical conduct. The board also may decide issues relating to a worker's conduct, responsibility, and scope of practice when necessary. Many health care occupations are regulated by state agencies. Some workers hold a license that determines which actions may be performed. Licensed professionals are legally responsible for their actions when performing as employees or in their own practice.

Malpractice and Liability

Health care workers are legally responsible, or liable, for the care that is given to their patients. The scope of duties that may be legally performed by a health care worker depends on the level of training and education of the worker. Some functions such as giving medications are regulated by laws and require a license. It is important that the health care worker understands the limits or scope of his or her practice. A written job description is useful in defining the scope of practice for a job.

It is considered to be malpractice to perform skills that are beyond the level of health care worker's education and training. It is also malpractice to neglect to do something that is considered to be common practice such as leaving the patient in an unsafe situation. Malpractice or liability insurance may be purchased by the health care worker for financial protection in the event that a patient questions the quality or scope of care. The cost of the insurance varies with the level of responsibility of the position and may be included as part of the worker's compensation or benefit package.

Confidentiality

Information regarding the patient in health care is considered **confidential** or private. The health care worker is ethically responsible to maintaining the patient's privacy. Breaking confidentiality may also be a legal violation if the information causes the patient financial or personal damage. The health care worker must share information regarding the patient with only the appropriate personnel involved in the care.

In 1996 Congress passed the Health Insurance Portability and Accountability Act (HIPAA) to try to reduce administrative overhead of health care providers and pro-

tect individually identifiable health information that might be accessible through use of electronic technology. In April 2001 standards for "Privacy of Individually Identifiable Health Information" were established by the Department of Health and Human Services (HHS). The rule applies to all agencies sharing, or transiting, personal health information whether it be paper, oral, and electronic. This covers people who are insured privately or by public programs, or who are uninsured. The standards protect medical records and personal health information. Life insurance and workers compensation programs are not covered by the regulations. These providers are allowed to use and reuse patient information without prior consent. An exception to the right of the patient to privacy is when there is imminent danger to another individual that can be foreseen by the practitioner. This "duty to warn" requires the health care practitioner to disclose the patient's relevant personal health information when such a threat exists.

Patient Rights

In addition to the guidelines set by the American Hospital Association, the patient also has the rights of any citizen of the United States and the state. Some of these rights include confidentiality and personal privacy. All patients must be given quality care without mistreatment, neglect, or abuse. The patient also has the right to voice grievances without fear of retaliation. The patient's personal possessions must be cared for and secured while care is being given.

Legal Directives

Advance directives and living wills are legal documents that allow patients to express their wishes about their health care and treatment. Two types of advance directives are the living will and power of attorney. An advance directive takes effect only when a patient loses ability to make his or her own decisions (Box 4-3). A living will allows a person to state in advance whether to receive and what life-support procedures to withhold if the person is terminally ill and permanently unconscious. A durable power of attorney for health care allows another person or agent to make decisions if the person is unable to make them. The person does not need to be terminally ill or permanently unconscious for the durable power of attorney to take effect. Advance directives are not "do not resuscitate (DNR)" orders. DNR orders are written by doctors to indicate that the patient is not to be resuscitated.

Box 4-3   Elements of Advance Care Directives

Some of the choices that may be addressed in an Advance Health Care Directive include the following:
- Choice to prolong or not to prolong life in the event of terminal conditions to include or exclude the following:
  Artificial nutrition through a conduit
  Hydration through a conduit
  Cardiopulmonary resuscitation (CPR)
  Mechanical respiration
- Choice to prolong or not to prolong life in the case of unconsciousness for a specified length of time or if determined that the state is vegetative or irreversible
- Relief from pain
- Designation of a power of attorney for health care to make these and other decisions
- Anatomical gift declaration to specify components to be donated, if any, and to whom for what purpose

Health Care and the Internet

Use of the Internet to access health care information and products has introduced a new set of issues and concerns. Patients can find information, join chat groups, purchase drugs and other medical items, and consult a health care practitioner online. There is not clear legal jurisdiction for health care that is provided over the Internet as it may cross state or even country boundaries. In the fall of 2000, the Joint Commission on Accreditation of Healthcare Organizations (JCAHO) adopted new credentialing standards for hospitals that are using telemedicine.

Documentation

Records of health care (charting) must be precise, clear, and concise to record the activities of care. The chart is the main technique used for health care workers to communicate about the patient's care. The chart is the written documentation that serves as the legal record of the care given

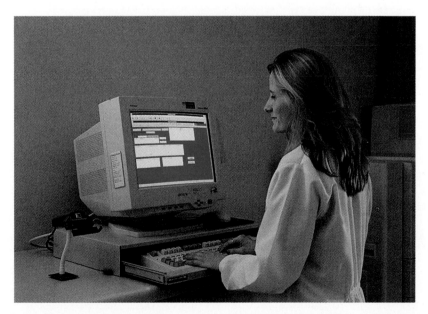

Figure 4-1   Computers and the Internet have become helpful tools in the health care field.

to the patient. It is divided into sections according to the service being provided for easy reference. Policies of the facility determine who records each type of treatment and the acceptable method for charting. Two general guidelines for good charting include (1) charting only for oneself and not for another person and (2) keeping any information contained in the chart confidential.

Reporting (telling) and recording (charting) observations and vital or life signs are the methods by which communication about the patient's status is made. Accurate and timely communication is necessary to ensure the best care possible. Abnormal vital signs should be reported immediately to the appropriate supervising personnel. Vital signs and other documentation may be entered directly into a computer, providing rapid information access (Figure 4-1), or may be recorded on graphic sheets and flow sheets (Figure 4-2). The handwriting on graphic sheets must be easy to read and the information accurate. Information should be written on paper soon after the assessment is made so that it is not forgotten.

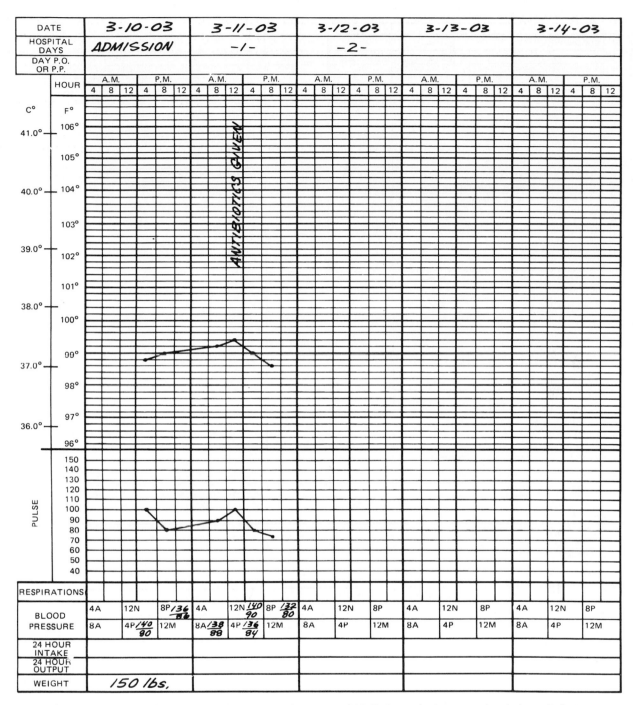

Figure 4-2   **A,** The graphic sheet is used to record vital signs during a patient's hospital stay.

Continued

DATE: _**3-11-03**_

		7-3	3-11	11-7	
SKIN	COLOR: PINK	—	—		
	PALE	B SMITH, RN	RDAVIS - RN		
	JAUNDICE	—	—		
	CYANOTIC	—	—		
	MOISTURE: WARM	—	R. DAVIS - RN		
	DRY	—	—		
	COOL	—	—		
	DIAPHORETIC	SLIGHT - B SMITH	R. DAVIS - RN		
LEVEL OF CONSCIOUSNESS	ALERT & COOPERATIVE	B. SMITH	R. DAVIS - RN		C/O HEADACHE, MD NOTIFIED 13:00 - R. DAVIS - RN
	RESPOND TO PAINFUL STIMULI	—	—		
	RESPOND TO VERBAL STIMULI	—	—		
	ALERT & UNCOOPERATIVE	—	—		
	COMATOSE	—	—		
	INCOHERENT	—	—		
	SLURRED SPEECH	—	—		
ABDOMEN	BS – PRESENT	B. SMITH	—		
	BS – ABSENT	—	—		
	FLAT – SOFT	B. SMITH	—		
	DISTENDED	—	—		
	NG TUBE	—	—		
	COLORS	—	—		
RESPIRATORY	O$_2$ – VIA/RATE	—	—		
	TRACH CARE	—	—		
	IPPB/UPDRAFT	—	—		
	TRI FLOW	—	—		
	COUGH & DEEP BREATHE	—	—		
		—	—		
IV'S	IV TYPE & FLOW RATE	—	B. SMITH		IV INSERTED PER MD ORDER BS, RN
	SITE/CONDITION	—	B. SMITH		IV INSERTED 14:30 - B. SMITH, RN
	IMED	—	—		
	HEP LOCK	—	—		
	IV DSG	—	—		
	IV TUBING	—	—		
ELIMINATION	VOIDING QS	B. SMITH	R. DAVIS - RN		
	FOLEY PATENT	—	—		
	COLOR	—	—		
	CATH CARE/TAPED	—	—		
	FOLEY DC	—	—		
	STOOL	+ FORMED BRN	—		
SAFETY PRECAUTIONS	SEIZURE PRECAUTIONS				
	SIDE RAIL UP				
	RESTRAINTS CHECKED				

B

Figure 4-2 (cont'd)   **B,** Nurse's notes provide a quick and effective way to document the care provided *(front).*

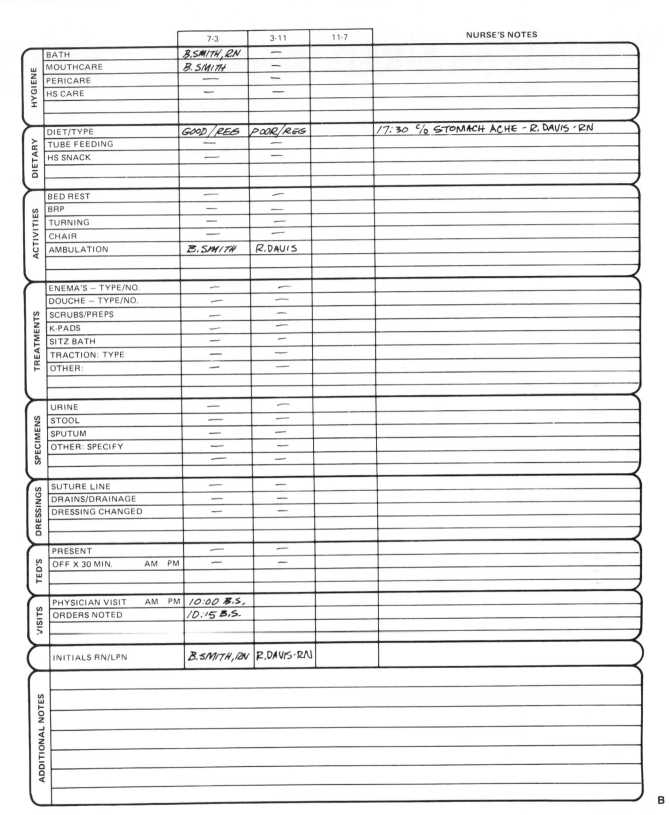

		7-3	3-11	11-7	NURSE'S NOTES
HYGIENE	BATH	B. SMITH, RN	—		
	MOUTHCARE	B. SMITH	—		
	PERICARE	—	—		
	HS CARE	—	—		
DIETARY	DIET/TYPE	GOOD/REG	POOR/REG		17:30 c/o STOMACH ACHE - R. DAVIS - RN
	TUBE FEEDING	—	—		
	HS SNACK	—	—		
ACTIVITIES	BED REST	—	—		
	BRP	—	—		
	TURNING	—	—		
	CHAIR	—	—		
	AMBULATION	B. SMITH	R. DAVIS		
TREATMENTS	ENEMA'S — TYPE/NO.	—	—		
	DOUCHE — TYPE/NO.	—	—		
	SCRUBS/PREPS	—	—		
	K-PADS	—	—		
	SITZ BATH	—	—		
	TRACTION: TYPE	—	—		
	OTHER:	—	—		
SPECIMENS	URINE	—	—		
	STOOL	—	—		
	SPUTUM	—	—		
	OTHER: SPECIFY	—	—		
		—	—		
DRESSINGS	SUTURE LINE	—	—		
	DRAINS/DRAINAGE	—	—		
	DRESSING CHANGED	—	—		
TED'S	PRESENT	—	—		
	OFF X 30 MIN. AM PM	—	—		
VISITS	PHYSICIAN VISIT AM PM	10:00 B.S.			
	ORDERS NOTED	10:15 B.S.			
	INITIALS RN/LPN	B. SMITH, RN	R. DAVIS - RN		
ADDITIONAL NOTES					

B

Figure 4-2 (cont'd)   **B,** Nurse's Notes provide a quick and effective way to document the care provided *(back)*.

Review Questions

1. Use the following terms in one or more sentences that demonstrate their relationship to each other.
   Legal
   Malpractice
   Negligent

2. Use the following terms in one or more sentences that demonstrate their relationship to each other.
   Ethics
   Moral

3. Use the following terms in one or more sentences that demonstrate their relationship to each other.
   Libel
   Slander

4. List two examples of patient's rights based on every citizen's rights.

Critical Thinking

1. Investigate the code of conduct or rules of ethics for a health care profession.

2. Explain why each of the following is a legal or ethical consideration of health care.
   a. The patient is restrained in a wheelchair without a physician's order.
   b. The patient requests to attend church services in the hospital chapel and is permitted to go.
   c. The health care worker charts that the patient is "an old battle-ax."
   d. The health care worker does not change the linen for two patients as was assigned
   e. The health care worker eats leftovers from a patient's dinner tray.
   f. The patient requests a room change to a nonsmoking area.

3. Describe the importance of confidentiality in health care.

4. Investigate the extent of use of computers for documentation in a local health care facility.

5
Employability Skills

Learning Objectives

Define at least 10 terms relating to seeking a career in health care.

Describe the purpose of a professional organization.

List three benefits of membership in a student organization.

List at least three reasons to use parliamentary procedure during an organization meeting.

Identify the use of three motions of parliamentary procedure.

Describe the purposes of the job application, resumé, interview, and resignation letter.

List at least five rules for completing a job application form.

Provide a positive response for at least five questions that might be asked in a job interview.

Complete a job application.

Prepare a resumé or personal data sheet.

Identify the components of a personal budget.

Key Terms

Adjourn
(uh-JERN) To suspend a session to another time or permanently

Agenda
(uh-JEN-duh) List of things to be done or considered, program of work

Budget
(BUD-jit) Summary of projected income and expenses

Debate
(di-BAYT) Discuss a question

Initiative
(in-ISH-uh-tiv) Energy or aptitude for action, enterprise

Motion
(MO-shen) Proposal for action

Organization
(or-guh-ni-ZAY-shen) A structure through which individuals cooperate systematically to conduct business

Resumé
(REZ-oo-may) Brief summary of professional and work experience

Tax
(taks) Contribution to the support of government, fee, or dues of an organization to pay its expenses

Professional Organizations

In an **organization,** a group of individuals join together to reach a goal by cooperation and division of tasks among themselves. Groups can accomplish goals faster and more easily than individuals. An organizational chart shows the relationships among and the roles of the members (Figure 5-1).

Organizational frameworks may be planned using management practices and theories. This is usually called *organizational development.* The goal of organizational development is to increase worker satisfaction and lead to increased productivity and quality. The health care worker plays an important part in the health care organization by setting goals, meeting challenges, and implementing ideas.

Work is a means of self-fulfillment and a method to earn a salary and establish economic security. Careful examina-

tion of the type of occupation may determine if it will be satisfying and meet the needs and goals of the prospective health care worker. The choice of a career should be based on an individual's interests, abilities, and character.

Student Organizations

Student organizations provide a means to learn the behavior and skills needed to succeed in school, on the job, and as citizens. Each student member is responsible for the effectiveness and success of the student organization. Two national organizations that may be part of a health careers program include the Health Occupations Students of America (HOSA) and SkillsUSA-VICA, formerly the Vocational Industrial Clubs of America (SkillsUSA-VICA) (Figure 5-2). HOSA is open to students in health occupations programs only. It was founded in 1976 and has chapters in 34 states. SkillsUSA-VICA is open to students in all trade and industrial programs. It has chapters in 54 states and territories.

STUDENT ORGANIZATION FRAMEWORK*

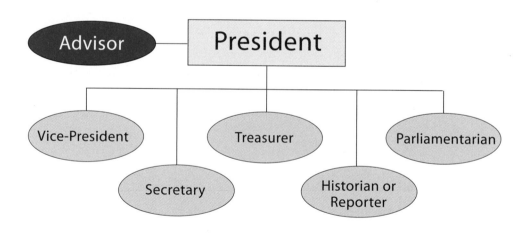

* The leadership of student organizations may vary.

Officer Responsibilities:

President: Chairs the meetings. Prepares the agenda with the assistance of the secretary.

Vice-President: Chairs the meeting in the absence of the President. Co-chairs all committees.

Secretary: Takes the minutes of the meetings. Prepares the agenda with the assistance of the President.

Treasurer: Maintains the financial books for the organization.

Historian/Reporter: Provides historical records and publicity for the organization using print and photographic media.

Parliamentarian: Ensures that parliamentary procedure is used during meetings. Answers procedural questions.

Advisor: Provides assistance as needed for organizational activities. Not a voting member.

Figure 5-1   As with the health care facilities, student organizations maintain levels of organization to protect each member's rights and expedite business.

Benefits of membership in a student organization include the exchange of information with others who have similar interests, an opportunity to sharpen skills through competition, and a way to develop leadership ability. Health care workers need leadership skills to provide better care. Many styles of leadership may be effective in different situations and may be practiced in student organization meetings (Table 5-1). Through organization membership, students develop programs and activities that build character, good citizenship, and a respect for ethical practices (Figure 5-3). Confidence gained by assuming responsibility may lead to self-actualization. Student organizations promote and recognize individual and group achievements.

Table 5-1   Leadership Style

Style	Description
Autocratic	The leader makes all of the decisions; discourages creativity; allows quick decision making and decisive action
By example	Leader is a role model for participants
Coaching	Leader explains decisions, asks for suggestions, and supervises projects
Delegating	Responsibility for decisions is given to others
Democratic	Participation is encouraged; decisions are made jointly; everyone is considered equal; may result in "tyranny of the majority" in which the minority never gets its way
Directing	Leader provides instruction and supervision
Laissez-faire	Nobody is in charge. Decision making is scattered; encourages creativity; may lead to lack of action
Situational	Leader adapts and changes styles depending on the matter at hand
Supporting	Leader facilitates and shares decision making

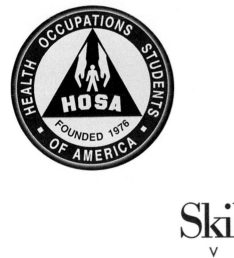

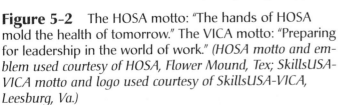

Figure 5-2   The HOSA motto: "The hands of HOSA mold the health of tomorrow." The VICA motto: "Preparing for leadership in the world of work." *(HOSA motto and emblem used courtesy of HOSA, Flower Mound, Tex; SkillsUSA-VICA motto and logo used courtesy of SkillsUSA-VICA, Leesburg, Va.)*

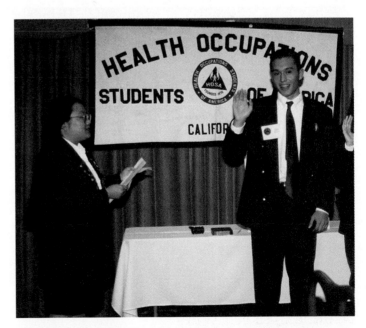

Figure 5-3   Officers of student organizations swear an oath of office as a sign that they understand the responsibilities and importance of their positions.

One of the elements of an effective group is a clear understanding of its purposes and goals. The group must be flexible in the methods used to meet the goals. The members need to practice good communication skills and be able to initiate and carry out effective problem solving. An effective group shares the leadership responsibilities among its members and uses the abilities of all members.

In meetings members make decisions and develop a sense of belonging to the organization. A good meeting develops a sense of pride and enthusiasm for activities. Good meetings are possible when all members feel a sense of ownership of the decisions. Leadership ensures that the meeting is planned, organized, and conducted to cover all ideas in a fair manner. Following through with plans after the meeting is also important to reach goals and develop a sense of community within the group.

Parliamentary Procedure

Parliamentary procedure is a set of rules for conducting a meeting in an organized and efficient manner. Robert's Rules of Order is the basis for these rules and serves as the guide or authority for business procedures in many groups and organizations. Parliamentary procedure maintains a sense of order during meetings and ensures that all members have a chance to participate equally. The procedure is designed to simplify matters by allowing only one person to speak at a time and by discussing only one idea at a time. Decisions are reached through a process of **motions, debate,** and voting that ensures that all members can be heard (Table 5-2). The vote of the majority determines the course of action, but the minority also has the right to be heard.

The **agenda** lists activities for the meeting (Box 5-1). The agenda for the first meeting should include establishing a yearlong calendar of activities, based on goals set by the group. Motions are made to propose action for the group. There are several types of motions used in parliamentary procedure, including main, subsidiary, privileged, and incidental ones. The type of motion determines when a person may speak. When the meeting is finished, a motion to **adjourn** ends it. Election of officers is determined by the constitution and bylaws of the organization. Parliamentary procedure can be learned by practice.

Table 5-2 Parliamentary Procedure: Motions Used to Conduct Meetings

Motion	Can Interrupt Speaker?	Second Required?	Debatable?	Amendable?	Type of Vote Required	Purpose
Main	No	Yes	Yes	Yes	Majority	To introduce business
Refer to Committee	No	Yes	Yes	Yes	Majority	To refer the matter to a committee
Approve minutes	No	Yes	Yes	Yes	Majority	To accept the minutes of a previous meeting
Amend a main motion	No	Yes	Yes	Yes	Majority	To change a motion
Table a motion	No	Yes	No	No	Majority	To wait to consider the matter
Adjourn	No	Yes	No	No	Majority	To end the meeting
Question of privilege	Yes	No	No	No	No vote	To give immediate attention to a problem
Division	No	Yes	No	Yes	No vote	To call for the vote to be verified
Point of order	Yes	No	No	No	No vote	To raise a parliamentary question

Box 5-1   Agenda

I. Call to order
II. Invocation
III. Pledge of allegiance
IV. Roll call and establish quorum
V. Minutes of previous meeting
VI. Treasurer's report
VII. Officers' reports
VIII. Committee reports
   A. Standing
   B. Special
IX. Unfinished business
X. New business
XI. Program
XII. Announcements
XIII. Adjournment

Career Planning

Each person seeks different things from a job (Figure 5-4). Approximately one third of a person's life is spent working, so the job should meet as many of the person's needs as possible. After deciding on the type of job preferred, the applicant must apply for available positions. Available jobs may be found through newspaper advertisements, employment agencies, and through friends. Other resources for job opportunities may include teachers, counselors, professional journals, and job posting boards at the place of employment. Employers look for the best person to fill the vacancy. They use the application, **resumé,** and interview to determine who is the best applicant.

Application

Some positions may require a letter of application (Figure 5-5). The letter of application requests a chance to apply for a position and should be brief (Skill 5-1).

Applications are often used to determine which candidates get an interview. The prospective employee should consider the application to be an example of the work the employer might expect (Figure 5-6). It should be filled in neatly, leaving no blank spaces. The application must be honest, but should present the applicant in the best light possible (Box 5-2). If possible, the applicant should obtain two blank application forms for the position. The first should be completed in pencil and then proofread and cor-

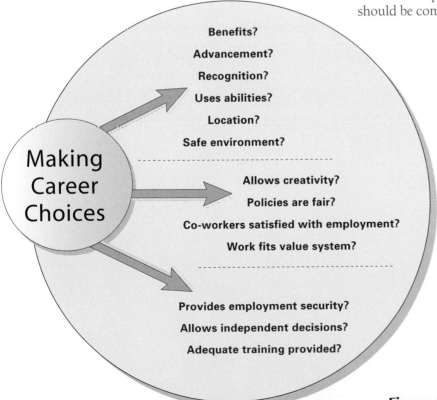

Figure 5-4   Career choice considerations.

Date

Ms./Mr. _____
Human Resource Manager
Agency Name
Address
City, State, Zip Code

Dear Ms./Mr. _____

Mr./Ms. _____ , my health occupations education teacher, suggested that I contact you about the position you currently have open in the area of _____ . Please consider me an applicant for this position.

I will graduate from _____ High School in June of this year. My courses have included training and work that support my desire to be employed in the health care field. I have reached competency levels in many of the basic health care skills, such as assessing vital signs and understanding medical terminology. I am enclosing a personal data sheet that lists these courses and competencies.

I plan to continue my education by taking classes during the hours I am not working. May I have an interview at your convenience? Please call the number noted below at any time and a message will be taken for me. Thank you for your time and consideration of my application.

Sincerely,

Student Name
Address
City, State, Zip Code

Phone Number

enclosure

Figure 5-5   Letter of application.

Skill 5-1

Preparing a Letter of Application

1. Address the letter to the person who will conduct the interview or make the hiring decision.

2. Type the letter using a standard business correspondence format.

3. Proofread and correct any errors of spelling or grammar.

4. Include three paragraphs. Express interest in applying for the position, supply brief information regarding qualifications, and provide a method by which you may be reached to schedule an interview.

5. Include your name, mailing address, phone number, and email address in the closing.

6. Include a personal data sheet or resumé with the letter.

---

rected. The final application can then be recopied in ink or typed, proofread, and returned to the employer. It may, however, be necessary to complete the application at the time it is obtained, so the applicant should have all necessary information at hand.

Resumé

The personal data sheet or resumé provides additional information that is not found on the application (Figure 5-7). It includes skills and achievements presented in an easily read and neat format. As with the letter of application and application form, the resumé should be without error, concise, and present the prospective employee in the best manner (Skill 5-2). At least three copies of the personal data sheet or resumé should be prepared for the job interview (Skill 5-3).

Interview

Many prospective employees do not recognize that the first interview occurs when the application is obtained from the receptionist. The appearance and behavior of the applicant during this part of the procedure may determine whether an interview is granted with the person who actually makes the hiring decision (Box 5-3).

Box 5-2 Application Guidelines

- Print or type all items accurately and neatly. Read every line carefully. If possible, have someone review the application for errors.
- Do not leave any blank spaces or lines. The phrase "not applicable," "N/A," or a dash indicates that the question was read but does not apply.
- Account for any periods of time not working or termination of employment in a positive manner. For example, a termination might have been caused by a "reduction in force" or "seeking better employment opportunity."
- Answer the question of salary as "open" if an amount is not known.
- Use a phone number that will be answered promptly. That may be the number of a family member or a friend who would take a message.

Application for Employment

Date _____

Name _____   Social Security # _____

Address _____ Zip _____   Telephone Number _____

If employed and you are under 18 can you furnish a work permit?   ☐ Yes   ☐ No

Are you legally eligible for employment in the U.S.A.?   ☐ Yes   ☐ No

Have you worked here before?   ☐ Yes   ☐ No   If Yes, when? _____

Are there any hours, shifts or days you cannot or will not work? _____

Are you willing to work overtime if required?   ☐ Yes   ☐ No

List friends or relatives working here. _____

Have you ever been convicted of a crime?   ☐ Yes   ☐ No   (A conviction record will not necessarily be a bar to employment)

EDUCATION

Circle Highest Grade Completed	Grade School 1 2 3 4 5 6 7 8	High School 9 10 11 12	College 1 2 3 4	Graduate 1 2 3 4	Degree Received	Course of Study
High School	Name and Address					
College(s)						
Graduate/Professional						
Specialized Training, Apprenticeship, Skills						
Honors and Awards and Accreditations						

MILITARY SERVICE RECORD   Have you served in the U.S. Armed Forces? _____   Dates of duty _____

POSITION(S) APPLIED FOR: 1) _____   2) _____

You must indicate a specific position. Applications stating "ANY POSITION" will not be considered.

Wage or salary requirements $ _____   When can you start? _____

Figure 5-6 Application for employment.

Application for Employment—continued

WORK HISTORY

If presently employed, may we contact your employer?   ❑ Yes   ❑ No

(1) **Present or Most Recent Employer**	Address	Phone
Date Started	Starting Salary	Starting Position
Date Left	Salary on Leaving	Position on Leaving
Name and Title of Supervisor		
Description of Duties		Reason for Leaving
(2) **Previous Employer**	Address	Phone
Date Started	Starting Salary	Starting Position
Date Left	Salary on Leaving	Position on Leaving
Name and Title of Supervisor		
Description of Duties		Reason for Leaving
(3) **Previous Employer**	Address	Phone
Date Started	Starting Salary	Starting Position
Date Left	Salary on Leaving	Position on Leaving
Name and Title of Supervisor		
Description of Duties		Reason for Leaving

Figure 5-6, cont'd   Application for employment.   *Continued*

ADDITIONAL INFORMATION

OTHER QUALIFICATIONS

Summarize special job-related skills and qualifications acquired from employment or other experience.

_____

_____

_____

SPECIALIZED SKILLS   (CHECK SKILLS/EQUIPMENT OPERATED)

_____ CRT	_____ Fax	Other (list):
_____ PC	_____ Lotus 1-2-3	_____
_____ Calculator	_____ PBX System	_____
_____ Typewriter	_____ WordPerfect	_____

State any additional information you feel may be helpful to us in considering your application.

_____

_____

_____

_____

Note to Applicants: DO NOT ANSWER THIS QUESTION UNLESS YOU HAVE BEEN INFORMED ABOUT THE REQUIREMENTS OF THE JOB FOR WHICH YOU ARE APPLYING.

Are you capable of performing in a reasonable manner—with or without a reasonable accommodation—the activities involved in the job or occupation for which you have applied? A description of the activities involved in such a job or occupation is attached.   ❑ Yes   ❑ No

REFERENCES

1. _____
   (Name)   Phone #

   _____
   (Address)

2. _____
   (Name)   Phone #

   _____
   (Address)

3. _____
   (Name)   Phone #

   _____
   (Address)

UNDER MARYLAND LAW, AN EMPLOYER MAY NOT REQUIRE OR DEMAND, AS A CONDITION OF EMPLOYMENT, PROSPECTIVE EMPLOYMENT, OR CONTINUED EMPLOYMENT, THAT AN INDIVIDUAL SUBMIT TO OR TAKE A LIE DETECTOR OR SIMILAR TEST. AN EMPLOYER WHO VIOLATES THIS LAW IS GUILTY OF A MISDEMEANOR AND SUBJECT TO A FINE NOT EXCEEDING $100.00.

By my signature below, I certify that I have read the above and understand it completely.

_____   _____
Signature   Date

Figure 5-6, cont'd   Application for employment.

Skill 5-2

Completing a Job Application

1. Obtain the application form from the employing agency. If applications do not need to be completed on site, take two. The first one may be completed as a draft and reviewed by another person before submitting a final version.

2. Print in black ink or type all items on the application accurately and neatly. Be consistent with the type of lettering used.

3. Do not leave any blanks or spaces to demonstrate thoroughness in the application completion. Draw a single line "emdash" or write "Not applicable" or "N/A" if the item does not apply to you.

4. Use positive language to account for any periods of time not working or attending school.

5. Account for any employment termination in a positive manner. For example, "reduction in force" or "better employment opportunity" would be more positive than "laid off" or "quit."

6. Answer questions on acceptable salary as "open" if the amount is negotiable or unknown.

7. Provide a phone number that will be answered by someone promptly. The employer will not make many attempts to contact a new applicant for an interview or to offer employment.

8. Submit the application before the deadline or closing of the position offering.

The interview provides the employer a chance to evaluate the applicant. It also provides the applicant with an opportunity to find out more about the job and employer. The applicant should prepare for an interview by anticipating questions and forming answers that are clear and concise (Box 5-4). Before the interview, the applicant should gather as much information as possible about the prospective employer. Minimally, the applicant should know the name and position of the interviewer, the basic job expectations, and a little about the employing agency. When the employer has finished questioning the applicant, it is appropriate to ask questions. These questions should reflect a real interest in knowing about the position (Skill 5-4).

Job Satisfaction

One criterion or need for a job satisfaction is the ability to pay for the wants and needs of life. To determine whether an employment opportunity will provide for these needs, a personal **budget** may be used to determine whether these financial goals can be met (Figure 5-8). The gross income is the money earned as a salary or wage. The net income is the amount that actually appears in the check after **taxes,** social security, and other deductions are made. A budget is a plan for the use of resources and expenditures. Once a budget is established, it may be adjusted as necessary.

When income is received, a checking and savings account may be the best way to store and distribute money (Figure 5-9). Banks provide varied incentive programs for their accounts and may offer "free" services, interest, or checks for investing with their company. A personal financial statement is also a tool that can be used for planning a budget (Figure 5-10).

Some taxes are taken directly from the check before it is received. This may include city, county, state, and federal taxes. Social security taxes or FICA wages are taken out of the check as well. Social Security is a retirement fund that was established to provide funds for the disabled, elderly,

Personal Data Sheet

Student Name
Address
City, State, Zip Code

Phone number

Personal data:

Date of birth	Weight
Marital Status	Height

Course work:

Typing	Health Occupations I
Computers	Health Occupations II

Activities:

President, Health Occupations Organization
Chairperson, March of Dimes Walk-a-Thon

Skills:

Have knowledge of medical terminology
Able to assess vital signs
Certified in cardiopulmonary resuscitation
Able to apply body mechanics safely

Work experience:

Volunteer at hospital weekly, 3 years
Student assistant in science, 1 year

References:

List three in alphabetical order. Include
name, address, and telephone number.
A reference should be asked prior to
including the name.

Figure 5-7   Personal data sheet.

Box 5-3   Guidelines for the Interview

1. Know the name of the interviewer and his or her position within the organization.
2. Know about the organization and the position desired.
3. Bring all information regarding references, social security number, past employment, and education needed to complete the application form. If permitted to complete the application away from the site, take two to use one for practice.
4. Present yourself for the interview in a positive and confident manner.
5. Arrive 5 minutes early for the appointment, not earlier or later.
6. Do not chew gum, eat candy, or smoke before or during the interview.
7. Wear appropriate clothing for the position desired. Be neat and clean.
8. Shake hands firmly with the interviewer when introduced. If you must introduce yourself, call the interviewer by title and name.
9. Remain standing until the interviewer asks you to sit down.
10. Place any personal items, such as a purse, on the floor. Keep a pencil and some paper at hand in case it is needed.
11. Be enthusiastic but not overbearing. Answer all of the questions in a positive manner without criticizing yourself or others.
12. Think about each question before responding to it. Look at the interviewer when speaking.
13. After the interviewer has completed his or her questions, ask any questions that remain unanswered for you.
14. Thank the interviewer for his or her time. Ask when the decision regarding the position will be known.

and unemployed. Other taxes such as property tax must be sent or paid annually to an agency such as the state. Indirect taxes are those paid every day, such as sales taxes and those on gasoline, cigarettes, and liquor. All citizens of the United States must prepare a federal income tax statement each year if the income reaches the specified amount.

Insurance costs may be deducted from the paycheck as well. Some types of insurance include health, life, unemployment, personal property, automobile, and worker's compensation. Some of these costs may be paid by the employer alone or together with the employee.

Resignation

Maintaining employment or keeping a job is accomplished by performing well and showing the favorable characteris-

Skill 5-3

Preparing a Resumé

1. Use only the information that presents you in the best light for the personal data sheet or resumé.

2. Head the resumé with your name, address, phone number, and email address.

3. Divide the resumé into categories of information. For example, categories may include course work, activities, skills, work experience, awards, and career goals. Use only one side of one sheet of paper.

4. List any chronological information, such as work dates, in order with the most recent listed first.

5. Type the resumé neatly without any errors. Center information from the top to the bottom of the paper.

6. Include three references in alphabetical order by last name. Include name, address, telephone number, and email address.

7. Make additional copies of your resumé to send with letters of application and to take to interviews.

Box 5-4 Interview Questions

Interviewer

1. What are your future goals?
2. What can you tell me about yourself?
3. Why did you choose our company for possible employment?
4. For what type of position are you applying?
5. Have you ever been dismissed from a job?
6. Why did you leave your last place of employment?
7. Why do you feel qualified for this position?
8. What do you feel are your strong points?
9. What do you feel are your weak points?
10. Do you have any plans for further education?
11. How many days of school/work did you miss last year?
12. What skills do you have that would be useful in this position?
13. Who is your favorite teacher, and why?
14. How do you get along with your family?
15. What do you like to do in your free time?
16. Why do you think you are a better applicant than the others applying for this position?
17. What motivates you?
18. How well do you do in school?
19. How do you rate yourself as a leader?
20. What would you say are your most important accomplishments to date?

Interviewee

1. How is the department or company organized for supervision?
2. With whom would I be working?
3. Are there opportunities for advancement in this position?
4. What is the performance evaluation procedure?
5. Is additional on-the-job-training possible?
6. Does the supervisor encourage initiative and creativity?

Skill 5-4

Interviewing

1. Dress appropriately for the interview. The type of dress will depend on the job being sought but should be neat, clean, and conservative. Come prepared with information such as social security number and employment history to complete the application form.

2. Arrive 5 minutes early to the interview. The interviewer may have other appointments scheduled. If the application must be completed at the time of the interview, allow additional time for that before the scheduled interview time.

3. Greet the receptionist politely. Many employers consider the receptionist's opinion of applicants in making a hiring decision.

4. Present yourself in a positive and confident manner. Always go alone to the interview.

5. Remain standing until asked to sit down. Shake hands firmly with the interviewer during introductions. Place any materials on the floor or on your lap, not on the interviewer's desk.

6. Sit comfortably but conservatively, with a straight back and feet on the floor or legs crossed at the ankles.

7. Answer questions completely, in a positive manner, using more than one-word responses. The interview allows the applicant to demonstrate the ability to communicate well.

8. Maintain eye contact when answering questions. Be enthusiastic but not overbearing.

9. Ask questions if some were unanswered during the interview. Questions show the interviewer that the applicant is interested and has been thinking during the interview. Before leaving, ask when the position will be determined and how you will be notified.

10. Thank the interviewer for his or her time, and shake hands upon leaving.

11. When the interview is finished, leave the building. The interviewer may be expecting other applicants.

Cost-of-Living Budget

Regular or Fixed Monthly Payments*

Mortgage or rent	$
Automobile payment	$
Automobile insurance	$
Appliances	$
Loan	$
Health insurance	$
Personal property insurance	$
Telephone	$
Utilities (gas or electric)	$
Water	$
Other non-emergency expenses	$

Discretionary or Variable Payments

Clothing, laundry, cleaning	$
Medicine	$
Doctor and dentist	$
Education	$
Dues	$
Gifts and donations	$
Travel	$
Subscriptions	$
Automobile maintenance and gas	$
Spending money and entertainment	$

Food Expenses

Food—at home	$
Food—away from home	$

Taxes

Federal and state income tax	$
Property	$
Other taxes	$

Other

Other	$

Total Monthly Payments

	$

Sample Recommended Budget Expenditures

Shelter (Rent or mortgage)	20%
Food	25%
Clothing	12%
Transportation	12%
Medical and dental	6%
Dues and charities	9%
Education and entertainment	10%
Savings	6%*

* Financial advisors recommend that savings should cover expenses for at least three months.

Figure 5-8   A personal budget ensures that money earned will meet the needs of life.

CHECK NO.	DATE	CHECK ISSUED TO OR DEPOSIT RECEIVED FROM	AMOUNT OF CHECK	AMOUNT OF DEPOSIT	BALANCE
1	1/1	Apartments R Us	500.00		250.00

Figure 5-9   Accurate records for income and expenditures is made easier with written records.

Personal Financial Statement

Assets		Debts	
Cash	$	Household bills unpaid	$
Securities (stocks, bonds, CDs)	$	Installment payments:	
Real Estate	$	Automobile	$
Automobile	$	Appliances	$
Furniture	$	Loans	$
Receivables (money owed to you)	$	Real estate payments	$
Other	$	Other	$
Value should be determined by the amount that could be obtained from a "quick" sale.		Insurance:	
		Automobile	$
		Personal property	$
		Health	$
Total Owned	$	Other	$
		Taxes	$
		Other debts	$
		Total Owed	$
		Total Owned Minus Total Owed = Total Worth	$

Figure 5-10   A person's financial standing is determined by the difference between the amount owned (assets) and the amount owed (debts).

tics of a health care worker. Some of these characteristics include a positive attitude, enthusiasm, an open mind, and constant efforts to improve performance. Poor interpersonal relations, lack of technical knowledge, and lack of dedication to work ethics such as promptness, honesty, and good grooming often cause job termination. Most people who lose a job after being hired do so because of attitude rather than ability to do the job. Advancement is earned by doing the job better and more quickly and showing the attributes of **initiative**, loyalty, and responsibility. Improvement in performance is expected over time from a new employee.

When a better opportunity or other personal considerations cause termination, there is a proper way to end the association. It is not advisable to end employment until another job has been secured. The time needed to "give notice" of termination depends on the level of responsibility of the job. Two weeks is usually long enough for the employer to make arrangements to fill the vacancy. A letter of resignation is submitted to the employer before telling other employees or patients (Figure 5-11). The letter should contain the date

on which the employment will end and express appreciation for the opportunity of having worked with the establishment. It is not necessary to give the reason for termination if this information might leave bad feelings.

If dismissed, fired, or laid off from a job, the worker is at a disadvantage in finding new employment. It is important to respectfully determine the reason for termination. In future interviews for employment, the applicant can use this information to demonstrate an effort to improve. Most employers will hire a person who has made a mistake but is willing to learn from it and improve.

Continuing Education

Continuing education refers to the training, courses, and study that are completed after the health care worker begins to practice. In many of the health care professions, continuing education is required for the health care worker to continue to practice or be relicensed.

Letter of Resignation

Date

Ms./Mr. _____
Supervisor
Agency Name
Address
City, State, Zip Code

Dear Ms./Mr. _____

It is now necessary for me to terminate my employment with the _____ agency. I have learned a great deal from my association with the organization and appreciate having had the opportunity to work with you and the other staff members.

To allow 2 weeks for hiring a replacement, I will be glad to work until _____ . If there is any way I can help with the transition, please let me know.

Sincerely,

Employee Name
Address
City, State, Zip Code
Phone Number

Figure 5-11   Letter of resignation.

Review Questions

1. Explain two purposes of a professional organization.

2. List three advantages of using parliamentary procedure during organizational meetings.

3. Use Table 5-2 to determine the correct way to interrupt a speaker during a meeting.

4. List at least five important items of information needed on a job application.

5. Compose at least five questions that might be asked during a job interview and outline appropriate responses.

6. List two reasons why an employee might be offered advancement on a job.

7. List two reasons why an employee might be dismissed from a job.

8. Make a personal budget for 1 month and 1 year.

Critical Thinking

1. Write a paragraph that describes your present choice in a career and its benefits.

2. Describe two ways that a person might think about being rejected for a job.

3. Write a paragraph that describes the benefits of one type of leadership style.

4. Attend a meeting of a professional organization or legislative body to view the procedures used and behavior of group members. Write a paragraph that describes whether the behavior was beneficial for conducting business.

5. Practice using parliamentary procedure by holding a meeting of the student organization.

6
Foundation Skills

Learning Objectives

Describe elements of basic health assessment.

Identify normal and abnormal vital sign values.

Describe the importance of the values for normal vital signs.

Perform basic mathematical skills related to health care.

Use basic medical terminology and abbreviations.

Identify risk factors for cardiac arrest.

Key Terms

Apical
(AYP-i-kul) Pertaining to the apex or pointed end of the heart

Auscultation
(os-kuhl-TAY-shen) Act of listening for sounds within the body

Blood Pressure
Pressure of circulating blood against the walls of the arteries

Cardiac Arrest
(KAR-dee-ak uh-REST) Sudden stopping of heart action

Diastolic
(die-uh-STAHL-ik) Blood pressure during ventricular relaxation

Palpation
(pal-PAY-shen) Technique used to feel the texture, size, consistency, and location of parts of the body with the hands

Percussion
(per-KUSH-en) Technique of tapping with the fingertips to evaluate size, borders, and consistency of internal structures of the body

Systolic
(sis-TOL-ik) Blood pressure during ventricular contraction

Vital
(VY-tul) Necessary to life

Skill 6-1

Admitting, Transferring, and Discharging the Patient

1. Maintain medical asepsis by using the guidelines provided in the Standard and Transmission-Based Precautions, including good handwashing technique and use of gloves as needed.

2. Gather the necessary equipment and supplies including clean linens, an admission kit, an admission checklist, and a pen.

3. Prepare the room as necessary with clean, appropriate equipment and supplies.

4. Greet the patient by name and introduce yourself. Patients are usually admitted to the unit of the hospital by a nurse, but other personnel may be assigned this duty if the patient does not need immediate care.

5. Assist the patient as necessary to put on a gown or pajamas.

6. Complete the admission checklist.

7. Explain the facility routine procedures and policies. The patient may not understand such regulations as the use of side rails for safety, removal of jewelry for safe storage, or use of a signal light to summon someone.

8. If transfer of the patient is necessary, explain the reason for the change. The patient may feel disoriented and insecure by being moved to another location.

9. Transport the patient in a wheelchair, on a stretcher, or in a bed.

10. When discharge from the facility is ordered, assist the patient to gather belongings in containers for transport.

11. Assist the patient to dress for discharge.

12. Accompany the patient to the car or other method of transport. The patient may need assistance to arrange adequate transportation to the home or another facility.

Health Assessment

Patient Interview and Examination

The basic health assessment may include an interview and physical examination to determine functional, cultural, spiritual, and physical characteristics. Basic health assessment may be the responsibility of many health care workers. The type and extent of assessment is determined by the role of the worker and the type of care being given. The patient interview may include the medical history, nature of the current complaint, and medication record. Some health care workers such as the Nurse Assistant and Licensed Practical Nurse may collect data that will be analyzed and evaluated by another health care worker such as the Registered Nurse (Skill 6-1).

Vital Signs

Vital signs, or life signs, are values that can be used to measure changes in body function, general health, and the response to treatment. Vital signs include **blood pressure** (BP) and temperature, pulse, and respiration (TPR). The value of vital signs is affected by many factors including age, activity, nutrition, emotion, fitness, medication, and illness. Height (ht), weight (wt), and fluid balance or intake and output (I&O) also may be used to assess the patient.

Vital signs are ordered with different frequency depending on the type of service being provided. Common orders for assessment include twice a day (bid.), three times a day (tid.), four times a day (qid.), or routinely once a day (qd). Vitals may be ordered at regular intervals such as every 4 hours (q4h) or every 15 minutes (q15m).

Blood Pressure

Blood pressure is a measurement of the force of the blood against the walls of the arteries as it circulates through the body. It reflects the effort the heart exerts to circulate the blood to the tissues. Two units or values for blood pressure are measured. They are the maximum pressure at which the pulse can be heard **(systolic)** and the minimum pressure at which it is audible **(diastolic)**. The systolic reading occurs while the ventricles of the heart are contracting. The diastolic reading occurs during relaxation of the ventricles. Instruments that are used to determine the blood pressure are the stethoscope and sphygmomanometer (Figure 6-1).

The stethoscope amplifies the sound. The sphygmomanometer is an inflatable cuff that measures pressure using air (aneroid) or mercury.

Blood pressure varies greatly among people. It is affected by the diameter and flexibility (elasticity) of the blood vessels, force of the heart contraction, and amount of blood in the vessels (Figure 6-2). Pressure on the area of the brain that controls blood pressure can also change its value. Limits of the usual blood pressure for most individuals have been set. The "normal" blood pressure is said to be 120/80 (systolic/diastolic) (Box 6-1). Generally, a range is acceptable from a systolic of 100 to 160 and a diastolic less than 100 (Skill 6-2).

Box 6-1   **Blood Pressure**

Normal value: 120/80
Abnormal parameters:
  Systolic >160
  Systolic <100
  Diastolic >100

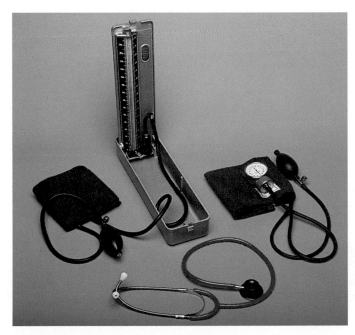

Figure 6-1 The aneroid sphygmomanometer measures blood pressure using air. This stethoscope has a flat diaphragm to hear shallow sounds. Sphygmomanometers also may contain mercury to measure the pressure.

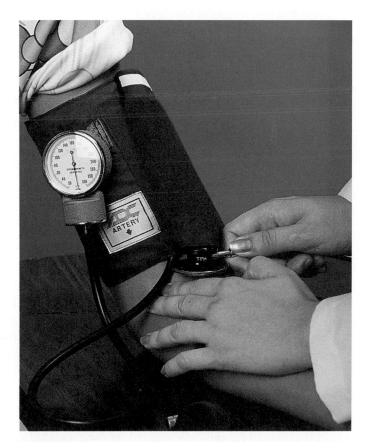

Figure 6-2 The brachial artery is found to determine the correct placement of the stethoscope.

Skill 6-2

Taking a Blood Pressure

1. Maintain medical asepsis by using the guidelines provided in the Standard and Transmission–Based Precautions, including good handwashing technique and use of gloves as needed.

2. Gather all necessary equipment including a stethoscope, sphygmomanometer, alcohol pledget, pen, and paper.

3. Identify the patient and explain the procedure. Identification of the correct patient and explanation of the procedure prevents errors and misunderstanding.

4. Position the patient in either a sitting or lying position with the upper arm exposed and supported above the level of the heart. Clothing must allow exposure of the upper arm completely without binding. Privacy should be provided if necessary. Either arm may be used, but arms with injuries, intravenous lines, or other treatments should be avoided because the procedure may cause injury or pain or the reading may be inaccurate.

5. Wrap the cuff of the sphygmomanometer around the arm 1 inch above the bend of the elbow *(antecubital space)*. The cuff should be tight enough that two fingers may be placed under the edge comfortably. If the cuff is too tight or too loose, the reading will be inaccurate. The cuff is placed 1 inch above the level of the bend of the elbow to allow room for the flat placement of the stethoscope.

6. While palpating the radial artery, tighten the thumbscrew of the sphygmomanometer and inflate until the pulse disappears. This reading is an approximate systolic pressure.

7. Deflate the cuff completely and allow the arm to rest for 30 seconds.

8. Clean the earplugs of the stethoscope with alcohol and place them into the ears with the opening pointing toward the nose.

9. Locate the brachial pulse with the tips of two fingers and place the flat part *(diaphragm)* of the stethoscope on the location of the pulse. Placement over the brachial artery allows the pulse to be heard more easily *(audible)* when the cuff is inflated.

10. Tighten the thumbscrew valve by turning it clockwise and inflate the cuff to 20 to 30 mm Hg above the approximate systolic value.

11. Deflate the cuff, slowly noting the location on the scale at which the first *(systolic)* and last *(diastolic)* pulse are heard. The last distinct beat is considered to be the diastolic pulse. Soft muffled or thumping sounds are not counted.

12. Deflate the cuff completely after the blood pressure is assessed and remove the cuff from the arm. The blood pressure can be reassessed using the same arm a second time. If a third reading is necessary, the cuff should be removed briefly between reading or moved to the other arm because tightening the cuff repeatedly may change the pressure.

13. Record the results. Report any unusual findings to the supervisor immediately. An elevated or low blood pressure may signal an emergency situation.

14. Store equipment in the designated area and discard the alcohol pledget in an appropriate container.

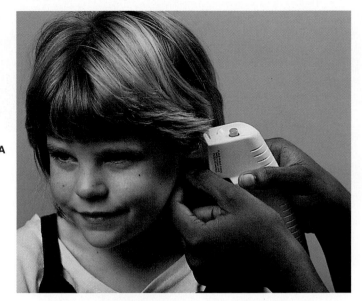

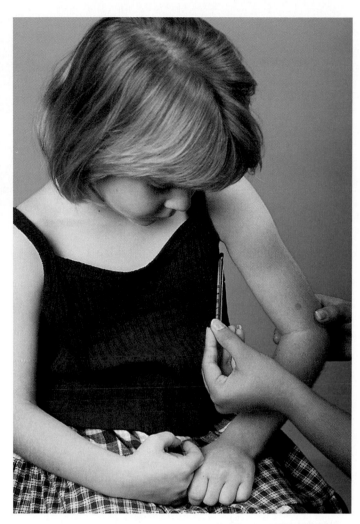

Figure 6-3   A, A tympanometer may be used to assess temperature. **B,** Axillary temperature may be needed for young, uncooperative, or unconscious patients. If the person is in the supine position, crossing the arm over the chest helps to maintain placement of the thermometer.

Temperature

Temperature is the measurement of the balance between the heat produced and lost by the body. Four methods are commonly used to measure temperature. They are the mouth (oral), armpit (axillary), rectum (rectal), and ear (temporal) (Figure 6-3). The skin above the temporal artery also can be used to assess the temperature. Temperature may be measured with the Fahrenheit or Celsius (Centigrade) scale. The normal reading for temperature depends on the location used to assess it (Table 6-1). An elevation of temperature (fever) may indicate infection or inflammation in the body (Skills 6-3 through 6-5).

There are several types of thermometers available for measuring temperature. The most common type is made of glass with an expandable mercury filling. Glass thermometers are designed differently for oral or rectal use. The bulb of the rectal thermometer is rounded to prevent injury to the tissues of the rectum. The tip of the stem of the rectal thermometer is red and that of the oral thermometer is blue or silver for easy identification (Figure 6-4). Rectal thermometers should never be used in the mouth. Mercury thermometers are used with less frequency because of environmental and health hazard resulting from the possibility of a mercury spill. Electronic and disposable chemical thermometers more commonly are used.

Table 6-1	Temperature	
Method	**Time**	**Normal**
Oral	3 min*	97.6°-99.0° F (98.6° F = 37.0° C)
Axillary	10 min*	96.6°-98.0° F (97.6° F = 36.4° C)
Rectal	3-5 min*	98.6°-100.0° F (99.6° F = 37.5° C)
Temporal	*	96.4°-100.4° F (98.4° F = 36.9° C)

*Time required to take temperatures may vary with the electrical instruments used for assessment and is usually signaled by a sound from the device.

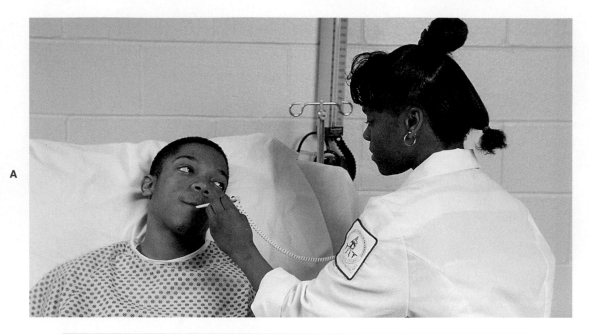

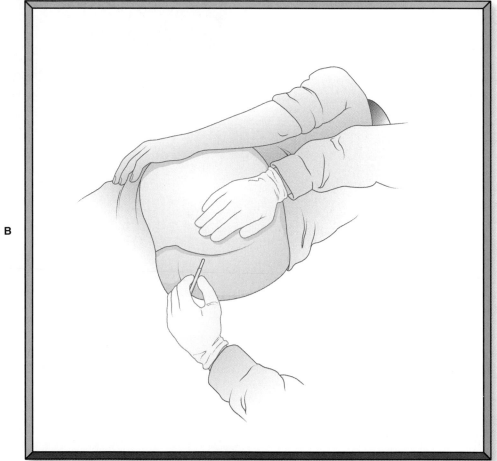

Figure 6-4   **A,** During the assessment of an oral temperature, the mouth should remain closed. **B,** Privacy is a primary consideration during assessment of the rectal temperature.

Skill 6-3

Taking an Oral Temperature

1. Maintain medical asepsis by using the guidelines provided in the Standard and Transmission-Based Precautions, including good handwashing technique and use of gloves as needed.

2. Gather necessary supplies and equipment, including a thermometer, tissue, alcohol swab or pledget, pen, and paper.

3. Clean an oral thermometer with disinfectant solution before use. Wash it with cool, soapy water and rinse to remove the disinfectant. The disinfectant may irritate the tissues of the mouth.

4. Shake the mercury level of the thermometer down with a sharp movement of the wrist until the reading is 96.0° F or lower. The shaking movement causes the mercury to fall to the bulb end of the thermometer. Activate the electronic thermometer if it is being used.

5. Cover the thermometer with a plastic sheath or wipe with alcohol from stem to bulb. The stem is considered cleaner than the bulb.

6. Identify the patient and explain the procedure. Determine that the patient has not consumed any hot or cold food or beverage or smoked for at least 5 minutes before taking the temperature. The temperature of the food or beverages and smoking will affect the reading.

7. Place the bulb end of the thermometer under the patient's tongue and instruct the patient to keep the lips closed for 3 minutes, taking care not to bite on the thermometer. If bitten, the thermometer could break and harm the patient. Electronic thermometers are held in place for 45 seconds. The mouth must be closed to obtain an accurate reading.

8. Remove the thermometer by holding it by the stem, and wipe it with alcohol from stem to bulb to prevent the spread of microorganisms. Discard alcohol pledget or swab in the proper container immediately. If a sheath or cover is used, remove it and discard it in the proper container immediately.

9. Read the thermometer by holding it at eye level and twisting the stem until the mercury can be seen. Record the result on paper. Readings that are between two lines on the thermometer are considered to be the higher reading.

10. Report any unusual findings to the supervisor immediately.

11. Clean the thermometer with disinfectant and store it in the designated area. Deactivate an electronic thermometer and place it in the recharging element.

12. Maintain medical asepsis by washing your hands when the procedure is completed.

Skill 6-4

Taking an Axillary Temperature

1. Maintain medical asepsis by using the guidelines provided in the Standard and Transmission-Based Precautions, including good handwashing technique and use of gloves as needed.

2. Gather the necessary supplies including an oral thermometer, tissue, dry wash cloth, alcohol pledget or swab, pen, and paper.

3. Clean an oral thermometer with disinfectant solution before use. Wash it with cool, soapy water and rinse to remove disinfectant. The disinfectant may irritate the skin.

4. Shake the mercury level of the thermometer down with a sharp movement of the wrist until the reading is 96.0° F or lower. Activate an electronic thermometer if it is to be used.

5. Cover the thermometer with a plastic sheath or wipe with alcohol from stem to bulb.

6. Identify the patient and explain the procedure. Provide for privacy.

7. Position the patient so that the area under the arm (axilla) is exposed. Pat the axilla dry with a clean cloth. Patting the area dry removes moisture and excess heat. Avoid rubbing and creating friction that may raise the temperature.

8. Place the thermometer with the end bulb in the middle of the axilla and cross the patient's arm on the chest to keep thermometer in place for 10 minutes.

9. Remove the thermometer and wipe it with alcohol from stem to bulb. Discard the alcohol swab and any sheath or covering in an appropriate container.

10. Read the thermometer by holding it at eye level and twisting the stem until the mercury can be seen. Record the result on paper. Readings that are between two lines on the thermometer are considered to be the higher reading. Report any unusual findings to the supervisor.

11. Reposition the patient for comfort and privacy.

12. Clean the thermometer with disinfectant solution and store it in the designated area. Deactivate an electronic thermometer and replace it in the recharging element.

Pulse and Respiration

Pulse is the heartbeat that can be felt (palpated) on surface arteries as the artery walls expand. The pulse is usually assessed using the radial artery near the wrist, but it may be found in other locations (Figure 6-5).

The rate of the heartbeat must be adequate to supply blood and its nutrients to all parts of the body. The pulse of an infant is significantly faster than that of an adult (Table 6-2). The normal adult pulse rate can range between 60 and 100 beats per minute. In addition to the rate, it is

Skill 6-5

Taking a Rectal Temperature

1. Maintain medical asepsis by using the guidelines provided in the Standard and Transmission-Based Precautions, including good handwashing technique and use of gloves as needed.

2. Gather all necessary equipment and supplies including a rectal thermometer, lubricating jelly, toilet tissue, disposable gloves, pen, and paper.

3. Clean a rectal thermometer with alcohol from stem to bulb or cover with a protective sheath. Rectal thermometers may be tipped with red and have rounded bulbs. Confusing oral with rectal thermometers is not sanitary and may cause illness.

4. Shake the mercury level of the thermometer down with a sharp movement of the wrist until the reading is 96.0° F or lower. Activate an electronic thermometer if it is to be used.

5. Lubricate 2 inches of the bulb end of the thermometer with lubricating jelly.

6. Identify the patient and explain the procedure. Arrange the unit to provide privacy.

7. Wear disposable gloves to prevent the spread of microorganisms.

8. Position the patient on one side and raise the patient's upper leg slightly toward the head.

9. Expose the anus by raising the upper buttocks. Gently insert the thermometer 1½ inches if the patient is an adult. The rectum of a child is shorter than that of an adult, and special care is needed when taking a rectal temperature.

10. Remain with the patient while holding the thermometer in place for 3 to 5 minutes. Accidental injury may occur if the patient is left alone with a rectal thermometer in place.

11. Remove the thermometer and wipe with tissue from stem to bulb to remove any fecal material. Discard the tissue and any cover used on the thermometer in the appropriate container immediately.

12. Reposition the patient for comfort, privacy, and safety.

13. Read the thermometer by holding it at eye level and twisting the stem until the mercury can be seen. Record the result on paper. Readings that are between two lines on the thermometer are considered to be the higher reading. Report any unusual findings to the supervisor.

14. Clean the thermometer with disinfectant and store it in the designated area. Deactivate an electronic thermometer after use and replace it in the recharging unit.

15. Discard gloves in an appropriate container.

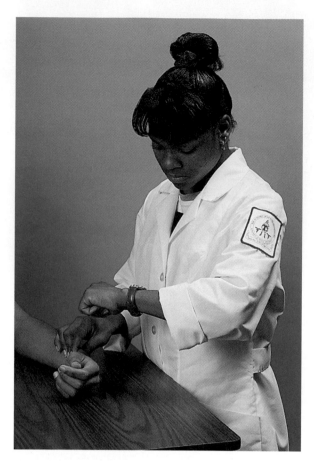

Figure 6-5 Pulse and respiration are assessed at the same time.

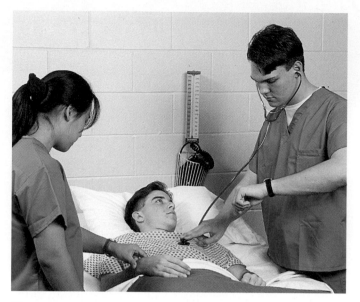

Figure 6-6 Taking of an apical and radial pulse at the same time may be needed to assess circulatory disorders.

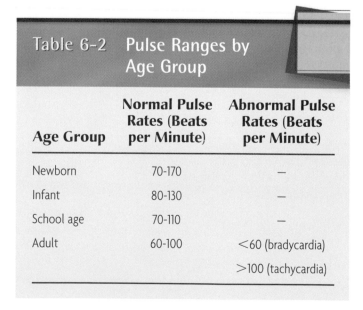

Table 6-2	Pulse Ranges by Age Group	
Age Group	**Normal Pulse Rates (Beats per Minute)**	**Abnormal Pulse Rates (Beats per Minute)**
Newborn	70-170	—
Infant	80-130	—
School age	70-110	—
Adult	60-100	<60 (bradycardia)
		>100 (tachycardia)

Box 6-2   Respiration in Adults

Rate per minute: 14-20
Rhythm: Regular
Character: Effortless, deep, quiet
Abnormal parameters:
Tachypnea >24
Bradypnea <10
Shallow
Stertorous (snoring)
Apnea
Cheyne-Stokes

important to assess the rhythm and character of the pulse. A regular rhythm is evenly paced. An irregular pulse may be fast or slow or may skip beats. Character, describing the force of the pulse, may be strong, weak, bounding, thready, feeble, or fleeting.

The pulse can be counted by listening to the heart through a stethoscope placed on the chest. This pulse is called an **apical** pulse (Figure 6-6). The apical pulse may differ from the radial pulse in some conditions that affect the peripheral blood flow.

Skill 6-6

Taking a Radial Pulse and Measuring Respiration

1. Maintain medical asepsis by using the guidelines provided in the Standard and Transmission-Based Precautions, including good handwashing technique and use of gloves as needed.

2. Gather the necessary supplies and equipment including a watch with a second hand, pen, and paper.

3. Identify the patient and explain the procedure.

4. Place the tips of your first two fingers over the radial artery. The thumb is not used because it has a pulse of its own, which may cause confusion.

5. Using a watch with a second hand, count the pulse beats for 1 minute. The pulse may instead be assessed for 30 seconds and doubled. An assessment less than 30 seconds can lead to error of four beats per minute or more. An irregular pulse must be counted for the complete 1 minute.

6. While still palpating the radial artery, count respirations for 1 minute. If the wrist is held, the patient will remain quiet so that respirations may be assessed. If coughing, talking, or other verbal reaction occurs during the counting of respirations, the count must be reassessed. The result may be affected if the patient is aware that the respirations are being counted.

7. Record the time, rate, and character of pulse and respirations.

8. Report any unusual findings to the supervisor immediately.

One respiration includes the inspiration and expiration of a breath. The normal rate for respiration is more rapid in infants than adults (Box 6-2). The rhythm and character of respiration are important observations. The rhythm of respiration describes its regularity. Character describes the depth and quality of the sound. Respirations that are difficult to see may be assessed by feeling the rise (expansion) and fall (contraction) of the chest or by using the stethoscope to listen for the respiratory or breath sounds (Skill 6-6).

Height and Weight

The weight that is recommended by health professionals is determined usually by using charts that are developed by insurance companies (Figure 6-7). The insurance companies determine at which weight for a specific height an in-

dividual is predicted to live the longest (Figure 6-8). The American Heart Association recommends desired weight be considered in relation to other risk factors of heart disease such as blood pressure and cholesterol levels.

Physical Assessment

Physical assessment uses techniques of inspection, **auscultation, palpation,** and **percussion** (Table 6-3). Inspection is done by using visual and auditory observation (Skill 6-7). Auscultation means listening to sounds, often with a stethoscope. Palpation is using the hands to observe structures by touch. Percussion is striking the body to assess the sound made. The patient is positioned according to physician orders and for comfort during assessment (Figure 6-9).

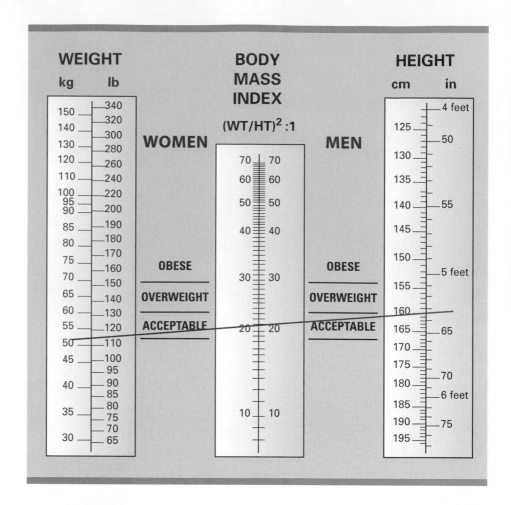

Figure 6-7 A height and weight chart.

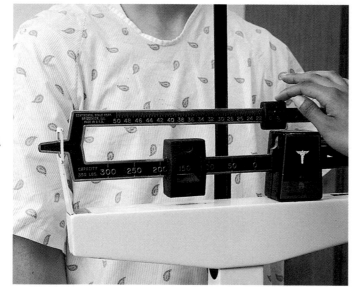

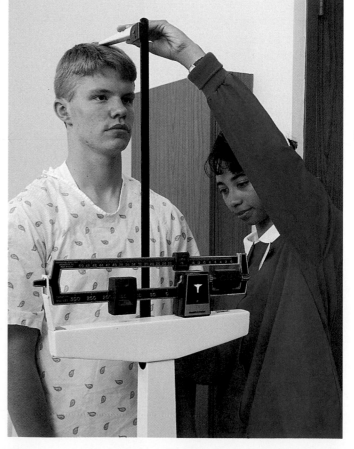

Figure 6-8 This patient is being measured for **A**, weight and **B**, height.

Table 6-3   Physical Assessment

Assessment	Observations
Appearance	Physical, developmental, social development; general health; significant features; height; weight; posture; communication skills; grooming; hygiene
Hair	Color; texture; cleanliness; distribution
Nails	Color; texture; markings; shape; size
Skin	Color; temperature; turgor; lesions; mucous membranes; injury; edema
Neurological	Pupil reaction to light; motor and verbal responses; reflexes; gait; orientation
Musculoskeletal	Range of motion; gait; posture; injury
Cardiovascular	Heart rate and rhythm; peripheral pulses; temperature
Respiratory	Rate; rhythm; quality; breath sounds; sputum production or cough
Gastrointestinal	Abdominal contour; bowel sounds; nausea or vomiting; defecation frequency and consistency
Genitourinary	Urine color; amount; frequency; odor; clarity

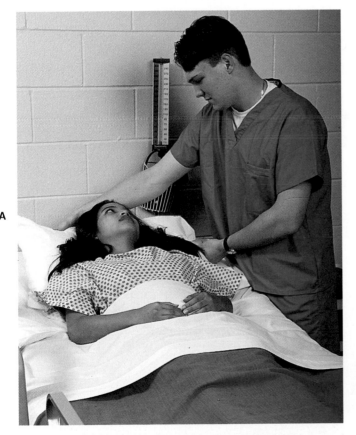

A

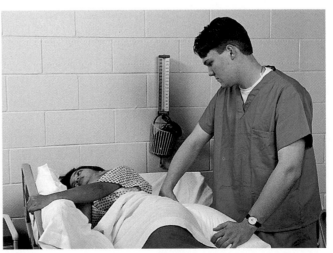

B

Figure 6-9   **A,** Always explain the procedure to the patient before performing it. **B,** The bed is raised to a comfortable working height while assisting the patient to turn, but is returned to the lowest level before leaving the bedside.

Skill 6-7

Recording Observations

1. Report any unusual findings to a supervisor before charting observations.

2. Use black ink and print information legibly.

3. Chart observations promptly after making them.

4. Follow all the rules for good charting.

5. Return the chart to the designated location when finished.

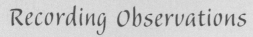

Information Exchange

Basic Math

Many of the procedures performed by the health care worker include the use of concepts of mathematics. For example, the conversion of medication dosages to calculate the correct dosage may be one of the responsibilities of the personnel administering them. The health care worker must be able to use the traditional, apothecary, and SI (metric) systems of measurement to measure time, temperature, distance, capacity (volume), and mass.

Addition and subtraction are methods for counting, resulting in a sum or difference between amounts. Multipli-

---

Box 6-3   Metric Conversion and Using Ratios

1. A tablet is marked as 5 gr of medication. The order is to give 15 gr. How many tablets are given?

   Step 1: $\dfrac{5 \text{ gr}}{1 \text{ tab}} = \dfrac{15 \text{ gr}}{? \text{ tab}}$

   Step 2: Multiply each fraction by ? tab

   5 gr × ? = 15 gr

   Step 3: Divide each fraction by 5 gr

   ? = 3

   The dosage would be 3 tablets. (Note that the units "gr" and "tab") cancel.

2. A patient's temperature is read as 36° Celsius. The patient asks if the temperature is high. What should the health care worker tell the patient?

   Step 1: Substitute the known value (36° C) in the formula for temperature conversion.

   F = 9/5 (36) + 32

   Step 2: Complete multiplication and division functions prior to addition and subtraction un-

less the addition or subtraction is in parentheses.

(9 × 36) / 5 = 64.8

   Step 3: Complete addition after multiplication and division functions are completed.

   F = 64.8 + 32 = 96.8

The health care worker should assure the patient that the temperature is within normal limits.

3. If a patient is to be assisted to walk qid. (four times a day) and the health care worker does not want to wake the patient during the night, when could the patient be assisted to walk?

   Step 1: 24 hours per day – 8 hours per night = 16 hours

   Step 2: $\dfrac{16 \text{ hours}}{4 \text{ walks}} = \dfrac{4 \text{ hours}}{1 \text{ walk}}$

The patient would be walked every 4 hours during the day.

Skill 6-8

Constructing a Line Graph

1. Draw a vertical and a horizontal axis.

2. Determine which of the two types of data to be compared varies the least. Place this information on the horizontal axis.

3. Label the point of intersection of the two axes as zero for each.

4. Divide each axis of the graph into portions that will include all of the data.

5 Chart the first point where the value of the first data intersects on the graph.

6. Chart the second point where the next value intersects on the graph.

7. Draw a straight line to connect the two points together.

8. Chart the third point where the third set of data intersects on the graph.

9. Join the second point to the third point with a straight line.

10. Continue charting and joining points on the graph until all data have been noted.

11. Label each axis with the units of measurement.

12. Label the graph.

cation and division perform addition and subtraction more quickly and result in a product or quotient. A fraction is a comparison of part of a whole to the entire unit. For example, $\frac{1}{4}$ indicates that the quantity being considered is 1 of 4 equal parts of the whole. Fractions may be "reduced" by dividing the top number (numerator) and bottom number (denominator) by the same number. For example, $\frac{2}{4}$ is equal to $\frac{1}{2}$. In health care, fractions or ratios often are used to calculate medications, determine temperature, or determine a schedule for the patient's care (Box 6-3).

There are three systems of measurement used in health care. They are the apothecary, SI (metric), and household units. The health care worker should be familiar with all three systems to be able to convert from one to another when necessary (Table 6-4).

Military Time

Some countries, the military, and the health care industry use a 24-hour system to measure time. In this system, the hours are numbered from 0 to 24 with noon being 12:00 (Figure 6-10). There is no need to use the morning (AM) and evening (PM) designation because there are no times with the same number. For example, 15:00 is the same as 3:00 PM. The use of a 24-hour time system in health care eliminates many chances for error in treatment.

Graphing

Graphs may be used to interpret data visually. Four types of graphs are the bar graph, pie chart, pictograph, and line graph (Figure 6-11). The line graph is commonly used to

Table 6-4	Liquid and Solid Systems of Measurement		
Metric	**Apothecary**	**Household**
Liquid Measurement		
.06 milliliters (mL)	1 minim (min)	1 drop (gtt)
5 mL	1 fluid dram (fl dr)	1 teaspoon (tsp)
15 mL	3 fl dr	1 tablespoon (tbs)
30 mL	1 fluid ounce (fl oz)	2 tbs
240 mL	8 fl oz	1 glass or cup
473 mL	16 fl oz	1 pint (pt)
1 liter (L)	32 fl oz	1 quart (qt)
Solid Measurement		
1 gram (g)	15 grains (gr)	15.4 grains (gr)
28.35 g	480 gr	1 ounce (oz)
31 g	1 ounce (oz)	437.5 gr
373 g	1 pound (lb)	0.75 pound (lb)
454 g	1.33 lb	1 lb
1 kg	2.7 lb	2.2 lb

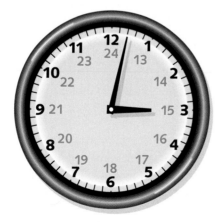

Figure 6-10 Using the 24-hour clock helps to prevent confusion regarding the time when care is given.

chart vital signs in health care (Skill 6-8). To read a graph, it must first be analyzed. The title tells what information is being depicted in the graph. The value or scale of each of the measurements is shown on the vertical and horizontal axis of the graph.

Computer Literacy

Computers are electronic equipment that store, manipulate, and retrieve information according to a program (software). The program is placed or loaded into the working space (memory) of the equipment. Computer hardware is the physical equipment including the keyboard, central processing unit (CPU), viewing screen (monitor), disk drive, and disks.

The computer may have two types of memory available to store information (data). They are read only memory (ROM) and random access memory (RAM). Magnetic recording tapes or disks (floppy disks) may be used to store information outside the computer. When connected to a printer, computers can output paper files. The combination of the hardware and software is generally referred to as the computer system.

Computers are used in all aspects of health care. Laboratory tests and respiratory ventilators are run by computerized equipment. Magnetic resonance imagery (MRI) and heart monitoring equipment are computer driven. Information about patient services and charges for services are maintained on computer systems in most facilities. The health care worker must be able to input and retrieve data from the computer to provide efficient care. Although each computer system has its own specifications for use, some basic rules apply to all units and programs (Box 6-4; Skill 6-9).

Medical Terminology

Medical terminology as it is used today dates to 300 BC in the writings of Hippocrates and Aristotle. The vocabulary is based on Latin and Greek roots for common words. Medical terminology allows health care workers to communicate in a precise and clear manner, so accurate pronunciation and correct spelling are important.

At first, medical terminology appears difficult and confusing. However, each word can be divided into parts that are reused to form new terms. The parts are word roots and combining vowels, prefixes, and suffixes. The root is the central part and determines the main meaning. The root usually is modified by a prefix or suffix to make it more specific. The prefix is the first part and the suffix is the last part. Not all medical terms have all three parts. It may be necessary to use a combining vowel between the parts of the term for easier pronunciation. By memorizing the parts, many word combinations can be formed (Figure 6-12).

Abbreviations and symbols are used by health care workers to save time in conveying information. Some abbreviations are considered standard and are used in all areas of care. Others may be used in only one facility, and they may cause confusion. Abbreviations are learned most

A

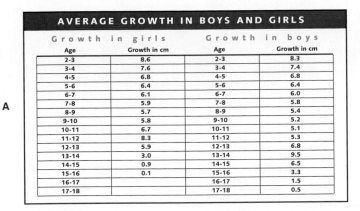

AVERAGE GROWTH IN BOYS AND GIRLS			
Growth in girls		Growth in boys	
Age	Growth in cm	Age	Growth in cm
2-3	8.6	2-3	8.3
3-4	7.6	3-4	7.4
4-5	6.8	4-5	6.8
5-6	6.4	5-6	6.4
6-7	6.1	6-7	6.0
7-8	5.9	7-8	5.8
8-9	5.7	8-9	5.4
9-10	5.8	9-10	5.2
10-11	6.7	10-11	5.1
11-12	8.3	11-12	5.3
12-13	5.9	12-13	6.8
13-14	3.0	13-14	9.5
14-15	0.9	14-15	6.5
15-16	0.1	15-16	3.3
16-17		16-17	1.5
17-18		17-18	0.5

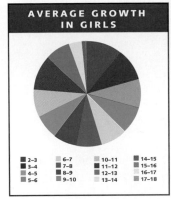

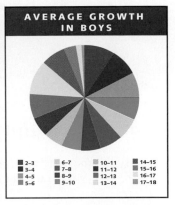

B

C

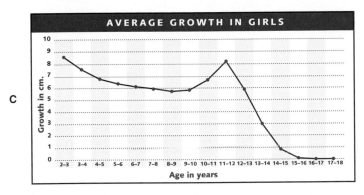

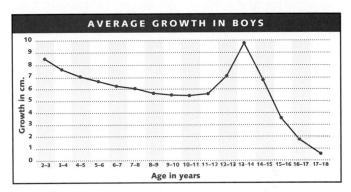

D

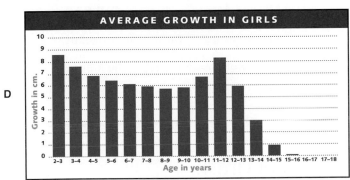

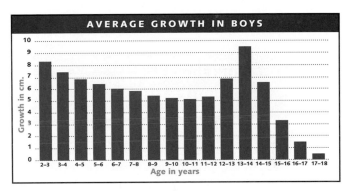

Figure 6-11 Graphing makes it easier to compare data and see changes. **A**, Data chart. **B**, Pie chart. **C**, Line graph. **D**, Bar graph.

easily by use. They may be divided into categories for easier reference. Some categories of abbreviations that may be used include the following:

1. Treatments and tests
2. Conditions and diagnoses
3. Titles (associations and personnel)

Common word roots, prefixes, suffixes, abbreviations, and symbols used in health care are found in the appendix of the textbook.

Most of the communication among health care professionals involves the use of medical terminology. To provide safe and accurate care to the patient, all health care workers must have knowledge of the basic terms of anatomy and physiology and of tests and treatments.

It may also be necessary to know the type of care or precautions that are necessary when a specific test or treatment is ordered by a physician. Some diagnostic tests require special diets or physical preparations before the test can be performed. For example, a barium enema (BE) allows the health care provider to view the large intestine, and the patient must have nothing to eat or drink (NPO) for several hours before the test.

Skill 6-9

Using the Computer

1. Identify the monitor, central processing unit, and disk drive for the computer. Information may be obtained in the central processing unit or on a removable or "floppy" disk.

2. Turn the computer on as indicated by the manufacturer's directions.

3. Initiate, or "boot," a program according to the manufacturer's instructions.

4. Input information as needed according to the program instructions.

5. Save information to the disk according to the program instructions.

6. Turn the computer off according to the manufacturer's instruction.

Box 6-4   Guidelines for Computer Users

Computers use very little electricity. If the interval between periods of use is only 20 to 30 minutes, it is better to leave the hardware on than to turn it off.

Computers and liquid do not mix. Beverages should be restricted from the computer area.

Computers "boot," or start programs, best from an off position. Although many computers may be instructed to reboot with control keys, it is better to use the power switch.

Floppy disks must be handled with care. The information stored on the disk may be damaged by:

- Excessive heat or cold
- Fingerprints on the recording surface or imprints made by writing on the disk label
- Bending
- Magnets placed close to the surface
- Dust, lint, and electrical static
- Removing the disk from the drive when the light indicates that it is being read or written on.

NEPHR + ECTOMY

| Prefix = Kidney | Suffix = Removal of |

Nephrectomy = Removal of the kidney

Figure 6-12   Nephrectomy means the removal of the kidney.

Physician Orders

Most descriptions of the care that is to be given are written by the physician. These directions for care are called the *physician orders* and are written in the chart. Some examples of physician orders follow:

ac & cl ½ hr ac and hs

Perform acetest and clinitest one-half hour before meals and at bedtime. The order probably would include directions for the administration of insulin if sugar or ketone is present in the urine test.

MOM 30 cc hs po PRN constipation

This order allows the patient to have 30 cc of milk of magnesia by mouth at bedtime, as needed, to relieve constipation. Although medications may be given (administered) only by licensed personnel, the health care assistant may be able to help by knowing what the order means.

Upper Gl, GB series in am

The patient will have radiographs, or x-rays, of the gallbladder, stomach, and upper part of the intestine in the morning. The test may require some physical preparation such as dietary restrictions or special treatments to clear the intestines.

pt scheduled for TAH, BSO in am. NPO p̄ MN.

Surgery is scheduled for the patient in the morning. The patient is not to have anything to eat or drink after midnight. The procedure will be a total abdominal hysterectomy with a bilateral removal of the fallopian tubes and ovaries. It is much quicker to write "TAH, BSO" than the words that mean the same thing. The correct terminology for the procedure is "total abdominal hysterectomy, bilateral salpingo-oophorectomy."

Emergency First Aid

First aid is the immediate care given to the victim of injury or sudden illness. The purpose of first aid is to sustain life and prevent death. It includes the prevention of permanent disability and the reduction of time needed for recovery. First aid provides basic life support and maintenance of vital functions.

Certification in first aid is awarded by several accredited agencies including the American Red Cross (ARC) and the American Heart Association (AHA). The American Red Cross course includes basic first aid for injuries, illness, and cardiopulmonary resuscitation (CPR) procedures. The American Heart Association teaches the cardiopulmonary resuscitation procedures only. In 2000 the American Heart Association revised its guidelines for emergency care (Box 6-5).

Cardiac Arrest

More than 15 million people worldwide have learned how to perform cardiopulmonary resuscitation (CPR). Cardiopulmonary resuscitation is a combination of mouth-to-mouth breathing and chest compressions that supply oxygenated blood to the brain. Cardiopulmonary resuscitation may be necessary when **cardiac arrest**, drowning, respiratory failure, electrical shock, head injury, or drug overdose occur.

Cardiac arrest also may result from blockage of an artery that supplies the heart or from insufficient supply of oxygen to the heart tissue. Signs and symptoms of a heart attack vary greatly. There may be more than one symptom present or none at all (Box 6-6). Risk factors for cardiac arrest have been identified (Box 6-7). The presence of more than one factor multiplies the risk greatly. Some risk factors can be changed through a prudent lifestyle, which includes regular exercise and a low-fat diet. Other risk factors such as heredity, gender, and age cannot be changed. Additional information about emergency care may be found in Chapter 31.

Review Questions

1. Use the following terms in one or more sentences that correctly relate their meaning.
   Blood pressure

   Diastolic

   Systolic

2. Use the following terms in one or more sentences that correctly relate their meaning.
   Auscultation

   Palpation

   Percussion

3. Describe the elements of a health assessment.

4. Describe the normal parameters for vital signs indicating what each measures.

5. Describe the risk factors of developing a heart attack.

Critical Thinking

1. Describe a personal action or lifestyle change that might be taken to eliminate each of the risk factors for cardiac arrest that can be changed.

2. Describe three activities that might change a person's vital signs.

3. Use the abbreviations in the appendix to write physician orders that would indicate that the patient was not supposed to eat after 12 midnight because of surgery scheduled in the morning for a total abdominal hysterectomy.

7
Wellness, Growth, and Development

Learning Objectives

Define at least 10 terms relating to wellness, growth, and development.

List at least three factors that may be used to determine a level of wellness.

List the function of each of the five nutrients.

Construct a food pyramid with recommended daily servings for each category.

Describe the relationship of calories to weight loss and gain.

Describe five types of therapeutic diets used to meet individual nutritional needs.

Identify at least five events that may lead to a reaction of stress.

Describe at least five health conditions that may result from stress.

Describe at least four methods that may be used to manage stress.

Compare the physical development of the body through the life span.

Describe the psychosocial development through the life span.

Describe each of the five stages of death acceptance.

Key Terms

Addiction
(uh-DIK-shen) Dependence on some habit; may be physical, psychological, or both

Anabolism
(ah-NAB-o-lizm) Any constructive process by which simple substances are converted by living cells into more complex compounds

Calorie
(KAL-o-ree) Unit of heat

Carbohydrates
(kar-bo-HI-drayts) Starches, sugars, cellulose, and gums

Catabolism
(kah-TAB-o-lizm) Breaking-down process by which complex substances are converted by living cells into simple compounds

Cholesterol
(ko-LES-ter-ol) Pearly, fatlike steroid alcohol found in animal fats and oils; precursor of bile acids and hormones

Fat
Adipose tissue; reserve supply of energy

Megadose
(MEG-uh-dos) Overdose, 10 times the recommended dose

Metabolism
(me-TAB-o-lizm) Sum of all the physical and chemical processes by which living organized substance is produced, maintained, and transformed to produce energy

Mineral
(MIN-er-ul) Nonorganic solid substance

Nutrients
(NOO-tree-ents) Proteins, carbohydrates, fats, vitamins, and minerals necessary for growth, normal functioning, and maintaining life

Nutrition
(noo-TRISH-un) Process of taking in nutrients and using them for body function

Protein
(PRO-teen) Group of complex organic compounds that are the main part of cell protoplasm

Terminal
(TER-min-ul) Illness or injury for which there is no reasonable expectation of recovery

Vitamins
(VIE-tuh-minz) Organic compounds needed by the body for metabolism, growth, and development

Wellness and Prevention

Wellness may be defined as a state of health on a continuum from a level of high energy and feeling of well-being to illness or death. Optimal wellness reflects a balanced relationship between the individual's physical, mental, and social health. Wellness is determined by the lifestyle choices a person makes. These choices include the amount of sleep, type of diet, exercise plan, personal habits, social relationships with others, and so forth. Many models have been designed to describe the type of lifestyle and personal habits that promote wellness (Figure 7-1). They interrelate the body, mind, and spirit. The body refers to physical health and development. The mind refers to intellectual and emotional development. The spirit includes inner and personal reflection.

Fitness may be evaluated by considering muscle strength and endurance, cardiorespiratory endurance, body composition, and flexibility. Some indicators that may be measured to evaluate optimal physical fitness include the following:
- Percentage of body fat (20% to 23% for women and 13% to 16% for men)
- Muscle strength
- Joint flexibility
- Balance and coordination
- Oxygen uptake
- Vital capacity

Some of the laboratory blood tests that may be used to indicate levels of wellness include the following:
- Cholesterol level
- Glucose level

An optimal state of wellness emphasizes self-care, personal responsibility, prevention of illness, and management

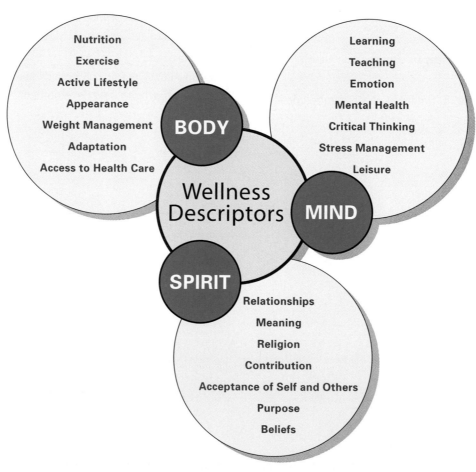

Figure 7-1   This model details different descriptors necessary for wellness.

of health through lifestyle choices. Concepts that may improve wellness include nutrition, stress reduction, counseling, habit cessation, and exercise.

Nutrition

Nutrients

Metabolism is the physical and chemical processes that produce energy. The energy used by the body for growth and activity comes from the food that is eaten. Body cells metabolize or process food in two ways. **Anabolism** is the process of building tissues from small compounds, and it requires energy to occur. **Catabolism** is the breaking down of tissues into materials that may be reused or excreted. Catabolism releases energy that may be used for other activities of the cell.

Nutrition is the study of the food that is eaten and how it is used in the body. **Nutrients** are chemical materials in

food and are vital to the body functions. Good nutrition is important in maintaining the best health possible.

Five nutrients have been identified as being essential to the maintenance of good health. They are carbohydrates, proteins, fats, vitamins, and minerals. Additionally, the body's cells need sufficient water to metabolize these nutrients. Effective use of one nutrient depends on the presence of all of the other nutrients in the body.

Since May 1994 all producers of processed foods have been required to comply with the Nutrition Labeling and Education Act. Labels on foods must be consistent and meet guidelines set by the Food and Drug Administration. Figure 7-2 lists the contents of processed food that must appear on the label. Additionally, foods that make health claims such as "low in . . . ," "good source of . . . ," or "lean" must meet specific guidelines before these statements and claims can be made. There are only seven categories for the claims.

The Reference Daily Intake (RDI) was developed by the Food and Drug Administration to be used for indicating the nutrient value of processed foods and supplements. It

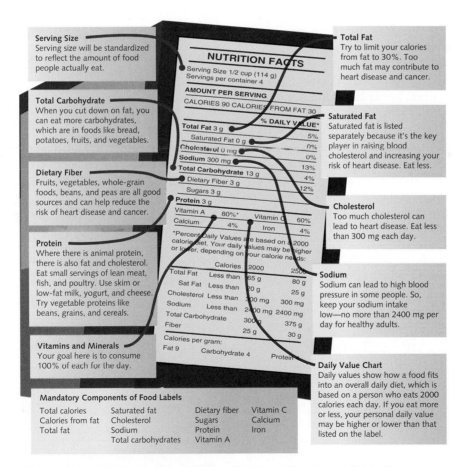

Figure 7-2   Food labels provide nutritional information that reflects the content of the food.

replaced the term *Recommended Daily Allowance* that was previously used for labeling.

The phrase *Recommended Dietary Allowance (RDA)* now indicates the amount of nutrients that should be consumed daily to meet the nutritional needs of almost all healthy people. The Recommended Dietary Allowance guidelines are established by a committee of the National Research Council. The committee, made up of nutritional scientists, has been providing these estimates since 1934 and revises its recommendations every 5 years.

Carbohydrates are found in all plants that are used as food sources. Carbohydrates are the main source of quick or immediate energy used by the body. Sugar and starch are the two main forms of carbohydrate. Foods that provide carbohydrates include cereal, potatoes, dried beans, corn, bread, and sugar. Carbohydrates found in fruit and vegetables also provide fiber or bulk to help with elimination of wastes. Carbohydrates also are needed to use fat. If carbohydrates are not present in the diet, proteins are used as the alternate energy source.

Proteins are found in food from animal sources such as eggs, milk, meat, fish, and poultry. Additionally, dried beans, peas, and cheese provide this nutrient. Protein contains the compounds (amino acids) needed to build muscle, bone, blood, and antibodies. Strict vegetarians who do not eat eggs or milk may combine legumes and whole grain products such as red beans and rice to obtain the nine essential amino acids. Amino acids that are called "essential" cannot be synthesized from other food sources.

Fats are found in the marbling or white part of meat, cooking oils, salad dressings, and in some milk products such as butter. Fat provides the most concentrated form of energy. Fat is needed to repair cells and to make hormones. Fats also supply essential fatty acids and fat-soluble vitamins. Fats are classified as saturated or unsaturated. Saturated fats are found in animal products and are solid at room temperature. Unsaturated fats are found primarily in vegetables and contain less cholesterol than saturated fats. **Cholesterol** is a waxy compound found in fats and is produced by the body. It is used by the brain to transmit nerve impulses and forms part of cell membranes. Cholesterol is needed in the skin to produce vitamin D and is used in formation of bile acids and reproductive hormones. Cholesterol is sticky and may deposit in the walls of blood vessels when too high a level accumulates in the blood. Because high cholesterol levels are linked to heart disease, unsaturated fats are believed to produce fewer health risks than saturated fats.

Vitamins are organic compounds that regulate cell metabolism. Each vitamin has specific functions (see Appendix III). Vitamins are divided into two groups depending on whether they dissolve in water or in fat. Vitamin supplements are not necessary if a varied or balanced diet,

which contains all the nutrients, is eaten. Vitamins, especially Vitamin C, may be destroyed when overcooked.

Minerals are simple compounds that regulate body processes. Nineteen minerals are used by the body. Seventeen are considered to be essential (see Appendix III). Minerals are found in many food sources. Ten times the recommended daily allowance of vitamins and minerals is considered to be an overdose, or **megadose** (Table 7-1).

Food Groups

In May 1992 the US Department of Agriculture established a pyramid of six food groups to help plan meals that provide all of the nutrients needed in a daily diet (Figure 7-3). A diet that includes all of the recommended servings of the food groups provides all of the nutrients. The food groups include milk equivalents, meat or protein equivalents, vegetables, fruits, and bread equivalents. Servings of fats, sweets, and oils are not recommended because they contain calories but no nutrients. Additionally, they are found in a natural form in many other foods.

The average person in the United States consumes 493 cans of soft drinks and 56 kg (123 lb) of sugar a year. Although the recommended daily allowance of salt is

Table 7-1	Effects of Vitamin and Mineral Megadosing	
Vitamin or Mineral	**Effect of Megadose**
Vitamin A	Blurred vision, hearing loss, liver damage, headache
Vitamin B$_6$	Physiological dependency*
Vitamin C	Physiological dependency, kidney stones
Calcium	Drowsiness, impaired absorption of other minerals and vitamins
Iron	Toxic build-up in liver, pancreas, and heart
Zinc	Nausea, vomiting, premature birth, stillbirth

*Physiological dependency has occurred when the dosage is reduced to normal levels and symptoms of deficiency appear.

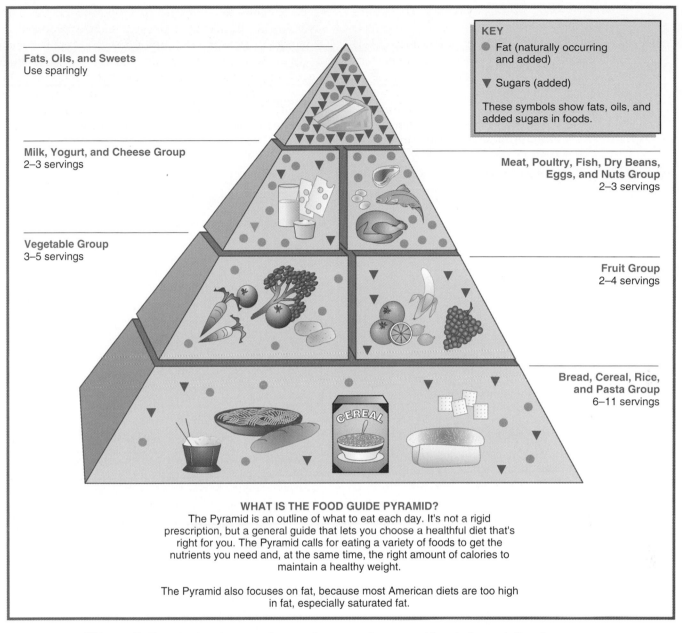

Fats, Oils, and Sweets
Use sparingly

Milk, Yogurt, and Cheese Group
2–3 servings

Vegetable Group
3–5 servings

KEY
● Fat (naturally occurring and added)
▼ Sugars (added)

These symbols show fats, oils, and added sugars in foods.

Meat, Poultry, Fish, Dry Beans, Eggs, and Nuts Group
2–3 servings

Fruit Group
2–4 servings

Bread, Cereal, Rice, and Pasta Group
6–11 servings

CEREAL

WHAT IS THE FOOD GUIDE PYRAMID?
The Pyramid is an outline of what to eat each day. It's not a rigid prescription, but a general guide that lets you choose a healthful diet that's right for you. The Pyramid calls for eating a variety of foods to get the nutrients you need and, at the same time, the right amount of calories to maintain a healthy weight.

The Pyramid also focuses on fat, because most American diets are too high in fat, especially saturated fat.

Figure 7-3   The food pyramid is used as a guide to provide a balanced diet. *(From Kinn ME, Woods M: The medical assistant, ed 8, 1999, Philadelphia, WB Saunders.)*

Table 7-2   Therapeutic Diets

Diet	Description	Use
Clear liquid	Minimal residue, dissolved sugar	Postsurgical, replace lost fluid
Full liquid	Strained, semi-liquid, clear liquid	Progression to regular diet, digestive system upset
Soft	Chopped, strained, pureed, little fiber	Inability to chew, difficulty swallowing
Regular	No restrictions	
Low calorie	800-2000 calories	Overweight, arthritis, cardiac condition
High calorie	More than 2000 calories	Anorexia nervosa, hyperthyroidism, underweight
Bland	No highly seasoned foods, low fiber	Ulcer, colitis
Low sodium	No salt added on tray	Kidney disease, cardiovascular disorder, edema, hypertension
Restricted residue	Low in bulk, low fiber	Rectal disease, colitis, ileitis
Low carbohydrate	Sweets not allowed	Diabetes
Low cholesterol	Restricted saturated fat	Coronary disease, atherosclerosis
Low fat	High carbohydrates, low protein	Gallbladder disease, obesity, heart condition, liver disease
Lactose free	Lactose-free milk products, nondairy creamer, soy milk	Alactasia
High protein	Low carbohydrate, high protein	Pregnancy, postsurgical, children in growing years, burn victims
Diet substitutes	Intravenous therapy, tube feeding	Dehydration, anorexia, poor nutrition, unconsciousness
Force fluids	Offer 8 oz of liquid every hour	Elderly, dehydration
Kosher	Separate utensils for meat and milk products	Observation of Jewish tradition

2200 mg or about 1 teaspoon, most people in the United States consume two to four times that amount. Most people in the United States could improve their nutrition by reducing the intake of fat, sugar, and salt. The amount of fruits and vegetables should be increased. Through adolescence, about 1 quart of milk daily is needed to supply the minerals necessary for bone growth.

Calories

Another method used to measure the amount of food needed to perform the body functions is counting calories. A **calorie** is the measurement of the amount of energy needed to raise 1 g of water 1° C. The amount of calories needed daily depends on sex, age, size, general condition, and daily activity. In general, the caloric need can be estimated by multiplying the desired weight in pounds by 15 calories per pound per day (Box 7-1). A balanced diet

provides 15% of the calories from protein sources. Fat sources should provide 30% of the daily calories with the remaining 55% provided by carbohydrates.

Weight can be regulated by counting calories. One pound (0.45 kg) of fat tissue is the equivalent of 3500 calories. Carbohydrates and protein provide 4 calories per g. Fat provides 9 calories per g. Vitamins and minerals do not contain any calories. Fad diets that limit the variety of foods eaten usually do not work on a permanent basis. One reason that quick weight loss is unsuccessful is that the body, when deprived of the essential nutrients, stores additional energy in the form of fat. Controlling weight is a balance between the number of calories taken in and the number of calories used as energy. The most successful method of weight loss is a gradual increase in caloric output by additional exercise and a decrease in the caloric intake of food. Weight loss of 1 to 2 pounds per week is considered safe and effective.

Box 7-1 Estimating Caloric Needs

Desired weight in pounds × 15 calories per pound per day = Necessary calories to maintain weight

Example: 150 lb × 15 calories per pound per day = 2250 calories per day

To lose 1 pound each week, subtract 500 calories each day.

Example: 500 calories per day × 7 days = 3500 calories (1 lb)

Diet Therapy

Special diets are used to treat specific health conditions (Table 7-2). In addition to providing a balanced diet with adequate calories, the needs of special populations must be considered. Food habits are influenced by nationality, race, culture, religious beliefs, and personal preferences. Special diets must consider these factors as well as nutrient requirements.

Stress Reduction

Identifying Stress

Stress is the body's nonspecific reaction to demands of everyday life. It affects a person physically and psychologically (Table 7-3). Stress is not the result of events that occur, but rather the attitudes that are formed about the events. Individual responses to the same event may differ, and stress may result from a perceived threat that is not a real event. Some people do not take responsibility for the effects of stress in their own life because they believe that others control it.

Everyday stresses include pressures of urban life such as traffic, major life changes such as birth and death, and management of a family and career. Social isolation may lead to stress when a person does not have an opportunity to express feelings or share in relationships with others. Financial concerns may also lead to the feelings of tension, frustration, and anxiety associated with stress.

Some of the common signs and symptoms of stress include the following:

- Increased heart rate
- Floating feeling of anxiety
- Trembling
- Indigestion
- Pain in the neck or back

Stress experienced for long periods of time has been linked to physical disorders including the following:

- Hypertension
- Headache

Table 7-3	Stress-Related Illness
Body Process	**Effect of Stress**
Cardiovascular system	Heart attack (myocardial infarction)
	High blood pressure (hypertension)
	Heart pain (angina)
	Migraine headache
	Stroke (cerebrovascular accident)
Digestive system	Ulcer
	Colitis
	Constipation
	Diarrhea
Skeletal system	Arthritis
Muscular system	Headache
	Backache
Respiratory system	Asthma
Endocrine system	Diabetes (type 2)
Nervous system	Accident proneness (decreased attention)
Immune process	Increased rate of infection
	Allergies
	Autoimmune disorders
Psychosocial process	Fighting
	Conflicts
	Alcoholism
	Drug abuse

Table 7-4   Personality Types*

Description	Type A Personality	Type B Personality
Movement	Walks, eats, and talks rapidly	Lacks sense of urgency, enjoys relaxing without guilt
Action	Does two or more things at a time	Does one thing at a time
Temperament	Competitive, impatient, aggressive, achievement oriented, hostile, status-conscious, focus on quantity more than quality, approval-seeking	Patient, easy-going, passive, noncompetitive, little need for advancement, focus on quality, self-reflecting

*These descriptors are extremes of the characteristics.

- Atherosclerosis
- Back pain
- Ulcers
- Colitis
- Substance abuse
- Obesity
- Insomnia
- Accident proneness
- Skin disorders
- Rheumatoid arthritis
- Decrease in immune system efficiency

Stress Theory

In the 1950s Franz Alexander proposed that some specific illnesses resulted from the stress of life events. His theory introduced the concept of psychosomatic disorders or illness that results from actions of the emotions on the body. Also called *psychophysiologic disorders, psychogenic disease,* or *organ neuroses,* this condition does not mean that the person is not ill, rather that the illness is caused by the person's own mind. Alexander proposed that certain specific personality traits combined with certain life events cause specific disorders of the body. Although Alexander's theory is now generally considered to be too rigid, the concept of many illnesses being caused at least in part by emotional factors is well accepted. For example, the action of tightening muscles of the neck and back when under stress may lead to a headache.

One of many theories on personality types was developed by two cardiologists, Meyer Friedman and Ray Rosenman in 1959 (Table 7-4). They proposed that, of two main personality types, people with Type A personalities were more prone to cardiovascular disorders and sudden

Box 7-2   Stress Management Techniques

- Plan and organize your workload.
- When possible, do things one at a time to completion.
- Occasionally, plan to escape and have fun.
- Be positive about things and avoid criticizing others.
- Avoid unnecessary competition.
- Learn to negotiate.
- Get regular exercise.
- Tolerate, forgive, and learn to accept others.
- Talk to someone about things that are troubling you.
- Relax with methods such as biofeedback, yoga, and meditation.
- Use time management techniques.
- Take mini-breaks during the day to relax and breathe.
- Practice acceptance of things that cannot be changed.
- Take responsibility for your own actions.
- Set realistic goals and expectations for self and others.
- Eat sensibly.

death. Their theory has been supported by research that followed the health of men who were evaluated for behavior patterns. After 8½ years, the Type A personalities in the study group had twice the incidence of coronary heart disease as the Type B personalities. It has been shown that when the "fight or flight" response is triggered repeatedly, a resulting abnormal level of adrenaline and cortisol increases the level of cholesterol and fat in the bloodstream. A Type C personality has been described as a person who can use the characteristics and behaviors of the Type A personality without triggering a stress response.

Stress Management

Some methods used to manage stress include proper nutrition, exercise, relaxation techniques, and personal behavior changes. Another stress management technique includes methods of time management (Box 7-2). Because stress builds, intervention to decrease stress should be practiced regularly. The goal of stress management is lower rates for blood pressure, pulse, and respiration, as well as a refreshed feeling of peacefulness or calm.

Methods to help manage stress include the following:
- Identify the cause of stress
- Make conscious choices to control stress
- Develop coping and relaxation techniques
- Practice good health habits
- Plan ahead
- Laugh
- Use energy (adrenaline) in another manner (exercise)
- Relax
- Seek emotional support
- Maintain good nutrition
- Avoid caffeine
- Practice meditation, biofeedback, guided imagery, prayer, or hypnosis
- Decrease alcohol or drug intake
- Sleep
- Take a warm bath
- Walk
- Decrease sugar intake
- Play games or enjoy hobbies
- Perform yoga

Counseling

Guidance or counseling may be given by professionals for emotional concerns and for career decisions. As society has become more complex, the need for more specific types of counseling has emerged. Some of the signs and symptoms of a disorder of mental health include sadness, violent or erratic moods, an inability to make decisions, sleep disturbances, self-destructive behavior, physical disorders, fear, anger, anxiety, or a sense of hopelessness. Although friends can provide emotional support by listening, professional counselors including psychologists, psychiatrists, and others use specific techniques to help people cope with and solve their own problems (Table 7-5).

Habit Cessation

Addiction may be physical, psychological, or both. In a chemical addiction, the substance produces a feeling of pleasure similar to that produced by the brain's own endorphins and enkephalins. The regular use of narcotics can change the ability of the brain to produce these chemicals, leading to increase dependence on the narcotic. However, many other common habits or addictions may affect a person's level of wellness in a negative manner. For example, according to the *New England Journal of Medicine,* the lifetime medical cost for smokers is one third higher than nonsmokers, even though smokers have a shorter life span.

Many methods or treatments have been developed to treat addiction problems. No one method is considered to be effective in all cases. Some examples of treatment methods include the use of aversion therapy, support groups, and acupuncture. It is generally accepted that a long-term recovery program is necessary for any treatment to succeed. Many programs also use behavioral training and coping techniques in addition to the specific habit cessation method.

Excercise

The benefits of exercise are both emotional and physical. A regular exercise program reduces the risk of cardiovascular disease and improves emotional outlook. Some specific physical benefits of exercise include increased bone density, decreased blood levels of cholesterol, improved ability to use glucose, and improved cardiac performance. The result of these effects is a decrease in the risk of developing heart disease, osteoporosis, diabetes, hypertension, and obesity. Exercise also causes the release of the brain's endorphins leading to a feeling of well-being. It has been associated with an improvement in self-image and a reduction of depression, stress, and anxiety. Even a person with a sedentary lifestyle or limited mobility must maintain a certain amount of activity so that the body is able to function. Without some activity, the body begins to dysfunction or become disabled. For example, when a cast is applied to allow a fracture to heal, the muscles begin to atrophy and must be rebuilt to establish normal activity after the cast is removed.

Aerobic exercise programs are designed to improve cardiac performance. To achieve aerobic benefits, it is recommended to raise the heart rate, or pulse, to approximately 70% of the individual's maximum heart rate and maintain the elevated rate for 30 minutes at least three times each week. To calculate the maximum heart rate, the person subtracts his or her age from 220 and then multiplies the remainder by 70% (Box 7-3). Any exercise program should

Table 7-5   Family Counseling Techniques

Technique	Description
Patient control	The individual is taught to control the problem with specific directives of actions to be taken when situations occur.
Communication skill building	Focus on improvement of communication techniques such as listening, brainstorming, and relating in a nonjudgmental manner.
Family floor plan	Participant draws a floor plan of the generational or nuclear family information. Space and territory allotted to family members is evaluated.
Family photos	Discussion and observation of family members viewing family photos may be used to diagnose family relationships, rituals, communication, and roles.
Empty chair	An empty chair may be used to express feelings and thoughts to a family member. The role of the family member may also be played by the one expressing feelings.
Family choreography	Family members are asked to arrange the family as they believe it relates and then rearrange members in a manner that would be preferred.
Family counsel meeting	Rules are outlined and specific times are set for the family to meet and interact to provide structure for participation and communication.
Family sculpting	Family members represent their perceptions of the others to communicate in a nonverbal manner.
Genogram	An informational and diagnostic tool developed by the therapist showing the family structure.
Prescribing indecision	A directive is given to the family member who usually makes decisions to let another member make decisions or to take a specified amount of time before a decision is made.
Reframing	Framing an action that is perceived as negative into a positive category.
Special days	Mini-vacations may be used to assist families to communicate or appreciate others.
Strategic alliance	One member of the family is given the role of helping another to implement behavioral change.
Tracking	The therapist listens to, records, and stores family events to identify possible interventions.

Box 7-3   Calculation of Heart Rate for Cardiovascular Exercise

Formula: $(220 - \text{Age}) \times 0.7 =$
Maximum heart rate
Example: $(220 - 20) \times 0.7 = 140^*$

---

*For a 20-year-old person, the recommended heart rate to maintain for 30 minutes at least three times a week is 140. The 70% is an average and may be adjusted to 60% for a less athletic person or to 80% for a more athletic person.

be started gradually to allow the body to adjust to the new stresses resulting from it.

Growth and Development

The physical and psychological stage of a person changes rapidly from the moment of birth. Growth refers to the changes that can be measured in height and weight and in body proportions. Development describes the stages of change in psychological and social functioning.

Table 7-6   Developmental Steps Through the Life Span

Stage of Life	Developmental Changes
Infant (birth to 1 year)	Growth occurs in spurts, needs constant care, learns the differences in sensory input, sleeps in short periods, motor responses uncontrolled, plays with own hands and feet, vital signs not stable, may experience separation anxiety at 8 months
Toddler (1 to 2 years)	Takes first steps, mood changes quickly, begins to sense own energy and independence, learns to speak, coordination improves, suffers separation anxiety when away from family, self-loving, uninhibited, accidents and respiratory illness main threats to death
Preschooler (3 to 5 years)	Becomes a social being, recognizes peers, growth slows, has an excess of energy, needs clear-cut rules, can organize experiences into concepts, develops own self-concept and body image
School-age child (6 to 12 years)	Learns to channel energy, acquires knowledge and new skills quickly, peers become more important, growth is slow and steady, begins to reason about experiences, learns to compromise and cooperate
Adolescent (13 to 18 years)	Reaches puberty and sexual maturation, hormone levels increase, growth slows and stops, peers may assume primary importance, may rebel against family and society, forms own identity, needs limits, drug abuse and suicide may result from conflicts
Young adult (19 to 45 years)	Demonstrates place in society, establishes independence from family, may marry and start own family, plans for economic security, chooses lifestyle options
Middle-age adult (46 to 65 years)	Earns most of the money and makes most of the decisions for society, may question own life choices in self assessment, decrease in hormone secretion leads to changes in body, metabolic rate decreases, eye sight may decline, skin thins and loses elasticity, learns to use leisure time
Older adult (66 years and older)	Must learn to reconcile life experiences with value system, slower neurological responses lead to slower interpretation of sensory input, may suffer hearing loss, restriction in mobility, decreased ability to respond well to stress

Physical Growth and Development

Physical changes occur in spurts throughout the life span (Table 7-6). At birth the baby, or neonate, is about 19 to 21 inches in length and weighs 7 to 8 pounds. The head is one fourth the length of the body compared with the adult ratio of one eighth. For the first 4 weeks, the baby is referred to as a *neonate.* As the person grows, the body proportions change and develop into an adult appearance.

The study of aging is called gerontology. *Geriatrics* refers to the care of the elderly. Aging is a normal process that occurs gradually through the life span. The elderly have specific needs resulting from the changes in body function and structure (Table 7-7).

Psychosocial Growth and Development

The psychosocial needs of the individual change as life progresses from birth to death. Developmental changes and abilities determine the type of care that is given (Table 7-8). Characteristic behaviors for each stage of development have been identified (Table 7-9). As a result of psychosocial development, children may not understand the confinement and pain resulting from illness and hospitalization (Figure 7-4). In giving the care to the patient who is dying, at any age, it is important to consider psychosocial development.

Table 7-7 Physical Growth Through the Life Span

Stage of Life	Milestones of Development
Infancy (birth to 1 year)	Head large in proportion to body; movement uncoordinated; vision unclear; good hearing, smell, and taste senses; teeth begin to erupt at 6 months; physical growth is rapid; decline in amount of "baby fat;" lumbar curvature develops
	Learns to walk, communicate (talk), and understand some words; eats solid foods; forms relationships; sleeps and eats regularly
Toddler (1 to 2 years)	Muscles and nervous system become more coordinated, especially hands; physical growth continues less rapidly
	Learns to communicate with words; becomes less dependent and tolerates separation from person giving primary care; controls bowels and bladder; able to move by crawling, climbing, and running; plays in parallel (not together)
Early childhood (3 to 5 years)	Grows taller; gains little weight; increases coordination; begins to draw and write
	Ability to communicate increases; learns gender difference and modesty; learns right from wrong; plays with others; develops sense of family; provides some care of self
Middle childhood (6 to 8 years)	Grows in height and weight slowly; primary teeth are lost; hand coordination increases allowing cursive writing; permanent teeth erupt
	Develops skills to play games; gets along with others of same age; learns basic skills of language and math; develops self-image of gender and self-esteem
Late childhood (9 to 12 years)	Muscles increase in strength, coordination, and balance; develops physical skills; grows in height (girls taller than boys); permanent teeth appear; secondary sexual characteristics appear
	Becomes independent; develops peer relationships; develops interest in sexual information
Adolescence (13 to 18 years)	Rapid physical growth; changes of puberty begin; growth uneven (clumsiness); "wisdom" teeth appear
	Rapid psychosocial development; relationships with peers and dating experiences develop
Young adulthood (19 to 45 years)	Little physical growth; bone growth plates close
	Chooses occupation; develops family unit with marriage, children, or others
Middle adulthood (46 to 65 years)	Gradual slowing of metabolism; changes of aging occur
	Lives on own or with adjusted family as children leave and parents age or die; develops leisure activities
Late adulthood (66 years and older)	Declines in physical strength, endurance, and overall health condition
	Adjusts to retirement, reduced income, and death of spouse; accepts own death

Table 7-8   Changes of Aging

System or Aspect	Change
Skeletal	Decrease in size; decalcification; bones more porous
Integumentary	Dry, thin, inelastic, pigment changes; hair thins; decrease in ability to make Vitamin D
Urinary	Number of nephrons decreases; bladder wall and meatus muscle tone lost
Respiratory	Costals harden; decrease in efficiency of system
Cardiovascular	Fatty deposits in vessels; hardening of vessels
Sensory	Decrease in muscle tone of eyes; hardening of lens; clouding of lens; increase pressure in eye; decrease in number of hair cells in ear; eardrum less flexible; decrease in number of taste buds; presbyopia decreases ability to focus
Reproductive	Menopause; decrease in amount of lubricant secretion and muscle tone of reproductive organs
Neurological	Decrease in response time
Digestive	Decrease of water in body; less saliva; less absorption of nutrients; decrease in stomach acids, slowing digestion
Endocrine	Decrease in hormones, especially thyroid and sex hormones
Sociological loss	Family, friends and contemporaries die
Metabolic slowing	Drugs processed more slowly; weight gained more easily; less sleep needed; more sleeping difficulties

Table 7-9   Psychosocial Development Through the Life Span

Stage of Life	Typical Behavior
Infant (birth to 1 year)	Responds reflexively; completely self-centered; detects changes; remembers responses and their results
Toddler (1 to 2 years)	Quickly changing moods; forming sense of independence; jealous when not center of attention; attached to mother and senses separation anxiety
Preschooler (3 to 5 years)	Speaks meaningfully; asks many questions, controls impulses, interacts with others of own age; forms theories about experiences
School-age child (6 to 12 years)	Learns quickly; curious; realistic; likes to associate with others of own age
Adolescent (13 to 18 years)	Reaches sexual maturity; seeks independence; able to learn quickly; develops concepts about life; develops slang and behaviors of peer groups
Young adult (19 to 45 years)	Expects physical health; continues to learn quickly; chooses career, family, or alternate lifestyle
Middle-age adult (46 to 65 years)	Makes decision for family, business, and society; seeks security for later years; questions meaning of life; finds ability to learn changing; memorization more difficult and spoken presentation less effective
Older adult (66 years and older)	Memory loss of recent events occurs; thinking process slows but is not impaired; learns best when focusing on one thing at a time; vision and mobility impaired; reviews life experiences

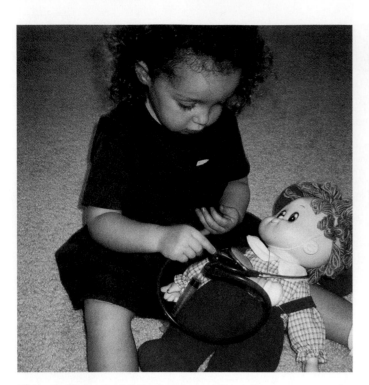

Figure 7-4 A child's understanding of treatments and tests can be improved through play.

Box 7-4 Bill of Rights for the Terminally Ill

I have the right to say what I feel about my death and express my own philosophy or religious beliefs about it.

I have the right to health care to provide comfort and lessen pain provided by caring and knowledgeable professionals.

I have the right to help in making decisions about my care and to have my questions answered honestly.

I have the right to maintain hope to meet the goals I set regarding my death.

I have the right to maintain dignity and individuality as a person and be treated as a living person until I die.

I have the right to die with my family or someone caring present and to die in peace with dignity.

I have the right to expect that my body will be treated with respect after my death.

Death and Dying

Death is a natural part of life. It is the end of life functions and results in the destruction of the body's cells. Biological death is the loss of cell function resulting in the absence of breathing and heartbeat. Clinical death, also called *brain death,* is the loss of function of the brain stem or the capacity for consciousness. Clinical death is defined legally as loss of brain activity for a specified amount of time. The study of death (thanatology) became an area of research in the twentieth century. Legal and ethical controversy surrounds the definition of death and the rights of the terminally ill to refuse life-prolonging treatments (Box 7-4).

Most people die in hospitals, long-term care facilities, or in hospices. In some cases, the dying person may stay at home until death, with occasional visits from hospice personnel. Death may occur suddenly or may be expected as a result of injury or **terminal** illness. Dying patients often represent failure to the health care professional. The attitude of the health care worker directly affects the dying patient and family (Box 7-5). Personal experience, religion, culture, and the ability to reason determine a person's attitude about death. Grief is the process that gradually resolves the sense of loss resulting from death.

Attitudes about death often change with circumstances and increased age. Before 5 years of age, most children do not view death as final. However, children between 8 and 11 years of age understand that death is personal and inevitable. Because the arrangements for the rituals after death are often made by a funeral director, the family is isolated from direct contact with the dead. This isolation may result in a sense of mystery or fright because of unknown elements about death.

One theory to explain the acceptance of death was developed by psychiatrist Dr. Elisabeth Kubler-Ross. She identified five stages of death. These stages are denial, anger, bargaining, depression, and acceptance. During denial, the individual refuses to believe that the death will or has occurred. Anger results as the person blames others or fate for the death or its prognosis. Bargaining with a higher power may occur to reconcile differences with a spiritual figure. Depression may occur when the person realizes the finality of the loss. The final stage is acceptance of the death or inevitability of dying.

Terminally ill individuals and their families do not always progress through all stages to acceptance. Psychological disorders may result as a failure to resolve this conflict. Dying people continue to have psychological, social,

Box 7-5   The Living Will

To My Family, My Physician, My Lawyer, and All Others Whom It May Concern,

Death is as much a reality as birth, growth, maturity, and old age—it is the one certainty of life. If the time comes I can no longer take part in decisions for my future, let this statement stand as an expression of my wishes and direction, while I am still of sound mind.

If at such a time the situation should arise in which there is no reasonable expectation of my recovery from extreme physical or mental disability, I direct that I be allowed to die and not be kept alive by medications, artificial means, or "heroic measures." I do, however, ask that medication be mercifully administered to me to alleviate suffering even though this may shorten my remaining life.

This statement is made after careful consideration and is in accordance with my strong convictions and beliefs. I want the wishes and directions here expressed carried out to the extent permitted by law. Insofar as they are not legally enforceable, I hope that those whom this Will is addressed will regard themselves as morally bound by these provisions.

and spiritual needs. There is usually a need to communicate and resolve conflicts when death is expected. The health care worker provides quality care by allowing the patient to express his or her thoughts and feelings without judgment.

Some physical signs that indicate that death is approaching include loss of muscle control, slowing of gastrointestinal functions, rise in body temperature, respiratory irregularities, and decrease in pain. The pulse rate is rapid, weak, and irregular. The patient may complain of feeling cold and have pale, cool skin caused by a decrease in circulation. Signs that death have occurred include absence of pulse, respiration, and blood pressure. The "death rattle," caused by mucus collecting in the throat and bronchial tubes, may be heard. Only a physician can legally pronounce a person dead.

Review Questions

1. Use each of the following terms in one or more sentences that correctly relate their meaning.
   Anabolism
   Calorie
   Catabolism
   Metabolism

2. List three factors that may be used to determine a level of wellness.

3. Describe the function of each of the five nutrients. Explain why water may also be considered a nutrient.

4. Draw the food pyramid including the groups and number of servings recommended for each.

5. Explain the relationship of calories to weight loss and gain.

6. List five therapeutic diets and the conditions for which each might be required.

7. Describe five body reactions resulting from stress.

8. Describe four methods that may be used to manage stress.

9. Compare physical development of a 1-year-old, 10-year-old, and adult.

10. Compare the psychosocial development of a 1-year-old, 10-year-old, and adult.

11. Describe the five stages of death acceptance.

Critical Thinking

1. Investigate the chemical differences between and uses of the following forms of sugar:

Brown	Mannitol
Corn syrup	Raw
Dextrose	Sorbitol
Fructose	Sucrose
Honey	Xylitol
Lactose	

2. Investigate the interaction of common drugs and foods.

3. Investigate the requirements for health claims on labeling such as the percentage of fat that can be contained in a food labeled "low fat."

4. Keep a diary of daily food consumption and activity. Calculate the calories for each and determine if weight will be lost or gained.

5. Investigate the diet of special populations found in the geographic area. Hypothesize about the success of several of the therapeutic diets with the local population.

6. Write an essay describing the meaning of death including any personal experiences that may help determine its meaning.

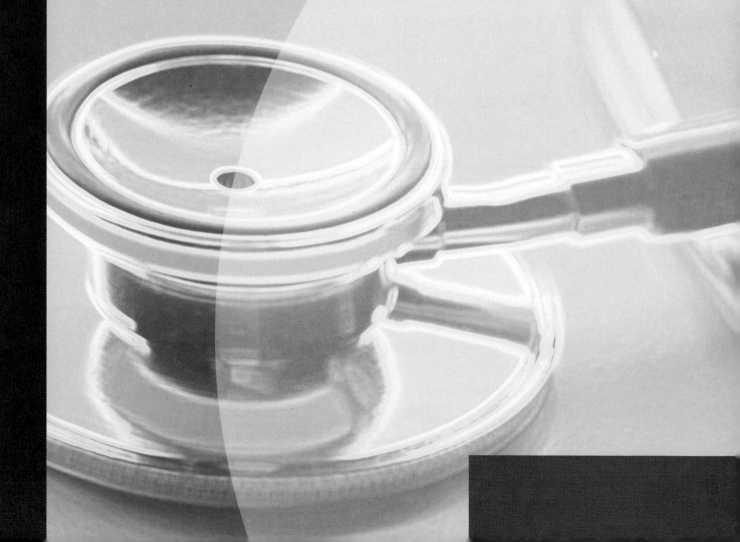

unit Two

Anatomy and Physiology

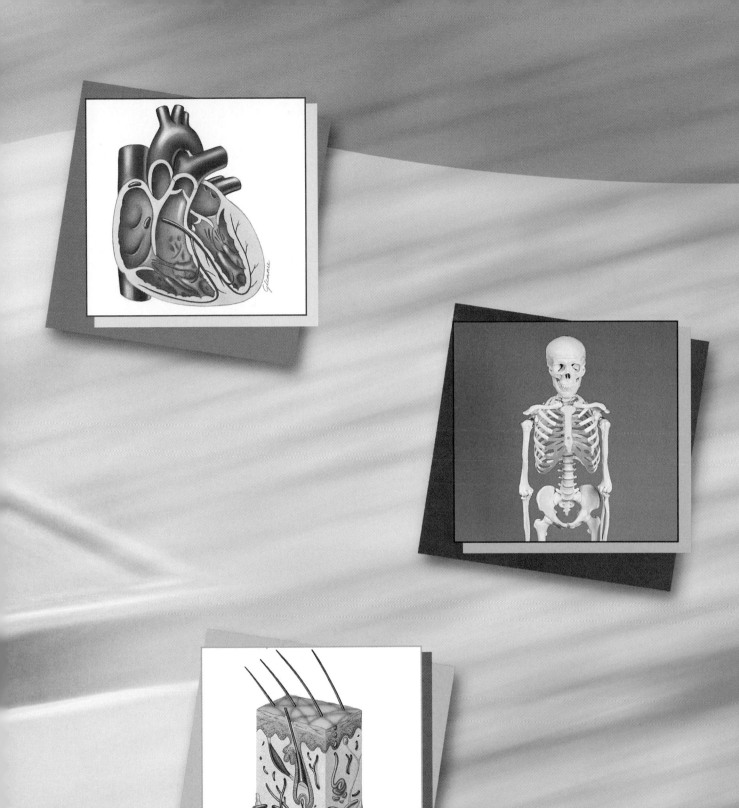

8

Body Organization

Learning Objectives

Identify the meaning of 10 or more terms relating to the organization of the body.

Describe the properties of life.

Label the structures of the cell and describe the function of each.

Describe the organization of the body from the smallest unit to the largest.

Describe organs of the body in relation to the plane, region, or cavity of location.

Describe five or more disorders resulting from defects in cell organization.

Key Terms

Autosome
(AW-toe-zome) Any chromosome except the X or Y

Condition
(kun-DISH-un) Change from normal function that cannot be cured

Congenital
(kon-JEN-i-tal) Referring to conditions that exist at birth regardless of cause

Disease
(di-ZEEZ) Interruption of normal function of the body, usually caused by microorganisms; can be treated

Dominant
(DOM-i-nant) Gene trait that appears when carried by only one in the pair of chromosomes

Electrolyte
(e-LEK-tro-lite) Substance that separates into ions in solution and is capable of conducting electricity

Genotype
(JEEN-o-tipe) Genetic pattern of an individual

Heredity
(he-RED-i-tee) Genetic transmission of trait or particular quality from parent to offspring

Homeostasis
(ho-me-o-STAY-sis) Tendency of an organism to maintain the "status quo" or the same internal environment

Mutation
(myoo-TAY-shun) Permanent change in a gene or chromosome

Organism
(OR-gah-nizm) Individual living thing, plant, or animal

Phenotype
(FEE-no-tipe) Physical, biochemical, and physiological configuration of an individual determined by genes

Recessive
(re-SESS-iv) Gene trait that does not appear unless carried by both members of a pair of chromosomes

Syndrome
(SIN-drome) Set of symptoms that occur together

Body Organization Terminology

TERM	DEFINITION	PREFIX	ROOT*	SUFFIX
Abduct	Draw away from the center	ab	duct	
Adduct	Draw toward the center	ad	duct	
Congenital	Born with	con	gen/it	al
Chemotherapy	Treatment by a chemical agent	chem/o	therapy	
Cytoplasm	Non-organelle material contained in cells		cyt/o	plasm
Dysfunction	Impairment of function	dys	function	
Genetic	Pertaining to genes		gen/et	ic
Genotype	Genetic makeup of an organism		gen/o	type
Physiology	Study of function		physi	ology
Semipermeable	Allowing only some materials to enter and exit	semi	permeable	

*A short transition phrase or vowel may be added to or deleted from the word parts to make the combining form.

Abbreviations of Body Organization

ABBREVIATION	MEANING
A&P	Anatomy and physiology
ant	Anterior
CA++	Calcium ion
Cl−	Chlorine ion
CVS	Chorionic villus sampling
DNA	Deoxyribonucleic acid
LUQ	Left upper quadrant
Na+	Sodium ion
post	Posterior
RLQ	Right lower quadrant

Anatomy and Physiology

The human body, like all living **organisms,** has four basic properties of life:

- Reception is the ability of the organism to control its actions and respond to changes in the environment.
- Metabolism is the process of taking in and using nutrients to produce energy and growth.
- Reproduction is the ability to reproduce offspring to continue the species.
- Organization divides the organism into distinct parts to perform these functions.

The two major types of study of the human body are called *anatomy* and *physiology.* Anatomy is the study of body structures and their location. Body structures are organized on five levels:

- Cells are the smallest unit of life.
- Tissues are combinations of similar cells.
- Organs are collections of tissues working together to perform a function.
- Body systems consist of organs that work together to provide a major body function.
- Organisms are the beings that result when the body systems work together to maintain life.

Cell Structure

The major structures, called organelles, of the cell are shown in Figure 8-1. These structures are as follows:

- The nucleus controls the activity of the cell and directs reproduction.
- The cytoplasm is a semifluid material that surrounds the cell parts and transports chemicals and nutrients within the cell.
- Mitochondria produce the energy used for cellular processes.
- The cell membrane surrounds the cell and controls which substances enter and leave the cell.

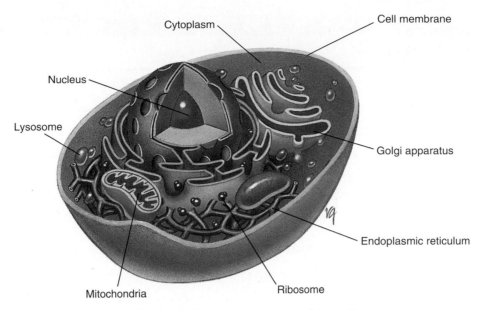

Figure 8-1   The structures of the cell.

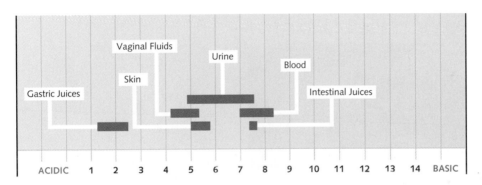

Figure 8-2   pH of the body. The body must maintain normal pH levels to function properly.

- Lysosomes help to break down, or digest, molecules.
- Ribosomes attached to the endoplasmic reticulum work to produce protein for the cell structures.
- The Golgi apparatus helps to transport proteins made by the ribosomes out of the cell by making glycoproteins.

Homeostasis is the tendency of a cell or the whole organism to maintain a state of balance. Molecules pass into and out of the cell to maintain this balance. The cells of the body constantly adjust to preserve a balance of fluids, temperature, oxygen, electrolytes, and nutrients.

Electrolytes are compounds made of charged particles called *ions*. These ions can conduct electrical current in water or in the cytoplasm of the cell. A positive charge, or cation, creates an acid. A negative charge, or anion, creates a base. The pH of a fluid is a measurement of how much acid or base is present. Each body tissue has a normal pH.

The cells do not function properly if the normal pH is not maintained for the area of the body (Figure 8-2). Different electrolytes also have specific functions, as shown in Table 8-1.

Tissue Types

There are four main groups of tissue in the body (Figure 8-3).

- Epithelial tissue covers the body, forms glands, and lines the surfaces of cavities and organs.
- Connective tissue, formed by a protein, includes soft tissue such as fat and blood cells and hard tissues such as bones, ligaments, and cartilage.
- Muscle tissue, made of protein fibers, has the unique property of shortening in length to produce movement.

Table 8-1   Electrolytes of the Body

Ion	Function
Cations(⁺)	
Sodium (Na⁺)	Controls water distribution by increasing ability of fluid to pass through cell membrane
Potassium (K⁺)	Maintains fluid balance, promotes growth of cells, nerve conduction, muscle contraction, and heart activity
Calcium (Ca⁺⁺)	Controls neuromuscular irritability, muscle contraction, blood clotting, building bones and teeth
Magnesium (Mg⁺⁺)	Maintains neuromuscular system, activates enzymes, regulates level of phosphorus
Hydrogen (H⁺)	Needed for cell and enzyme functions, binding of oxygen to hemoglobin
Anions (⁻)	
Bicarbonate (HCO₃⁻)	Maintains acid-base balance
Phosphate (HPO₄⁼)	Maintains fluid and acid-base balance
Chloride (C⁻)	Maintains fluid balance
Sulfate (SO₄⁼)	Maintains fluid balance

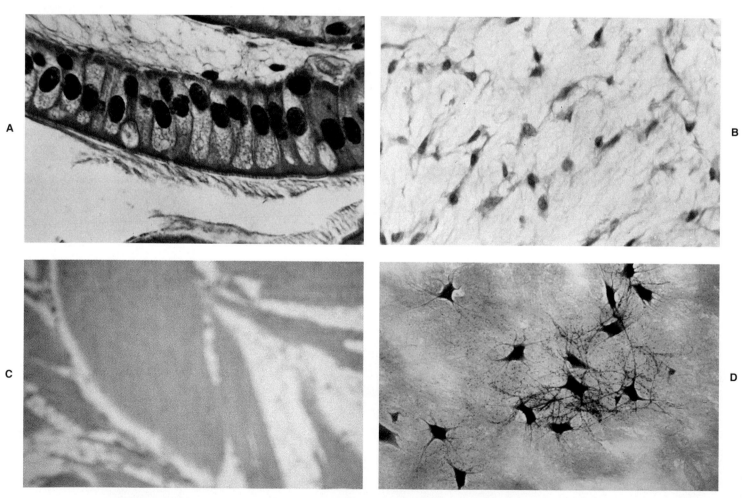

A

B

C

D

Figure 8–3   Tissues of the body. **A,** Epithelial. **B,** Connective. **C,** Muscle. **D,** Nervous.
*(**A, B,** and **D,** Courtesy Ward's Natural Science Establishment, Rochester, NY.)*

- Nervous tissue, composed largely of specialized cells called *neurons,* is found in the eyes, ears, brain, spinal cord, and peripheral nerves. Nervous tissue transmits communications.

Body Systems

The study of the functions of the body is called *physiology.* Functions are studied according to body systems. A body system is a group of related organs that together accomplish functions necessary to maintain and support life. The 12 body systems are as follows:

- The integumentary system covers the body and protects other body systems.
- The cardiovascular system transports oxygen and nutrients to all body parts and removes waste products.
- The circulatory system includes the blood and lymph that move throughout the body.
- The respiratory system exchanges gases between the air and blood.
- The muscular system allows the body to move and controls movements within the body.
- The skeletal system provides body support and protection.
- The digestive system processes food and eliminates food waste.
- The urinary system filters the blood and removes liquid wastes.

- The endocrine system coordinates body activities through hormones.
- The nervous system regulates the environment and directs the activities of other body systems.
- The sensory system perceives the environment and sends messages to and from the brain.
- The reproductive system provides for human reproduction.

The following 12 chapters discuss the body systems in more detail.

Describing the Body

Body Planes

Structures of the body can be located and described in relation to planes that divide the body (Figure 8-4). Three planes are used to describe the body:

- The coronal or frontal plane separates the front and back of the body.
- The transverse plane divides the upper and lower body.
- The sagittal plane divides the body into right and left sides.

The location of organs is described in relation to these planes. For example, an organ or growth may be below (inferior) or above (superior) the transverse plane. It may be close to (medial) or away from (lateral) the sagittal plane.

A   B   C

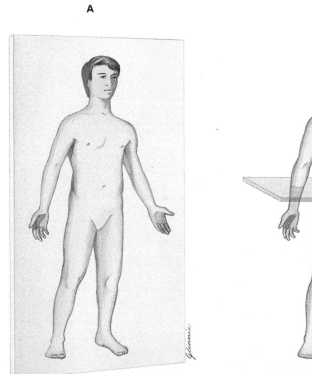
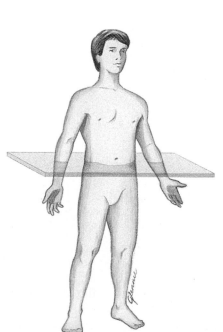
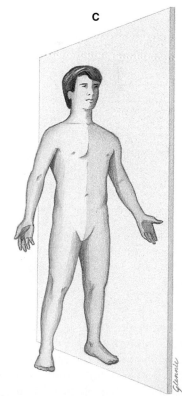

Figure 8-4   Body planes. **A,** Coronal. **B,** Transverse. **C,** Sagittal.

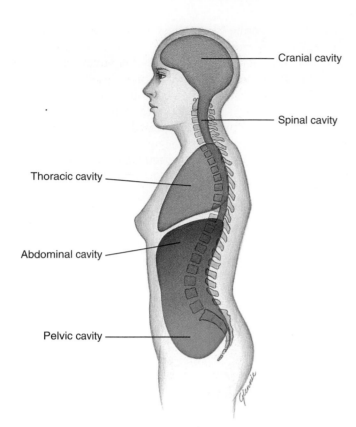

Figure 8-5   Cavities of the body.

It may be in front of (anterior or ventral) or behind (posterior or dorsal) the coronal plane. Other terms for location include close to (*proximal*) or away from (*distal*) a point where one organ attaches to another.

Body Cavities

There are five cavities in the human body (Figure 8-5):

* The thoracic cavity contains the lungs, heart, esophagus, trachea, and major blood vessels.
* The abdominal cavity contains the stomach, gallbladder, pancreas, intestines, liver, spleen, adrenal glands, and kidneys.
* The pelvic cavity contains the reproductive organs, bladder, and rectum.
* The cranial cavity contains the brain, ventricles, and some glands.
* The spinal cavity houses the spinal cord and nerves.

Body Regions

Locations within the abdominal and pelvic cavities are described in terms of nine regions (Figure 8-6). The abdomen is also sometimes sectioned into four quadrants: the right upper, right lower, left upper, and left lower quadrants (Figure 8-7).

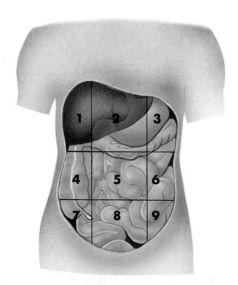

Figure 8-6   Body regions. *1,* Right hypochondriac. *2,* Epigastric. *3,* Left hypochondriac. *4,* Right lumbar. *5,* Umbilical. *6,* Left lumbar. *7,* Right inguinal. *8,* Hypogastric. *9,* Left inguinal. *(From Thidodeau GA, Patton KT: Anatomy & physiology, ed 5, St Louis, 2003, Mosby.)*

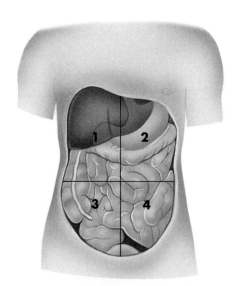

Figure 8-7   Division of the abdomen into four quadrants. Diagram shows relationship of internal organs to the four abdominopelvic quadrants: *1,* right upper quadrant (RUQ); *2,* left upper quadrant (LUQ); *3,* right lower quadrant (RLQ); *4,* left lower quadrant (LLQ). *(From Thibodeau GA, Patton KT: Anatomy & physiology, ed 5, St Louis, 2003, Mosby.)*

Cell Function

Cell Reproduction

Mitosis is the process by which a cell divides to reproduce, creating an identical replica with the same chromosomes. Each cell of an organism carries all of the genetic information of the organism. In humans, there are 46 chromosomes in each cell except the gametes (sperm and egg). With the exception of the sex chromosomes (X and Y), all of the chromosomes are paired and called *homologous* **autosomes**.

In the process of meiosis the cell divides into two parts each with only one half of the chromosomes. Meiotic cell division is part of the reproduction process and results in the formation of sex cells (gametes). The combination of two gametes with chromosomes from different parents into one cell is called *fertilization*. The offspring inherits any abnormal gene found on the chromosome of either parent. Figure 8-8 compares the processes of mitosis and meiosis.

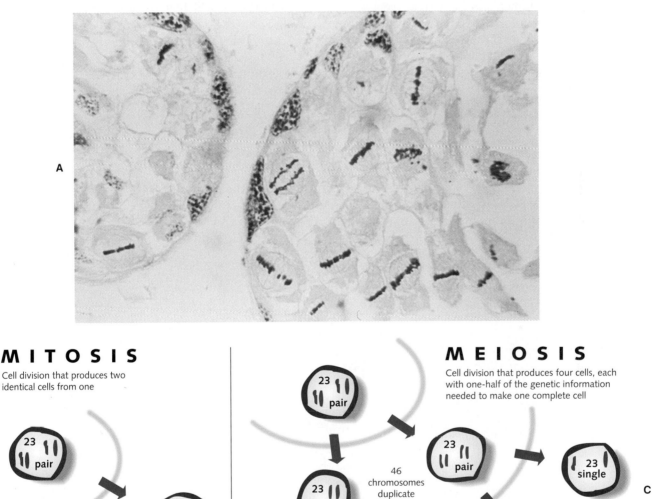

Figure 8-8   **A** and **B**, Mitosis produces two cells that are identical and complete. **C**, Meiosis results in four cells, each with one half of the genetic material of the cell.

Heredity

Heredity is the passing on of genetic information that determines the characteristics of an individual person. The arrangement of genetic material determines many characteristics, such as blood type, physical appearance, and gender.

Genes contain the hereditary information in the cell. They are made up of protein chains in a molecule called *deoxyribonucleic acid (DNA)*. Threadlike strands of DNA make up structures called *chromosomes.* Chromosomes contain between 50,000 and 100,000 genes that determine the person's general human and individual traits. A microscopic photograph (karyotype) of the 46 chromosomes in the cell shows the chromosome composition (Figure 8-9). The human genetic sequence (genome) has been completely "mapped" (sequenced, or identified), but the function of all of the genes has not yet been determined.

The configuration of genetic information in the chromosome is called the **genotype.** The trait or appearance that results from the genotype is called the **phenotype.** The characteristic of a **dominant** gene appears even when only one gene is inherited. Traits caused by **recessive** genes appear only when the gene is inherited from both parents and is present on both paired chromosomes. When two genes are alike on the chromosome pair, the combination is called *homozygous.* When they differ, they are called *heterozygous.*

The genetic information carried by the chromosomes is responsible for the development of all body cells and the formation of tissues, organs, and body systems. Chapter 34 provides more information regarding biotechnology, the study of genetic manipulation.

Genetic Disorders

Abnormal genes or chromosomes cause many disorders, which are therefore called *inherited, hereditary,* or *genetic* disorders. The terms **congenital** and **condition** are used to describe these disorders as opposed to the terms *contagious* and **disease,** which are used when a disease is contagious and caused by an organism such as a virus or bacteria. Some of these disorders affect only one body part or system, but others cause defects or symptoms in two or more body systems. When symptoms of a genetic disorder appear, the condition may be called a **syndrome.**

Common genetic disorders are included in the following body system chapters, according to the system primarily affected. The following are some of the most common genetic disorders:

- Cleft lip or palate (see Chapter 9)
- Clubfoot (see Chapter 13)
- Cystic fibrosis (see Chapter 12)
- Down syndrome (see Chapter 18)
- Huntington's chorea (see Chapter 18)
- Klinefelter's syndrome (see Chapter 20)

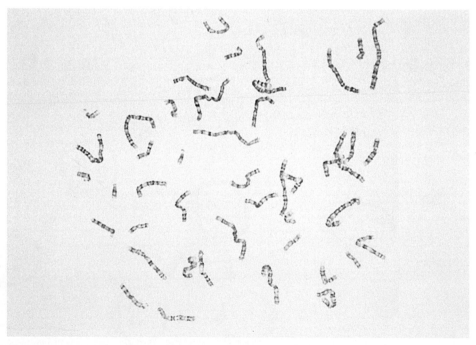

Figure 8-9   The karyotype is an organized picture of the chromosomes. *(Courtesy Ward's Natural Science Establishment, Rochester, NY.)*

- Neural tube defect (see Chapter 18)
- Neurofibromatosis (see Chapter 18)
- Phenylketonuria (see Chapter 15)
- Sickle cell anemia (see Chapter 11)
- Spina bifida (see Chapter 18)
- Tay-Sachs disease (see Chapter 15)
- Thalassemia (see Chapter 11)

Cancer

Cancer is the uncontrolled growth of abnormal cells that tend to spread (metastasize) and invade the tissue around them. A new growth of cells or neoplasm may be benign or malignant. Cancer cells are able to grow rapidly because they create their own blood vessels to take the oxygen and nutrients from the body. Common sites for development of cancer include the lungs, breast, colon, uterus, oral cavity, and bone marrow. Many malignancies are curable if detected early. Warning signs of cancer vary with the area affected.

Although the specific cause of cancer is not known, it results from a mistake in one single cell's division (**mutation**). Cancer cells have properties similar to embryonic cells during fetal division. The DNA message that directs embryo cells to divide rapidly is chemically repressed when the fetal development is complete. In cancer, this uncontrolled cell division begins again. It is theorized that this change is brought on by exposure to something that induces or starts it (carcinogen). More than 80% of the cases of cancer are related to smoking or exposure to chemicals, radiation, and ultraviolet light such as the sun. Some cancers are related to viral infections such as hepatitis B and Epstein-Barr. Genetic susceptibility in certain cancers is a factor in breast and basal cell skin cancer. More than 12 cancers are believed to be directly inherited. Genes that cause cancer are called *oncogenes*.

In 1999 scientists at Emory University discovered enzymes that generate abnormal cell growth in both cancer and some forms of cardiovascular disease. The enzymes appear to change oxygen into a reactive form that has been theorized to cause damage to DNA and lead to an acceleration of the aging process. The reactive oxygen has been proven to cause cells to divide more rapidly. The scientists hypothesize that reactive oxygen may be a cause rather than a byproduct of cancer. New approaches to cancer treatment resulting from this research may include agents that block the enzymes or that destroy the reactive oxygen in cancer cells.

The body fights cancer by forming antibodies against the abnormal cells. It is believed that small groups of cancer cells develop in the body continually without detection. These "silent cancers" are successfully removed by the body's immune processes.

Issues and Innovations

Genetic Engineering

At least 3000 disorders are known to result from genetic abnormalities. Research now shows that other disorders with no known cause may also be genetically linked, including some forms of retardation and cancer (Table 8-2). Chromosomes also can be damaged by drugs, radiation, toxins, viruses, and other environmental agents. In all, approximately 1 of every 150 to 200 births involves a serious chromosomal defect.

Using advanced techniques, new procedures can now identify abnormal genes in the unborn fetus. Chorionic vil-

Table 8-2	Mapped Genetic Disorders*	
Gene	**Chromosome**	**Description**
AD3	X	Alzheimer's disease, type 3
AD4	1	Alzheimer's disease, type 4
SOD1	21	Amyotrophic lateral sclerosis
APOE	19	Apolipoprotein E
BRCA1	17	Breast cancer, type 1
BRCA2	13	Breast cancer, type 2
CFTR	7	Cystic fibrosis
DMD	X	Duchenne muscular dystrophy
HD	4	Huntington disease
IDDM1	6	Type 1 diabetes
CDKN2	9	Malignant melanoma
NF2	22	Neurofibromatosis
OBS	7	Obesity
PAH	12	Phenylketonuria
DPC4	18	Suppressor of pancreatic carcinoma
FMR1	X	S-linked mental retardation

*In some cases, the presence of the gene for a disorder does not guarantee that it will occur.

lus sampling (CVS) is a method of examining the chromosomes, using a small sample of placental tissue, at about the seventh to eighth week of pregnancy. Amniocentesis, a procedure that examines the fluid that surrounds the fetus in the uterus, can detect genetic defects in the sixteenth or seventeenth week of pregnancy. More than 200 disorders can be identified by amniocentesis. Some researchers are developing techniques to identify fetal disorders using maternal blood samples that contain fetal cells. These fetal cells are present in the mother's blood after they have leaked through the placenta.

Preimplantation diagnosis combines the biotechnology of in vitro fertilization and genetic testing. In this procedure, embryos are created outside of the body in petri dishes. A single cell sample is taken from the embryo when it has grown to 8 cells in a process called *embryo biopsy*. The single cell is then examined for genetic defects. Only the embryos that are free from genetic error are then implanted.

Research teams are now investigating the possibility of correcting defective genes in humans. Gene splicing, the transplanting of genes, has been conducted successfully in "test tube" animal embryos. Procedures are also being developed to implant a normal gene in a defective one, by using a retrovirus to carry the normal gene into the cells of the affected individual after birth.

Genetic screening of potential parents can help determine the risk of a genetic disorder occurring. Special counseling then provides parents with information about their options before and after conception if a defect is expected or found. The couple's family medical and genetic histories are charted to determine the potential for chromosomal defects.

Ethical decisions resulting from increased knowledge about genetics are a growing concern of health care workers now and in the future. Hospitals have ethics committees to decide what type of care should be given to babies born with genetic defects. Genetic research has raised ethical questions never before faced. Emergent techniques of genetic engineering will create new challenges and new ethical decisions. Chapter 34 provides more information regarding genetic engineering and biotechnology.

Cancer Treatments

Using the theory that the body's immune system can treat cancer, scientists are developing cancer vaccines. Immunotherapy involves using chemicals that are isolated from bacteria infected with the cancer, killed suspensions of bacteria, and some biological substances that harm tumors. The biological substances include interferon, interleukin, tumor necrosis factors, and growth factors. Other scientists are researching the possibility of replacing the genetic message of cancerous cells that causes the rapid cell division to occur.

In some cases, lasers are used to destroy cancerous cells. Fiberoptic technology called *photodynamic therapy* is used to place a destructive wavelength of laser directly into the tumor. Hyperthermia, or an increase in temperature, is being used in combination with radiation to treat some tumors. The cells of the tumor can be raised to temperatures high enough to kill them without killing the surrounding body cells.

Review Questions

1. Use the following terms in one or more sentences that correctly relate their meaning.
   Autosome
   Dominant
   Genotype
   Phenotype,
   Recessive

2. Describe four properties of living organisms.

3. List the four units of organization of the body from the smallest to the largest.

4. Describe the structure and location of the four types of tissue of the body.

5. Complete the following phrases using directional terms to describe the location of each body part. List the plane that is used to section the location.

   The eyes are located _____ to the nose. Plane: _____

   The head is located _____ to the neck. Plane: _____

   The spine is located _____ to the sternum. Plane: _____

   The stomach is located _____ to the heart. Plane: _____

   The fingers are located _____ to the hand. Plane: _____

6. List one body organ or structure located in each of the following sections of the body:
   right upper quadrant   epigastric region
   thoracic cavity   spinal cavity
   left upper quadrant   abdominal cavity
   hypogastric region   right inguinal region
   umbilical region   left lumbar region

7. Differentiate between the genotype and phenotype of an individual.

8. Identify three tests used to detect genetic abnormalities of a fetus.

9. Describe two areas of research dealing with correcting genetic defects.

Critical Thinking

1. Investigate and compare the cost of at least three tests used to diagnose disorders relating to body organization.

2. Investigate at least five common medications used in treatment of body organization disorders.

3. List at least five health care occupations involved in care of disorders of the body organization.

4. Investigate advanced techniques used in genetic engineering.

9
Integumentary System

Learning Objectives

Define at least 10 terms relating to the integumentary system.

Describe the function of the integumentary system.

Identify at least five integumentary system structures and the function of each.

Describe at least five disorders of the integumentary system.

Identify at least three methods used to assess the function of the integumentary system.

Describe three methods that can be used to maintain healthy skin.

Identify three types of skin cancer and at least five methods for prevention.

Key Terms

Adipose
(AD-i-pose) Of a fatty nature, fat

Biopsy
(BI-op-see) Removal and examination of living tissue

Ceruminous
(se-ROO-min-us) Pertaining to earwax

Dermatitis
(der-muh-TY-tis) Inflammation of the skin

Dermis
(DER-mis) Corium, or layer of skin beneath the epidermis

Epidermis
(ep-i-DER-mis) Outermost and nonvascular layer of skin

Follicle
(FOL-i-kul) Sac or pouchlike depression or cavity

Lunula
(LOO-nyuh-lah) General term for a small crescent- or moon-shaped area of fingernail

Melanin
(MEL-uh-nin) Dark, shapeless pigment of the skin

Papilla
(pah-PIL-uh) Small, nipple-shaped projection or elevation

Pilus
(PIE-lus) Hair

Sebaceous
(se-BAY-shus) Pertaining to sebum or a greasy lubricating substance

Subcutaneous
(sub-kyoo-TAY-nee-us) Beneath the skin

Sudoriferous
(soo-doe-RIF-er-us) Conveying sweat

Integumentary System Terminology*

TERM	DEFINITION	PREFIX	ROOT	SUFFIX
Cheilorrhaphy	Suture of the lip		cheil/o	rrhaphy
Cutaneous	Pertaining to the skin		cutan	eous
Cyanoderm	Blue skin	cyan/o	derm	
Dermatitis	Inflammation of the skin		derm/at	itis
Melanoma	Tumor that is black		melan	oma
Psoriasis	Condition of the skin characterized by itching		psor	iasis
Rhinoplasty	Plastic repair of the nose		rhin/o	plasty
Sarcoma	Tumor of the flesh		sarc	oma
Sebaceous	Pertaining to oil		seb/ac	eous
Stomatitis	Inflammation of the mouth		stoma/t	itis

*A short transition phrase or vowel may be added to or deleted from the word parts to make the combining form.

Abbreviations of the Integumentary System

ABBREVIATION	MEANING
bx	Biopsy
CA	Cancer
C & S	Culture and sensitivity
etiol	Etiology
LE	Lupus erythematosus
mm	Millimeter
oint	Ointment
PABA	Paraaminobenzoic acid
sc	Subcutaneous
SLE	Systemic lupus erythematosus

Structure and Function of the Integumentary System

The integumentary system is composed of the skin and accessory structures (Figure 9-1). Accessory structures of the system include the hair, nails, specialized glands, and nerves. The main function of the integumentary system is to protect the other body systems from injury and infection. A second function is to help the body maintain homeostasis by regulating temperature, retaining body fluids, and eliminating wastes. The skin also helps to perceive the environment with sensory receptors. The skin stores energy and vitamins and produces vitamin D from sunlight. Some hormones, fat-soluble vitamins, and drugs may be absorbed through the skin.

Skin

The skin, covering 17 to 20 square feet (1.6 to 1.9 m²), is the largest organ in the body. It varies in thickness from $\frac{1}{50}$ inch (0.5 mm) in the eyelids to $\frac{1}{4}$ inch (6.3 mm) in the soles of the feet. Changes in the skin often indicate the presence of other body system disorders, including anemia, respiratory disorders, liver disorders, cancer, and shock (Figure 9-2).

The **epidermis,** or cuticle, is the outermost layer of the skin and is composed of a surface of dead cells with an underlying layer of living cells. Water repellent cells made of protein (keratinocytes) make up 90% of the epidermis. Oil (**sebaceous**) and sweat (**sudoriferous**) glands and hair follicles lie in the epidermis. Melanocytes, which produce **melanin,** are located in this layer. Melanin is the pigment that gives skin its color. The surface of the epidermis is covered with a film composed of sweat, oil, and epithelial cells that lubricates, hydrates, provides antibacterial protection, and blocks toxic agents from entering the body.

The **dermis,** or corium, is called the "true" skin. The dermis contains the blood vessels and nerves. Each square inch of skin contains 15 feet of blood vessels.

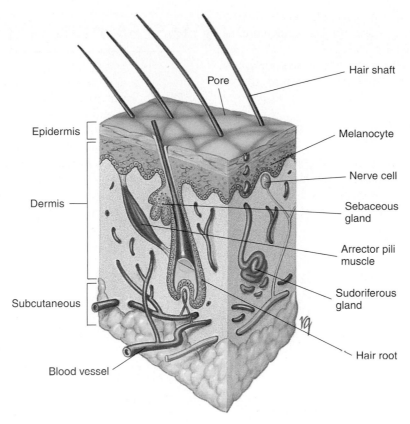

Figure 9-1   Structures of the skin.

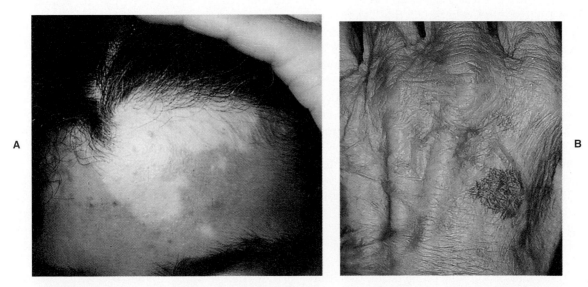

Figure 9-2   **A**, Vitiligo, a pigmentation disorder, has no known cause. **B**, Lentigo, a form of melanoma, is often found in people with extensive sun exposure. (**A**, *Courtesy Jamie Tschen MD;* **B**, *from* Mosby's medical, nursing, and allied health dictionary, *ed 6, St Louis, 2002, Mosby.*)

The innermost layer of the skin is called the **subcutaneous** layer. Fatty (**adipose**) tissue of the subcutaneous layer cushions and insulates the body's organs.

The nerve endings in the skin allow it to be sensitive to environmental stimuli. Skin senses pain, pressure, touch, and changes in temperature.

Hair and Hair Follicles

Skin normally has hair (**pilus**) in all areas except the soles of the feet and palms of the hands. Some hair blocks foreign particles from entering the body through structures such as the nose and eyes. Each hair root originates in the dermis. The visible portion is called the *shaft*. The hair **follicle** is the root with its covering. One or two oil (sebaceous) glands are attached to each hair follicle. A tiny muscle (arrector pili) is attached to the hair shaft and causes "goose bumps" or the hair to "stand on end" in response to cold or fear. Hair color and texture are inherited. The color depends on the amount of melanin in the cells.

Glands

The three types of glands in the skin are the sebaceous glands (oil), sudoriferous glands (sweat), and the ceruminous glands of the ear canal.

Sebaceous glands are located everywhere in the skin except the palms of the hands and the soles of the feet. Each square inch of skin has about 2000 sebaceous glands. Sebum, or oil, causes the skin to be soft and waterproof.

Sudoriferous glands originate in the subcutaneous layer of the skin. Some of these glands (apocrine) are attached to hair follicles and others (eccrine) empty directly onto the skin. Apocrine glands are located in areas such as under the arms (axilla), the breasts, and pubic area. In some areas of the skin, each square inch contains about two million sudoriferous glands. Sudoriferous glands help regulate body temperature and excrete body wastes. The skin loses at least 500 ml of water each day; more water is lost through sweating caused by exercise or heat.

Ceruminous glands are located only in the auditory canal of the ear. These glands secrete wax that helps to protect the ear from infection and prevents entry of foreign bodies.

Nails

The function of the nails is to protect fingers and toes from injury. Fingernails and toenails are formed from dead, keratinized epidermal cells. The root or area of nail growth is covered by skin at the area of attachment to finger or toe. The crescent-shaped white area near the root is the **lunula.**

Assessment Techniques

Dermatology is the study of skin. **Dermatitis** is the general term for inflammation of the skin. Skin disorders are usually uncomfortable and unattractive but not life-threatening.

Skin lesions can usually be seen with visual inspection. The size, shape, texture, and color of a lesion often helps reveal its cause. A **biopsy** or culture may be used to identify the causative organism.

The uppermost part of the dermis is composed of **papillae,** or ridges. The papillae form regular patterns in the fingers, palms of the hands, and soles of the feet where the skin is thick. Fingertip and toe prints are unique to each person. In addition to forming a surface that permits gripping, the fingerprints allow the identification of each individual. The patterns of ridges in fingerprints and toe prints may also be linked to disorders such as Down syndrome.

Disorders of the Integumentary System

Acne vulgaris (AK-nee vul-GAYR-is) usually appears in adolescence and may continue into adulthood. Acne often is caused by the increased secretion of oil (sebum) related to increased hormones during puberty. Bacterial growth and blockage of the hair follicles cause papules, pustules, and blackheads. Acne tends to run in families. Contrary to popular belief, diet does not cause or affect the severity of acne. Treatment may include exposure to ultraviolet light, oral or topical antibiotics, or removal of the top layers of skin that has scarred (dermabrasion).

Albinism (AL-bin-izm) is an inherited disorder in which the melanocytes do not produce melanin. Lack of melanin leads to pale skin, white hair, and pink eyes. People with albinism are prone to severe sunburn and light may damage unprotected structures of the eyes.

Alopecia (al-o-PEE-shee-uh), or baldness, is the inherited tendency to lose hair from the head. Production of androgenic (an-dro-JEN-ik) hormones beginning at puberty initiates the loss. Baldness is more common in men, but it may occur in women. Temporary hair loss may be caused by drugs, radiation, pregnancy, high fever, anorexia, and cosmetics.

Athlete's foot, or epidermophytosis (ep-i-DER-mo-fi-TOE-sis), is a fungal infection. The skin may itch, blister, and crack, especially between the toes. Athlete's foot is very contagious and can be transmitted on wet floors, such as in gym showers. Treatment includes application of antifungal medication and keeping the area clean, ventilated, and dry.

Cellulitis (sel-yoo-LIE-tis) is a bacterial infection of the dermis and subcutaneous layer of the skin. It occurs in people with low resistance to infection such as the elderly, children, and chronically ill. The person may experience fever, chill, and vesicles (VES-i-kulz) on a reddened, warm area of the skin. It can lead to impaired circulation and permanent lymphedema (lim-feh-DEE-muh) in the extremities. Treatment includes rest, immobilization of the infected area, and antibiotics.

Chloasma (klo-AZ-muh) is a patchy discoloration of the face caused by high hormone levels that occur during pregnancy and by prolonged use of oral contraceptives. It may disappear at the end of the pregnancy or with stopping birth control pills. Chloasma also may be a sign of problems with the liver. Treatment is often not necessary, but nonprescription cosmetic products can minimize the discoloration.

Cleft lip or *cleft palate* (kleft PAL-ut) occurs in 1 of 700 babies born in the United States each year. In this condition, the upper lip has a cleft or space where the nasal processes or palate does not meet properly. Heredity appears to be the direct cause in 25% of the cases, and environmental factors and premature birth also may cause the condition. Treatment includes surgical and dental correction, speech therapy, and sometimes psychological counseling.

Contact dermatitis is an allergic reaction that may occur after initial contact or as an acquired response. Some substances that frequently cause acquired dermatitis include poison ivy, nickel in jewelry, and preservatives in cosmetics. Redness, itching, swelling, and blisters may result from contact with the irritating substance. Treatment may include washing the affected area, applying antiinflammatory creams, and avoiding exposure to the irritating substance.

Dandruff (DAN-druf), characterized by itching of the scalp, produces white flakes of dead skin cells. Dandruff can be controlled by massaging the scalp and brushing and shampooing the hair. Medicated shampoos designed to control dandruff often help.

Decubitus ulcers (de-KYOO-bit-us UL-serz), or decubiti, are sores or areas of inflammation that occur over bony prominences of the body due to prolonged pressure and hypoxia to the affected tissues. These "bedsores" are seen most often in elderly and immobilized persons. Frequent change in position, good nutrition, and massage to the area help to prevent decubiti. Decubiti are described in four stages by their severity. Decubiti often are resistant to treatment, which may include application of antibiotics, removal of necrotic tissue, and frequent cleaning of open sores. Larvae (maggots) of blowflies, which feed only on dead tissue, have been used in some severe cases to clean sores. In addition to removing the dead tissue, the maggot larvae provide stimulation of the affected area with their movement and produce compounds that are lethal to bacteria that cause gangrene and similar infections.

Eczema (EK-ze-muh), a form of dermatitis, is a group of disorders caused by allergic or irritant reactions. Eczema is characterized by swelling, redness, and itching and weeping, crusted skin lesions. Although it is not contagious, it seems to run in families. Treatment of eczema includes removing the irritant and keeping the affected skin clean.

Fungal (FUN-gul) skin infections live only on the dead, outer surface or epidermis. Some may cause no symptoms. Others may produce irritation, scaling, redness, swelling, or blisters. Most fungal infections occur in areas of the body that provide moisture and are named by the area in which they appear. Examples include athlete's foot (see above), jock itch, and scalp, nail, body, and beard ringworm. Treatment by the use of antifungal creams usually cures these skin conditions. In severe cases, oral antifungal medication may be necessary.

Furuncle (FER-ung-kl), commonly called a *boil,* is a bacterial infection of a hair follicle. A carbuncle is several boils that join together. Recurring boils may indicate diabetes or an immune disorder. Boils are infectious, but the spread can be controlled with careful cleanliness and handwashing. Treatment includes hot compresses, antibiotics, and sometimes drainage by lancing.

Hirsutism (HER-soot-izm), or hypertrichosis (hy-per-tri-KO-sis), is an abnormal amount of hair growth in unusual places. In women, hair may appear on the face, back, and chest. Hirsutism may be caused by hormone supplements or may be a hereditary condition. Unwanted hair may be removed temporarily by shaving, waxing, or depilatories, or it may be removed permanently by electrolysis.

Impetigo (im-puh-TI-go) is a very contagious bacterial skin infection that occurs most often in children. It begins with small vesicles, which become pustules and form a crust. Itching and burning may occur. Impetigo may lead to kidney infection, but lesions usually clear without causing lasting damage. It can be fatal in infants. Treatment includes antibiotics and isolation to prevent spread of the infection.

Kaposi's sarcoma (Figure 9-3) is a form of cancer that originates in blood vessels and spreads to the skin. Kaposi's sarcoma appears as a round or oval spot on the skin that may be red, purplish, or brown in color. It has two forms. One form affects older people and rarely spreads to other parts of the body. The second form is associated with diabetes, lymphoma, and AIDS. It grows more quickly and may spread to the lungs, liver, and intestines. Treatment for Kaposi's sarcoma has not been very successful but may include chemotherapy or interferon.

Lupus erythematosus (LOO-pus air-ith-uh-mah-TOE-sis) may be a benign dermatitis or a chronic systemic disorder. Its cause is unknown. As dermatitis, it appears as a scaly rash and may lead to baldness. When systemic, lupus affects the vascular and connective tissues and also appears as a rash on the skin. Treatment includes protection from exposure to the sun and antiinflammatory drugs.

Psoriasis (so-RY-uh-sis) is a chronic skin disorder in which too many epidermal cells are produced. Psoriasis appears as red, thick areas, or plaques (plaks), covered with scales, which may be gray or silver. Although the cause is unknown, psoriasis may be triggered by stress and other factors. The disorder seems to run in families and appears in adolescence or early adulthood. Treatment includes topical medication, removal of the scales, and application of ultraviolet light.

Rashes may result from viral infection, especially in children (Table 9-1). Treatment is usually symptomatic, designed to prevent scratching that may result in scars. Complications from diseases that cause childhood rashes are possible but unlikely.

Scleroderma (skle-ro-DER-muh) is a rare autoimmune disorder that affects the blood vessels and connective tissues of the skin and other epithelial tissues. Hard, yellowish lesions are formed. Scleroderma usually remains localized but may become systemic. Treatment may include use of antiinflammatory medication and physical therapy to prevent muscle contracture and deformity.

Skin cancer has three basic forms, called *basal* (BAY-zuhl) *cell,* *squamous* (SKWAY-mus) *cell,* and *melanoma* (mel-uh-NO-ma) (Figure 9-4, *A* to *C*). Basal cell cancer is the most common type. If detected early, it usually can be treated successfully by removing the lesions by burning, freezing, or surgery. Radiation may be required.

Although skin cancer is the most common form of cancer, it is also the most treatable, particularly if diagnosed early. Early signs of skin cancer include a spot or growth that does not heal or a mole or birthmark that changes size, color, thickness, or texture (Box 9-1).

Skin lesions differ in texture, color, location, and rate of growth. Skin lesions are usually uncomfortable but are seldom life-threatening. They may result from irritation or infection. They may also indicate a condition of the body as a whole (Table 9-2).

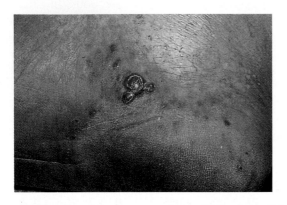

Figure 9-3   Kaposi's sarcoma. *(From Thibodeau GA, Patton KT:* Anatomy & physiology, *ed 5, St Louis, 2003, Mosby.)*

Box 9-1   Warning Signs of Melanoma

- Change in size of a pigmented spot or mole
- Change in color of an existing mole (white, red, or blue pigmentation of the surrounding skin)
- Change in consistency or shape of the skin over a pigmented spot
- Inflammation of the skin around an existing mole

Table 9-1   Viral Infections Causing a Rash

Infection	Period of Incubation	Period of Contagiousness	Site of Rash	Nature of Rash
Measles (rubeola)	7-14 days	2-4 days before rash appears, plus 5 days	Ears, neck, face, trunk, arms, legs	Irregular, flat, red rash lasts 4-7 days
German measles (rubella)	14-21 days	Shortly before onset of symptoms until rash disappears	Face, neck, trunk, arms, legs	Pinkish, flat, begins 1-2 days after symptoms appear, lasts 1-3 days
Chickenpox	14-21 days	Before onset of symptoms until all vesicles have crusted	Trunk, face, neck, arms, legs, infrequently palms and soles	Small, flat red spots from fluid-filled blisters followed by crusting, lasting a few days to 2 weeks

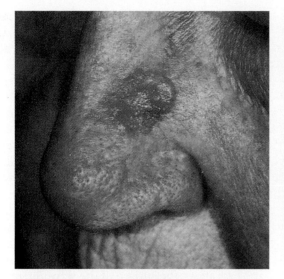
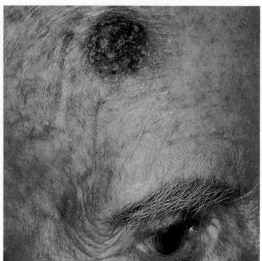
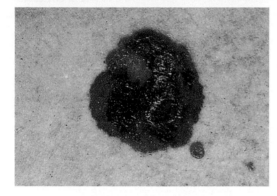

Figure 9-4   The three most common forms of skin cancer. **A**, Squamous cell. **B**, Basal cell. **C**, Malignant melanoma. *(From Thibodeau GA, Patton KT: Anatomy & physiology, ed 5, St Louis, 2003, Mosby.)*

Table 9-2   Skin Lesions

Lesion	Description	Possible Cause
Crust	Dry pus, lymph, or blood covering injury, secondary skin lesion	Scab on abrasion; eczema
Cyst	Sac of fluid or dead cells, solid to the touch	Plugged oil gland
Fissure	Deep groove in skin, crack	Athlete's foot
Keloid	Progressively enlarging scar	Burn
Macule	Discolored spot on skin; not raised or depressed	Measles, mononucleosis, freckles
Papule	Raised, solid area, less than 1 cm in diameter	Warts, moles, pimples
Pustule	Pus-filled, raised area, white, yellow, greenish-yellow	Pimples, acne
Ulcer	Open sore, may bleed or have discharge	Bedsore
Venous star	Bluish, spiderweb-like veins	Pressure in peripheral veins
Vesicle	Raised fluid-filled pouch, specific location	Burns, scabies, shingles, chickenpox

Streptococcus species (strep-to-KOK-us) are nonmotile bacteria that affect many parts of the body. Each year 500 to 1500 cases of group-A strep infections appear as a skin disorder. Streptococci infections may become "flesh eating" in nature, destroying up to 1 cm² of skin each hour. If treated within 3 days, this bacterial infection can be cured easily with antibiotics. The condition may be fatal if not treated promptly.

Vitiligo (vit-il-EYE-go) is a condition that causes loss of pigment of the skin that results in irregular white patches. The condition may appear at any time and has an increased incidence in some families. The cause of vitiligo is unknown but may be the result of an autoimmune response. Most vitiligo goes untreated. Although some areas may repigment, new patches may appear.

A *wart* is a papule (PAP-ool) caused by a viral infection of the skin. Plantar, common, and flat warts are typical, and they may disappear after a few weeks or may last for years. They can usually be permanently removed by chemicals, freezing with liquid nitrogen, or burning. Chapter 20 provides information about how warts affect the reproductive system.

Issues and Innovations

Skin and Hair Care

People in the United States spend approximately $6 billion dollars for skin and hair products each year. The major contribution to a clear complexion and attractive hair is good overall health. Cleanliness, nutritious meals, and exercise reduce the risk of skin disorders. With conditions such as acne, some commercial products lead to additional skin problems rather than solutions.

Regular washing is the best way to prevent skin eruptions caused by excessive oil. A drying agent (astringent) applied after washing can remove excess oil from the skin. Products such as cleansing creams, which contain oil, do not help individuals with excessive oil but may help people with dry skin.

Cosmetics manufacturers use many advertising techniques (gimmicks) to sell their products. Products are promoted as "imported," "scent free," "organic," "never rinse," "smell away," and "industrial strength," but none of these properties is beneficial to the cleanliness and health of skin. Creams that "reduce wrinkles" often contain alpha-hydroxy acids, which cause sloughing (loss) of dead cells and thickening of underlying tissues. A chemical peel or application of a strong exfoliant contains a greater percentage of this acid compound. The FDA has no record of serious injury from use of dewrinkling creams, although some reports of rashes and burns have been made. The FDA does not test cosmetics for effectiveness but establishes that the creams are safe in the doses currently being sold.

All soaps work by emulsification; they surround and bind to the dirt so that it can be rinsed off. It is important that the soap be completely rinsed off to remove the dirt from the skin. Acne soaps may include antibacterial ingredients or abrasive materials to remove dead skin. One of the most effective antibacterial compounds is benzoyl peroxide. Antibacterial compounds are most effective when applied before a blemish appears. Hypoallergenic soaps contain no chemicals or fragrances that may irritate sensitive skin.

Many products are available to remove unwanted hair or add desired hair. Some of the more common ways to remove unwanted hair are shaving, waxing, and depilatory creams. Depilatory creams work by chemically destroying the hair above the surface of the skin. There is no evidence that removal by shaving or with creams changes the pattern of growth or the texture of the hair. Hair can be removed permanently by electrolysis, which is the electrical destruction of each undesired hair follicle. There is no reliable evidence that any cosmetic product stimulates the regrowth of hair. Minoxidil is a drug being used by some physicians to treat hair loss conditions. Hair transplants and hairpieces are effective ways to add desired hair.

Sun and Skin Cancer

The skin defends against the damaging ultraviolet radiation of the sun by producing melanin. Melanin accumulates in the cells of the skin and causes a tan, but the skin is easily damaged by excessive sunlight. Ultraviolet light of the sun causes damage to cells of the dermis and loss of moisture that results in wrinkled, dry, and tough skin. Mild sunburn is actually a first-degree burn. A more serious second-degree burn with blister formation can also result. Newer skin products contain PABA (paraaminobenzoic acid), which is effective in blocking the ultraviolet rays of the sun.

Ultraviolet rays in sunlight may change the DNA structure in skin cells. Such changes may lead to mutations in the cells, or skin cancer. Ultraviolet radiation is considered to be the main cause of skin cancer. According to the American Cancer Society, more than 1,000,000 nonmalignant skin cancers occur each year in the US, with more than 50,000 cases of melanoma in 2002. Damage to the skin from the sun is cumulative, or adds up over the years, increasing the risk of developing skin cancers with each sun exposure.

Basal cell carcinoma is the most common type of skin cancer. It starts in the lowest layer of the epidermis and appears as waxy, pearly growths or red, scaly patches and is most often found on the face, arms, and hands. The cancer lesions may alternate bleeding and healing. Basal cell carcinoma is treated by scraping, burning, or cutting out the lesion.

Squamous cell carcinoma is the second most common type and originates in the middle layer of the epidermis. It spreads more quickly than basal cell and also appears on areas of skin most often exposed to the sun. This cancer looks like red, scaly patches that do not heal. Eventually, the cancer grows into the underlying tissues if not treated. Squamous cell carcinoma is removed with the same techniques used to treat basal cell carcinoma.

Melanoma is the third and most serious form of skin cancer. It originates in the pigment-producing or melanin cells of the skin. It is most often caused by exposure to the sun. It appears as a brown or black molelike growth on the back, legs, or torso. One half of the cases develop from existing pigmented moles. When treated early, cure rates are close to 100%. If not treated early, melanoma may be fatal. Melanoma is treated by removal of the growth. If the melanoma cells have spread, cure rates are low. Malignant melanoma has been treated with some success by using gene therapy. A marked gene is inserted into the tumor and can be recognized for attack by the body's immune system. Another treatment called *extracorporeal photo chemotherapy* (photophoresis) separates and irradiates white blood cells, which are then washed and reinserted. These cells act as a vaccine against the existing cancer.

Review Questions

1. Use the following terms in one or more sentences that correctly relate their meaning.
   Adipose

   Dermis

   Epidermis

   Subcutaneous

2. Describe five functions of the integumentary system.

3. Describe the location and function of each of the following parts of the integumentary system.

Ceruminous glands	Nerves
Dermis	Sebaceous gland
Epidermis	Shaft
Hair follicle	Subcutaneous gland
Nails	Sudoriferous gland

4. List three disorders of the integumentary system that are caused by a pathogen.

5. List three signs that might indicate a cancerous growth.

6. Describe three precautions that may be used to avoid skin cancer.

7. List five diseases or conditions in other body systems that might be detected by changes in the skin.

Critical Thinking

1. Investigate and compare the cost of at least three tests used to diagnose disorders of the integumentary system.

2. Investigate the function of at least five common medications used to treat the integumentary system.

3. List at least five occupations involved in the health care of integumentary system disorders.

4. Describe three commercials that are used to sell skin and hair products. Identify the technique or claim in each that is used to sell the product.

10
Cardiovascular System

Learning Objectives

Define at least 10 terms relating to the cardiovascular system.

Describe the function of the cardiovascular system.

Identify at least 10 cardiovascular system structures and the function of each.

Describe at least five disorders of the cardiovascular system.

Identify at least three methods of assessment used to evaluate the cardiovascular system.

Key Terms

Cardioversion
(kar-dee-o-VER-zhun) Restoration of normal heart rhythm by electrical shock

Contract
(kon-TRAKT) Shorten, reduce in size

Coronary
(KOR-uh-nair-ee) Pertaining to the heart; coronary arteries supply blood to the heart muscle

Diastole
(di-AS-to-lee) Dilation of the heart; resting phase or filling of the ventricles, alternating with systole

Infarction
(in-FARK-shun) An area of tissue death (necrosis) caused by loss of oxygen (ischemia) as a result of obstruction of circulation to the area

Pulmonary Circulation
(PUL-muh-nayr-ee ser-kyuh-LAY-shun) Carrying venous blood from the right ventricle to the lungs and returning oxygenated blood to the left atrium of the heart

Rate
(rayt) Expression of speed or frequency of an event in relation to a specified amount of time, number of contractions of the heart per minute

Rhythm
(RITH-um) Measured movement, recurrence of an action or function at regular intervals, interval of heart contractions

Stenosis
(ste-NO-sis) Narrowing or stricture of a duct or canal

Stethoscope
(STETH-o-skope) Instrument used to listen to body sounds (auscultation), such as the heartbeat

Systemic Circulation
(sis-TEM-ik ser-kyuh-LAY-shun) General circulation; carrying oxygenated blood from the left ventricle to tissues of the body and returning the venous blood to the right atrium of the heart

Systole
(SIS-toe-lee) Filling of the atria and contraction of the ventricles of the heart, alternating with diastole

Vessel
(VES-el) Any one of many tubules in the body that carry fluid

Cardiovascular System Terminology*

TERM	DEFINITION	PREFIX	ROOT	SUFFIX
Atherosclerosis	Condition of hardening of the arteries		ather/o	sclerosis
Cardiology	Study of the heart		cardi/o	ology
Congenital	Born with	con	gen	ital
Electrocardiography	Recording of the electrical activity of the heart	electro	cardi/o	graphy
Hypertension	High blood pressure	hyper	tension	
Myocardial	Pertaining to the muscle of the heart	myo	card	ial
Pericardial	Around the heart	peri	card	ial
Phlebitis	Inflammation of the veins		phleb	itis
Subclavian	Below the clavicle	sub	clav	ian
Thrombitis	Inflammation of a clot		thromb	itis

*A transition phrase or vowel may be added to or deleted from the word parts to make the combining form.

Abbreviations of the Cardiovascular System

ABBREVIATION	MEANING
AP	Apical
BP	Blood pressure
CHF	Congestive heart failure
chol	Cholesterol
EKG	Electrocardiogram
HB	Heartbeat
HDL	High-density lipoprotein
LDL	Low-density lipoprotein
MI	Myocardial infarction
PVC	Premature ventricular contraction

Structure and Function of the Cardiovascular System

The structures of the cardiovascular system are the heart and the blood **vessels.** The heart beats more than 100,000 times a day, circulating approximately 5 L of blood. The functions of the cardiovascular system are the following:

- Transport nutrients and oxygen to the body
- Transport waste products from the cells to the kidneys for excretion
- Distribute hormones and antibodies throughout the body
- Help control body temperature and maintain electrolyte balance (homeostasis)

Heart

The heart is a two-sided, double pump. It weighs less than a pound and is slightly larger than a fist. The heart is located between the lungs in the thoracic cavity, positioned partially to the left of the sternum. The base or topmost (superior) part of the heart is flatter in shape than the tapered apex or lower (inferior) portion.

The right side of the heart pumps oxygen-poor (deoxygenated) blood to the lungs, where carbon dioxide is exchanged for oxygen. This is referred to as **pulmonary circulation.** The left side pumps the oxygen-rich (oxygenated) blood to the rest of the body. This is referred to as **systemic circulation.** The blood returns to the right side of the heart from the body to complete the cycle (Figure 10-1).

Hepatic circulation refers to the path of the blood from the intestines, gallbladder, pancreas, stomach, and spleen through the liver. The liver stores and modifies nutrients in the blood for use by the body. It also removes or alters toxic substances so that they may be eliminated by the urinary system. The nutrient-rich blood, which has been filtered by the liver, is returned to the heart through the inferior vena cava for use throughout the body.

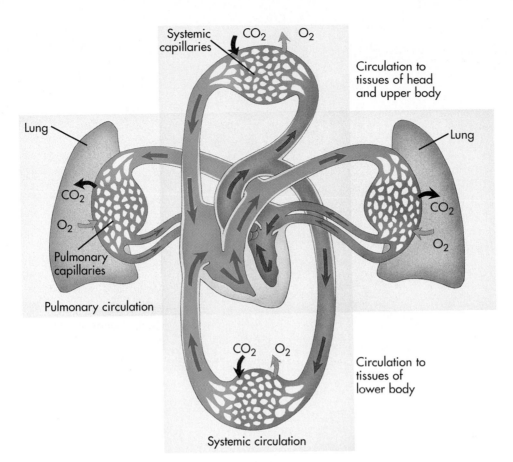

Figure 10-1   Blood flow through the circulatory system. *(From Thibodeau GA, Patton K: Anatomy & physiology, ed 5, St Louis, 2003, Mosby.)*

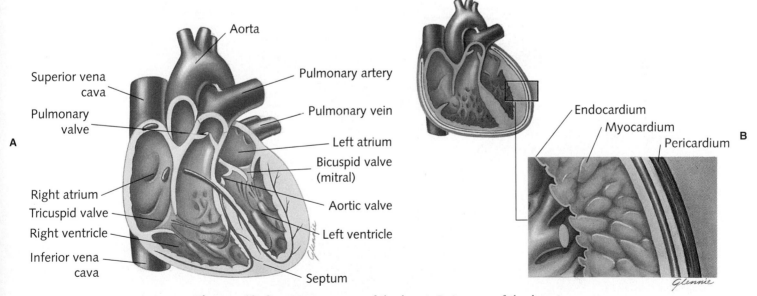

Figure 10-2   **A**, Structures of the heart. **B**, Layers of the heart.

The heart has four chambers (Figure 10-2). The top chambers are called *atria*. The lower chambers are called *ventricles*. The blood enters the heart through the atria and leaves the heart from the ventricles. The septum divides the right and left sides of the heart. Four valves prevent the blood from flowing backward through the system. Two of these valves are called *atrioventricular valves*. They separate the atria and ventricles on each side of the heart. The semilunar valves separate the ventricles from the outgoing vessels (pulmonary artery and aorta). The valves are named

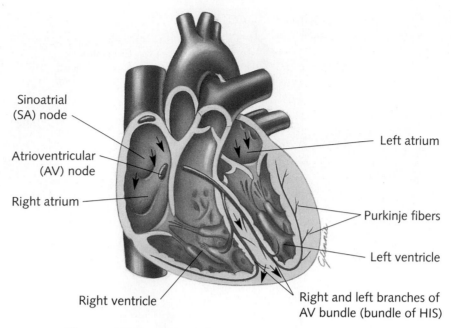

Sinoatrial
(SA) node

Atrioventricular
(AV) node

Right atrium

Left atrium

Purkinje fibers

Left ventricle

Right ventricle

Right and left branches of
AV bundle (bundle of HIS)

Figure 10-3 Path of electrical conduction in the heart.

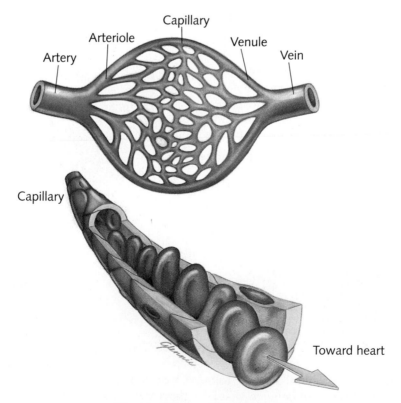

Capillary

Arteriole

Artery

Venule

Vein

Capillary

Toward heart

Figure 10-4 Blood vessels.

according to their structure (semilunar) and location (pulmonary or aortic).

The heart has three layers of tissue. The endocardium is a smooth layer of cells lining the inside of the heart and forming the valves. The smoothness of the endocardial tissue helps prevent damage to blood cells circulating through the system. The myocardium is the thickest layer, consisting of muscle tissue. This part of the heart pumps blood through the system. The pericardium is a double membrane that covers the outside of the heart, providing lubrication between the heart and surrounding structures to prevent tissue damage. The pericardial sac is made up of the inner serous (watery) and outer fibrous layers.

The activity of the heart muscle is controlled largely by the nervous system but is affected also by the action of hormones and other mechanisms such as fluid balance. Additionally, the heart contains the only muscle tissue that can stimulate its own contractions. Specialized sinoatrial cells in the right atrium (SA node) act as a pacemaker to start a heart contraction (Figure 10-3). The change in the electrical potential of these cells stimulates another group of cells, called the *atrioventricular node* (AV node), to send the impulse into the lower portions of the heart. The impulse of the AV node stimulates specialized bundles of muscle called the *AV bundle* or *bundle of HIS*. These fibers then stimulate the Purkinje fibers, which surround the lower portions of the ventricles. The Purkinje fibers cause the ventricles to **contract.** Another unique property of the heart is the ability to adjust the strength of the contractions based on the amount of blood in its chambers. Without the influence of the nervous system and other controls, the heart would contract only 40 times each minute instead of the normal 60 to 90 times.

Blood Vessels

There are three main types of blood vessels in the body (Figure 10-4):

- Arteries carry blood away from the heart.
- Veins carry blood back to the heart.
- Capillaries are microscopic vessels that carry blood between the arterial and venous vessels.

Blood is pumped from the heart to the body by the largest artery in the body, the aorta. Figure 10-5 shows the principal arteries of the body. The aorta branches into other arteries, which in turn branch into smaller vessels called *arterioles*. The blood moves from arterioles to microscopic capillaries. Gases, nutrients, and wastes are exchanged through the thin walls of the capillaries. The blood, which has now given up its oxygen, flows from the capillaries into tiny veins called *venules*. Venules branch together to form larger veins (Figure 10-5). The blood is re-

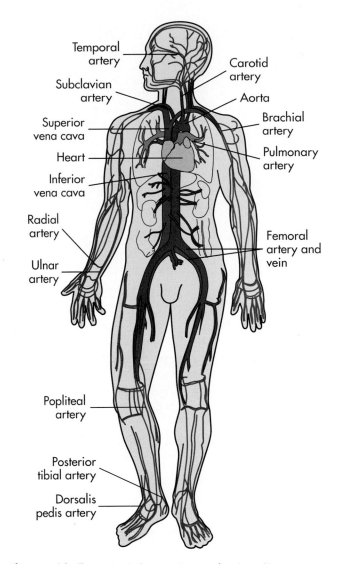

Figure 10-5   Principle arteries and veins. *(From Sorrentino S: Mosby's textbook for nursing assistants, ed 5, St Louis, 2000, Mosby.)*

turned to the heart in the body's largest veins, the superior vena cava and inferior vena cava. With the exception of the pulmonary artery, blood in the arteries is oxygenated. Except for the pulmonary vein, blood in veins is deoxygenated.

Arteries have a muscular layer of tissue that helps pump blood out to the body. Veins have a much thinner muscular layer. Gravity and the movement of the muscles surrounding the veins help deliver blood back to the heart. Veins also have valves that prevent blood from flowing back, away from the heart, once it has moved forward.

Path of the Blood Through the Heart

Tracing the path of a blood cell through the heart is one way to learn the heart's structures and understand its functions (Table 10-1). Although the heart is considered a two-sided pump to differentiate the systemic and pulmonary circulation, the two atria contract at the same time, then the ventricles contract. Deoxygenated blood enters the right atrium of the heart from the body through the inferior and superior vena cavae. Additionally blood from the heart muscle itself returns through a structure called the *coronary sinus*. The blood then passes through the tricuspid valve into the right ventricle. This valve closes as the pulmonary valve opens, allowing the passage of blood from the right ventricle to the pulmonary arteries. The pulmonary valve closes as the blood enters the lungs for the diffusion of oxygen and carbon dioxide. The oxygenated blood then travels through the pulmonary veins to the left atrium. From the left atrium the blood travels through the bicuspid or mitral valve to the left ventricle. The mitral valve closes as the blood leaves the left ventricle through the aortic valve. The blood then travels through the aorta to the rest of the body. As the ascending aorta leaves the heart, it branches in three directions to supply blood to the head and upper limbs. Two **coronary** arteries, which supply blood to the heart, branch off of the ascending aorta. The descending portion of the aorta supplies blood to the abdominal area and lower extremities. Deoxygenated blood is returned to the heart through the inferior and superior vena cavae from the body to complete the path.

Table 10-1	Path of the Blood Through the Heart
Structure	**Oxygen Content**
Body	Exchange of carbon dioxide and oxygen
Superior and inferior vena cavae	Deoxygenated
Right atrium	Deoxygenated
Triscupid valve	Deoxygenated
Right ventricle	Deoxygenated
Pulmonary valve	Deoxygenated
Pulmonary artery	Deoxygenated
Lungs	Exchange of carbon dioxide and oxygen
Pulmonary vein	Oxygenated
Left atrium	Oxygenated
Mitral valve	Oxygenated
Left ventricle	Oxygenated
Aortic valve	Oxygenated
Aorta	Oxygenated
Body	Exchange of carbon dioxide and oxygen

Assessment Techniques

Health care workers assess the activity of the heart as an indicator of overall body condition. Methods to assess the heart's condition include the following:

- Measuring pulse and blood pressure
- Listening to heart sounds
- Determining cardiac output
- Measuring muscle activity with electrocardiography
- Inserting a cardiac catheter
- Using echocardiography

Pulse

With each heartbeat, blood surges against the walls of arteries. That surge, called a *pulse,* can be felt and counted in arteries close to the skin. There are eight body locations where the pulse can be counted (Figure 10-6). The most commonly used site is the radial artery of the wrist. The large carotid artery in the throat is used in emergency situations. The brachial artery is used to measure the blood pressure. Other locations include the temporal, femoral, popliteal, posterior tibial and pedal arteries. The normal pulse range for adults is from 60 to 90 beats per minute, depending on the person's age, weight, fitness level, and emotional state. A pulse rate outside the normal range may indicate a disorder.

Blood Pressure

Blood pressure is the force of the blood against the walls of the arteries. The systolic blood pressure, or **systole,** occurs when the ventricles of the heart contract, pushing blood through the arteries. The diastolic pressure, or **diastole,** occurs when the ventricles relax. Normal blood pressure is written as 120/80 (systolic/diastolic). However, blood pressure varies greatly among people. A healthy systolic pressure is usually less than 140 and greater than 90. The diastolic pressure should be less than 100. A blood pressure outside this range may indicate a disorder such as hypertension or renal failure.

Heart Sounds

The "lub-dup" sound of the heart can be heard using a **stethoscope.** This characteristic sound results from the opening and closing of the valves in the heart as the blood is pumped from the atria to the ventricles and then to the lungs and then throughout the body. Abnormal or extra sounds are called *murmurs.* Murmurs are classified by the

timing, intensity, location, pitch, and quality of the sound. Some heart murmurs are benign (causing no ill effect), but other murmurs may indicate a disorder. A vibration caused by an abnormal flow of blood can sometimes be felt by touching over an artery and is called a "thrill."

Cardiac Output

The heart regulates the **rate** at which the blood circulates to the tissues. This measurement is called the *heart rate.* The stroke volume is the amount of blood contained in the ventricles. This blood is pumped into the arteries with each heartbeat. The volume of blood that is pumped from the heart by each contraction, multiplied by the heart rate, is called *cardiac output:*

$$\text{Stroke volume (mL/beat)} \times \text{Heart rate (beats/min)} = \text{Cardiac output (mL/min)}$$

For example, the cardiac output of an individual with a heart rate of 70 beats/min and a stroke volume of 70 mL/beat is 4.9 L. The normal cardiac output ranges from 4 to 8 L of blood per minute. The cardiac output affects the blood pressure. An abnormally high or low cardiac output may indicate a disorder of the cardiovascular system.

Electrocardiogram

The pattern of electrical activity in heart contractions can be measured graphically with an electrocardiogram (EKG) (Figure 10-7). Electrodes attached to different sites on the body measure electrical changes occurring during heart

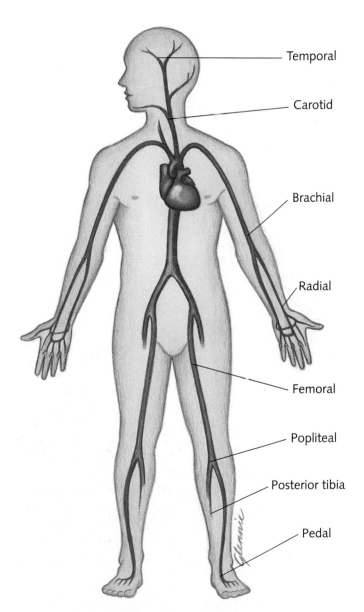

Temporal

Carotid

Brachial

Radial

Femoral

Popliteal

Posterior tibia

Pedal

Figure 10-6 Peripheral pulse points.

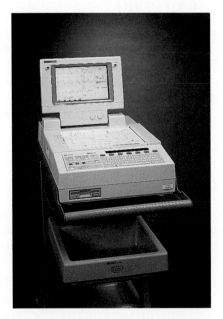

Figure 10-7 An electrocardiogram (EKG) machine. *(Courtesy Philips Medical Systems, Andover, Md.)*

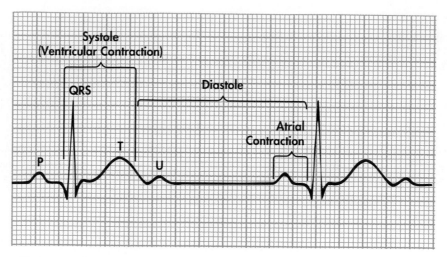

Figure 10-8 A normal electrocardiogram (EKG) pattern with descriptions. *(From Grauer K: A practical guide to ECG interpretation, ed 2, St Louis, 1998, Mosby.)*

contractions. Each section of the EKG pattern indicates a specific part of the heart's electrical activity (Figure 10-8). Normal and abnormal heart activities have characteristic wave patterns (Figure 10-9).

Some heart problems appear only during strenuous or specific activities. These can be diagnosed using stress testing with electrocardiography or by wearing a portable electrocardiograph to compare heart activity with a log of activities during a specified time period.

Echocardiography

Echocardiography (ECG) is a procedure using ultrasonic waves which shows the structures and motion of the heart. This procedure sends high-pitched sounds, which cannot be heard by the human ear, into the body. The echoes of these sounds are plotted by a special instrument called a *transducer* to produce a graphic picture of the heart and valves. Echocardiography is used to detect conditions such as mitral valve defects and atrial tumors.

Cardiac Catheterization

Cardiac catheterization is a procedure in which a tube is inserted through a blood vessel into the heart. A dye is then released through the catheter and traced using x-ray. This procedure is called *contrast coronary angiography.* Cardiac catheterization is used to measure the pressure in the chambers of the heart, to take blood samples, and to view obstructions in the vessels. Ultrasound transducers also have been inserted into the tip of catheter to allow viewing of an image of the inside of the arteries.

Disorders of the Cardiovascular System

An *aneurysm* (AN-yoo-rizm) is an area of a blood vessel that bulges because of a weakness in the wall. Most aneurysms occur in the aorta, but they also can occur in other vessels. The condition can be congenital and may cause no symptoms. But if an aneurysm ruptures, the person may have a life-threatening drop in blood pressure because blood is released into the body cavities. An aneurysm may be diagnosed if it displaces other body structures. Abnormal blood flow caused by an aneurysm may sometimes be heard with a stethoscope over the area. The sound of this abnormal blood flow is called a *bruit.* Aneurysms often can be corrected surgically by replacing the weak section of vessel.

Atherosclerosis (ath-er-o-skle-RO-sis) is a narrowing of blood vessels caused by deposits of fatty material containing calcium and cholesterol. This condition is sometimes called "hardening of the arteries" because the vessels lose their elasticity. When this narrowing occurs, the tissue that is deprived of blood will die. The exact cause of atherosclerosis is not known, but poor diet and lack of exercise increase the risk of developing it. Atherosclerosis can occur in any area of the body, but often it is found in the coronary arteries of the heart or in the arteries of the brain. Tissue death in the brain caused by atherosclerosis is called a *stroke.* Blockage of the blood vessels of the heart results in a heart attack (see following section on myocardial infarction). A person with atherosclerosis may experience short-

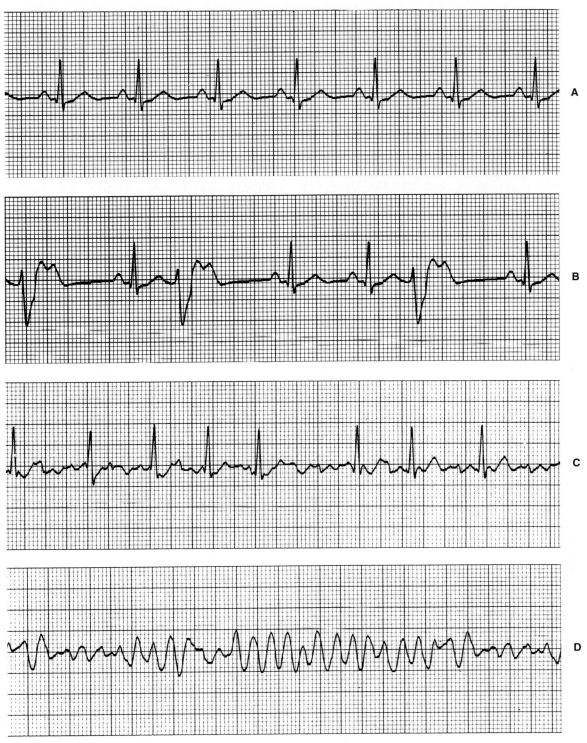

Figure 10-9   Electrocardiogram (EKG) patterns. **A**, Normal sinus rhythm. **B**, Unifocal PVCs. **C**, Atrial fibrillation. **D**, Ventricular fibrillation (V-fib). *(From Tait C: EZ ECGs booklet, ed 2, St Louis, 2001, Mosby.)*

ness of breath, fainting, and other indications of insufficient blood supply. Atherosclerosis can be treated by controlling risk factors, such as diet and exercise. Surgical removal of fatty deposits is possible in some vessels. Other treatments include drug therapy and surgery to alleviate symptoms of the condition.

Cardiac arrhythmia (uh-RITH-mee-uh) is a disturbance of the heart's **rhythm** caused by a defect in the heart's pacemaker cells or by damage to heart tissue. The person may experience dizziness, changes in heart rate, and poor blood circulation. Treatment may include insertion of an artificial pacemaker, the procedure of **cardioversion,** or medication.

Cardiovascular disease is a general term for the combined effects of arteriosclerosis, atherosclerosis and several related conditions, which are collectively called *coronary artery disease* (CAD). It is responsible for more than 50% of all deaths in the United States and is three times more common than cancer. It might appear as a heart attack or stroke. Health care for cardiovascular disease is directed toward prevention, including a healthy diet, exercise, and avoidance of tobacco products. Treatments for coronary artery diseases are numerous (Table 10- 2).

Congenital (kon-JEN-i-tal) *heart* disease is a group of disorders that affect about 25,000 newborns each year in the United States. Although the exact causes of many abnormalities in fetal heart development are not known, genetic influences or exposure of the mother to environmental factors may be causes. Common defects include narrowing, or **stenosis,** of vessels to the heart, atrial or ventricular septal defects. Coarctation (ko-ark-TAY-shun) of the aorta and patent ductus arteriosus (PA-tent DUK-tus ar-tee-ree-O-sus), a condition in which the opening between the pulmonary artery and aorta does not close at birth, may also occur. Individuals with a heart defect often experience shortness of breath and bluish discoloration of the skin, called cyanosis (si-uh-NO-sis). This is caused by inadequate perfusion of oxygen to the tissues. Heart defects often can be corrected surgically.

Congestive (kon-JES-tiv) *heart failure* (CHF), usually caused by disease in another body system, is the inability of the heart to pump blood adequately to meet the body's needs. CHF may occur suddenly or develop over time. It leads to inadequate respiratory and kidney function. The person usually experiences shortness of breath, rapid heartbeat, called *tachycardia* (tak-ee-KAR-dee-uh), and fluid retention. Treatment includes medication to lessen the symptoms and lifestyle changes to reduce risk factors.

Hypertension (hy-per-TEN-shun), also called *high blood pressure,* affects about 35 million people in the United

Table 10-2   Treatment of Coronary Artery Disease and Angina*

Procedure	Description	Characteristics
Coronary artery bypass graft (CABG)	A blood vessel from another part of the body (often the leg) is grafted in front of and beyond the artery blockage to provide a new route for blood flow.	Preferred if there are three or more blocked arteries, when the main artery is blocked more than 50%, and in diabetics.
Percutaneous transluminal coronary angioplasty (PTCA)	A camera is used to guide catheter into the blocked artery. The artery is opened by inflating a balloon. A mesh tube may be inserted (stent) to reinforce the opening.	Less invasive than CABG narrowing or reclosing of the artery occurs in about 50% of the patients, requiring reopening.
Enhanced external counter-pulsation (EECP)	An air pump inflates and deflates cuffs around the legs causing blood to be pushed to the heart.	Used in China and in clinical trials in the United States; will not replace CABG or PTCA.
Ultrasound thrombolysis	High-frequency sound waves are used to dislodge and dissolve fatty plaques in coronary arteries.	Experimental; initial cases have low incidence of restenosis.
Endoscopic transthoracic sympathicotomy	Nerves that cause chest pain are blocked to relieve angina.	Experimental; blocks symptoms of heart attack if it occurs.
Angiogenesis	A gene is injected into heart to cause growth of new blood vessels.	Experimental; genetic therapy.

*No surgical procedure cures coronary artery disease. A healthy lifestyle and possible medication will still be necessary after surgery.

States. The cause of most cases of high blood pressure is not known. Some cases may result from other conditions such as kidney disease and adrenal gland disorders. A tendency toward high blood pressure may be inherited. High blood pressure is one of the major risk factors for development of a heart attack, stroke, heart failure, and kidney failure. Because most people with high blood pressure have no symptoms at all, hypertension is sometimes called "the silent killer." The person may sometimes experience headaches, dizziness, and shortness of breath. Treatment for hypertension may include exercise, diet modification, avoiding tobacco products, and regular use of medication.

Myocardial **infarction** (my-o-KAR-dee-al), known as heart attack, can begin with a buildup of fatty deposits in the lining of the coronary arteries that feed the heart muscle. If the delivery of oxygen is obstructed, a heart attack occurs. It can also result from blockage of the blood vessels to the heart by a clot called an *embolus*. The area of the heart that is deprived of oxygen quickly dies. The victim of a heart attack usually experiences chest pain called *angina pectoris*. The person may experience chest pain, dizziness, sweating, nausea, shortness of breath, or a combination of these effects. In some cases, there are no symptoms at all. The damaged areas of the heart form scar tissue, making the heart less efficient in delivering blood to the body. If a large area of the heart is affected, it may stop functioning entirely. This situation is called *cardiac arrest*. Treatment begins with reestablishing a pulse and then immediate and complete rest to minimize the damage to the heart muscle. In addition, drugs may be given to dissolve or prevent clotting of blood or to increase the heart's ability to work. This treatment is followed by rehabilitation and lifestyle changes to reduce the risks. These may include control of blood pressure, a diet low in cholesterol and saturated fats, avoidance of tobacco products, weight reduction, and regular exercise.

Phlebitis (fle-BY-tis) is inflammation of a vein, often with formation of a clot (thrombus). If the thrombus breaks free, then called an *embolus* (EM-bo-lus), it may lodge in a smaller artery and cause tissue damage or sudden death. Phlebitis often results from damage to the vessel wall or prolonged sitting or standing. The person may experience swelling, stiffness, and pain in the affected part. Treatment of phlebitis includes administration of blood-thinning medications (anticoagulants) and elevation of the affected limb. Treatment may also include surgical removal of the clotted vein or injection of dissolving drugs to remove the clots.

Rheumatic (roo-MAT-ik) *heart disease* is a condition in which the heart muscle and valves are damaged by a recurrent bacterial infection that usually begins in the throat. The bacteria produce a toxin that causes inflammation and damage to the heart valves. Rheumatic fever is most common in children 5 to 15 years of age. The person experiences swelling of the joints, fever, shortness of breath, and

chest pain (angina). The damaged heart valves may harden (sclerosis) and not close completely, allowing blood to leak through the valves. If the damage is great, affected valves may be replaced surgically.

Varicose (VAYR-ih-kos) *veins* is a condition in which veins become enlarged and ineffective. This commonly occurs in the leg veins of people who stand for long periods. Varicose veins may also be caused by congenitally malformed valves, pregnancy, or obesity. The person may experience swelling, visible bluish veins, redness, and pain. Treatment includes increased exercise and elevation of the affected part. Support hosiery is often helpful. If the condition warrants, surgery can be performed to remove the veins.

Issues and Innovations

Heart Replacement

The first artificial heart was implanted in a human being in 1982 by Dr. William DeVries. The Jarvik-7 was connected to an external power source and pump. It, along with newer versions of this type of device, is considered a temporary bridge to stabilize a person waiting for a donor heart. Currently, it takes more than 6 months to obtain a heart for transplant once the recommendation has been made for the procedure. Most transplant recipients live for more than a year and can return to work.

In May 1991 the Texas Heart Institute in Houston began using a portable heart-assist device to decrease the workload of the heart. Another development is the use of an implantable defibrillator that senses an abnormal electrical activity in the heart and delivers an immediate shock to resume a normal rhythm or prevent sudden death.

In July 2001 the AbioCor self-contained artificial heart was used for the first time by developer Dr. O. H. Frazier (Figure 10-10). The first recipient, Mr. Robert Tools, lived 151 days with the heart. Five people were recipients of this heart by December 2001. The AbioCor clinical trial that Mr. Tools and the other recipients participated in was designed to test whether the AbioCor Implantable Replacement Heart could extend life for people with end-stage heart failure who have no other clinical option and provide them with a good quality of life. To be accepted into the trial the person had to be ineligible for heart transplantation and have a high probability of dying within 30 days.

According to the Organ Procurement Transplantation Network (OPTN), in 2000, more than 4000 people are on a waiting list for a heart transplant. About 2300 receive a heart each year. The demand for heart transplant is growing at a rate of about 15% each year. One of the most far-reaching programs to meet this demand is called *Living Implants From Engineering* (LIFE). Michael Sefton began this consortium in 1988 with the goal of producing an unlim-

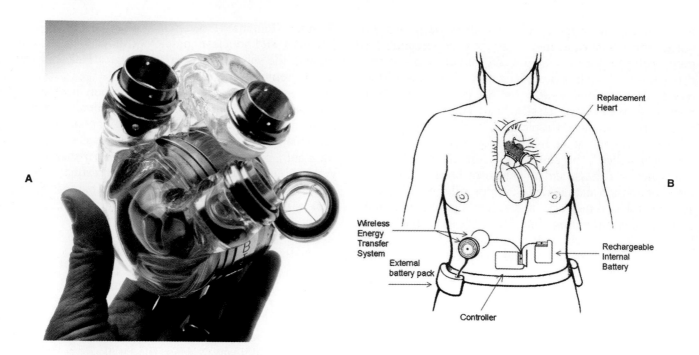

Figure 10-10   **A,** AbioCor heart. **B,** Placement of AbioCor heart in the body. *(Courtesy ABIOMED, Inc, Danvers, Mass.)*

ited supply of human organs for transplantation. An artificial heart made of human tissue is their 10-year goal. The procedure being used is to design a scaffold or model of the heart with biodegradable materials. On this model, human tissue will be grown. Whole organs have been created with similar techniques, including a bladder for dogs that was designed at Harvard Medical School.

Cholesterol Controversy

Cholesterol, which is found in all animal cells, is used in the body to make cell walls and hormones and in some body functions. The liver makes enough cholesterol for all these needs. Cholesterol does not mix in water, so it is carried in the blood in proteins (lipoprotein). Cholesterol is found in both low-density lipoprotein (LDL) and high-density lipoprotein (HDL) forms. The HDL form takes cholesterol to the liver, whereas the LDL form blocks the arteries. Elevated blood cholesterol is one of the major risk factors for development of heart disease.

Guidelines given to the public for the recommended types and amount of cholesterol have been confusing and disputed in the past. Currently, the emphasis is placed on the ratio of LDL to HDL in the blood as well as an overall value of less than 200 mg/dL (milligrams of cholesterol to deciliters of blood). The HDL portion should make up at least 20% to 30% of the combined total. The National Cholesterol Education Program, part of the National Heart, Lung, and Blood Institute, states that an HDL level of 60 mg/dL might even protect against heart disease. In the last 30 years, the national average of blood cholesterol has been lowered from 220 to 205 mg/dL.

Losing excess weight, exercising, and not smoking increase the overall HDL value. A diet with low-cholesterol foods such as fruits and vegetables is the best method for reducing the values. Some medications are used to reduce the level of cholesterol in the blood. Recently, claims have been made that vitamins that prevent the oxidation (chemical breakdown) of cholesterol helps prevent heart disease. However, this type of treatment is not recommended because of the harmful effects of large doses of these vitamins. Some research done in England has indicated that smaller, more frequent meals lower the amount of LDL produced.

Review Questions

1. Use the following terms in one or more sentences that relate their meaning.
   Cardioversion

   Infarction

   Rhythm

   Vessel

2. Describe the four functions of the cardiovascular system.

3. Explain the differences in structure of the arteries, veins, and capillaries.

4. Identify the location of the following parts of the cardiovascular system.

Carotid artery	Mitral valve
Endocardium	Pericardium
Femoral artery	Radial artery
Inferior vena cava	Sinoatrial node
Left ventricle	Tricuspid valve

5. Explain the action of the heart during systolic and diastolic contraction.

6. Which disorder of the cardiovascular system is called the "silent killer"?

7. Describe the location of eight pulse points that can be used to assess the rate of the heart.

8. Draw and identify a normal and three abnormal electrocardiogram patterns. Note the heart activity that is indicated by each peak of the normal graph.

Critical Thinking

1. Investigate and compare the cost of at least three tests used in diagnosing disorders of the cardiovascular system.

2. Investigate the function of at least five common medications used in treatment of the cardiovascular system.

3. List at least five occupations involved in the health care of cardiovascular system disorders.

4. Investigate the way potential candidates are chosen for heart transplant surgery and its benefits and drawbacks.

11
Circulatory System

Learning Objectives

Define at least 10 terms relating to the circulatory system.

Describe the two functions of the circulatory system.

List the five functions of the blood.

Describe the function of lymph.

Describe at least five disorders of the circulatory system.

Identify at least three methods of assessment of the circulatory system.

Key Terms

Allergen
(AL-er-jen) Substance capable of inducing specific hypersensitivity

Anemia
(uh-NEE-mee-uh) Below normal number of red blood cells

Antibody
(AN-tih-bod-ee) Molecule that interacts with specific antigen

Coagulation
(ko-ag-yoo-LAY-shun) Process of clot formation

Erythrocyte
(e-RITH-ro-site) Red blood cell or corpuscle

Immunity
(ih-MYOO-nih-tee) Security against a particular disease

Inflammation
(in-fluh-MAY-shun) Localized protective response to injury or destruction of tissue resulting in pain, heat, redness, swelling, and loss of function

Leukocyte
(LOO-ko-site) White blood cell

Plasma
(PLAZ-muh) Fluid portion of blood

Serum
(SEER-um) Fluid portion of blood with clotting proteins removed

Spectrophotometry
(spek-tro-fo-TOM-uh-tree) Measurement of quantity of matter in solution by passing light through spectrum

Thrombocyte
(THROM-bo-site) Blood platelet

Circulatory System Terminology*

TERM	DEFINITION	PREFIX	ROOT	SUFFIX
Anemia	Without blood	a/n	emia	
Erythrocyte	Red blood cell	erythro	cyte	
Hemogram	Record of blood	hemo	gram	
Leukocyte	White blood cell	leuk/o	cyte	
Lymphedema	Swelling of the lymph	lymph	edema	
Phagocyte	Eating cells	phag/o	cyte	
Polycythemia	Abnormal increase in the number of blood cells	poly	cyt/h	emia
Septicemia	Condition of poisoning of the blood		sept/ic	emia
Splenomegaly	Enlargement of the spleen		splen/o	megaly
Thrombocyte	Blood platelet	thromb/o	cyte	

*A transition phrase or vowel may be added to or deleted from the word parts to make the combining form.

Abbreviations of the Circulatory System

ABBREVIATION	MEANING
ABG	Arterial blood gas
AIDS	Acquired immune deficiency syndrome
alb	Albumin
bl	Blood
CBC	Complete blood cell count
FBS	Fasting blood sugar
hct	Hematocrit
H&H	Hematocrit and hemoglobin
RBC	Red blood cell count
WBC	White blood cell count

Structure and Function of the Circulatory System

The circulatory system includes the blood and lymph that move through the body. Both blood and lymph are tissues that function to maintain homeostasis and give the body **immunity.**

Blood

Hematology is the study of blood. The body contains approximately 4 to 5 L of blood, making up about 8% of the body's weight. The functions of blood include the following:
- Transporting nutrients, oxygen, and hormones
- Removing metabolic wastes and carbon dioxide
- Providing immunity (resistance to disease) through antibodies
- Maintaining body temperature and electrolyte balance
- Clotting to prevent bleeding from a wound

Blood divides into solid and liquid portions when spun in a centrifuge (Figure 11-1). The solid parts, called *formed elements,* are red blood cells, white blood cells, and platelets (**thrombocytes**). Table 11-1 shows the formed elements of blood. The remaining liquid portion is composed of the buffy coat and **plasma.** The buffy coat is a mixture of the white blood cells and platelets.

Red Blood Cells

More than 25 trillion red blood cells (RBCs), also called **erythrocytes,** circulate in the body's 4 to 5 L of blood (Figure 11-2). Erythrocytes contain a protein called *hemoglobin* that carries oxygen to all cells and removes carbon dioxide. Each red blood cell lives only 90 to 120 days. New cells are manufactured by the red marrow or myeloid tissue in bones (see Chapter 13). A few million new red blood cells are made each second in a process called *hemopoiesis.* The liver and spleen remove dead red blood cells and reuse the material.

Table 11-1   Formed Elements of Blood

Cell Type	Description	Function
Erythrocyte	Biconcave disk; no nucleus; 7 to 8 μm in diameter	Transports oxygen and carbon dioxide
Leukocyte		
Neutrophil	Spherical cell; nucleus with connected filaments; cytoplasmic granules stain light pink to reddish-purple; 12 to 15 μm in diameter	Phagocytizes microorganisms
Basophil	Spherical cell; nucleus with two indistinct lobes; cytoplasmic granules stain blue-purple; 10 to 12 μm in diameter	Releases histamine, which promotes inflammation, and heparin, which prevents clot formation
Eosinophil	Spherical cell; nucleus often with two lobes; cytoplasmic granules stain orange-red or bright red; 10 to 12 μm in diameter	Releases chemicals that reduce inflammation; attacks certain worm parasites
Lymphocyte	Spherical cell with round nucleus; cytoplasm forms a thin ring around the nucleus; 6 to 8 μm in diameter	Produces antibodies and other chemicals responsible for destroying microorganisms; responsible for allergic reactions, graft rejection, tumor control, and regulation of the immune system
Monocyte	Spherical cell; nucleus round, kidney or horseshoe shaped; contains more cytoplasm than lymphocytes; 10 to 15 μm in diameter	Phagocytic cell in the blood leaves the blood and becomes a macrophage, which phagocytizes bacteria, dead cells, fragments, and debris within tissues
Platelet	Cell fragments surrounded by a cell membrane and containing granules; 2 to 5 μm in diameter	Forms platelet plugs; releases chemicals necessary to blood clotting

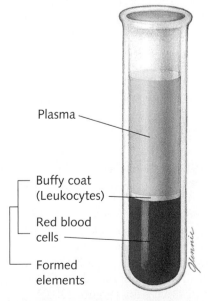

Plasma

Buffy coat
(Leukocytes)

Red blood
cells

Formed
elements

Figure 11-1   Hematocrit.

White Blood Cells

White blood cells (WBCs), also called **leukocytes,** fight disease and infection. There are fewer white blood cells than red and they are larger. Leukocytes live about 9 days and can move out of the blood vessels as part of the immune process. White blood cells remove foreign particles, fight infection, and help prevent disease. Pus consists of white blood cells mixed with bacteria.

There are five types of white blood cells (see Table 11-1):
- Neutrophils (NOO-truh-filz) engulf and digest bacteria in a process called *phagocytosis.*
- Basophils (BAY-suh-filz) contain the anticoagulant substance heparin and participate in the inflammatory response of the body.
- Eosinophils (EE-uh-sin-uh-filz) defend the body from allergic reactions and parasitic infections and may help remove toxins from the blood.

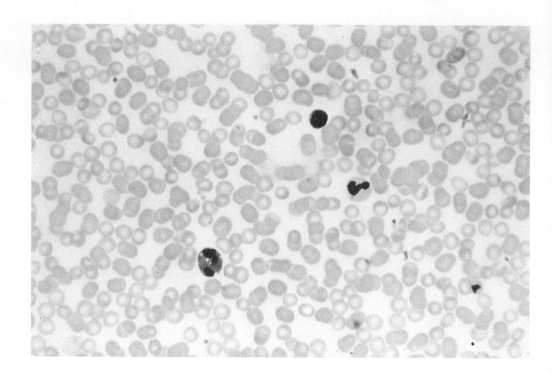

Figure 11-2 Erythrocytes circulating in the blood. *(Courtesy Ward's Natural Science Establishment, Rochester, NY.)*

- Lymphocytes (LIM-fuh-sites) participate in the production of antibody and plasma cells and help destroy foreign particles.
- Monocytes (MON-uh-sites) help remove foreign materials and bacteria in the process of phagocytosis.

Platelets

Platelets, also called *thrombocytes,* are the smallest blood cells. They promote clotting to prevent blood loss. As platelets pass over a rough spot in a vessel, they become sticky. They may form a plug to seal small vessels by themselves or start the clotting process. To form a clot, platelets combine with a protein, called *prothrombin,* and calcium to form thrombin. This mass combines with another protein called *fibrinogen* to form a gel-like substance called *fibrin,* which forms the clot. Thrombocytes usually are produced in red bone marrow and live for about 5 to 9 days.

Plasma

Plasma is a pale yellow liquid that is left when the formed elements are removed from blood. Whole blood is 55% plasma. Plasma is 90% water and approximately 10% proteins. It also contains nutrients, electrolytes, oxygen, enzymes, hormones, and wastes. The proteins help fight infection and assist in the clotting (**coagulation**) of blood. **Serum** is plasma without the clotting proteins. Serum may be used for identification and research of antibodies.

Blood Typing

A person's blood type is an inherited characteristic of the blood. Before a transfusion is given, many factors are checked to prevent an adverse reaction in the person receiving the blood. Blood type is determined by antigens located on the surface of the red blood cell. Clumping of the blood cells may occur when the antigens of donated blood react with antibodies in the plasma of the person receiving it. This clumping of incompatible cells blocks the blood vessels and may cause death.

There are four major blood types: A, B, AB, and O (Table 11-2). Type AB blood is called the *universal recipient* because it has no antibodies in the plasma to react with other blood cells and can receive any type of blood safely. Type O blood is the universal donor because the blood cells have no antigens to react with the antibodies in the plasma of the other blood types. Therefore type O blood can be given safely to a person of any blood type.

Another important aspect of blood typing is the identification of the antigen known as the *Rh factor.* The Rh factor is found in the red blood cells. About 85% of North Americans have this factor and are said to be Rh-positive (Table 11-3). If Rh-positive blood is given to someone with Rh-negative blood, that person's blood considers the Rh-positive blood a foreign particle and tries to combat it by forming antibodies. A second transfusion of Rh-positive blood can be fatal to an Rh-negative person. The Rh factor also becomes important in the Rh-negative mother having a second Rh-positive baby (Figure 11-3).

Table 11-2   Blood Types

Blood Group Components

Group	Antigen Marker*	Antibody†	Compatible Donor
A	A	Anti-B	A,O
B	B	Anti-A	B,O
AB	A,B	None	A,B AB,O
O	None	Anti-A Anti-B	O

*Found on RBC.
†Found in plasma.

Table 11-3   Approximate Distribution of Blood Types in the U.S. Population

Blood Type	Prevalence
O Rh-positive	38%
O Rh-negative	7%
A Rh-positive	34%
A Rh-negative	6%
B Rh-positive	9%
B Rh-negative	2%
AB Rh-positive	3%
AB Rh-negative	1%

Data from American Association of Blood Banks, 2002.
Distribution may differ for specific racial and ethnic groups.

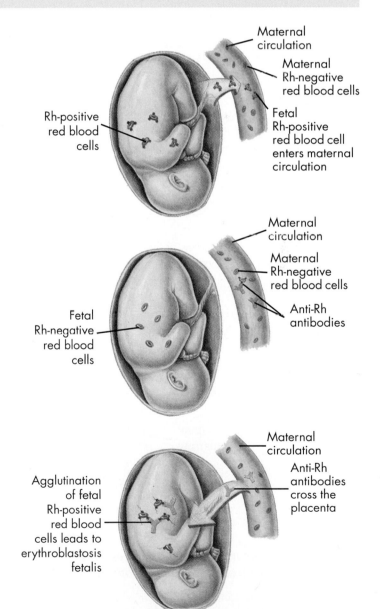

Figure 11-3   Erythroblastosis fetalis. When an Rh⁻ mother delivers an Rh⁺ baby, some of the baby's blood may contact the blood of the mother. The mother's blood then forms antibodies against Rh⁺ red blood cells. If the mother has another Rh⁺ pregnancy, her antibodies will attack the baby's blood, causing erythroblastosis fetalis. (*From Thibodeau GA, Patton KT:* Anatomy & physiology, *ed 5, St Louis, 2003, Mosby.*)

Lymph and Lymphatic Tissues

Lymph has two important functions. The first is maintaining the body's fluid balance. Lymph is a watery substance formed from fluid that filters into the body tissues or interstitially. This fluid is returned to the body through the lymph vessels, which operate independently from the circulatory vessels. Lymph capillaries are more porous than blood capillaries, allowing the fluid in the tissues to collect and be returned to the circulatory system. Fats, protein molecules, and some cancerous cells may also use this method of transportation in the body. Unlike blood, lymph flows in only one direction—toward the heart. Lymph moves from the tissues into capillaries that drain into lymphatic ducts that lead into the blood. Unlike blood, lymph circulates very slowly. Movement of the body muscles surrounding the lymph vessels keeps the lymph flowing.

The lymphatic tissues consist of the tonsils, thymus, spleen, nodes, and the lymph vessels. There are three sets of lymphoid tissue considered to be the tonsils: palatine,

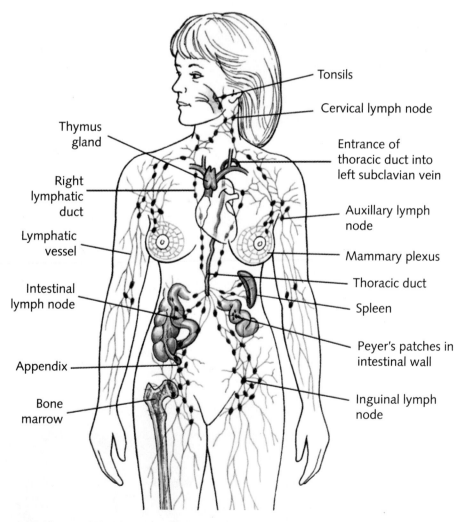

Tonsils

Cervical lymph node

Entrance of thoracic duct into left subclavian vein

Auxillary lymph node

Mammary plexus

Thoracic duct

Spleen

Peyer's patches in intestinal wall

Inguinal lymph node

Thymus gland

Right lymphatic duct

Lymphatic vessel

Intestinal lymph node

Appendix

Bone marrow

Figure 11-4   Lymph vessels and nodes. *(From Seeley RR, Stephens TD, Tate P: Anatomy & physiology, ed 3, St Louis, 1995, Mosby.)*

pharyngeal (adenoids), and lingual. The thymus, located in the chest, is a source of lymphocytes before birth and through puberty. At that time, this organ is gradually replaced by fat and connective tissue in a process called *involution.* The thymus is considered by some to be the "biological clock" that indicates the progress of the aging process. The thymus also has endocrine functions (see Chapter 17).

The spleen is the largest lymphoid mass in the body and an important part of the circulatory system. In addition to storing approximately 1 pint of blood, the spleen filters bacteria and foreign substances so that they may be destroyed by phagocytic leukocytes. The spleen also makes lymphocytes and monocytes. Worn red blood cells are broken apart and the iron is retrieved for further use by the spleen.

Lymph vessels are located in all body tissues except the brain and placenta (Figure 11-4). Lymph nodes, located in clusters along the path of lymph vessels, are biological filters that remove bacteria and cancerous cells from the body. Nodes are small, about 0.5 to 1 cm in diameter, but may swell during an infection as they filter bacteria and produce additional leukocytes.

Immunity

Lymph is also very important in the process of immunity. The immune response takes two forms—specific and nonspecific. The nonspecific, or innate, reaction provides general protection. It includes the barrier of the skin, mucous membranes, tears, and the leukocytes. The leukocytes form antibodies in response to antigens or foreign materials that enter the body.

The inflammatory response, a type of nonspecific defense, may be a localized or systemic reaction. The usual progression of a localized response occurs following tissue damage by bacteria or infection. The response of the injured cells is the release of chemicals, which cause vascular dilation and an increase in blood flow. This vascular dilation allows other molecules to enter the area, walling off the injured tissue. The bacteria are then destroyed by phagocytic action of white blood cells. The area appears reddened and is warm and painful. It often causes swelling and decreased function.

Another nonspecific response is the systemic inflammatory response that affects the entire body. In addition to all of the signs and symptoms of a localized response, it also includes an increase in neutrophil production, elevated temperature, and fluid loss into the tissues. This reaction may lead to shock and death if not stopped.

There are two types of specific immunity that protect the body at the cellular level. These are acquired and inherited immunity. Inherited immunity develops before birth and is a genetic trait. For example, humans are not susceptible to some diseases that affect dogs or cats.

Acquired immunity can be either natural or artificial depending on how it is attained. Natural immunity is caused by exposure to the agent unintentionally. For example, the formation of antibodies to prevent the reoccurrence of measles is natural immunity. Immunity that is obtained by the fetus from the mother or in breast milk is an example of passive natural immunity.

Artificial acquired immunity is obtained intentionally. For example, vaccination against poliomyelitis is a form of active, artificial immunity. Injection of gamma globulin taken from one person and given to another is an example of passive artificial immunity.

An immune response resulting in tissue damage may be triggered by hypersensitivity to an antigen. There are four main types of hypersensitivity. Type I occurs when plasma and memory cells are produced on first exposure to an **allergen.** On the second exposure, an immediate anaphylactic response occurs. A Type II or cytotoxic response occurs when antibodies react with foreign or normal cells causing the destruction of cells. An example is the reaction of an incompatible blood transfusion or Rh incompatibility reaction. In Type III hypersensitivity, phagocytes are released to remove antigen-**antibody** complexes that are deposited in the tissues. The by-products of the phagocytic action to remove these complexes damage the tissues. More than 12 hours after exposure to the antigen, a Type IV, or delayed hypersensitivity, reaction occurs. It also results in tissue destruction as a result of both phagocytic and cytotoxic cells that are produced.

Table 11-4 Blood Components and Values

Blood Component	Normal Values*	
	Male	**Female**
Hemoglobin (hgb)	13.5-17.5 g/dL	12.5-15.5 g/dL
Hematocrit (hct)	36%-48%	36%-48%
Leukocyte (WBC)	5000-10,000 mm^3	5000-10,000 m^3
Neutrophil	60%-70%	60%-70%
Eosinophil	1%-4%	1%-4%
Basophil	0%-0.5%	0%-0.5%
Lymphocyte	20%-30%	20%-30%
Monocyte	2%-6%	2%-6%
Erythrocyte (RBC)	4,600,000-6,200,000 mm^3	4,200,000-5,400,000 mm^3
Mean corpuscular volume (MCV)	80-94 μm	80-94 μm
Mean corpuscular hemoglobin (MCH)	27-32 μg/cell	27-32 μg/cell
Mean corpuscular hemoglobin concentration (MCHC)	33%-38%	33%-38%
Platelet	200,000-350,000 mm^3	200,000-350,000 mm^3
Reticulocyte	0.5-1.5% of RBCs	0.5%-1.5% of RBCs
Erythrocyte sedimentation rate (ESR)	0-9 mm/hr	0-20 mm/hr
Bleeding time	30 sec-6 min	30 sec-6 min
Partial thromboplastin time (PTT)	20-45 sec	20-45 sec
Glucose		
Fasting	60-100 mg/dL	60-100 mg/dL
2 hours after eating (2 hr pp)	65-140 mg/dL	65-140 mg/dL
Cholesterol	150-300 mg/dL	150-300 mg/dL
Total protein	6-8 mg/dL	6-8 mg/dL
Uric acid	2.5-8 mg/dL	2.5-8 mg/dL
Total bilirubin	0.1-1 mg/dL	0.1-1 mg/dL
Fibrinogen	200-400 mg/dL	200-400 mg/dL
Blood urea nitrogen (BUN)	10-20 mg/dL	10-20 mg/dL
Serum creatinine	0.7-1.4 mg/dL	0.7-1.4 mg/dL
Alkaline phosphatase	30-115 mU/mL (adult)	30-115 mU/mL (adult)
Aspartate aminotransferase (AST; formerly SGOT)	10-40 U	10-40 U
Creatinine phosphokinase isoenzyme (CPK)	12-70 U/mL	10-55 U/mL
Lactic dehydrogenase isoenzyme (LDH)	100-225 mU/mL	100-225 mU/mL
Calcium (Ca)	8.5-10.5 mg/dL	8.5-10.5 mg/dL
Chloride (Cl)	95-105 mEq/L	95-105 mEq/L
Potassium (K)	3.5-5 mEq/L	3.5-5 mEq/L
Sodium (Na)	135-145 mEq/L	135-145 mEq/L

*Varies with technique, laboratory, and type of blood sample.

Abbreviations: *g/dL*, Grams per deciliter; *mm^3*, cubic millimeter; *μm^3*, cubic micrometer; *μg/cell*, micromicrogram; *mm/hr*, millimeter per hour; *mg/dL*, milligram per deciliter; *mU/mL*, milliunit per milliliter; *U*, unit; *mEq/L*, milliequivalent per liter.

Assessment Techniques

Blood and lymph can be assessed by direct examination, chemical tests, and coagulation studies. Table 11-4 shows the normal values of some blood components. Some common tests for direct examination of the blood include the following:

- The hemoglobin test (Hgb) measures the amount of oxygen-carrying ability of the blood.
- The hematocrit (Hct) measures the volume of erythrocytes in the blood.
- Sedimentation rates measure how long it takes for erythrocytes in the blood to settle to the bottom of a container.
- Reticulocyte studies measure the number of immature red blood cells.
- Red blood cell (RBC) counts determine the number of circulating red blood cells in 1 mm^3 of blood.
- Platelet or thrombocyte counts measure the number of platelets in 1 mm^3 of blood to determine clotting ability.
- Aspiration biopsy cytology (ABC) studies examine bone marrow from the iliac crest of the hip.

Chemical tests use a process called **spectrophotometry** to measure the exact chemical make-up of a blood sample. Spectrophotometry calculates the concentration of substances in solution by measuring the amount of light it absorbs. Chemical tests measure proteins, glucose, uric acid, cholesterol, enzymes, and electrolyte ions. Two routine blood tests include several of these tests combined:

- Complete blood cell count (CBC) measures at least six tests, including the number of red and white blood cells and the proportional difference between the number of white and red blood cells (differential).
- Sequential multiple analysis (SMA) includes both the cell counts and the chemistry tests.

Two kinds of coagulation studies assess the ability of the blood to clot:

- Bleeding time is the amount of time an incision takes to clot.
- Prothrombin time (PT) uses an anticoagulant to measure the blood sample's clotting rate.

Disorders of the Circulatory System

Acquired immunodeficiency syndrome (AIDS) is a dysfunction of the immune system caused by a virus. It is the fifth leading cause of death of people 25 to 44 years of age in the United States. A person infected with the human immunodeficiency virus (HIV) may not show any severe symptoms for up to 6 years. During this time, the person may experience fatigue, weakness, painful joints, and diarrhea. This condition is known as *AIDS related complex* (ARC) syndrome. The virus eventually uses the cell's own materials to make viral DNA, damaging the host cell. The damaged T-lymphocytes of affected white blood cells allow disease to enter the body. Victims of AIDS generally die from sarcoma or protozoal pneumonia (Figure 11-5). The HIV virus is transmitted by the exchange of body fluids such as blood and semen. There is no cure. Research is being conducted to develop a vaccine against the HIV virus and to stop it from reproducing in the body. Treatment in-

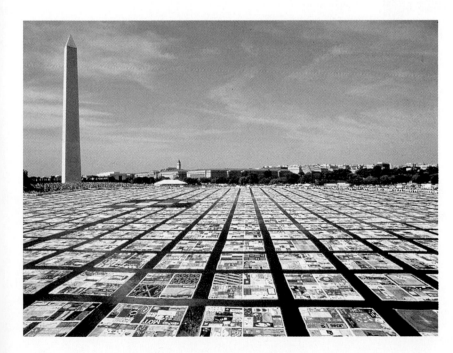

Figure 11-5 The AIDS Quilt. *(Courtesy The NAMES Foundation, Atlanta, Ga; Photographer Mark Theissen.)*

cludes the use of several experimental antiviral medications as well as alternative treatments such as ozone and oxygen therapy.

Allergy (AL-er-jee) is a hypersensitive response by the immune system to an outside substance. An otherwise harmless substance becomes an allergen in the body. Then antibodies are formed in the blood to combat the allergen. Common allergens include pollen, dander, feathers, and plant oils. The allergic person may experience **inflammation** of the respiratory, gastrointestinal, and integumentary systems. In severe cases the condition may be life threatening. Treatment may include desensitization to the allergen or administration of antiinflammatory drugs.

Anemia is the most common blood disorder. The blood has an inadequate amount of hemoglobin, red blood cells, or both. Anemia may have several different causes. Pernicious anemia involves inadequately developed red blood cells. It results from poor absorption of vitamin B_{12}, which is needed in the formation of red blood cells. Iron-deficiency anemia involves an inadequate amount of hemoglobin caused by a shortage of iron. Aplastic anemia occurs when bone marrow is destroyed by radiation, chemicals, or medications. This type of anemia is often the result of cancer treatment. Two types of hemolytic anemia include sickle cell and thalassemia (see below). A person with anemia may experience fatigue, shortness of breath, pallor, and rapid heart rate. The treatment of anemia may include dietary supplements or blood replacement.

Autoimmune (aw-toe-im-YOON) diseases are conditions in which the immune system of the body turns against itself (Table 11-5). Systemic lupus erythematosus (LOO-pus er-i-thuh-muh-TOE-sus) affects connective tissue. It may also affect the kidneys, lungs, and heart. Hashimoto's disease results in destruction of the thyroid. Myasthenia gravis (my-as-THEE-nee-uh GRA-vis) affects the nerves and causes paralysis. The treatment of these disorders includes immunosuppressive drugs and steroids to relieve inflammation.

Elephantiasis (el-uh-fun-TIE-uh-sis), a form of lymphedema, is a massive accumulation of lymphatic fluid in body tissues, causing an abnormally large growth of tissue or hypertrophy (hy-PER-tro-fee). Elephantiasis is caused by obstruction of the lymph vessels by tiny worms (filariae) that are common in tropic and subtropic areas. The larvae of the worms enter the lymph system through an insect bite such as a mosquito. Early on, the person experiences fever, chills, and ulcer formation. Individuals with elephantiasis are more susceptible to infections. No cure is known for this condition. Exposure can be prevented with mosquito control measures, and treatment includes the use of oral medications.

Erythroblastosis fetalis (e-rith-ro-blas-TOE-sis) is a condition in an unborn baby in which the mother forms antibodies against the antigens in the baby's blood. This condition may result in an Rh-positive child of an Rh-negative mother and Rh-positive father. The condition may cause brain damage in the baby. The treatment includes monitoring of bilirubin levels during pregnancy and intrauterine blood transfusion if needed (see Figure 11-3). An exchange transfusion of blood may be required at the time of birth.

Hemophilia (hee-mo-FIL-ee-uh) is a rare, sex-linked genetic blood disease in which the blood is missing a clotting factor. The person may have uncontrolled and prolonged internal and external bleeding. Bleeding under the skin may appear as extensive bruising. The treatment includes giving plasma that contains the missing clotting factor. There is no cure for this condition. Experimental gene therapy has been tested at Boston's Beth Israel Deaconess Medical Center, where researchers inserted the missing normal genes into skin cell samples of hemophiliacs. The cells were then reinjected into the fatty tissue of the abdomen with a modest increase in the production of blood-clotting proteins.

Hepatitis is a viral infection of the blood (Table 11-6). Two forms, hepatitis B and hepatitis C, can be transmitted through body fluids including blood. People usually do not get sick when first infected with hepatitis C and may not show symptoms for up to 20 years, at which time the liver damage is severe. About 10,000 people in the United

Table 11-5	Autoimmune or Autoimmune-Related Disorders
Disorder	**Body System Affected**
Addison's disease	Endocrine
Dermatomyositis	Integumentary and muscular
Diabetes mellitus	Endocrine
Graves' disease	Endocrine
Hashimoto's thyroiditis	Endocrine
Multiple sclerosis	Nervous and muscular
Myasthenia gravis	Nervous and muscular
Pernicious anemia	Circulatory
Rheumatoid arthritis	Muscular and skeletal
Systemic lupus erythematosus	Multiple systems

States die from hepatitis C each year. One in five patients develop cirrhosis of the liver and may develop liver cancer. Treatment is injection of alpha interferon. Since a test was developed in 1990, blood donations are tested routinely for hepatitis C.

Hodgkin's disease is a malignant cancer of the lymph system that usually appears in people between the ages of 15 to 30. The person experiences painless enlargement of the lymph nodes (lymphoma), itching, weight loss, fever, anemia, and difficulty swallowing. Hodgkin's disease appears most often in men. Hodgkin's is one of the most curable cancers. Treatment may include chemotherapy, radiation of the lymph nodes, or blood marrow transplant.

Leukemia (loo-KEE-mee-uh), also called *blood cancer,* is an abnormal malignant increase in the number and longevity of white blood cells. The leukemia cells, which are immature and less effective in fighting disease, replace red blood cells. The person experiences anemia and bleeding gums, and the condition is often life threatening. Treatment may include radiation, chemotherapy, or bone marrow transplantation. The person may also be isolated to prevent infection.

Lymphosarcoma (lim-fo-sar-KO-muh) is a group of malignant cancers of lymph tissues other than Hodgkin's disease. Lymphosarcoma may develop at any age but commonly appears in middle age. The person has a painless enlargement of the lymph nodes. The disease spreads to the bone marrow and causes anemia, weight loss, and skin lesions. The treatment of lymphosarcoma may include chemotherapy and radiation.

Polycythemia (pol-ee-sie-THEE-mee-uh) is an abnormal increase in the number of blood cells, making the blood thicker and slower flowing. The person experiences increased blood pressure, dizziness, an enlarged spleen, and reddened skin. Polycythemia results from excessive development of the bone marrow but the cause is unknown. It has no cure but the treatment may include removing blood.

Septicemia (sep-tih-SEE-mee-uh), commonly called *blood poisoning,* is an infection that occurs when pathogens enter the blood. The person experiences nausea, vomiting, fever, chills, shortness of breath, and an increased leukocyte count. The treatment includes antibiotics, oxygen therapy, and plasma transfusion. A recombinant form of human protein, called *Xigris,* has been approved by the FDA for treatment of this condition. Septicemia can lead to shock and death.

Sickle cell (SIK-el sel) *anemia* is a genetic condition that results in malformed red blood cells. The "sickled" cells are more fragile and cause pain as the vessels are blocked and less oxygen is delivered. Sickle cell anemia occurs in 8 of 100,000 African Americans. The condition may result in no symptoms when only one gene (allele) is affected. The gene is found in 1 of every 600 African Americans and 1 of

Table 11-6   Hepatitis*

Type	Transmission	Symptoms	Prevention and Treatment
A	Ingestion of feces contaminated object, food, or water	Flulike symptoms, jaundice	Vaccine available; immune globulin on exposure, bed rest
B	Direct blood contact with infected body fluids or contaminated objects such as needles. Babies may be infected during birth	Flulike symptoms, cirrhosis and cancer of the liver, jaundice	Vaccine available; interferon reduces chance of recurrence
C	Direct blood contact with infected body fluids or contaminated objects such as needles. Babies may be infected during birth	Chronic liver damage, cirrhosis and cancer of the liver; most people have no symptoms	No vaccine; interferon, ribavirin
D	Direct blood contact with infected body fluids or contaminated objects such as needles. Babies may be infected during birth	Flulike symptoms, cirrhosis and cancer of the liver, jaundice; more severe than hepatitis B	Hepatitis B vaccine; interferon
E	Ingestion of feces or contaminated water	Liver inflammation, flulike symptoms; many people have no symptoms	No vaccine; bed rest, fluids

*More information about hepatitis infections may be found in Chapter 15.

every 1000 Hispanics. Sickle cell anemia can lead to death in severe cases. There is no cure for sickle cell anemia, although transplant of bone marrow from a nonaffected sibling has been tried with some success.

Splenomegaly (splee-no-MEG-uh-lee) is an enlargement of the spleen caused by an acute infection such as mononucleosis or anemia. The person experiences symptoms similar to those of anemia and leukemia. The treatment may require removal of the spleen (splenectomy).

Thalassemia (thal-ah-SEE-mee-uh) is one of the most common genetic blood disorders. It appears in two forms, called *alpha* and *beta,* which are identified by which gene is involved. Thalassemia affects the production of hemoglobin and may cause anemia. Beta thalassemia occurs most often in people of Mediterranean origin. In the most severe form, it is called *thalassemia major* or *Cooley's anemia.* At age 1 or 2 an infant with this form may experience listlessness, poor appetite, and infections. The condition leads to yellow skin (jaundice), enlarged spleen, and car-

diac malfunction. The treatment includes blood transfusions to lessen the effects. Gene manipulation and bone marrow transplants are new treatments, but they have achieved only minor success.

Thrombocytopenia (throm-bo-sie-toe-PEE-nee-uh) is a decrease in the number of platelets in the blood. This condition can be caused by a drug reaction, radiation, chemotherapy, or an autoimmune disorder. The person experiences symptoms similar to those of leukemia: skin rash, nosebleed, bleeding, and bruising. The treatment method chosen depends on the original cause of the platelet decrease.

Thrombosis (throm-BO-sis) is a condition in which a blood clot, called a *thrombus,* forms in the blood vessels. The clot slows the flow of blood to the tissues. If the clot breaks away, it is called an *embolus.* The embolus may lodge in a blood vessel and cause tissue death in the area (Figure 11-6). The person feels pain in the area of the clot because of a lack of oxygen in the tissues. The treatment includes elevation of the affected part and may include anticoagulants. In severe cases, surgery may be necessary to remove the clot.

Issues and Innovations

Transfusion

According to the National Blood Data Resource Center, hospitals in the United States transfused 12.4 million units of whole blood and red blood cells to 4.5 million patients in 1999. Transfusions are given to improve the blood's ability to carry oxygen to the cells, increase blood volume, improve immunity, and correct clotting problems. New methods of transfusion have been developed to minimize the risk of this procedure. These methods, as well as improved methods for testing blood transfusions, have reduced the risk of an adverse reaction or infection by a blood borne organism. The risk of contracting HIV from a blood transfusion is approximately 1 in 420,000. Some facilities offer a service called direct donation. In this procedure, blood is donated to a specific person from family and friends. Blood supply testing is regulated by the Food and Drug Administration.

Autologous transfusion is the collection and transfusion of a person's own blood. For example, up to one unit of blood may be given each week for 6 weeks before an elective surgery is planned. Whole blood can be refrigerated safely for up to 35 days or frozen for several months before use. Hemodilution or blood dilution is the removal of one or more units just before surgery for transfusion at the end of surgery. Fluids are given to the person to dilute the remaining blood.

When a person is bleeding after an accident, his or her own blood may be collected and returned to the person in

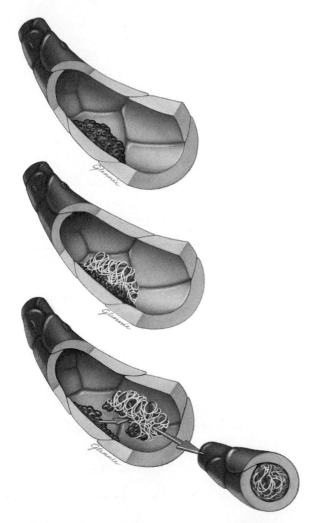

Figure 11-6 Development of an embolus.

a process called intraoperative salvage. Autotransfusion prevents complications of blood transfusion such as mis-matched blood types, the risk of disease transmission, and tissue rejection.

Platelets may be donated through a process called apheresis to be used for patients undergoing bone marrow transplant, surgery, chemotherapy, radiation treatment or organ transplant. Platelets have five day storage life. Before apheresis, platelets for one transfusion required donations from 5 to 10 people. In apheresis, the donated blood is separated into parts using a centrifuge. The platelets are re-covered separately and the rest of the blood is returned to the donor. With this technique, a single donation provides a complete platelet transfusion.

Interferon

Interferon is a protein that prevents a virus from reproduc-ing. It is made in the body by T-lymphocyte cells (white blood cells). Synthetic interferon is now being manufac-tured using gene-splicing techniques with bacteria. It is being used to fight viruses and some cancers. Interferon is being tested in prevention of many viral diseases including AIDS and the common cold. It has also been used in treat-ment of leprosy and malaria. Interferon can also be used to diagnose tumors and hepatitis.

Monoclonal Antibodies

Monoclonal antibodies are proteins with unique abilities in the blood. Specific antibodies can be "harvested" and fused to new cells in laboratory tissue cultures. These "hy-bridomas" can be used to treat some cancers and some specific viruses. Monoclonal antibodies are being used in organ transplants to prevent rejection, to slow the progress of autoimmune diseases, and to help diagnose malignant tumors, leukemia, and some sexually transmit-ted infections. Monoclonal antibodies are found in some over-the-counter products to test for pregnancy, ovula-tion, and blood in the stool. Research is now beginning to find other uses of these proteins for circulatory system disorders.

Review Questions

1. Use the following terms in one or more sentences that correctly relate their meaning.
   Allergen
   Antibody
   Immunity
   Inflammation

2. Describe the two functions of the circulatory system.

3. Describe the five functions of the blood.

4. Describe the role of lymph in the circulatory system.

5. Describe the function of each of the white blood cells.

6. Describe three tests used to assess the function of the circulatory system.

7. Describe two types of autotransfusion. List three benefits of autotransfusion.

Critical Thinking

1. A test to detect HIV was introduced in blood banks in 1985. The first hepatitis C test was not utilized until 1990. Hepatitis C has infected four times as many people as HIV. Describe a plan that would not cause panic or discrimination against victims but could inform the public about the risks of contracting or not treating hepatitis C.

2. Investigate and compare the cost of at least four tests used in diagnosing circulatory system disorders.

3. Investigate the function of at least five medications used in treatment of circulatory system disorders.

4. List at least five occupations involved in the health care of circulatory system disorders.

12
Respiratory System

Learning Objectives

Define at least 10 terms referring to the respiratory system.

Describe the three functions of the respiratory system.

Identify at least 10 respiratory system structures and the function of each.

Describe at least five disorders of the respiratory system.

Describe at least three methods of assessment of the respiratory system.

Key Terms

Apnea
(AP-nee-uh) Cessation of breathing

Bradypnea
(brayd-IP-nee-uh) Abnormally slow rate of breathing

Chronic
(KRON-ik) Persisting over a long period of time

Cilia
(SIL-ee-uh) Hairlike projections from the surface of a cell

Dysphagia
(dis-FAY-jee-uh) Difficulty swallowing

Dyspnea
(DISP-nee-uh) Difficult or labored breathing

Eupnea
(YOOP-nee-uh) Easy or normal breathing

Expiration
(ek-spih-RAY-shun) Act of breathing out, exhalation

Inspiration
(in-spih-RAY-shun) Act of drawing air into the lung, inhalation

Mediastinum
(mee-dee-uh-STY-num) Thoracic space between the two lungs

Phlegm
(flem) Thick mucus secreted by the tissues in the respiratory passages and usually discharged through the mouth

Pulmonary
(PUL-mo-nayr-ee) Pertaining to the lungs

Respiration
(res-pih-RAY-shun) Exchange of oxygen and carbon dioxide between the atmosphere and the cells of the body, also called *ventilation*

Tachypnea
(tak-IP-nee-ah) Excessively fast respiration

Respiratory System Terminology*

TERM	DEFINITION	PREFIX	ROOT	SUFFIX
Apnea	Without breathing	a	pnea	
Bronchitis	Inflammation of the bronchus		bronch	itis
Dysphagia	Difficulty swallowing	dys	phag	ia
Eupnea	Normal breathing	eu	pnea	
Laryngitis	Inflammation of the voice box (larynx)		laryng	itis
Pleuritis	Inflammation of the lining of the lung		pleur	itis
Pneumonectomy	Removal of the lung		pneumon	ectomy
Tachypnea	Fast respiration	tachy	pnea	
Tonsillitis	Inflammation of the tonsils		tonsill	itis
Tracheotomy	Incision into the windpipe (trachea)		trache	otomy

*A transition phrase or vowel may be added to or deleted from the word parts to make the combining form.

Abbreviations of the Respiratory System

ABBREVIATION	MEANING
ABG	Arterial blood gases
BS	Breath sounds
CF	Cystic fibrosis
CO_2	Carbon dioxide
COPD	Chronic obstructive pulmonary disease
ENT	Ears, nose, and throat
TB	Tuberculosis
TCDB	Turn, cough, deep breathe
trach	Tracheotomy
URI	Upper respiratory infection

Structure and Function of the Respiratory System

The respiratory system brings oxygen into the body through the breathing process. With **inspiration**, or inhaling air, oxygen is brought into the lungs. With **expiration**, or exhalation, carbon dioxide is removed from the lungs.

The respiratory system functions in three ways:
- It exchanges gases between the blood and the lungs.
- It helps regulate body temperature by cooling or warming the blood.
- It helps maintain the blood's electrolyte balance.

There are three processes of **respiration:**
- External respiration, or ventilation, brings oxygen into the lungs.
- Internal respiration exchanges oxygen and carbon dioxide between blood and body cells.
- Cellular respiration changes acid produced during metabolism into harmless chemicals in the cells.

Both the voluntary and involuntary nervous systems control respiration. How fast (rate) and how deep (depth) the breaths are, is regulated chemically. If the concentration of gases in the blood changes, the brain adjusts respiratory rate and depth to counteract the changes to maintain homeostasis.

Air enters the respiratory system (Figure 12-1) through the nose (nasal cavity). The nasal cavity is lined with hairs called **cilia** to help filter out any foreign particles. It also helps to warm and moisten the air. Air also enters through the mouth (oral cavity), when the nasal cavity is blocked. The tonsils and adenoids at the back of the throat help the body resist infection.

The sinuses are hollow spaces in the bones of the skull that open into the nasal cavity. Sinuses help regulate the temperature of air before it reaches the sensitive lungs. They also humidify and filter the air. The spaces act as chambers for vibration of the air producing "vocal resonance" or the sound quality of the voice.

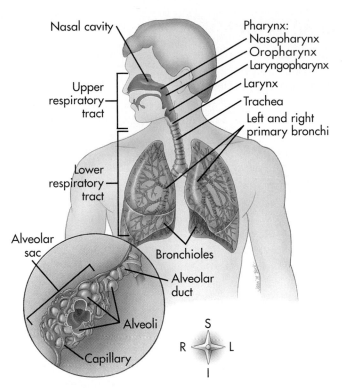

Figure 12-1   Structure of the respiratory system. *(From Thibodeau GA, Patton K: Anatomy & Physiology, ed 5, St Louis, 2003, Mosby.)*

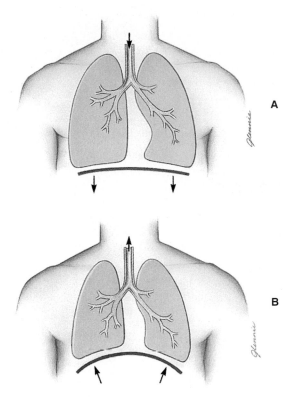

Figure 12-2   The mechanics of breathing. **A,** The diaphragm contracts to pull air into the lungs. **B,** As the diaphragm relaxes, the air is released.

The air from the nose or mouth is then funneled through the throat (pharynx) and into the windpipe (trachea). The pharynx is divided into three portions, the nasopharynx (nose), oropharynx (mouth), and laryngopharynx (larynx).

The trachea or windpipe is lined with rigid cartilage to keep the passageway open. Sometimes an opening is made into the trachea as an alternative method for the exchange of gases (tracheotomy).

The voice box (larynx) is located below the pharynx. Voice sounds are made when air moves through it. A flap of tissue called the *epiglottis* covers the voice box or larynx during swallowing to prevent food and liquid from entering the bronchi and lungs. The pharynx also contains the opening for tubes through which air reaches the middle ear to adjust for pressure changes (eustachian tubes).

The trachea branches into two tubes called *bronchi.* Each bronchus enters one of the lungs and then branches into smaller tubes called *bronchioles.* The bronchi and bronchioles are lined with tiny hairs called *cilia* and sticky mucus called **phlegm** to catch dust and germs. The respiratory system produces approximately 125 mL of mucus each day that is removed by the movement of the cilia.

The bronchioles have small sacs at their ends called *alveoli.* Capillaries in the walls of the alveoli exchange oxygen and carbon dioxide by the process of diffusion. Each alveolus is lined with a liquid called *surfactant* through which the diffusion occurs.

The large number of alveoli, nerves, lymph tissues, and capillaries give the lungs a spongelike texture. The lungs are divided into sections called *lobes.* The right lung has three lobes and the left lung has two lobes. The space separating the lungs (**mediastinum**) contains the esophagus, heart, and bronchi.

Each lung is surrounded by a double membrane called *pleura.* The pleurae separate and lubricate the delicate lung tissues. The pleurae are slippery, allowing a gliding motion of the lungs during respiration. The ribs support and protect the chest cavity (thorax). During breathing, muscles lift and separate the ribs to help the lungs expand.

The diaphragm is a large flat muscle that separates the thoracic cavity from the abdominal cavity. The diaphragm contracts and moves downward during inhalation. This creates suction, and air is pulled in from outside the body. Exhalation occurs when the diaphragm relaxes (Figure 12-2).

Assessment Techniques

Different aspects of respiratory function can be assessed. These include the respiration rate, character, sounds, lung volume, and blood gases.

Rate

The normal rate of respiration varies with age, gender, posture, exercise, temperature, and other factors. Children breathe more than 20 times a minute, adults breathe 16 to 20 times, and the elderly often breathe less than 16 times. Normal respiration is called **eupnea**. Painful or difficult respiration is **dyspnea**. **Tachypnea** is an abnormal respiratory rate greater than 24, and **bradypnea** is less than 10.

Character

Respirations should have a regular rhythm, occurring at regular intervals. Irregular rhythms of respirations may occur in different patterns, such as a rapid series followed by a pause or by no respiration, called **apnea**. Respirations may also be dry, which is normal, or wet. They can also be characterized as deep or shallow.

Sounds

Breath sounds can be heard by using a stethoscope. The quality of the sound varies with the location of the stethoscope over the bronchial tree but should all be dry and clear. Wheezing or other abnormal or misplaced (adventitious) sounds in the upper respiratory tract may indicate an abnormal condition.

Lung Volume

The amount of air that can be brought into the lungs is called respiratory capacity. It is measured with a spirometer. Lung capacity depends on age and physical condition. The measurement of respiratory capacity is called *lung volume* (Figure 12-3). The vital capacity includes the tidal volume, inspiratory reserve, and expiratory reserve.

The tidal volume is the amount of air normally exchanged with each cycle of inspiration and expiration. Inspiratory reserve is an additional amount of air that can be inhaled with conscious effort. Expiratory reserve is the additional amount of air the person can exhale beyond the normal amount with conscious effort.

The sum of these three values is called the *vital capacity*. This is the total amount of air that can be exchanged by that person. A certain amount of air is always in the lungs to maintain their shape. This is called *residual volume*.

Blood Gases

Blood gas studies measure the amount of gases such as oxygen (O_2) and carbon dioxide (CO_2) are in the blood and the blood's pH. These tests provide an accurate assessment of respiratory function (Table 12-1).

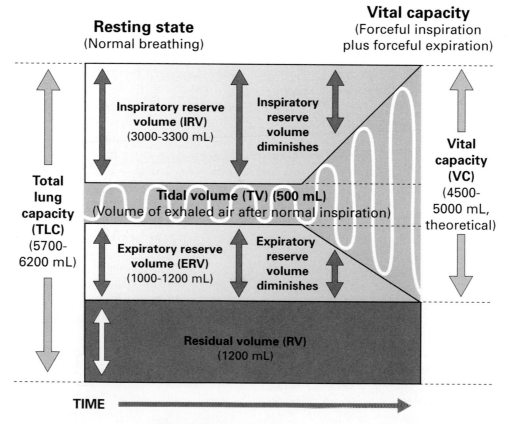

Figure 12-3   Respiratory capacity.

Table 12-1   Blood Gas Analysis

Test	Normal Range*	Description
Arterial O$_2$ saturation (SaO$_2$)	93% to 98%	Ratio of oxygen content and capacity
Arterial O$_2$ tension (PaO$_2$)	80 to 104 mm Hg†	Partial pressure of oxygen
pH (arterial)	7.38 to 7.44	Hydrogen ion concentration
Arterial CO$_2$ tension (PaCO$_2$)	36 to 42 mm Hg	Partial pressure of carbon dioxide
Total CO$_2$ (venous)	26 to 30 mEq/L	Measurement from all compounds containing CO$_2$ in plasma
Bicarbonate HCO$_3^-$ (venous)	25 to 28 mEq/L	Concentration bicarbonate ion in plasma
Base excess (arterial)	$^-$2.4 to $^+$2.3 mEq/L	Excess of basic ions, value should be zero

*Value may vary with differing laboratories.
†*mm Hg,* Millimeters of mercury.

Disorders of the Respiratory System

Anthrax (AN-thraks) is caused by spores of the bacteria *Bacillus anthracis.* The spores may be present in the soil for years and occasionally infect grazing animals. In humans, anthrax may appear as an infection of the skin, digestive system, or respiratory system. Inhalation anthrax has a death rate of more than 80%. In 2001 anthrax spores were sent through the U.S. postal system as a type of biological terrorism, which resulted in the death of five people. A vaccine for anthrax has been developed. After exposure, treatment with antibiotics may prevent infection.

Asthma (AZ-muh) affects 26 million people, 5 million of whom are 17 years old or younger. The conventional belief is that asthma is an allergic reaction. However, recent studies indicate that cells in the airway may trigger the attack, not the immune system. It is known that asthma attacks may result from exposure to an allergen, cold temperature, exercise, or emotion. The bronchi narrow and contract in spasms, and the person may experience wheezing and difficulty exhaling. Treatment includes relaxation and medication to clear air passages. If the cause is determined to be the airway cells, treatment might include inhalation of genes that stop the reaction. There is no known cure for asthma, but half of all children outgrow the condition by their teens.

Atelectasis (at-uh-LEK-tuh-sis) is collapse of part or all of a lung, caused by a tumor in the thoracic cavity, pneumonia, or injury. The person feels severe pain and shortness of breath, or dyspnea. Treatment corrects the cause and reexpands the lung with **pulmonary** suction.

Bronchitis (bron-KIE-tis) is an infection of the bronchi. Inflammation causes the bronchial walls to thicken, and less air can be exchanged. Bronchitis often results in a heavy cough and much mucus eliminated as sputum. Treatment may include the use of expectorant medications and postural drainage.

Carbon monoxide poisoning occurs from breathing carbon monoxide, usually from automobile exhaust fumes. Breathing too much carbon monoxide can be life threatening because the body cells are deprived of oxygen. Carbon monoxide poisoning first causes nausea and drowsiness. The person should be removed from the area of the gas, and oxygen should be administered.

Chronic obstructive pulmonary disease (COPD) is a group of **chronic** respiratory disorders including asthma, chronic bronchitis, and pulmonary emphysema. These conditions have similar symptoms and treatments. The symptoms include shortness of breath (dyspnea) and tissue overgrowth called *hyperplasia* (hi-per-PLAY-zhee-uh). Treatment includes giving oxygen, an antidiuretic (an-tie-die-uh-RET-ik), a medication used to increase the amount of fluids excreted by the body, and a bronchodilator (brong-ko-die-LAY-ter), a medication used to dilate the bronchi and bronchioles for easier breathing.

A *cold* is a respiratory infection, caused by 1 of more than 200 viruses. It lasts from 1 to 2 weeks. It may cause a sore throat, sneezing, aches, pains, a runny nose, and fever. Cold medications may relieve the symptoms, but there is no cure.

Cystic fibrosis (SIS-tik fie-BRO-sis) is a genetic disorder of the exocrine (EK-so-krin) glands, usually diagnosed before the age of 6 months. The mucus in the respiratory system becomes thicker (more viscous), and excess salt appears on the skin. The condition requires intensive pulmonary care to prevent chronic disorders.

Emphysema (em-fuh-SEE-ma) results when the alveoli lose elasticity, usually after 50 years of age. The alveoli become dilated and do not exchange gases well. Emphysema can result from smoking or several disorders of the respiratory system. Treatment includes use of "pursed lip breathing," the very slow exhalation of air to allow alveoli to respond.

Hanta virus is a respiratory condition spread by breathing in materials contaminated by urine or saliva of infected rodents such as deer mice and chipmunks. The symptoms appear like influenza including fever, cough, muscle ache, and inflamed, reddened eyes. This virus has a rapid onset and is often fatal. Treatment is supportive to assist the infected person with respiratory function.

Hay fever is a respiratory inflammation caused by allergens such as plants, dust, and food. It may cause headache, nausea, and watery drainage from the eyes and nose. Treatment includes medication for the symptoms or desensitization therapy.

Lung cancer is directly linked to smoking and smoke products. After cardiovascular disease, lung cancer is the second leading cause of death in smokers. The cancer is usually not detected until it is widespread. The cancer may spread to many parts of the body through the lymph nodes. Treatment may include surgical removal of lung segments as well as chemotherapy and radiation.

Pleural effusion (PLER-uhl e-FYOO-zhun) is a condition in which air or fluid enters the pleural cavity. The space for respiration becomes limited. Pleural effusion is usually caused by cancer, infection, or congestive heart failure. The person may feel shortness of breath and pain. Treatment may include thoracentesis (tho-rah-sen-TEE-sis), which removes the fluid with a needle, or a suction drainage tube.

Pleurisy (PLOO-rih-see) is an inflammation of the membranes that line the lungs. It is usually a complication of a severe respiratory infection such as pneumonia. The person experiences difficulty breathing, pain, and grating breath sounds, also known as *crepitus* (KREP-ih-tus).

Pneumonia (noo-MO-nee-ah) is an inflammation of the lungs, in which a buildup of excessive moisture impairs breathing. It may be caused by bacteria, viruses, or chemical irritants. Aspiration pneumonia is caused by foreign substances, such as vomitus, entering the respiratory passage. Treatment is directed at the original cause, including medication to decrease the moisture.

Pneumoconiosis (noo-mo-ko-nee-O-sis) is an inflammation in the lungs caused by inhaled irritants. These may include dust, asbestos, sand, iron, and coal particles. The lungs may have excessive fluid, and the person feels shortness of breath.

Respiratory acidosis (RES-per-uh-tore-ee as-ih-DO-sis) is a buildup of carbon dioxide in the blood, causing a lowered blood pH. The condition may result from COPD or drug overdose. The person may experience decreased mental functioning or delusions (delirium); death may also result. Treatment may include giving oxygen or providing ventilation with a respirator.

Respiratory alkalosis (RES-pir-uh-tore-ee al-kah-LOH-sis) is a deficiency of carbon dioxide in the blood. It is most often caused by hyperventilation, or rapid breathing, resulting from anxiety or exercise at high elevations. The person experiences extreme nervousness, tingling in the extremities, and muscle spasms (tetany). It is rarely life threatening. Treatment involves breathing slowly or breathing into a paper bag. These techniques increase the carbon dioxide level in the blood.

Respiratory distress syndrome is a condition that occurs when the alveoli do not inflate properly. Adult respiratory distress syndrome (ARDS) may result from inhaling foreign substances and swelling (edema) of respiratory tissues. Infant respiratory distress syndrome (IRDS) is the leading cause of death in premature births. Approximately 50,000 newborns are affected yearly with 5000 resulting in death. Treatment is the delivery of oxygen and, in infants, application of surfactant through tubes into the lungs.

Sinusitis (sine-us-I-tus) is an inflammation of one or more of the paranasal sinuses. It can result as a complication of an upper respiratory or dental infection, or changes in atmosphere such as in swimming or air travel. Symptoms include pain, pressure, headache, fever, and increased secretions. Treatment includes nasal decongestants, steam inhalations, and antibiotics if infection is present.

Sudden infant death syndrome (SIDS) is a respiratory disorder of newborns. More than 2500 babies in the United States die from SIDS each year. The SIDS diagnosis is given for the sudden death of an infant under 1 year of age that remains unexplained after a complete investigation. SIDS may be called "crib death," because it often occurs when the baby is sleeping. The cause of SIDS may be related to a defect in a part of the brain but environmental and metabolic factors are also considered as risk factors. Babies that are at high risk for SIDS may be monitored with heart and respiratory devices while sleeping. One new technique to prevent death is pajamas that have respiratory and heart monitors built into them.

Tuberculosis (tuh-ber-kyoo-LO-sis) is caused by bacteria that are difficult to destroy, and it can be transmitted through the air. It leads to excessive sputum production and coughing. Since 1991 more cases of tuberculosis have developed than in all previous time. It is the most common fatal infectious disease in the world today. Recently a strain of the bacteria that is resistant to the medications used previously has evolved. The incidence of this strain of infection is currently increasing. Treatment includes medication for up to 2 years and may require surgical removal of the affected tissue to destroy the bacteria. Respiratory isolation may be necessary to prevent the spread of tuberculosis.

An *upper respiratory infection* (URI) is caused by a virus or bacteria in the nose, pharynx, or larynx. Pharyngitis (fare-in-JIE-tis) is a sore throat often accompanied by difficulty in swallowing (**dysphagia**). Laryngitis (lare-in-JIE-tis) may cause hoarseness or loss of voice. Tonsillitis (ton-sil-I-tis) is painful inflammation of the lymph nodes and may require surgical removal of the tonsils. Treatment for all types of upper respiratory infections includes rest and medication to relieve pain, reduce fever, and combat the cause of the infection.

Issues and Innovations

Tobacco Issues

Cigarette smoking has been linked to many illnesses such as heart disease and cancer. Research shows that nonsmokers subjected to "passive," "secondhand," or "sidestream" smoke from the cigarettes of other people also face these risks. Studies have demonstrated that a person who works in a restaurant or bar where smoking is permitted has a 50% greater chance of developing lung cancer than someone who does not. The American Lung Association has reported that 20% of the U.S. population are at risk of developing lung disease from secondhand smoke. The U.S. Department of Health, Education, Welfare, and Public Health Services reports that secondhand smoke has higher levels of tar, nicotine, and carbon monoxide than is inhaled by the direct smoker.

The Federal Environmental Protection Agency has classified secondhand smoke as a Group A carcinogen along with asbestos and radon. In many regions new laws restrict smoking to designated areas to protect nonsmokers from exposure to the smoke. Insurance companies often have higher rates for smokers because of the greater health risks and problems of safety. Smoking has been an issue used to determine custody in divorce settlements.

Some advertisements of "smokeless" tobacco such as chew or tobacco powder imply that it does not involve the same health risks. But placing smokeless tobacco between the lower lip and teeth (dipping) is actually as dangerous as smoking and perhaps more so because the juice from tobacco causes a change in mouth tissue called *leukoplakia* (loo-ko-PLAY-kee-uh). These white, leathery patches become mouth cancer in 5% of cases (Figure 12-4). Damage to the taste buds on the tongue affects the person's sense of taste. Tobacco and the sweeteners in the smokeless tobacco products also damage the gums, which causes the teeth to decay and loosen.

Cancer may develop in the esophagus if the tobacco juices are swallowed. Ulcers may occur in the stomach from increased production of gastric acid. The nicotine habit develops with smokeless tobacco just as with cigarette smoking. Heart disease may result from an increase in

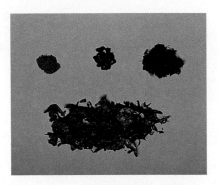

Figure 12–4   Leukoplakia is a precancerous tissue growth of the mucous membranes of the mouth. It is directly related to the use of smokeless tobacco products.

blood pressure and heart rate. Cancer of the bladder, pancreas, and kidney have been shown to occur more often in those using smokeless tobacco.

Environmental Health Risks

Various inhaled inorganic substances can be hazardous to one's health. For example, miners who inhale coal dust develop black lung disease (pneumoconiosis) or silicosis. Inhalation of asbestos leads to chronic scarring of the lung tissue. Berylliosis can result from inhalation of beryllium used in fluorescent light bulbs and the aerospace industry.

Inhalation of biological contaminants such as bacteria, fungus, and dust mites can lead to allergic rhinitis. Other items of concern in the environment include pesticides, particulates in air pollution, and combustible gases. New environmental risks are continually being identified. The 1987 annual report of the American Lung Association estimated that 65,000 people in the United States develop lung diseases from exposure to substances found in the workplace each year.

In a long-term study of 45 different neighborhoods, three areas in Pennsylvania were found to have three times the usual rate of lung cancer. In these areas a high level of sulfur dioxide was found in the air.

In the Silicon Valley area of California, hundreds of workers experienced symptoms apparently resulting from exposure to toxic chemicals used in the computer industry. The symptoms experienced include hypersensitivity to ordinary chemicals, memory loss, fatigue, impaired concentration, and violent mood swings.

Sick building syndrome includes several environmental conditions that may lead to sickness. Most often, sick buildings do not have windows that open to the outside and their heating and cooling ducts start at a common source. An elevated level of carbon dioxide in the building causes sickness. Specific types of sick building syndrome include "air-conditioner lung" and "humidifier fever."

Review Questions

1. Describe the three functions of the respiratory system.

2. Describe the function of each of the following structures of the respiratory system.
   Epiglottis
   Pleura
   Sinus
   Tonsil

3. Describe three tests used to assess the function of the respiratory system.

4. Describe five body systems that are affected by the use of tobacco in any form.

5. Describe two health hazards that have been attributed to inhalation of environmental materials.

Critical Thinking

1. Investigate the rate of tobacco use by adolescents. Design a public information poster that might be used to stop someone from using tobacco.

2. Investigate at least five common medications used in treatment of respiratory system disorders.

3. List at least five occupations involved in the health care of respiratory system disorders.

4. Investigate the current research being conducted about respiratory disorders that result from environmental factors.

5. Research and review an article regarding a recent development or treatment method relating to the respiratory system.

13
Skeletal System

Learning Objectives

Define at least 10 terms relating to the skeletal system.

Describe the five functions of the skeletal system.

Identify at least 10 structures of the skeletal system.

Describe at least five disorders of the skeletal system.

Identify at least three methods of assessment of the skeletal system.

Key Terms

Articulation
(ar-tik-yoo-LAY-shun) Joint; place of junction between two bones

Bursa
(BER-sah) Sac-like cavity filled with fluid to prevent friction

Cancellous
(KAN-seh-lus) Spongy or lattice-like structure

Cartilage
(KAR-tih-lij) Specialized, fibrous connective tissue

Collagen
(KOL-uh-jen) White protein fibers of the skin, tendons, bone, and cartilage (connective tissue)

Compact
(KOM-pakt) Having a dense structure

Degenerative
(de-GEN-er-uh-tiv) Having progressively less function

Extremities
(ek-STREM-ih-tees) Arms or legs

Ligament
(LIG-uh-ment) Band of fibrous tissue that connects bones and supports joints

Marrow
(MARE-o) Soft organic material filling the cavities of bones

Orthopedic
(or-tho-PEE-dik) Pertaining to the correction of deformities

Periosteum
(pair-ee-OS-tee-um) Specialized connective tissue covering all the bones of the body

Resorption
(re-SORP-shun) Loss of bone tissue caused by the action of specialized cells (osteoclasts)

Synovial
(sin-O-vee-uhl) Pertaining to transparent alkaline fluid contained in joints

Tendon
(TEN-dun) Fibrous cord by which a muscle is attached to a bone

Skeletal System Terminology*

TERM	DEFINITION	PREFIX	ROOT	SUFFIX
Arthritis	Inflammation of the joint		arthr	itis
Arthrodesis	Surgical union or fixation of the joint		arthr/o	desis
Arthroplasty	Plastic reconstruction of the joint		arthr/o	plasty
Cervical	Pertaining to the neck		cervic	al
Chondrectomy	Removal of the cartilage		chondr	ectomy
Intercostal	Between the ribs	inter	cost	al
Odontology	Study of the tooth		odont	ology
Orthopedics	Pertaining to correcting or straightening the bones	ortho	ped	ics
Osteoarthritis	Inflammation of the bones and joints	osteo	arthr	itis
Periodontal	Around the tooth	peri/o	dont	al

*A transition phrase or vowel may be added to or deleted from the word parts to make the combining form.

Abbreviations of the Skeletal System

ABBREVIATION	MEANING
AKA	Above knee amputation
amb	Ambulatory
bil	Bilateral
CAT	Computerized axial tomography
CXR	Chest x-ray
ext	Extremity
fx	Fracture
lat	Lateral
lt	Left
ortho	Orthopedics

Structure and Function of the Skeletal System

The human body has more than 200 bones (Table 13-1). The skeletal system works directly with the muscular system to perform many functions, including the following:

- Providing shape and support
- Protecting internal organs
- Storing minerals and fat
- Producing blood cells and platelets
- Assisting in movement

Bone tissue is composed of inorganic salts, particularly calcium phosphate, water, and organic material such as bone cells, blood vessels, nerves, and elastic material (**collagen**). Like other body cells, bone cells must continually receive food and oxygen. However, bones and their adjoining structures, ligaments and tendons, have fewer nerves and blood vessels than other body structures.

Bones continue to grow for the first 18 to 20 years of life. Even after growth stops, bone cells die and are replaced by new cells throughout life. Osteoblasts are cells in the bone tissue that produce new cells. Osteoclasts are cells that break bone cells down (**resorption**).

Bones may have **cartilage**, a fibrous connective tissue, on some surfaces to prevent friction. Bones are attached to other bones by **ligaments**. A sheet of fibrous tissue connecting bone to bone is called an *aponeurosis* (ap-o-noo-RO-sis). Bones are joined to muscles by **tendons**. Fascia (FASH-ee-uh) is a variable fibrous connective tissue that joins organs. Chapter 14 provides more information about the muscular system. The two major types of bone tissue are dense (**compact**) and loosely packed or spongy (**cancellous**).

Table 13-1   Bones of the Body

Part of Skeleton	Body Part	Body Part Division	Names of Bones
Axial skeleton	Skull (28)	Cranium (8)	Frontal (1), parietal (2), temporal (2), occipital (1), sphenoid (1), ethmoid (1)
		Face (14)	Nasal (2), maxillary (2), zygomatic (2), mandible (1), lacrimal (2), palatine (2), inferior concha (2), vomer (1)
		Ear bones (6)	Maleus (2), incus (2), stapes (2)
	Hyoid (1)		
	Spinal column (26)		Cervical vertebrae (7), thoracic vertebrae (12), lumbar vertebrae (5), sacrum (1), coccyx (1)
	Sternum and ribs (25)		Sternum (1), true ribs (14), false ribs (10)
Appendicular skeleton	Upper extremities (64)		Clavicle (2), scapula (2), humerus (2), radius (2), ulna (2), carpals (16), metacarpals (10), phalanges (28)
	Lower extremities (62)		Coxal bones (2), femur (2), patella (2), tibia (2), fibula (2), tarsals (14), metatarsals (10), phalanges (28)

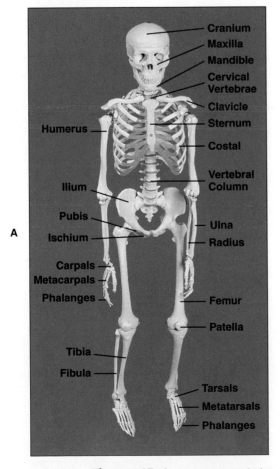
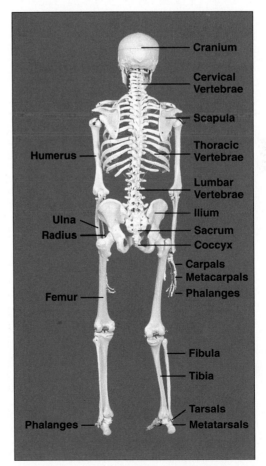

Figure 13-1   Common skeletal bones. **A**, Front view. **B**, Back view.

Types of Bones

The skeletal system consists of two major groups of bones (Figure 13-1):
- The axial skeleton includes the 80 bones of the head and trunk.
- The appendicular skeleton includes the 126 bones of the pelvis, shoulders, arms, and legs (**extremities**).

Bones are also classified by shape (Table 13-2):
- Long bones are longer than wide.
- Short bones have similar length and width.
- Flat bones have two layers with space between them.
- Irregular bones are those that do not fit into the other categories.

Skull

The skull includes the bones of the cranium, face, and ear. The cranium is made up of eight bones (Figure 13-2). The sinus cavities make the skull lighter and the voice sound stronger. At birth, the bones of the cranium have two openings called *fontanels*. These close by 2 years of age. The face is made up of 14 bones (Figure 13-3). The lower jaw (mandible) is the only movable bone of the skull.

Table 13-2	Bones by Shape
Shape of Bone	**Examples**
Long	Femur, humerus, radius, ulna, tibia, fibula
Short	Tarsal, carpal, metatarsal, metacarpal
Flat	Cranium, costal, scapula, sternum
Irregular	Vertebrae, mandible, ilium, ossicle, patella

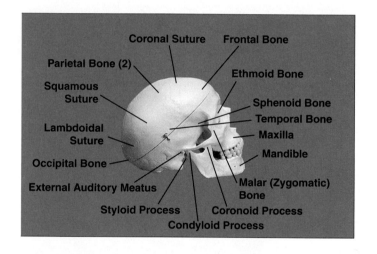

Figure 13-2 The bones of the skull include the cranium, face, and ears.

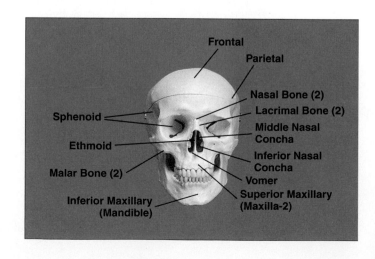

Figure 13-3 The skull includes the bones of the face. (The palate [2] and inferior turbinate [2] are not visible.)

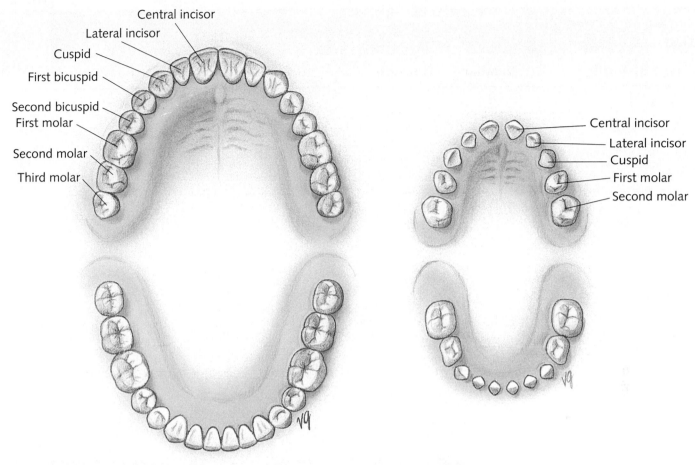

PERMANENT DENTITION   DECIDUOUS DENTITION

Figure 13-4   Tooth development.

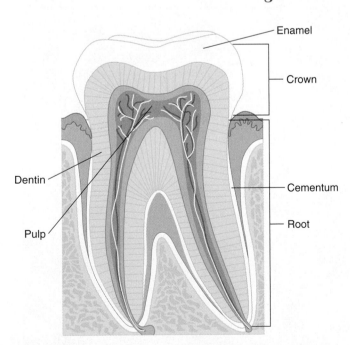

Figure 13-5   Parts of a tooth. *(From Bird DL, Robinson: Torres and Ehrlich modern dental assisting, ed 7, Philadelphia, 2003, WB Saunders.)*

Teeth

The adult has 32 teeth after the deciduous or primary teeth are replaced (Figure 13-4). Each tooth has a number of parts (Figure 13-5):

- The crown is the white section above the gum.
- The root is below the gum.
- Enamel, the hardest substance in the body, covers the crown.
- Cementum is the hard, bonelike substance covering the root.
- Dentin is located between the enamel and the pulp.
- The pulp is the soft living portion of the tooth, containing the nerves and blood vessels.

The four major types of teeth have different shapes and functions (Table 13-3 on p. 192).

Table 13-3 Teeth Types

Type of Tooth	Number	Function	Location	Description
Incisor	8	Cuts food	Front of mouth (central or lateral)	Broad, sharp edge
Cuspid (canines or eyeteeth)	4	Tears food	At angles of lips	Longest in mouth
Bicuspid (premolar)	8	Pulverizes or grinds food	Between cuspids and molars	Flat
Molar	12*	Grinds food	Back of mouth	Largest, strongest

*The third molar is called the "wisdom" tooth. It does not appear in every individual.

Thorax

The thorax is the part of the skeletal system that includes the ribs, sternum, and vertebral bones that protect the lungs and heart (Figure 13-6). The first seven pairs of ribs are called "true" ribs and are attached to the sternum. The lower five pairs of ribs are called "false" ribs and are not attached directly to the sternum. The costal cartilage of each false rib attaches it to the rib above it. The bottom two pair of false ribs are attached only to the spine and are called "floating" ribs. The area between the ribs is called *intercostal space*. It contains muscles, blood vessels, and nerves.

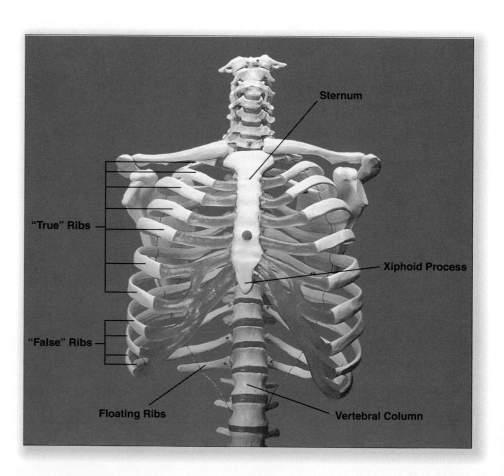

Figure 13-6 The thorax.

Vertebral Column

The adult vertebral (spinal) column consists of 26 vertebrae. It has five parts (Figure 13-7). The curvature of the vertebral column gives it strength and flexibility. Between the vertebrae are discs of cartilage that cushion the bones and allow movement.

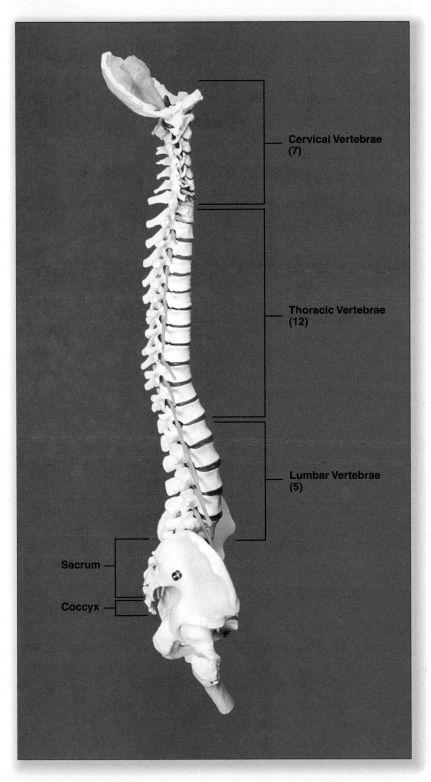

Figure 13-7   The lateral view of the vertebral column shows its five major parts. These five parts contain 26 vertebrae total.

Long Bones of the Extremities

The long bones of the arms and legs contain **marrow** that makes blood cells for the body. Long bones grow and lengthen from a layer of cartilage called the *epiphyseal plate*. This area becomes completely ossified when the bones stop growing. The different parts of the long bone are shown in Figure 13-8.

The diaphysis, or shaft, of the long bone contains fatty tissue and yellow marrow in its cavity. This fatty tissue provides stored energy. The epiphysis, or end of the long bone, contains the red marrow that produces red blood cells. The red marrow also destroys old red blood cells, forms all but one type of white blood cell, and produces platelets. Children have red marrow throughout the body. It is replaced by yellow marrow in all bones except the flat and long bones as they become adults.

The **periosteum**, or membrane that covers the bone, contains osteoblasts, special cells that form new bone tissue. In addition to arteries, nerves, and veins, the medullary cavity, or hollow inner tube of the diaphysis, also contains specialized cells called *osteoclasts*. Osteoclasts enlarge the diameter of the cavity by removing bone cells.

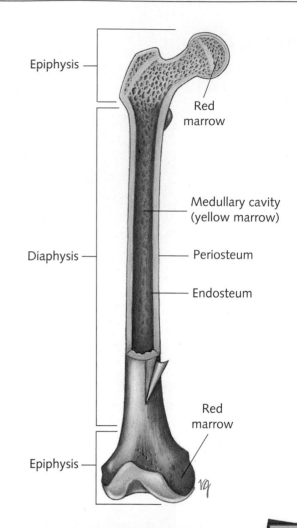

Figure 13-8   The anatomy of a long bone.

Table 13-4   Bone Markings

Type of Marking	Description	Example
Process		
Crest	Narrow ridge	Iliac crest
Condyle	Rounded process that articulates with another bone	Occipital condyle of skull
Tubercle	Small, rounded elevation that attaches muscles and ligaments	Proximal end of humerus
Tuberosity	Large rounded elevation that attaches muscles and ligaments	Ischial tuberosity
Trochanter	Very large projection	Greater trochanter of femur
Head	Rounded projection from neck of bone, articulates with cavity	Head of humerus
Depression		
Sinus	Chamber or cavity in bone	Frontal sinus of skull
Foramen	Opening for nerves and blood vessels	Foramen magnum
Fissure	Narrow slit, cleft, or groove	Inferior orbital fissure of the eye
Fossa	Shallow concave depression on bone surface	Acetabular fossa

Bone Markings

Bone markings are the shapes of different parts of bones (Table 13-4). There are four major types of bone markings:

- Projections bulge from a bone and attach to muscles, ligaments, and tendons.
- Openings are holes or spaces in bones.
- Depressions include openings and cavities in bone.
- Ridges are lines on a bone surface.

Joints

Two or more bones join together at a joint, also called an **articulation.** Joints are commonly named by the bones that are joined. For example, the sternoclavicular joint is between the sternum and clavicle. There are three types of joints:

- Immovable (synarthrosis)
- Slightly movable (amphiarthrosis)
- Freely movable (diarthrosis)

An example of an immovable joint is any one of the sutures of the cranium after they have ossified and closed. An example of a slightly movable joint is bones of the pelvis.

Movable joints are also called **synovial** joints. They contain a protective **bursa,** which is a sac filled with synovial fluid that cushions the moving parts. Bursae are found at the freely movable joints such as the elbows, knees, hips, shoulders, and ankles. The six types of diarthrosis joints are named according to how they move (Figure 13-9):

- Ball and socket joints of the shoulders and hips
- Hinge joints of the elbow and knee
- Gliding joints of the wrists
- Pivot joint at the base of the skull

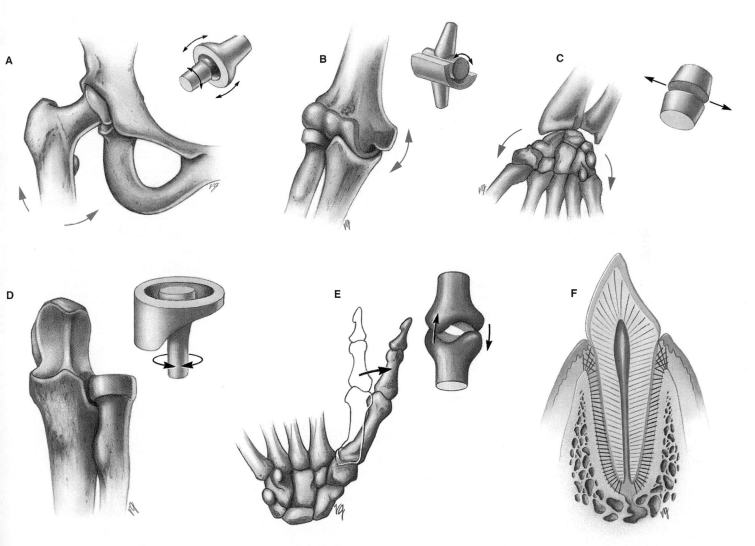

Figure 13-9   Types of joints. **A,** Ball and socket. **B,** Hinge. **C,** Gliding. **D,** Pivot. **E,** Saddle. **F,** Gomphosis.

- Saddle joint of the thumb
- Gomphosis, such as the attachment of a tooth into its socket in the jaw

The ball and socket joint allows the movements of flexion, extension, abduction, adduction, and a limited rotation. Hinge joints have limited movement in only one direction like a hinge. Gliding joints allow the bones to slide. The pivot joint at the base of the skull is unique, allowing rotation of the head. The saddle joint allows many movements such as the thumb touching the fingertips. Gomphoses are specialized joints that allow very slight movement and attach a peglike structure such as a tooth into a socket such as the jaw.

Assessment Techniques

X-ray images use electromagnetic energy that is absorbed by the body's tissues to produce images on photographic film. X-ray machines may be portable or stationary. They may be used to detect bone fractures, cancer, infection, arthritis, and deformities. They may also be used to determine bone age, congenital skull deformities, and injuries resulting from abuse in children. Although an x-ray has minimal risk and is painless, it is less sensitive than a bone scan in detecting bone destruction.

Bone marrow aspiration or sampling is accomplished by inserting a long needle into the spinal column to remove marrow. The sample is used to determine the cause of an abnormal blood test, unexplained blood disorders such as leukemia, to sample for pathogens or chromosome abnormality, and to evaluate response to cancer treatment. It may be performed in the hospital or as an outpatient procedure. Although there are relatively few complications to the procedure, it may cause discomfort.

A bone marrow biopsy is used to obtain a piece of bone containing intact marrow to identify abnormalities such as thrombocythemia. It is also used to diagnose tumors, lymphoma, and the cause of an unexplained fever. It may also be used if bone marrow aspiration is unsuccessful. The procedure is similar to the bone marrow aspiration except that a core of bone is removed for examination.

A radionuclide bone scan or bone scintigraphy is used to detect bone cancer when x-rays do not show any abnormalities but a malignancy is suspected. It may also be used to locate bone infection and other abnormalities. Stress fractures that do not show on an x-ray may be seen using a bone scan. The procedure involves injection of the radionuclide, which spreads through the bone. Increased concentration of the material indicates a diseased area.

A computerized tomogram (CT) scanner is a machine that sends several beams of x-rays simultaneously from different angles. A computer determines the relative density of the tissues examined by the strength of the beams. The technique of CT scanning was developed by Sir Geoffrey Hounsfield, who was awarded the Nobel Prize for his work. The CT scanner is used for taking pictures of every part of the body.

Magnetic resonance imaging (MRI) uses magnetic and radio waves to show computerized images of the body. There is no exposure to x-rays or any other damaging forms of radiation with an MRI. Because the MRI scan shows very detailed pictures, it is the best technique to identify tumors (benign or malignant) in the brain. The MRI scan can also show the heart and blood vessels. It is also used to examine the joints, spine, and sometimes the soft parts of the body, such as the liver, kidneys, and spleen.

About 1.3 million fractures that occur each year in the United States in people over 45 years of age are attributed to osteoporosis. Bone densitometry is used to measure bone mass density to determine the extent of osteoporosis and fracture risk. Common techniques include single-photon absorptiometry (SPA) and dual-photon or dual-energy x-ray absorptiometry. There is some controversy about the accuracy and effectiveness of this assessment technique.

Disorders of the Skeletal System

Ankylosing spondylitis (ang-kil-O-sing spon-dih-LIE-tis) is a hereditary chronic spinal disease of unknown cause. Some or all of the bones and joints of the spine fuse together as a result of this condition. It results in stiffness, decreased mobility, and possible back deformity. There is no cure, but treatment can slow the progression of the disease. Treatment includes a combination of rest, exercise, pain relievers, antiinflammatory medication, and heat applications.

Arthritis (ar-THRIE-tis) includes a group of disorders evidenced by inflammation of a joint, pain, and stiffness during movement. Arthritis, the number one crippling disease in the United States, affects more than 50 million people. Arthritis may be caused by joint disease, infection, gout, or trauma, but most cases are of unknown cause. Three forms of arthritis are ankylosing spondylitis, **degenerative** joint disease, and rheumatoid arthritis (each described separately here). There is no cure, but treatment can relieve discomfort and promote movement in the joint. Controlled activity, rest, diet, application of heat and cold, and medication are all used. Surgery to replace joints may be used in severe cases.

Avulsion (uh-VUL-shen) fractures occur when a ligament or tendon pulls off part of a bone during an injury. This type of injury may occur in the ankles, legs, hip, and upper arms. Small fractures may not need treatment and may not cause pain or discomfort. Large avulsion fractures may require surgical reattachment.

Bursitis (bur-SIE-tis) is inflammation of the sac around a joint and is caused by trauma or irritation. Bursitis results in swelling and restricted movement. Treatment includes protection of the joint, rest, medications, and removal of excess fluid. The condition can become chronic if the joint is injured repeatedly.

Caries (KARE-eez), also called *cavities,* are a major cause of tooth loss in young people. Dental caries are caused by bacteria. If the infection is extensive, the bone supporting the tooth can be damaged. Treatment may include "filling" the cavity with a restorative material such as amalgam or by removing the tooth.

Carpal (KAR-pul) *tunnel syndrome* is a common disorder caused by pressure on the median nerve of the wrist resulting from repetitive use or trauma. The person may feel numbness, burning, tingling, pain, and weakness in the hand. Treatment may include resting the affected wrist, splinting, antiinflammatory medication, or surgical correction.

Degenerative (de-GEN-er-ruh-tiv) *joint disease,* also called *osteoarthritis* (os-tee-o-ar-THRIE-tis), is usually associated with aging, but the cause is unknown. It is the most common form of arthritis. The condition has gradual onset as the cartilage in the joint softens. The person feels pain after exercise and stiffness after inactivity. Treatment includes medication for the pain and to reduce inflammation. In severe cases the joint may be surgically replaced.

A *dislocation* (dis-lo-KAY-shun) occurs when bones move out of their proper location, usually in the shoulder or hip. Dislocation is either congenital or the result of trauma. The person feels pain and loss of mobility. The bones may relocate by themselves or require surgery. Ligaments may be damaged.

A *fracture* (FRAK-chur) is a broken bone caused by trauma. A fracture may be open (the skin is broken) or closed (skin is not broken). Swelling, bruising, and pain may occur. Treatment includes use of casts, traction, and electrical stimulation to increase the rate of healing.

Gout is a painful swelling of a joint that results from the buildup of uric acid crystals, most commonly in the great toe. Fever and chilling may also occur. The condition is usually due to an inability to adequately remove uric acid from the blood. Signs and symptoms of gout can result as a complication of another disorder. Treatment includes the use of medications, weight loss, and diet therapy that restricts the intake of purine.

A *herniated* (HER-nee-ate-ed) *disc* is a ruptured or "slipped" disc between vertebrae. It results in pain and reduced mobility. Treatment includes pain medication, bed rest, and possibly surgical correction.

Kyphosis (kie-FO-sis), also called "hunchback" or "humpback," is an abnormal curvature of the thoracic part of the spine. The person may feel pain caused by affected nerves. Causes may include rheumatic arthritis, rickets, poor posture, or chronic respiratory diseases. Treatment may include exercise to strengthen the back and bracing.

Lordosis (lore-DOE-sis), also called "swayback," is an abnormal curvature of the lumbar spine. The cause may be obesity, pregnancy, or poor posture. The person may feel lower back pain. Treatment includes exercise and bracing.

Meningomyelocele (muh-ning-go-MIE-uh-lo-seel), also called *spina bifida* (SPY-na BIF-ih-da), is a congenital condition of the spinal column. It can cause paralysis and nervous system disorders because of pressure on the spinal nerves. Treatment includes surgery and the prevention of infection. Surgical correction of the opening has been done in utero in some cases.

An *osteoma* (os-tee-O-ma) is a bone tumor. It may be noncancerous (benign) or cancerous (malignant). Its symptoms depend on the location and size of the growth. A benign growth can be cured by surgical removal. Some malignant bone tumors may require chemotherapy or surgical removal.

Osteomalacia (os-tee-o-muh-LAY-she-a), also called *rickets* in children, is a softening of the bones caused by vitamin D and calcium deficiency. The person may experience pain, muscular weakness, anorexia, loss of weight, and deformity. Treatment includes adding nutrients to the diet.

Osteomyelitis (os-tee-o-my-uh-LIE-tis) is a bacterial infection of bone. Sudden fever and pain may occur. Treatment includes immobilization of the part and antibiotics.

Osteoporosis (os-tee-o-po-RO-sis) is a weakening of the bones that affects more than 20 million people in the United States. The bones become fragile and break usually in the hip, spine, and wrist. Women with a small, thin build are most likely to develop it, especially after menopause. Inadequate calcium in the diet, lack of exercise, and excessive use of caffeine and alcohol may also be associated with this condition. Lower back pain and abnormal curvature of the spine may result. There is no cure, but treatment to reduce symptoms includes dietary supplements of calcium and vitamin D. Estrogen and other hormone replacement therapies have been shown to improve bone density.

Paget's (PAJ-ets) *disease,* also called *osteitis deformans,* is a condition of unknown cause. It usually appears after the age of 35. Because of excessive destruction of bone cells, the long bones become bowed and the flat bones deformed. Although there may be no symptoms, bone pain, dizziness, headache, and deafness may result. Treatment, if necessary, includes medication, mild exercise and a high-protein diet.

Periodontitis (pair-ee-o-don-TIE-tis) affects 90% of adults in the United States and causes most tooth loss in people over age 35. Periodontitis is an inflammation of the tissues that keep teeth in place. It may start as sore, bleeding gums and may include persistent bad breath and tender, swollen, and receding gums. In advanced stages pus may form and teeth may loosen. Treatment may include removing the tooth, scraping the gums, and performing root canal surgery to remove the infected area.

Rheumatoid arthritis (ROO-mah-toid ar-THRIE-tis) is a condition that affects many parts of the body and joints. Its cause is unknown. It may lead to crippling deformity and atrophy of the muscle tissue. The synovial membrane thickens, causing pain and stiffness in the joints. Treatment includes physical therapy or **orthopedic** braces. Although there is no cure, antiinflammatory medications and rehabilitative care can slow the spread to other joints.

Rickets (RIK-ets) is a painless deformity at the epiphysis of the bones caused by insufficient vitamin D. In children the fontanels may close late and the arms and legs may be bowed in shape. Treatment includes dietary supplements of vitamin D.

Scoliosis (sko-lee-O-sis) is an abnormal lateral spinal curvature. It may cause one shoulder to become higher than the other. It may be congenital, but it develops in the early teens during the growth spurt. It also may be caused by rickets, shortening of one leg, or other spinal disorders. The person may feel discomfort in walking and experience lower back pain. Treatment includes corrective exercise, braces, possibly casting, and, in some cases, surgical correction.

Subluxation (sub-luk-SAY-shun) is partial dislocation of a joint, such as occurs in the neck in a "whiplash" injury. The person may feel mild or severe pain in areas affected by the spinal cord nerves. Treatment includes manipulation of the spine and may include bracing or surgery.

Talipes (TAL-I-pez) is a congenital deformity involving the foot and ankle. Clubfoot is one type of talipes in which one or both feet are turned, usually inward, affecting mobility. Treatment may include surgery, corrective (orthopedic) shoes, or both.

Issues and Innovations

Progress in Dental Care

Dental health care includes more than repair of caries and treatment of periodontal disease. Dentistry now offers corrective measures for damaged, discolored, and misplaced teeth. Innovations include bonding, porcelain facing, bleaching, bracing, and tooth replacement. Bonding is a process to correct the surface of a tooth that is damaged or discolored. Bonding uses adhesive materials such as epoxy and ceramic powder. Porcelain veneers, another method of correcting surfaces, use composite resins. These last longer than bonding but are more costly. Sealants or plastic coatings are used to fill spaces to prevent formation of caries.

New methods of bleaching are also used to remove stains from tooth surfaces. Gas plasma or blue light, pastes, and chemical strips are being used to whiten the surface of teeth. Exact coloration may be difficult with bleaching, and the process may weaken the tooth. Metal brackets, also called *braces,* traditionally worn by children, are now used by people of all ages. Other new methods to move teeth include plastic braces, which are less visible, and electrical stimulation.

Osteointegration is the process of placing implants into the bone to replace missing teeth. This process takes several months and more than one surgical treatment to place hardware made of inert substances such as titanium into the jaw bone (endosseus). Although there is a greater risk of infection than in other replacement techniques, the implants are more stable and last longer.

A chemical has recently been developed that softens areas of decay in a tooth. The decay dissolves and can be painlessly removed, reducing the need for traditional drilling of cavities. About 3000 dentists in the United States are now using this method. The chemical treatment usually costs more than drilling, and it takes longer to remove the decayed area. But this new chemical method may provide a better surface for bonding to the metals used for fillings. Amalgam fillings may be replaced by a composite material for patients who have a concern about the release of mercury into the body from fillings.

Bone Substitutes and Repairs

Several new materials have been found to replace missing or damaged bones. One type of material is called "organo-apatites," consisting of a mineral network that can mesh together with existing bone. This implant material has been shown to promote growth and repair of existing bone tissue in dogs.

Coral from the ocean is also being used to repair bones by grafting (Figure 13-10). This animal leaves a calcium deposit that is not rejected by the human body's immune system. Another advantage of using this material is its relative abundance.

Medical researchers are now using a process, called *stereolithography,* to make surgical implants for cranial and joint injuries. Stereolithography was adapted from the process used to make floor covering like linoleum. In the process, digital computer imaging is used to create an implant that is shaped with lasers and liquid plastic. The laser forms layer upon layer of the plastic until the implant matches the computer image.

Bone regeneration using the Ilazarov method was first introduced in the United States in 1987. The orthopedic surgical procedure involves making cuts in the affected bone surface without damaging the underlying nerves and blood vessels. Pins and a brace are placed around the bone allowing it to be pulled apart gradually. Natural bone tissue is allowed to regrow in the split area. Bones can be lengthened approximately 1 mm every 24 hours and reports have been made of lengthening up to 13 inches. The orthopedic surgery has been successful in treating bone deformities resulting from polio, trauma, and other degenerative conditions.

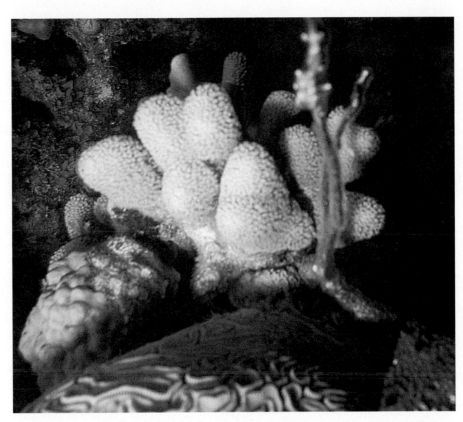

Figure 13-10   Coral is now being used in grafting procedures to repair human bones.

Review Questions

1. Use the following terms in one or more sentences that correctly relate their meaning.
   Collagen

   Ligament

   Synovial

   Tendon

2. Describe the five functions of the skeletal system.

3. In one or more sentences, identify the location of each of the following bones of the skeletal system and the characteristics these bones have in common.
   Femur

   Fibula

   Humerus

   Radius

   Tibia

   Ulna

4. Identify and explain how the effect of a disorder of the skeletal system is similar to kyphosis.

5. Describe the functions of red and yellow bone marrow.

6. Describe six types of joint movement.

7. Describe three methods of bone replacement or repair.

Critical Thinking

1. Investigate and compare the cost of at least three tests used to diagnose disorders of the skeletal system.

2. Investigate the function of at least five common medications used in treatment of skeletal system.

3. List at least five occupations involved in the health care of skeletal system disorders.

4. Investigate first-, second-, and third-class lever movement of joints.

5. Research the process of bone tissue formation after a fracture.

14
Muscular System

Learning Objectives

Define at least 10 terms relating to the muscular system.

Describe the six functions of the muscular system.

Identify at least 10 structures of the muscular system and the function of each.

Describe at least five disorders of the muscular system.

Describe at least three methods of assessment of the muscular system.

Key Terms

Antagonist
(an-TAG-uh-nist) Muscle that acts in opposition to the action of another muscle, its agonist

Atrophy
(AT-ro-fee) Wasting away, decrease in size

Contraction
(kon-TRAK-shun) Shortening or development of tension in muscle tissue

Contracture
(kon-TRAK-chur) Permanent shortening of tendons and ligaments of a joint resulting from atrophy of muscle

Dystrophy
(DIS-tro-fee) Muscle disorder resulting from defective or faulty nutrition, abnormal development, infection

Myalgia
(my-AL-juh) Muscle pain

Paralysis
(puh-RAL-ih-sis) Loss or impairment of motor function

Posture
(POS-chur) Attitude or position of the body

Prime Mover
(prime MOO-ver) Muscle that acts directly to bring about a desired movement, agonist

Range of Motion
(raynj uhv MO-shen) Active or passive movement of muscle groups to full extent possible, used to prevent contracture

Sarcomere
(SAR-ko-meer) Repeating units of muscle fibers with the ability to contract

Skeletal
(SKEL-e-tal) Pertaining to the framework of the body

Stimulus
(STIM-yoo-lus) Any agent, act, or influence that produces a change in the development or function of tissues

Tonus
(TO-nus) Slight, continuous contraction of muscle

Visceral
(VIS-er-al) Pertaining to any large interior organ in any one of the cavities of the body

Muscular System Terminology*

TERM	DEFINITION	PREFIX	ROOT	SUFFIX
Atrophy	Without growth, wasting away	a	troph	y
Biceps	Muscle with two heads	bi	ceps	
Blepharospasm	Uncontrolled muscle contraction of the eyelid		blephr/o	spasm
Dystrophy	Faulty growth	dys	troph	y
Fibromyositis	Inflammation of the muscle tissues	fibro	my/os	itis
Myalgia	Muscle pain		my	algia
Myoma	Tumor of the muscle		my	oma
Myometrium	Muscle of the uterus	my/o	metrium	
Quadriceps	Muscle with four heads	quadr/i	ceps	
Visceral	Pertaining to the inside		viscer	al

*A transition phrase or vowel may be added to or deleted from the word parts to make the combining form.

Abbreviations of the Muscular System

ABBREVIATION	MEANING
ATP	Adenosine triphosphate
Bx	Biopsy
CA++	Calcium
EMG	Electromyogram
IM	Intramuscular
LP	Lumbar puncture
MD	Muscular dystrophy
MI	Myocardial infarction
OT	Occupational therapy
PT	Physical therapy

Table 14–1 Types of Muscle Tissue

Muscles	Appearance	Manner of Control
Skeletal	Striated	Voluntary
Visceral	Smooth	Involuntary
Cardiac	Indistinctly striated	Involuntary

- Aid in movement
- Provide and maintain **posture**
- Protect internal organs
- Provide movement of blood, food, and waste products through the body
- Open and close body openings
- Produce heat

Muscle **contraction** is the movement of muscles when stimulated. **Tonus** is the muscle's ability to maintain slight, continuous contraction. Muscles can be stimulated electrically, mechanically, or chemically. Muscles are flaccid, or soft, when not contracted. Muscle tissue has several unique characteristics:

- Irritability or excitability is the muscle's ability to respond to a **stimulus** such as a nerve or hormone.

Structure and Function of the Muscular System

The human body has more than 600 muscles. The three types of muscle tissue are **skeletal, visceral,** and cardiac (Table 14-1). The functions of muscles are to do the following:

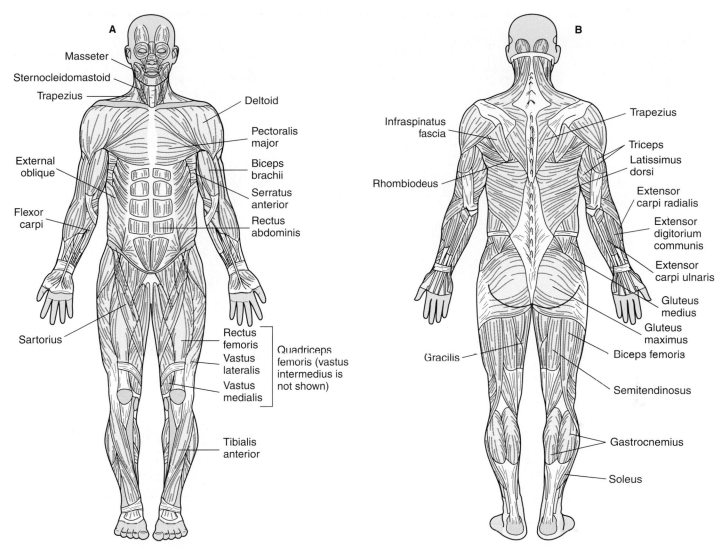

Figure 14-1   Common muscle groups. **A**, Front view. **B**, Back view. *(From Sorrentino S: Mosby's textbook for nursing assistants, ed 5, St Louis, 2000, Mosby.)*

- Contractility is the muscle's ability to shorten forcefully when stimulated.
- Extensibility is the muscle's ability to stretch and lengthen.
- Elasticity is the muscle's ability to recoil to its resting length when relaxed.

Types of Muscle Tissue

Skeletal Muscle

Skeletal muscles make up more than 40% of a person's body weight. They increase in size and weight with exercise and decrease with inactivity. Muscle size and strength vary among people because of genetic differences and nutritional and exercise habits. Muscles are attached to bones by tendons, which are narrow strips of dense connective tissue. Muscles are named according to their location, related bones, shape, action, or size (Figure 14-1).

Skeletal muscle tissue looks striated, or banded, under the microscope (Figure 14-2). Striated muscle is made of bundles of fine fibers. The number of muscle fibers does not increase much after birth. Increase in muscle mass is due to an increase in the size of the fibers. Fascia is a layer of fibrous connective tissue that separates individual muscles.

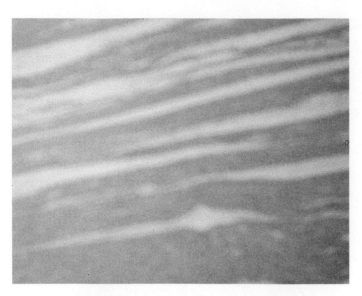

Figure 14-2   Skeletal muscle tissue.

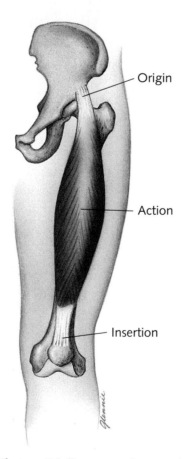

Figure 14-3   Parts of a muscle.

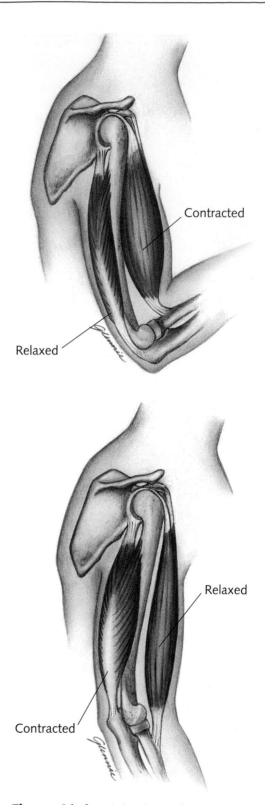

Figure 14-4   Skeletal muscle movement.

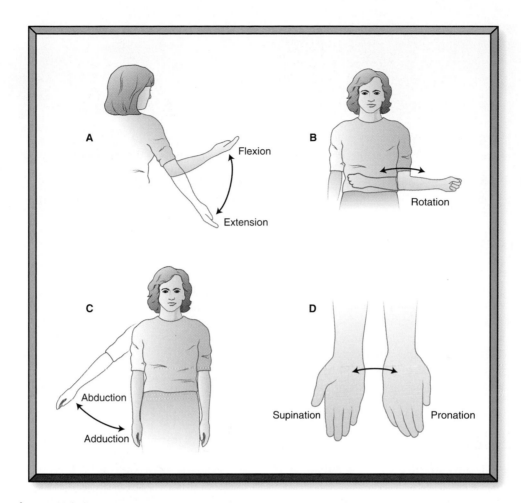

Figure 14-5   Types of muscle movement. **A,** Flexion and extension. **B,** Rotation. **C,** Abduction and adduction. **D,** Pronation and supination.

The basic unit of muscle fibers that causes muscle contraction is called a **sarcomere.** Sarcomeres are organized units made up of actin and myosin myofibrils. Most skeletal muscles contract under the person's voluntary control. Skeletal muscles have three parts (Figure 14-3):

- The origin is one end of the muscle, attached to the less movable part of the bone.
- The insertion is the other end of the muscle, attached to the more movable part of the bone.
- The acton or body is the thick, middle part of the muscle.

Skeletal muscles produce movement by pulling bones. Figure 14-4 shows how skeletal muscles work in pairs; one contracts and pulls while its counteracting muscle relaxes.

- The **prime mover,** or agonist muscle, pulls to cause the movement.

The **antagonist** muscle relaxes when the agonist contracts.

Other muscles, called *synergists* and *fixators,* help keep the muscle and bone stable during movement.

There are seven basic types of body movements that can be made by skeletal muscles (Figure 14-5). Flexion moves a bone closer to another bone, and extension moves a bone farther from another bone. Rotation is a circular or semicircular motion. Abduction is movement of a body part away from the midline, and adduction is movement toward the midline. Pronation is turning the hand or foot downward or backward, and supination is the opposite of pronation, turning the hand or foot upward or forward.

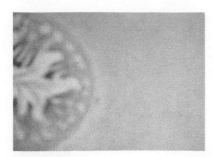

Figure 14-6   Visceral muscle tissue.

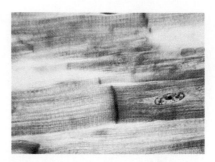

Figure 14-7   Cardiac muscle tissue. *(Courtesy Ward's Natural Science Establishment, Rochester, NY.)*

Visceral Muscle

Visceral muscle lines various hollow organs, makes up the walls of blood vessels, and is found in the tubes of the digestive system. Visceral muscle is smooth and has no striations like the bands of the skeletal muscle (Figure 14-6). Like skeletal muscle, it contracts when stimulated. Visceral muscles are controlled by the autonomic nervous system. One example of a visceral muscle is the sphincter (circular) muscles, which open and close the pupil of the eye.

Cardiac Muscle

Cardiac muscle is found only in the heart. It is indistinctly striated muscle (Figure 14-7). It is under involuntary control. Cardiac muscle has specialized cells that provide a stimulus for contraction. Because of this "pacemaker," the heart continues beating when not stimulated by neural impulses. Chapter 10 provides more information about the heart.

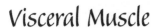

How Muscles Contract

When stimulated, a complex chain of molecular actions is responsible for muscle contraction. The sliding filament theory of muscle contraction explains this process (Figure 14-8). Proteins and other molecules in the muscle tissue interact, and the resulting molecules are shorter than they were originally, thereby making the tissue contract.

Muscle cells use a form of glucose (glycogen) to provide the energy used for contraction. The glucose is used to fuel the ADP-ATP cycle for energy production in the muscle cells. In the ADP-ATP cycle, adenosine diphosphate (ADP) combines with a phosphate to store energy as adenosine triphosphate (ATP) and breaks this bond to release energy for use by the muscle tissue. The ADP-ATP cycle provides the energy needed to combine the proteins actin and myosin into actomysin. Calcium is needed for the reaction

to occur. The lactic acid that is produced from the metabolism of glycogen is converted to water and carbon dioxide in the presence of oxygen. If oxygen is in short supply, lactic acid, a byproduct of this process, can build up in the muscle and cause soreness. Heat is produced by this action as another byproduct.

Types of Muscle Contraction

The strength of a muscle contraction depends on the strength of nerve impulses received in the muscle from the brain. Each muscle fiber either contracts completely or not at all. The stimulus must be strong enough to cause the contraction. This is the "all-or-none" law of skeletal muscle contraction. Not all muscle contractions are the same.

- Isotonic contraction is muscle shortening that produces movement such as skeletal muscle movement during exercise.
- Muscle tone or tonus is a state of partial contraction that maintains a person's posture.
- Isometric contraction does not cause muscle shortening or movement, such as in the motion of pushing against a fixed object like a wall.
- A twitch is a quick, jerky contraction of a whole muscle from one stimulus.
- Tetanic contraction is more sustained than a twitch and is caused by many stimuli in rapid succession. Tetany is continued contraction of a skeletal muscle.
- Fibrillation is uncoordinated contraction of muscle fibers.
- Convulsions are contractions of groups of muscles in an abnormal manner.
- Spasms are involuntary, sudden, and prolonged contractions.

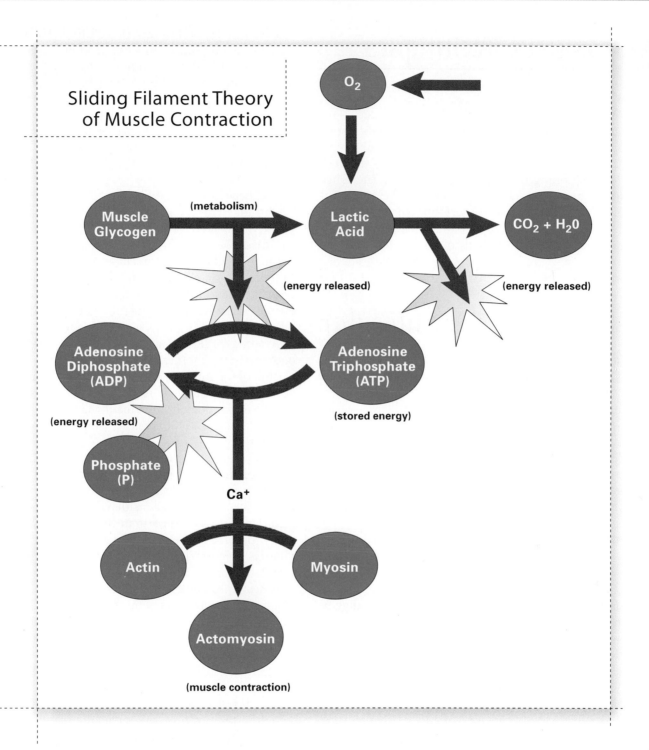

Figure 14–8   The sliding filament theory. The muscle cells use a form of glucose (glycogen) to produce energy used in conversion of ADP to ATP. When a stimulus to contract the muscle is received, the ATP cycle provides energy to combine the proteins actin and myosin into actomyosin. Calcium is needed for the reaction to occur. The lactic acid that is produced from the metabolism of glycogen is converted to water and carbon dioxide in the presence of oxygen.

Assessment Techniques

The muscular system can be assessed in a number of ways. With general inspection, the muscular system is assessed for asymmetry, deformity, swelling, or bruising. With systematic movement of body parts, muscle groups can be assessed for weakness. Reflex tests assess the neurological functioning of the muscular system. The range of joint motion produced by skeletal muscles can be measured using a protractor. Blood tests measuring enzymes may indicate muscular system damage. Electromyography tests individual muscles through needles inserted into the muscle. A muscle biopsy may be used to assess for tissue disorders.

Disorders of the Muscular System

Back pain, a common disorder, usually results from weakened muscles around the spine in the lower back. Recurrent back pain can be caused by a sedentary lifestyle, obesity, poor posture, or muscle tone. Back pain may also result from muscle strain or pressure on the sciatica nerve of the leg. The treatment includes bracing the back for support, heat applications, and exercises to strengthen the muscles. Medication may be used for pain or muscle spasm.

Contracture is a condition in which muscles remain contracted as a joint loses flexibility and ligaments and tendons shorten. Contractures result from gradual muscle wasting, called **atrophy** because of a lack of movement of the muscles. Contractures can be prevented with **range of motion** exercises. Treatment of severe contractures may involve surgical cutting of ligaments.

A *muscle cramp* is a sudden, involuntary contraction of a muscle producing pain. Cramps usually occur in the legs or feet. Cramps may result from exertion or unknown causes, as with the common cramps that occur at night. Treatment includes stretching and gentle pressure to relieve the pain.

Muscular dystrophy is a group of genetic diseases involving painless, gradual atrophy of muscle tissue. Duchenne muscular dystrophy, a severe X-linked form, occurs in 1 out of every 3000 to 5000 boys. It can be detected with 95% accuracy during pregnancy. Becker muscular dystrophy is a milder form. Severe forms cause total disability, and others cause a mild disability. No cure has been found. Treatment may include medication to slow the progression of the disease, braces, or corrective surgery. Research in gene therapy is being conducted as a treatment for this disorder.

Fibromyalgia (fie-bro-my-AL-jee-uh) includes a group of muscle disorders affecting the tendons, ligaments, and other fibrous tissues. Common sites of pain include the neck, shoulders, thorax, lower back (lumbago), and thighs. It does not cause inflammation. The person feels pain and tenderness after being exposed to cold, dampness, illness, or minor trauma. Generalized **myalgia** usually occurs in women. Treatment includes decrease in stress, rest, heat, massage, therapy to stretch the muscles, and exercise.

Gangrene (GANG-green) is caused by *Clostridium,* a bacterium that kills muscle tissue. Gangrene begins when the bacteria enter an area of muscle tissue that has died. The bacteria destroy the surrounding living tissue. The extremities are most often affected, but the gallbladder or intestines may become infected in some cases. Treatment includes removal of dead tissue, antibiotics, and medication against the toxins produced by the bacteria.

A *hernia* (HER-nee-uh) is the abnormal protrusion of a body part into another body area. An example is the protrusion of the intestine through abdominal muscles in the groin area. Hernias may result from weakness in the muscles of the abdomen. Treatment may include bracing, a surgical procedure to restore proper positioning, and medication.

Myasthenia gravis (my-us-THEE-nee-uh GRAV-is) is a condition in which nerve impulses are not transmitted normally from the brain to the muscles. Its cause is not known, although it is considered to be an autoimmune disorder. Muscle weakness in different body areas eventually becomes severe, although remission may occur. There is no cure. Treatment may include maintaining life support.

Poliomyelitis (po-lee-o-my-eh-LI-tis) is a viral infection that results in **paralysis** of muscles. Polio can be prevented by a vaccine. No cure has been found. Treatment is directed toward relieving symptoms.

Muscle sprain (sprane) is traumatic injury to the tendons, muscles, or ligaments of a joint. It causes pain and swelling. Treatment includes alternating application of heat and cold, rest, and ultrasound.

Muscle strain is torn or stretched tendons and muscles, causing pain. It may occur if muscles are exerted too suddenly or for too long. In severe cases, muscles may break in two pieces, leaving a gap in the middle. Treatment includes stopping the activity, elevating the arm or leg, and applying ice to minimize swelling. Some treatments alternate cold and hot applications.

Pes panus, also called "flatfoot" or "fallen arches," may be congenital or result from weakened foot muscles. It causes extreme pain. Treatment includes corrective shoes, massage, and special exercises.

Tetanus (TET-uh-nus), commonly called "lockjaw," is caused by a bacterial infection. Muscle spasms may be severe and can result in death. Tetanus can be prevented by vaccination. No cure has been found. Treatment involves preventing complications of muscle spasm and life support.

Trichinosis (trik-i-NO-sis) is a parasitic infection caused by eating undercooked pork. The parasites form cysts in muscle tissues, especially the diaphragm and chest muscles. Infection causes pain, tenderness, and fatigue. The infection can be fatal if it affects the brain or heart. Treatment includes fluids, nutritional support, and medication to relieve pain, reduce fever, and kill the parasites.

Issues and Innovations

Sports Medicine

Many people think of sports medicine as a new health field, but actually it has long existed as a medical specialty. In 1928 the International Sports Medicine Federation was organized. In 1954 the American College of Sports Medicine (ACSM) was formed. It is the primary organization for this specialty in the United States. Sports medicine is involved in all sports and athletics. More than just treating sports injuries, trainers and doctors also direct the healthful development and training of athletes. Chapter 30 provides more information about career opportunities in athletic training.

Athletic injuries include strains, sprains, cuts, bruises, and similar conditions, many affecting the muscular system. Such injuries can be very serious and take months to heal. Most sports injuries result from poor flexibility, overtraining, poor training methods, inadequate equipment, or muscle imbalance.

An innovation arising from sports medicine is the field of biomechanics, the study of muscles in movement. Other sports medicine innovations in treatment of injury include ultrasound and electrical stimulation to increase circulation and promote healing.

Fitness Fad

Recent surveys show that about two thirds of the people in the United States exercise regularly, an increase of more than 25 million people since 1984. However, only 37% of high school students exercise for 20 minutes at least three times a week. Regular exercise improves physical fitness and health and also promotes a feeling of well-being. People who exercise on a regular basis feel better about themselves and cope better with stress and tension.

In the last 10 years many new health clubs and spas have opened to provide facilities for exercise. When choosing an exercise club, some things to consider include the staff's credentials, how crowded or spacious the facilities are, the cleanliness of the club, and the contract terms.

It is possible to become too concerned with exercise. For some people, exercise may come to take priority over family, work, and friends. Psychologists believe that this obsession results from the person's becoming dependent on the "high" of exercise. This feeling results from a chemical called *endorphin* (en-DOOR-fin) that is released by the brain during exercise.

A person who has become obsessed with exercise feels he or she needs to work out daily to be even minimally functional. Such an "addicted" person feels withdrawal symptoms such as irritability and depression when not regularly exercising. It is a sign that there is a problem if the person continues to exercise when ill or injured.

Review Questions

1. Use the following terms in one or more sentences that correctly relate their meaning.
   Atrophy
   Contracture
   Posture
   Range of motion
   Skeletal

2. Describe the six functions of the muscular system.

3. Identify the functional and structural units of the muscular system.

4. Describe three muscular system disorders that are caused by infectious agents.

5. Describe three methods used to assess the function of the muscular system.

6. List three benefits of maintaining a regular exercise program.

Critical Thinking

1. Investigate and compare the cost of at least three tests used in diagnosing disorders of the muscular system.

2. Investigate the function of at least five common medications used in treatment of muscular system disorders.

3. List at least five occupations involved in the health care of muscular system disorders.

4. Classify the following muscle movements as voluntary or involuntary action.

Blinking	Laughing
Digestion	Pupil size
Eye movement	Respiration
Facial grimace	Snapping fingers
Heartbeat	Swallowing

5. Research rehabilitation training programs utilizing progressive-resistance and variable-resistance machines and other new treatments for sports injury.

6. Research and review an article regarding a recent development or treatment method relating to the muscular system.

15
Digestive System

Learning Objectives

Define at least 10 terms relating to the digestive system.

Describe the four functions of the digestive system.

Identify at least 10 digestive system structures and the function of each.

Describe at least five disorders of the digestive system.

Identify the location and function of three accessory organs of the digestive system.

Identify at least three methods of assessment of the digestive system.

Key Terms

Alactasia
(a-lak-TAY-zee-uh) Malabsorption of lactose caused by a deficiency of the enzyme lactase

Bile
(BY-uhl) Fluid that helps digest fat in the small intestine; produced by the liver and stored in the gallbladder

Bolus
(BO-les) Rounded mass of food

Bulimia
(buh-LEEM-ee-uh) Excessive binge eating, which may be followed by self-induced vomiting or purging

Cholecystectomy
(ko-le-sis-TEK-to-me) Surgical removal of the gallbladder

Chyme
(KIME) Thick, semiliquid contents of stomach during digestion

Defecation
(def-ih-KAY-shen) Evacuation of waste or fecal material from rectum

Deglutition
(dee-gloo-TISH-en) Act of swallowing

Emesis
(EM-eh-sis) Act of vomiting, vomit

Endoscopy
(en-DOS-ko-pee) Visual inspection of a body cavity using a scope

Enema
(EN-uh-muh) Liquid instilled into rectum

Flatulence
(FLACH-uh-lents) Excessive air or gas in stomach or intestines leading to distention of organs

Ingestion
(in-JES-chen) Taking food or medicine into the body through the mouth

Jaundice
(JAWN-dis) Yellow appearance resulting from bile pigment stored in the skin and sclera of the eyes

Mastication
(mas-tik-KAY-shen) Process of chewing food

Peristalsis
(per-ih-STOL-sis) Wavelike series of contractions of the digestive system that propels the contents

Sphincter
(SFINK-ter) Ringlike band of muscle that closes a passage or opening

Villus
(VIL-es) One of many tiny vascular projections on the surface of the small intestine

Digestive System Terminology*

TERM	DEFINITION	PREFIX	ROOT	SUFFIX
Appendectomy	Removal of the appendix		append	ectomy
Cholecystectomy	Removal of the gallbladder	chole	cyst	ectomy
Colocentesis	Surgical puncture into the colon		colo	centesis
Enteritis	Inflammation of the intestines		enter	itis
Hematemesis	Vomiting of blood		hemat	emesis
Hepatitis	Inflammation of the liver		hepat	itis
Laparotomy	Incision into the abdomen		lapar	otomy
Peptic	Pertaining to digestion		pept	ic
Proctoscopy	Examination of the rectum		proct/o	scopy
Visceral	Pertaining to the organs		viscer	al

*A transition phrase or vowel may be added to or deleted from the word parts to make the combining form.

Abbreviations of the Digestive System

ABBREVIATION	MEANING
abd	Abdominal
BE	Barium enema
BM	Bowel movement
Cal	Calorie
cl liq	Clear liquid
FDA	Food and Drug Administration
GB	Gallbladder
GI	Gastrointestinal
NPO	Nothing by mouth
PO	By mouth (per os)

Structure and Function of the Digestive System

The digestive system consists of the organs that make up the alimentary canal, or digestive tract, from the mouth to the anus (Figure 15-1). The digestive tract is about 30 feet long. It is not a sterile system like the other internal organs because it is open to the outside environment at both ends.

The main function of the digestive system, also called the *gastrointestinal system,* is to break down food to a form that can be used by body cells. The digestive process includes transportation of food and wastes, physical and chemical breakdown, absorption of digested food, and final elimination of wastes (Table 15-1). It also helps to maintain the proper amount of water, electrolytes, and other nutrients in the body.

Organs of the Digestive Process

Mouth

Food enters the alimentary canal at the mouth (**ingestion**). The teeth bite and chew the food to begin its physical breakdown. The tongue aids in tasting, chewing (**mastication**), and swallowing (**deglutition**) of food. The hard palate is the anterior roof of the mouth. Unlike the hard palate, the soft palate tissue is not attached to bone on the posterior portion of the mouth. The uvula is a small piece of tissue at the rear of the mouth that prevents food from entering the nasal cavity during swallowing.

As food is chewed it is mixed with saliva. Three salivary glands secrete an enzyme (amylase) that begins the chem-

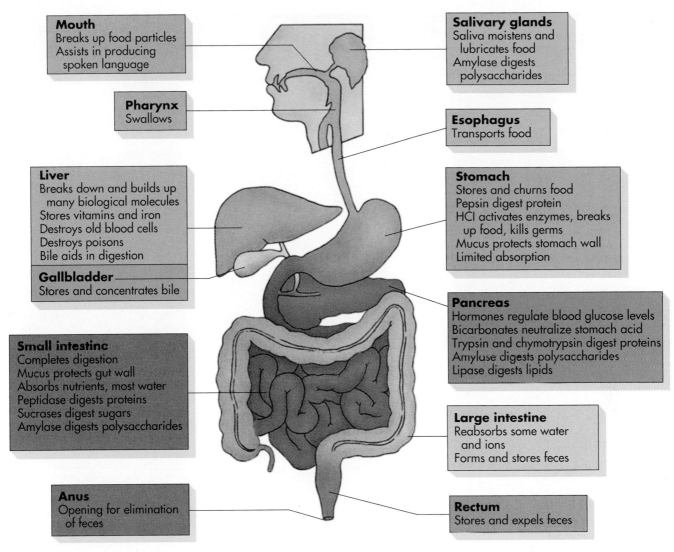

Mouth
Breaks up food particles
Assists in producing
spoken language

Pharynx
Swallows

Liver
Breaks down and builds up
many biological molecules
Stores vitamins and iron
Destroys old blood cells
Destroys poisons
Bile aids in digestion

Gallbladder
Stores and concentrates bile

Small intestine
Completes digestion
Mucus protects gut wall
Absorbs nutrients, most water
Peptidase digests proteins
Sucrases digest sugars
Amylase digests polysaccharides

Anus
Opening for elimination
of feces

Salivary glands
Saliva moistens and
lubricates food
Amylase digests
polysaccharides

Esophagus
Transports food

Stomach
Stores and churns food
Pepsin digest protein
HCl activates enzymes, breaks
up food, kills germs
Mucus protects stomach wall
Limited absorption

Pancreas
Hormones regulate blood glucose levels
Bicarbonates neutralize stomach acid
Trypsin and chymotrypsin digest proteins
Amylase digests polysaccharides
Lipase digests lipids

Large intestine
Reabsorbs some water
and ions
Forms and stores feces

Rectum
Stores and expels feces

Figure 15-1   The digestive system is approximately 30 feet long. *(From Thibodeau GA, Patton KT:* Anatomy & physiology, *ed 4, St Louis, 1999, Mosby.)*

ical portion of the digestive process. An enzyme is a protein that increases the rate of a chemical activity in the body. The three salivary glands are the parotid, sublingual, and submandibular (Figure 15-2). Amylase starts the transformation of starch to sugar. The portion of food mixed with saliva that is swallowed is called a **bolus.**

Pharynx

The pharynx or throat is divided into three portions called the *nasopharynx* (nose), *oropharynx* (mouth), and *laryngopharynx* (voice box). Food passes through the oropharynx from the mouth to the esophagus. The epiglottis is located at the junction of the esophagus and the oropharynx. The epiglottis is a small piece of tissue that closes off the

trachea to prevent food and moisture from entering the respiratory tract.

Esophagus

The esophagus is a tubelike structure that carries food from the mouth to the stomach. The bolus of food moves down the esophagus to the stomach with a slow, wavelike motion. **Peristalsis** is a wave of contraction by which food is moved through the digestive system.

Stomach

In the stomach, the food bolus mixes with hydrochloric acid and the enzymes pepsin and gastrin to become

Table 15-1 Digestive System

Organ	Size	Time for Food Passage	Enzymes Produced	Digestive Process
Mouth (salivary glands)		10-20 sec (voluntary control)	Salivary amylase Mucus*	Turn starch to glucose Lubricate
Pharynx			Mucus*	Lubricate
Esophagus	10-12 in (25-30 cm)	5-8 sec	Mucus*	Lubricate
Stomach		1-4 hr	Lipase	Digest fat
			Gastrin*	Stimulate hydrochloric acid
			Pepsinogen	Break down proteins
			Hydrochloric acid*	Dissolve minerals, kill bacteria
			Mucus*	Lubricate chyme, protect stomach lining
Pancreas			Pancreatin, trypsin	Break down protein
			Lipase	Break down fat
			Amylase, maltase	Break down starch
Liver	3 lb (1.4 kg)		Bile*	Break down fat
Small intestine		3-5 hr	Sucrase, maltase	Break down sugar
Duodenum	10 in (25 cm)		Lactase	Break down lactose
Jejunum	8 ft (2.4 m)		Lipase	Break down fat
Ileum	12 ft (3.6 m)			
Large intestine	5 ft (1.5 m)	8-24 hr	Mucus*	Lubricate
Appendix	3 in (7.5 cm)			Function unknown
Rectum	5 in (12.5 cm)	Voluntary control	Mucus*	Lubricate

*Not an enzyme.

chyme. The stomach is a saclike muscular organ that churns and squeezes food and continues its physical breakdown. Digestion of protein begins in the stomach. A few substances, such as glucose, some drugs, and alcohol, are absorbed directly into the blood through the stomach walls. The cardiac **sphincter** is a valve that prevents the chyme from flowing back into the esophagus. The pyloric sphincter controls the flow of the chyme into the intestines. It takes 1 to 4 hours for the stomach to empty the chyme into the intestines.

Small Intestine

From the stomach, the food enters the small intestine. The small intestine is longer and narrower than the large intestine. It is lined with tiny, threadlike projections of tissue called *villi* (singular, *villus*) that increase the area for absorption of nutrients. The three sections of the small intestine are the duodenum, the jejunum, and the ileum. The small intestine produces juices to aid the digestive process. Most absorption of digestive products occurs in the small

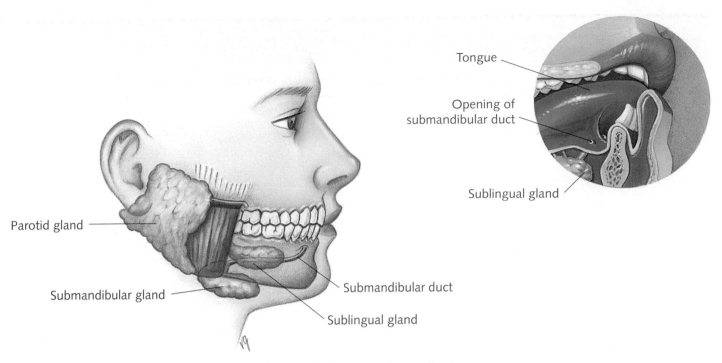

Figure 15-2   The salivary glands.

intestine. When digestion is completed, carbohydrates have been reduced to sugar (monosaccharide and disaccharide). Protein has been changed to amino acid and dipeptide. Fats have been reduced to fatty acid and glyceride.

Large Intestine

The large intestine has three major portions called the *ascending colon, transverse colon,* and *descending colon*. The appendix is a small tube of intestine descending from the side of the intestine with an unknown function in humans. Most of the water from ingested food is absorbed back into the blood through the walls of the large intestine, along with vitamins, electrolytes, and bile salts. The bacteria *Escherichia coli* normally resides in the large intestine and helps to form feces and to produce vitamin K.

The feces, or waste material, is collected in the rectum at the end of the large intestine and eliminated by **defecation** through the anus. Feces are composed of undigested food, bacteria, mucus, and water.

Peritoneum

The peritoneum is a flat serous (moist) membrane that surrounds the abdominal cavity. It lubricates and prevents friction between the organs. The mesentery is a fan-shaped projection of peritoneum that contains blood vessels and nerves. It provides support and helps to keep the abdominal organs in place by binding to them.

Accessory Organs of the Digestive System

The digestive system has three accessory organs, which aid the process of food breakdown. These exocrine, or ducted, organs carry digestive juices to the intestinal tract.

The pancreas is the only organ with both exocrine and endocrine functions. The exocrine function of the pancreas is to excrete digestive enzymes into the small intestine. The enzymes include pancreatin, trypsin, maltase, amylase, and lipase. Chapter 17 provides more information about the endocrine function of the pancreas.

The liver is the largest gland in the body. It has many important functions in addition to producing **bile** to assist in the digestion of fat. The liver converts glucose to a storage form called *glycogen*. It stores the fat-soluble vitamins (A, D, E, and K) and vitamin B_{12}. It also breaks down many of the toxins taken into the body, including alcohol. It destroys old red blood cells, reprocesses the products, and synthesizes blood proteins. The liver also produces cholesterol, coagulation products, and antibodies.

The gallbladder, located adjacent to the liver, stores bile until it is needed in the small intestine for digestion of fatty food particles.

Assessment Techniques

Five types of assessment are commonly performed on the gastrointestinal system: radiography, **endoscopy**, gastric analysis, fecal analysis, and palpation and auscultation.

Radiography

Barium is an opaque substance that, when swallowed before x-rays are taken, allows the structures of the esophagus, stomach, and small intestine to be seen. The rectum, colon, and lower portion of the small intestine can be evaluated on x-rays after a barium **enema.**

The gallbladder can be assessed using an ingested dye. The dye becomes part of the bile and aids visualization of the gallbladder on x-rays. Stones in the gallbladder may be seen as shadows.

Endoscopy

An endoscope is a small, flexible tube that can be inserted into body cavities, allowing the examiner to see body parts. Parts of the gastrointestinal system that can be assessed with an endoscope include the esophagus (esophagoscopy), stomach (gastroscopy), large intestine (colonoscopy), sigmoid colon (sigmoidoscopy), and rectum (proctoscopy) (Figure 15-3).

Gastric Analysis

Gastric analysis is the study of the gastric juices in the stomach. A nasogastric tube is used to remove stomach contents. High levels of acid may indicate an ulcer, and low levels may be caused by anemia. Gastric analysis also may be performed by administering a special dye. The rate at which the dye appears in the urine is a measurement of the amount of stomach acid. Paracentesis or insertion of a needle into the abdominal cavity to remove fluids also may be performed to sample fluids outside of the digestive tract.

Fecal Analysis

Stool specimens may be examined for the presence of microorganisms or blood (occult blood test). Watery or hard stools may indicate digestive disorders or an imbalance in diet and exercise. Black, tarry stools may indicate the presence of blood. Yellow, fatty stools may indicate a disorder of the liver.

Palpation and Auscultation

Feeling the abdomen (palpation) and listening to bowel sounds with a stethoscope (auscultation) are other methods of assessing the gastrointestinal system. A normal abdomen is flat and soft. Bowel sounds should be heard 5 to 35 times each minute.

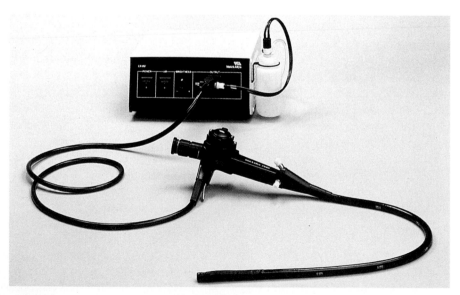

Figure 15-3 Endoscopy allows the health care worker to see inside the body. (*Courtesy Welch Allyn, Skaneateles Falls, NY.*)

Disorders of the Digestive System

Alactasia, also called "lactose intolerance," is a very common disorder. In individuals who do not produce enough of the enzyme lactase, unabsorbed lactose ferments in the intestines, leading to gas (**flatulence**), cramps, and diarrhea. Lactose is found in dairy products, such as milk. Treatment includes decreased lactose intake or dietary lactase supplements.

Appendicitis (ap-pen-dih-SI-tis) is the inflammation of the appendix for unknown causes. Appendicitis most often occurs between the ages of 10 and 30 with a lifetime risk of 7%. The signs and symptoms of appendicitis vary greatly. The person may experience fever, pain in the right lower quadrant, and a high white blood cell count. The treatment is surgical removal of the appendix, called an *appendectomy.*

Cholecystitis (ko-le-sis-TIE-tis) is inflammation of the gallbladder. It occurs when stones are formed in the gallbladder from crystallized cholesterol, bile salts, and pigments. The person feels abdominal pain. Treatment includes diet changes to reduce fats. Stones may be dissolved nonsurgically using bile acids or crushed with ultrasonic lithotripsy. In more severe cases, surgical removal of the gallbladder (**cholecystectomy**) is necessary. A laparoscopic cholecystectomy may be performed in some cases, preventing the need for major abdominal surgery.

Cirrhosis (ser-RO-sis) is a chronic degenerative condition of the liver accompanied by the formation of scar tissue. The person may experience **jaundice,** skin lesions, demineralization of the bones, enlargement of the liver, anemia, and bleeding disorders. It may result from alcoholism. The treatment is designed to relieve the symptoms, such as stopping any alcohol consumption and by diet modifications that allow the liver to rest. Cirrhosis can be fatal if the liver is severely damaged.

Colon (KO-lun) *cancer* is an abnormal growth in the large intestine. Warning signs of colon cancer include rectal bleeding, abdominal pain, and a change in bowel habits. An annual digital rectal examination and fecal occult blood test are recommended after the age of 50. Precancerous polyps can be removed to prevent cancer from occurring. Colon cancer may be treated by removal of the affected section and may require placement of an artificial anus or opening in the abdominal wall (colostomy).

Constipation (kon-stih-PAY-shun) is the inability to defecate. It is usually caused by a diet lacking in fiber or roughage, insufficient fluid intake, and lack of exercise. The person feels abdominal discomfort and distention. Treatment may include laxatives, but their frequent use may cause the bowel to become "lazy" and may be habit-forming.

Diarrhea (die-uh-REE-uh) is the passage of frequent and watery stools. It can be caused by infection, stress, or diet. Chronic diarrhea can lead to rectal tissue damage. Treatment includes a bland diet and medication (Table 15-2).

Diverticulitis (di-ver-tik-yoo-LIE-tis) is weakening of the colon wall leading to formation of a pouch (diverticula), causing infection or abscesses if fecal material is trapped. The cause is unknown. The person experiences constipation, abdominal pain, loss of bowel sounds, and sometimes fever and rectal bleeding. Surgery may be required to remove the affected part.

Food poisoning is very common and includes 300 illnesses transmitted by food. Examples include *Salmonella* species and *Listeria monocytogenes.* The person may experience headache, unrelenting diarrhea, vomiting (**emesis**), and fever. The treatment may include administration of antibiotics.

Gastritis is inflammation of the stomach lining, which may be caused by many factors including the bacteria, *Helicobacter pylori.* Symptoms of gastritis include stomach pain, heartburn, indigestion, and development of a peptic ulcer. Treatment for gastritis caused by *H. pylori* includes medications such as antibiotics to kill the bacteria and proton pump inhibitors to heal the stomach lining.

Gastroesophageal reflux disease (GERD) occurs in approximately 10% of Americans each day. Over time, this condition may lead to damage of the esophagus, difficulty swallowing, coughing, and an increased risk of throat cancer. Symptoms of GERD include frequent heartburn or chest pain, bitter taste in the mouth, difficulty swallowing, and frequent hoarseness or coughing. Treatment includes

Table 15-2   Bland Diet*

Eat	Avoid
Eggs	Raw fruits or vegetables
Meat	Carbonated beverages
Poultry	Spicy or seasoned foods
Fish	Rich desserts
Enriched fine cereals	
Milk	

*Mechanically, chemically, physiologically, and sometimes thermally nonirritating.

changes in the timing, type and amount of food eaten, and medications. If lifestyle changes and medication do not work, surgery may be used to improve the function of the esophageal sphincter that closes over the stomach.

Halitosis, or bad breath, is caused by anaerobic bacteria that produce foul-smelling sulfur compounds on the surface of the tongue and in the throat. These bacteria assist in digestion by breaking down proteins found in specific foods, mucous or phlegm, blood, and in diseased or "broken-down" oral tissue. Factors that increase the production of these sulfur compounds include dry mouth, postnasal drip, a high protein diet, and gum disease. Treatment of halitosis includes the use of compounds containing some combination of chlorine dioxide, oxychlorine, and zinc compounds and toothpaste that removes the odor. Treatment may also include scraping the tongue to remove the coating of white plaque.

Heartburn is a painful, burning sensation in the esophagus caused by the backflow of acidic chyme from the stomach. Losing excess weight, wearing loose clothing, and maintaining an upright position while eating can reduce this condition. Antacids may be used to neutralize the acid.

A *hemorrhoid* (HEM-o-royd) is a painful, dilated vein in the lower rectum or anus. Hemorrhoids may be caused by straining to defecate, the pressure of an enlarged uterus during pregnancy, insufficient fluid intake, refined food, and abuse of laxatives. The treatment includes soaking the area with a sitz bath, fecal softeners, medication, and sometimes surgery.

Hepatitis (hep-uh-TIE-tis) is a viral infection of the liver. Hepatitis A, or contagious hepatitis, is transmitted in food or water by the feces of an infected person. Hepatitis B, or serum hepatitis, is transmitted in blood, saliva, and other body fluids. Hepatitis C, D and E (non-A, non-B) have also been described by researchers. Inflammation from the hepatitis B virus is generally more severe than hepatitis A. Inflammation of the liver may also result from infection by the Epstein-Barr virus, rubella, herpes simplex, and other viral diseases. With all types of hepatitis the person experiences abdominal pain, discolored feces, and yellowed skin (jaundice). The treatment usually includes bed rest and a diet that is low in fat and high in vitamins.

Inflammatory bowel disease, including Crohn's (krohnz) disease and ulcerative colitis (UL-ser-uh-tiv ko-LIE-tis) is a common condition of unknown cause. Crohn's disease is inflammation and ulceration, usually affecting the ileum or colon or both. It causes cramping, diarrhea, and bloody stools. More than 500,000 Americans have Crohn's disease. Recently a genetic abnormality has been identified that makes some families more likely to have it. Ulcerative colitis involves the wall of the colon and rectum, leading to watery diarrhea containing blood, mucus, and pus. Emotion and stress can trigger the symptoms of inflammatory bowel disease. Treatment may include diet changes, med-

ication, and, in severe cases, surgery to remove portions of diseased bowel.

Mumps is a highly contagious viral infection of the parotid glands, most common in 5- to 15-year-olds. The person experiences a painful swelling of the parotid glands and fever. In older persons, infection may damage the testes and ovaries, leading to sterility. Treatment is directed toward relieving symptoms.

Pancreatitis (pan-kree-uh-TIE-tis) may be a mild, acute, or chronic condition resulting from gallbladder stone blockage, disease, injury, or alcoholism. Gallbladder disease and alcoholism account for 80% of the cases of acute pancreatitis. The condition causes pain, vomiting, abdominal distention, and fever. The treatment includes a low-fat diet, monitoring of blood sugar, pain relief, and sometimes surgery.

Peritonitis (per-ih-toe-NIE-tis) is an inflammation of the abdominal cavity, caused by bacteria. The bacteria may enter this normally sterile area when the bowel is injured. The person experiences vomiting and abdominal pain. The treatment includes antibiotics.

Phenylketonuria (fen-il-kee-toh-NOO-ree-ah) is an inherited disease that can lead to mental retardation if untreated. About 1 in 8000 babies born in the United States each year has this condition, which is linked to a recessive gene. Phenylketonuria causes abnormal metabolism of some proteins. The infant first experiences irritability and restlessness. Damage to the brain from this condition can lead to convulsions. Treatment includes diet modification and monitoring of the blood levels of the proteins. Newborns are routinely screened for this disorder.

Pyloric stenosis (pie-LOR-ik steh-NO-sis) is a birth defect in which a constricted pyloric sphincter does not allow food to pass easily into the small intestine. Approximately 1 in 4000 infants is affected. The baby experiences projectile vomiting, diarrhea, dehydration, and weight loss. This condition can be corrected surgically.

Tay-Sachs (tay-SAKS) disease is a recessive genetic disorder in which fat cells accumulate in the body and cause damage to normal cells. The enzyme that metabolizes lipids is not produced in the Tay-Sachs child. Symptoms appear between 3 to 6 months of age. The child experiences a progressive loss of muscle control, blindness, deafness, and paralysis as brain cells are destroyed by the accumulation of lipid compounds. There is no specific therapy for the condition although supportive measures may be given. Tay-Sachs always leads to death, usually before age 3. The condition appears more often in people of Eastern European Jewish origin.

Ulcer (UL-ser) is an open sore on the lining of the digestive tract, affecting about one of every four adults in the United States. Stomach (gastric) ulcers are called peptic ulcers. Ulcers can be caused by emotional stress that increases the secretion of stomach acid. Most duodenal ulcers are believed to be caused by a bacterial infection. The bacteria, *Helicobacter pylori*, digests the stomach lining and increases the amount of acid production. The presence of the bacteria can be determined by blood tests for antibodies, or a biopsy of stomach tissue. Ulcers can be aggravated by tobacco, caffeine, aspirin, and alcohol. The treatment includes a bland diet, reduced stress, and medication to decrease the amount of acid. If caused by bacteria, ulcers may be treated with antibiotics. Surgery to remove the affected tissue is sometimes necessary.

Issues and Innovations

Food-Borne Illness

The current trend of eating raw or rare fowl, fish, and beef is a serious health hazard. These foods are popularly sold as sushi, rare duck, steak tartare, and carpaccio. The U.S. Department of Agriculture (USDA) estimates that 37% of all fowl is infected with 1 or more of more than 2000 closely related *Salmonella* bacteria. The Food and Drug Administration (FDA) has found *Campylobacter* species in 20% of chickens and 83% of turkeys inspected. These bacteria cause diarrhea, vomiting, and fever. The condition may be mild or require medical attention. The USDA recommends that all meat be cooked to an internal temperature of 160° F to kill the bacteria. Another fad is to eat unpasteurized cheese. In 1985, 80 people in California died from eating cheese that contained *Listeria monocytogenes*. Although illegal, unpasteurized cheeses imported from Europe remain available in some stores. The Centers for Disease Control report that between 10,000 and 20,000 illnesses including from 200 to 300 deaths result each year from ingestion of the bacteria *Escherichia coli* in undercooked meat. Contaminated by feces during the slaughtering process, ground beef is the most frequent food vector of *E. coli*. Other outbreaks have been linked to contaminated apple cider, lettuce, mayonnaise, salad dressing, and water. The bacteria cause bloody diarrhea and the infection can lead to kidney failure and formation of blood clots.

Some people are sensitive to a preservative ingredient called *sulfite*, which is added to some foods. The sulfite-sensitive person experiences headache, abdominal discomfort, and diarrhea about 10 minutes after eating it. Sulfites may cause constriction of the bronchial tubes, from which more than a dozen deaths have been reported. In 1986 the FDA prohibited the use of sulfites on fruits and vegetables. Since 1987 manufacturers have been required to list sulfite content on the label of canned foods.

In 1995 the Food and Drug Administration approved irradiation of meat products for controlling disease-causing microorganisms. The approval applies to fresh and frozen red meats such as beef, lamb, and pork. The FDA concluded that irradiation does not compromise the nutritional quality of meat products. FDA had previously approved irradiation of poultry, pork, fruits, vegetables, grains, spices, seasonings, and dry enzymes used in food processing.

Eating Disorders

More than 60 million people in the United States are obese or at least 20% above the recommended weight for their age, sex, and height (Figure 15-4). In 1987 studies showed that obesity in children had risen 40% in the last 15 years, caused by increased time watching television, fast foods, and lack of exercise. Literally hundreds of diets and programs for weight reduction are now available. The healthiest and most successful programs include both calorie reduction and increased exercise.

A protein injection has been developed for use in mice that are missing a gene called *OB* (obese) that controls weight. The protein, called *leptin*, increases the mouse's metabolic rate and reduces appetite leading to weight loss. A similar gene for obesity has not yet been identified in humans. Leptin for human use has been developed with mixed results and is under clinical trial.

Bulimia is an eating disorder characterized by binge eating and purging. Binge eating, which is rapid and uncontrolled eating, may last a few minutes to several hours. Binge eaters have been known to consume more than 20,000 calories at one time. Binging is followed by self-induced vomiting (purging) or use of laxatives. Bulimia often affects teenage women but may occur in older women or men as well. It is often associated with anorexia nervosa. People with anorexia are often perfectionists who appear confident and in control. They actually lack confidence and perceive themselves as incompetent and overweight, even when significantly underweight.

Purging may cause rashes, dry skin, and swollen salivary glands. Eventually, bulimia can lead to destruction of the tooth enamel and tooth decay, irregular heart action, ulcers, colitis, muscle weakness and cramps, a perforated esophagus, and absence of a menstrual period. Resulting vitamin deficiencies and electrolyte imbalances lead to heart, liver, and kidney damage. Bulimia may result in death if untreated. Anorexia nervosa and bulimia are now considered to be addictions. They can be controlled with counseling and behavior modification programs.

Designer Foods

The Food and Drug Administration called the new biotechnologically engineered "Flav Savr" tomato as safe as tomatoes bred by conventional means. It was the first whole food to be genetically altered. The developing company, Calgene, began sales of the Flav Savr in 1994. Ge-

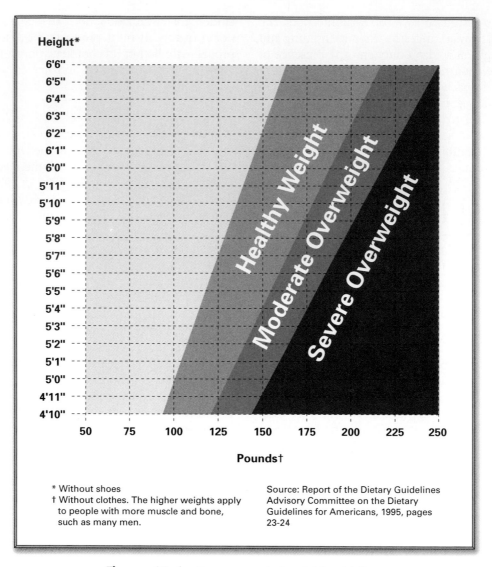

Figure 15-4 Recommended weight guidelines.

netic alteration of the tomato decreases production of the enzyme that causes ripening, causing the tomato to soften more slowly. The Flav Savr can be left on the vine longer than conventionally grown tomatoes, producing a more "homegrown" taste.

Low-fat and nonfat products are appearing in the grocery stores with increasing frequency as people become more conscious of the hazards of fat in the diet. In fact, fat-reduced items made up 7% of the processed food items introduced for sale in 1993. Most "fat substitutes" are made of water, air, protein, carbohydrates, and starches in varied combinations. Other agents such as emulsifiers and thickening agents are used to mimic the qualities of fat. The ideal fat varies for each product to produce some combination of texture, color, and taste. Substitution of fat in foods does not indicate a reduction of caloric content.

Review Questions

1. Use the following terms in one or more sentences that correctly relate their meaning.
   Bile

   Cholecystectomy

   Emesis

   Jaundice

2. Describe the four functions of the digestive system.

3. Identify the location and function of each of the following parts of the digestive system.
   Cardiac valve

   Colon

   Esophagus

   Small intestine

4. Describe three digestive system disorders.

5. List the function and organ of production for five enzymes used by the digestive system.

6. Describe the location and function of the three accessory organs of the digestive system.

7. Describe the usage of barium enemas, gastric analysis, and endoscopic procedures in assessing the function of the digestive system.

8. Describe the effects of anorexia and bulimia on the body.

Critical Thinking

1. Investigate and compare the cost of at least three tests used in diagnosing disorders of the digestive system.

2. Investigate the function of at least five common medications used in treatment of the digestive system.

3. List at least five occupations involved in the health care of digestive system disorders.

4. Use the phone book to investigate the prevalence of treatment programs for eating disorders in the community.

5. Research and review an article regarding a recent development of treatment method relating to the digestive system.

16
Urinary System

Learning Objectives

Define at least 10 terms relating to the urinary system.

Describe the two functions of the urinary system.

Identify four structures of the urinary system.

Identify the function of at least three structures of the kidney.

Identify at least five components normally found in urine.

Describe the possible cause of at least five abnormal components of urine.

Describe at least three methods used to assess disorders of the urinary system.

Key Terms

Albuminuria
(al-byoo-min-OO-ree-uh) Excess protein in the urine

Anuria
(uh-NYOO-ree-uh) Complete suppression of excretion by kidneys, absence of urine

Dialysis
(die-AL-ih-sis) Separating particles from a fluid by filtration through a semi-permeable membrane

Diuresis
(die-yoo-REE-sis) Increased excretion of urine

Dysuria
(dis-YOO-ree-uh) Painful or difficult urination

Glycosuria
(glie-ko-SOO-ree-uh) Presence of sugar in urine

Hematuria
(hem-uh-TOO-ree-uh) Presence of blood in urine

Micturition
(mik-tuh-RISH-en) Passage of urine, urination

Oliguria
(ol-ig-YOO-ree-uh) Excretion of diminished amount of urine in relation to fluid intake

Polyuria
(pol-ee-YOO-ree-uh) Passage of large amount of urine in given time

Pyuria
(pie-YOO-ree-uh) Pus in the urine

Urinalysis
(yer-rin-AL-ih-sis) Physical, chemical, or microscopic examination of urine

Urination
(yoo-ruh-NAY-shen) Discharge or passage of urine

Void
(voyd) To empty, urinate, or defecate

Urinary System Terminology*

TERM	DEFINITION	PREFIX	ROOT	SUFFIX
Cystocele	Tumor or swelling of the bladder		cyst/o	cele
Cystoscopy	Examination of the bladder		cyst/o	scopy
Lithotomy	Incision into a stone		lith	otomy
Nephrology	Study of the kidney		nephr	ology
Nephropexy	Fixation of the kidney		nephr/o	pexy
Nocturia	Urination at night	noct	uria	
Pyelonephrectomy	Removal of the kidney pelvis	pyel/o	nephr	ectomy
Pyuria	Pus in the urine	py	uria	
Renal	Pertaining to the kidney		ren	al
Renal calculus	Kidney stone		ren calculus	al

*A transition phrase or vowel may be added to or deleted from the word parts to make the combining form.

Abbreviations of the Urinary System

ABBREVIATION	MEANING
amt	Amount
BRP	Bathroom privileges
cath	Catheter
cysto	Cystoscopy
FF	Force fluids
I&O	Intake and output
IVP	Intravenous pyelogram
KUB	Kidneys, ureter, bladder
qns	Quantity not sufficient
sp gr	Specific gravity

Structure and Function of the Urinary System

There are two primary functions of the urinary system:
- To regulate the chemical composition of body fluids
- To remove body wastes by filtering blood

The urinary system filters about 180 liters of blood plasma daily. On the average, 1 to 1.5 L of urine is formed and excreted daily to remove waste products. The amount of urine formed is controlled largely by hormones. An increase in the antidiuretic hormone (ADH), from the pituitary gland, decreases the amount of water excreted by the kidneys. An increase in the amount of aldosterone, from the adrenal gland, conserves sodium in the plasma causing water to be retained. The urinary system consists of the two kidneys, the ureters, the bladder, and the urethra (Figure 16-1).

Kidneys

The basic structural unit of the urinary system is the kidney. Each kidney is about 4 inches (10 cm) long and 2 inches (5 cm) wide and weighs about 150 g. Each kidney contains about 1 to 2 million nephrons, the tiny structures that filter the blood (Figure 16-2). The nephron is the location of formation of urine and is the functional unit of the urinary system. The process by which the urine is filtered in the nephron is complex (Table 16-1). The kidney has three layers (Figure 16-3):
- The cortex, the outer layer, is composed of soft, granular, reddish-brown tissue.
- The medulla is deep red.
- The renal pelvis is the funnel-shaped innermost structure that collects and temporarily stores urine as it is formed.

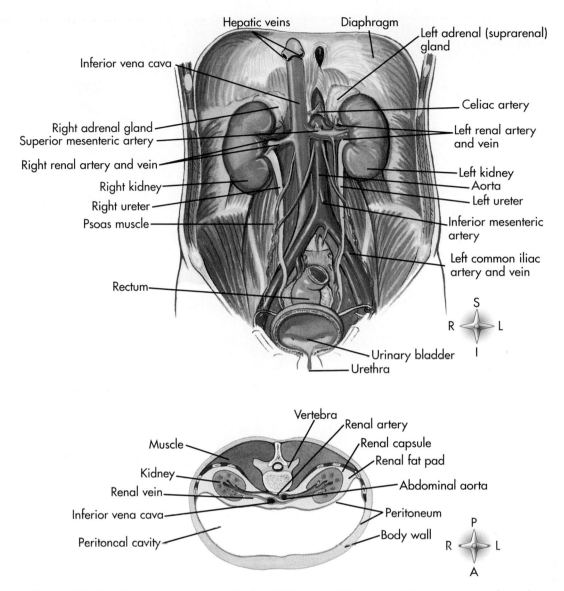

Figure 16-1   The urinary system. *(From Thibodeau GA, Patton KT: Anatomy & physiology, ed 5, St Louis, 2003, Mosby.)*

Inside the renal pelvis is the hilum, which serves as a passageway for lymph vessels, nerves, the renal artery, and renal vein.

Ureters

The ureters, small tubes composed of smooth muscle tissue, move the urine from the kidney to the bladder with peristaltic motion. Each ureter is about 10 to 12 inches (25 to 30 cm) in length. At the junction with the bladder, a valve-like narrow region of the ureter prevents urine from flowing back to the kidneys.

Bladder

The bladder, a smooth muscular sac that expands as it fills with urine, can hold up to 1 L. When the bladder fills, nerves in the muscular wall are stimulated and cause the urge to urinate. **Urination** is also called **voiding** or **micturition.**

Urethra

The urethra moves urine from the bladder to be excreted from the body. It is about 1 to 1½ inches (5 cm) in length in the female and runs through the vulva. In the male it is

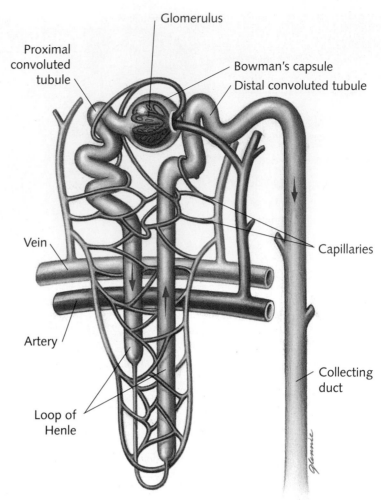

Figure 16-2 The nephron.

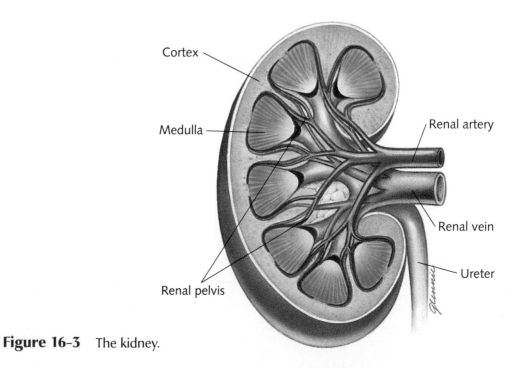

Figure 16-3 The kidney.

Table 16-1 Nephron Function

Section of Nephron	Function
Renal arterioles	Carries blood to nephron
Bowman's capsule	Filters out water, glucose, and electrolytes (Na^+, Cl^-)
Proximal tubule	Reabsorbs glucose, some electrolytes (Na^+, Cl^-) and water
Loop of Henle	Secretes urea, reabsorbs electrolytes (Na^+, Cl^-) and water
Distal tubule	Secretes ammonia, some electrolytes (K^+, H^+), and some drugs
Collecting duct	Reabsorbs electrolytes (Na^+) and urea; secretes ammonia and electrolytes (K^+, H^+)
Renal venules	Returns blood to the body

8 inches (20 cm) in length and runs through the penis. At the end of the urethra is an opening called the *urinary meatus,* through which urine passes to the outside of the body.

Urine Formation

Every minute about 600 mL of blood plasma enters the nephrons of each kidney through the renal arteries. In the glomerulus of the nephron, particles are filtered from the blood to be eliminated from the body. Water, glucose, vitamins, amino acids, and chloride salts are reabsorbed into the blood in the renal tubules. Ammonia, potassium, hydrogen ions, and some drugs are secreted into the urine by tubular cells using the process of active transport. The blood leaves the kidneys through the renal veins.

Urine normally consists of 95% water. The remaining 5% includes waste products from the breakdown of protein, hormones, electrolytes, pigments, toxins, and any abnormal components (Table 16-2). Urine is normally sterile in the kidneys and bladder.

Assessment Techniques

The primary methods of assessing the urinary system are urinalysis and examinations such as radiography and cystoscopy. Urodynamic testing, another method, measures the force of the urine flow through the system.

Urinalysis

Urinalysis is a series of tests determining urine composition. These tests can detect many body disorders. Urinalysis assesses the urine color, clarity, pH, specific gravity, odor, and volume. It can also determine the components that are not normally found in urine.

Urine color normally varies from yellow to amber or straw. Dark or red urine may indicate the presence of bile or blood. Some drugs may color urine, turning it blue, orange, or other colors.

The clarity of urine is normally clear. Cloudy composition may indicate mucus or bacteria in the urine. Alkaline urine contains calcium and may appear cloudy.

The pH of urine should be in the range of 4.8 to 7.4 (average 6) or slightly acidic. The acidity helps to prevent bacterial growth. Vegetarian diets may lead to a slightly more alkaline composition.

Specific gravity is a measurement of the density of a liquid. The normal specific gravity of urine is 1.002 to 1.040. Dehydration might lead to a higher measurement, and a condition such as diabetes insipidus would lead to a lower specific gravity.

Urine that is fresh should have no odor. An ammonia smell indicates that the specimen is old. A fruity odor may indicate the presence of sugar caused by uncontrolled diabetes mellitus. A foul or putrid smell indicates the presence of bacteria. The normal urine output in 24 hours is 1 to 1.5 L. **Anuria,** or no urine output, may indicate kidney malfunction or low blood pressure. **Oliguria,** or less than 0.5 L urine output daily, may be caused by retention of urine or dehydration. Output of more than 2 L is called **polyuria. Diuresis,** a temporary increase in the amount of urine output, can be caused by ingestion of certain beverages, drugs, or increased fluid intake.

Abnormal components of urine include sugar (**glycosuria**), proteins such as albumin or globulin (**albuminuria**), blood (hematuria), pus (**pyuria**), casts, and ketones. The presence of sugar and waste products of fat metabolism (ketones) may indicate uncontrolled diabetes mellitus. Proteins may appear during pregnancy. Urine may contain blood or pus as a result of infection or injury of the urinary system. Casts are dead cells and waste materials that indicate injury to the urinary tract.

Table 16-2   Characteristics of Urine

Characteristic	Normal	Abnormal
Volume	1-1.5 L/day	Polyuria (>2.0 L/day) Oliguria (<0.5 L/day)
Odor	None	Sweet (sugar) Ammonia (old) Offensive (bacteria)
Color	Yellow, straw, amber	Red (blood, infection, some drugs) Brown (bile) Orange, blue (drugs)
Turbidity	Clear	Cloudy (pus, bacteria, cells, fat, phosphates)
pH	4.8-7.4 (average 6)	Alkaline (phosphates, vegetarian diet)
Specific gravity	1.002-1.040	High (dehydration) Low (diuresis)

Abnormal Component	Possible Cause
Sugar (glycosuria)	Diabetes mellitus
Protein (albuminuria)	Renal disease
Ketones (ketonuria)	Incomplete fat metabolism, diabetes mellitus
Blood (hematuria)	Infection, injury
Pus (pyuria)	Infection
Bacteria (bacteriuria)	Infection
Casts	Dead cells, injury

Other Examinations

Radiological examination of the kidneys, ureters, and bladder (KUB) may be used to detect the presence of stones in the system. In a procedure called *intravenous pyelogram* (IVP), blockage in the urinary system can be seen. In this procedure, an opaque liquid called a *contrast medium* is injected into a blood vessel. A series of x-rays are then taken as the liquid passes through the system.

Another procedure used to examine the bladder is called *cystoscopy*. To view the inside of the bladder and urethra, a cystoscope is inserted in the urethra, and the bladder is inflated with water or air. Minor surgical procedures, such as taking tissue samples for biopsy, are performed using the cystoscope.

Urodynamic tests determine the force of the flow of urine through the system. The rate may be measured with uroflowmetry. Bladder and sphincter muscle control can be assessed with the use of electromyography (EMG).

Disorders of the Urinary System

Cystitis (sis-TIE-tis) is inflammation of the bladder caused by many different types of bacteria. Cystitis more commonly occurs in women than in men because of the shorter length of the urethra. The leading causative organism is *Escherichia coli*, or *E. coli*, which, through poor hygiene, may be carried from the rectum to the urinary tract. The person may experience painful urination or **dysuria**, the urge to urinate frequently, or blood in the urine, known as **hematuria.** Treatment usually includes an increase in fluid intake and antibiotics. Although cystitis may also be caused by tumors or calculi, many cases may be prevented by using good hygiene practices.

Edema (eh-DEE-ma) is an abnormal accumulation of fluid in the tissue intercellular space. This area may be swollen locally in one part of the body or throughout all tissues of the body (systemic). Edema caused by kidney (renal) failure is systemic. It may be treated by use of **dialysis** and diuretic medication.

Nephritis (neh-FRY-tis), which is inflammation of the kidneys, may occur as a result of illness or chronic cystitis. Pyelonephritis (pie-eh-lo-nef-RIE-tis) is an inflammation of the kidney pelvis and the nephron. Symptoms are similar to those of cystitis but more commonly involve back pain. Untreated nephritis may cause permanent damage to the kidney tissues. Treatment includes antibiotics and increased fluid intake.

Renal calculus (RE-nal KAL-kyoo-lus) is a kidney stone. Kidney stones occur in about 1 out of 1000 people. Calculi are composed of uric acid and calcium salts. Although the specific cause is not known, a lack of adequate fluid intake and large doses of vitamins, especially vitamin C, may lead to kidney stone formation. The person feels extreme pain when an area of the kidney or ureter is blocked by the stone. Treatment depends on the location and size of the stone and might include surgical removal. Lithotripsy (LITH-o-trip-see) has become an alternative treatment.

Renal (REE-nul) *failure,* the absence of urine formation, can be acute or chronic. When the kidneys fail, nitrogen wastes and fluids build up in the tissues, leading to many complications, such as congestive heart failure. It may be fatal. Acute renal failure may result from trauma, toxins, or hemorrhage. It is often treated with restriction of fluids, antibiotics, and diuretic medications. Acute renal failure is often reversible. Chronic renal failure may result from other conditions such as high blood pressure, diabetes mellitus, and autoimmune disorders. Chronic renal failure develops slowly and may have initial symptoms of sluggishness, fatigue, and mental slowness. The condition is eventually called *end-stage renal disease* (ESRD) when the kidneys have lost all function. Renal failure results in 80,000 deaths in the United States each year. Treatment includes special diet considerations, diuretic medications, dialysis, and transplant. In children, chronic renal insufficiency (CRI) is treated with growth hormone.

Uremia (yoo-REE-mee-uh) is a condition in which the kidneys do not filter the blood. Waste products and urea stay in the blood and tissues, preventing nutrients and oxygen from entering the cells. Uremia may result from trauma, hypotension, nephritis, renal failure, and other conditions. The person may experience nausea, vomiting,

headache, and coma. White crystals, called *uremic frost,* may form on the skin as the body attempts to excrete the uremic waste. Treatment may include a restricted diet and dialysis to remove the waste products.

Urethritis (yoo-rih-THRIE-tis) is acute or chronic inflammation of the urethra. It may be caused by bacteria or chemical irritation from agents such as bubble bath. The person experiences frequent, painful urination, and a red and painful urinary meatus (mee-AY-tus) and surrounding tissues. Urethritis can lead to a narrowing or stricture of the urethra resulting from the formation of scar tissue. Treatment may include antibiotics, sitz baths, and an increase in fluid intake.

Urinary incontinence (in-KON-tih-nens) is the inability to control urination. A number of factors, including lack of muscle control, immobility, or spinal cord or neurological damage, may cause urinary incontinence. Treatment may include retraining the bladder, drugs, or surgery.

Urinary retention is the inability to urinate when the urge is felt or the bladder is full. Retention may result from an obstruction, drugs, trauma, or neurological disorders. The person may experience abdominal pain, distention, and excretion of small amounts of urine. Treatment focuses on the underlying cause and may include inserting a tube (catheterization) to empty the bladder.

Urinary tract infections (UTI), usually caused by bacteria, may affect the bladder, kidneys, or prostate. The person may experience fever, lower back pain, and frequent, painful, and bloody urination. Antibiotics and sitz baths may be used to relieve the infection and discomfort.

Issues and Innovations

Dialysis

Dialysis is the filtration of body fluids through a semipermeable membrane or machine instead of the kidneys to remove excess water and waste. Hemodialysis is the filtration of the blood using an artificial membrane. Blood is removed from a vein, filtered slowly through the machine, and returned to the body. It may take several hours to complete the process. Hemodialysis may be required two or three times weekly to replace failed kidney function. The procedure is expensive and carries the risk of infection and damage to blood cells.

Another form of dialysis uses the peritoneal membrane of the abdomen as the filter to remove the wastes from body fluid. Continuous abdominal peritoneal dialysis (CAPD) requires insertion of a cannula into the abdominal cavity. A solute of glucose and salts is poured into the abdominal cavity to combine with the waste products. The fluid is then drained out of the cavity by gravity. Peritoneal dialysis can be performed in the home, although a risk of infection exists because of the opening into the body cavity. Other complications include the development of scar tissue in the abdomen called *adhesions*.

Kidney Transplant

Kidney transplant is another method of restoring kidney function. Drawbacks include the difficulty of matching tissues, high expense, and a shortage of donor kidneys. Although the cost of kidney transplant is high, $75,000 to $100,000, this is still less than the cost of treating a patient with kidney failure using dialysis over a period of 6 years (Table 16-3).

Kidney transplant is now routine and has a success rate of greater than 95%. Approximately 11,000 kidney transplants are completed each year. New drug treatments reduce the chance of rejection of the transplanted kidney. The shortage of donors, both living and cadaver, is a concern for health professionals. According to the National Institutes of Health, in 1999 there were 8839 cadaver, 3583 related donor, and 1061 unrelated donor kidney transplants. In comparison, more than 50,000 people were waiting for kidney transplants in 2001.

Lithotripsy

Extracorporeal shock wave lithotripsy uses high-energy pressure or sound waves sent through the kidney to disintegrate kidney stones. The "shock wave" may be sent

Table 16-3	Cost of Transplants*
Organ	**Cost**
Heart	$300,000
Heart/lung	$300,000-$350,000
Small bowel	$350,000
Kidney	$75,000-$100,000
Kidney/pancreas	$150,000
Liver	$250,000-$275,000
Lung	$200,000-$250,000
Pancreas	$100,000

*Costs cited from the National Foundation for Transplants. Costs include hospital and physician fees.

through water or air. Two fluoroscopic monitors are used to position the lithotripsy machine and target the stone precisely. Up to 2000 "shocks" may be needed to dissolve a stone. Although the procedure may infrequently cause bleeding or heart irregularities, it may prevent the need for surgery to remove the stone (Figure 16-4).

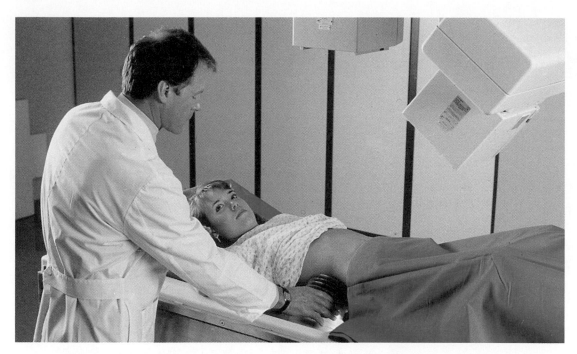

Figure 16-4   Lithotripsy allows removal of the kidney stones without surgery. *(Courtesy Siemens Medical Solutions USA.)*

Review Questions

1. Use the following terms in one or more sentences that correctly relate their meaning.
   Diuresis
   Glycosuria
   Polyuria
   Urination

2. Describe the two functions of the urinary system.

3. Describe the function of the four structures of the urinary system.

4. Describe the function of the structures of the kidney.

5. Describe the location and function of each of the following parts of the urinary system.
   Bladder
   Renal pelvis
   Cortex
   Ureter

6. List five components normally found in urine.

7. List five abnormal components of urine and one possible cause of each.

8. Differentiate between peritoneal dialysis and hemodialysis.

9. Describe three methods of assessment of the urinary system.

Critical Thinking

1. Investigate and compare the cost of at least three tests used in diagnosing disorders of the urinary system.

2. Investigate the function of at least five common medications used in treatment of the urinary system.

3. List at least five occupations involved in the health care of urinary system.

4. Investigate the recommended dietary needs after renal failure.

5. Investigate and compare the cost of dialysis and kidney transplant. What other factors might be considered in choosing the method of treatment for renal failure?

6. List five beverages that act as diuretics.

7. Investigate the function of each part of the nephron.

8. Research and review an article regarding a recent development or treatment method relating to the urinary system.

17
Endocrine System

Learning Objectives

Define 10 terms relating to the endocrine system.

Describe the function of the endocrine system.

Identify at least nine endocrine system structures.

Identify at least one hormone produced by each of the 10 endocrine glands.

Describe at least five disorders of the endocrine system.

Describe at least three methods used to assess the function of the endocrine system.

Key Terms

Basal Metabolic Rate
(BAY-sal met-uh-BOL-ik rayt) Minimal energy expended for respiration, circulation, peristalsis, muscle tone, body temperature, and glandular activity of the body at rest

Endocrine
(EN-do-krin) Glands that secrete internally into blood or lymph

Exophthalmos
(ek-sof-THAL-mus) Abnormal protrusion of eyeball

Gonadotropin
(go-NAD-o-trope-in) Any hormone that stimulates the reproductive organs

Hormone
(HORE-mone) Chemical substance produced in the body that has specific regulatory effect on the activity of a specific organ

Hyperglycemia
(hi-per-glie-SEE-mee-uh) Abnormally high sugar content in the blood

Hypoglycemia
(hi-po-glie-SEE-mee-uh) Abnormally low sugar content in the blood

Immunoassay
(im-yoo-no-AS-say) Quantitative determination of antigenic substances by examination of blood

Polydipsia
(pol-ee-DIP-see-uh) Excessive thirst persisting for long periods of time

Polyphagia
(pol-ee-FAY-jee-ah) Excessive hunger

Polyuria
(pol-ee-YOO-ree-uh) Passage of a large volume of urine in a given time

Prostaglandin
(pros-tah-GLAN-din) Lipid molecule that has hormonelike effect; tissue hormone

Puberty
(PYOO-ber-tee) Period during which the secondary sexual characteristics begin to develop and the capability of sexual reproduction is attained

Endocrine System Terminology*

TERM	DEFINITION	PREFIX	ROOT	SUFFIX
Acromegaly	Enlargement of the extremities		acro	megaly
Adenoma	Tumor of a gland		aden	oma
Adenomalacia	Softening of a gland		aden/o	malacia
Adrenalectomy	Removal of the adrenal gland		adrenal	ectomy
Endocrine	To secrete inside	endo	crine	
Hyperglycemia	Too much sugar in the blood	hyper	glyc	emia
Pancreatitis	Inflammation of the pancreas		pancreat	itis
Polyphagia	Excessive hunger	poly	phagia	
Polyuria	Excessive excretion of urine	poly	uria	
Thyroidectomy	Removal of the thyroid		thyroid	ectomy

*A transition phrase or vowel may be added to or deleted from the word parts to make the combining form.

Abbreviations of the Endocrine System

ABBREVIATION	MEANING
ADH	Antidiuretic hormone
ANS	Autonomic nervous system
BMR	Basal metabolic rate
DM	Diabetes mellitus
FSH	Follicle stimulating hormone
GH	Growth hormone
SIAD	Syndrome of inappropriate antidiuretic hormone
STH	Somatotropic hormone
TH	Thyroid hormone
TSH	Thyroid-stimulating hormone

Structure and Function of the Endocrine System

The primary function of the **endocrine** system is to produce **hormones** that monitor and coordinate body activities (Figure 17-1). Hormones are chemical messengers secreted by the endocrine glands. Each type of hormone moves through the blood to its own target cells, which react specifically to it. The endocrine glands secrete hormones directly into the blood stream. Hormones may be proteins, glycoproteins, polypeptides, amino-acid derivatives, or lipids.

Hormones may be divided into three categories based on their function:
- Tropic hormones target other endocrine structures to increase their growth and secretions.
- Sex hormones influence reproductive changes.
- Anabolic hormones stimulate the process of building tissues.

Hormones direct many body processes including growth, metabolism, and reproductive functions (Table 17-1). Hormones regulate the body's reaction to stress and maintain the internal environment (homeostasis). The importance of hormones in the body can be demonstrated by the numerous and diverse disorders that occur when the amount of hormone produced is either too great (hypersecretion) or too little (hyposecretion). The quantity of hormones in the blood is monitored through a negative-feedback mechanism, which stimulates more secretion when needed (Figure 17-2). Additionally, the autonomic nervous system controls and stimulates the secretion of the hormones of the adrenal gland.

Table 17-1   Endocrine Glands and Hormones*

Gland	Hormone	Function
Pituitary	Somatotropin (or growth hormone [GH])	Promotes tissue growth and development
Pineal	Melatonin	Supports biological clock
Thyroid	Thyroxine (TH)	Regulates metabolic rate
Parathyroid	Parathyroid hormone (PTH)	Regulates calcium and phosphates in blood stream and bones
Thymus	Thymosin	Stimulates development of T cells
Adrenal	Epinephrine	Regulates autonomic nervous system response
Pancreatic islets	Insulin	Regulates blood sugar
Ovaries	Estrogen	Regulates female sexual characteristics
Testes	Testosterone	Regulates male sexual characteristics

*Most of the endocrine glands secrete more than one hormone with functions not listed here.

Glands and Their Hormones

Hypothalamus

The hypothalamus is a structure located above the pituitary gland that translates nervous system impulses into endocrine system messages. It regulates the secretions of the pituitary adenohypophysis.

Pituitary

The pituitary gland (hypophysis) is sometimes called the "master" gland because the hormones that it produces regulate the secretion of other glands. It is located at the base of the brain and is divided into two parts, the anterior and posterior.

The anterior pituitary (adenohypophysis) produces seven hormones:

- Thyroid-stimulating hormone (TSH) stimulates the growth and secretion of the thyroid gland.
- Adrenocorticotrophic hormone (ACTH) stimulates the growth and secretion of the adrenal cortex.
- Follicle-stimulating hormone (FSH) stimulates the growth of the ovarian follicle, production of estrogen in females, and production of sperm in males.

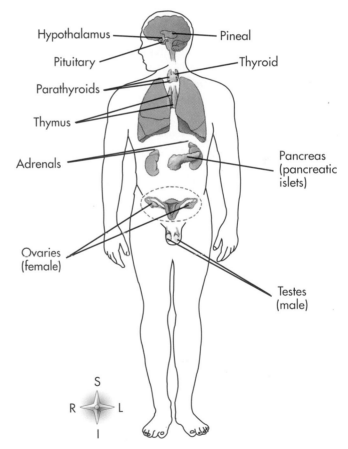

Figure 17-1   The endocrine system. *(From Thibodeau GA, Patton KT:* Anatomy & physiology, *ed 5, St Louis, 2003, Mosby.)*

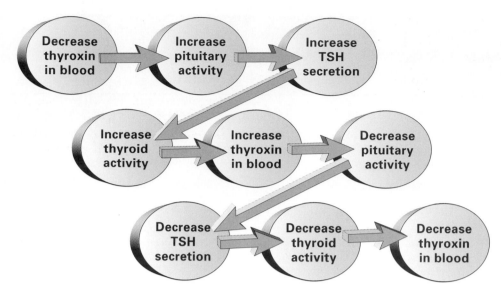

Figure 17-2 The triggered factor for the negative feedback mechanism of hormone control may be the concentration of a hormone or other substance such as calcium in the blood.

- Luteinizing hormone (LH) stimulates ovulation and the formation of the corpus luteum in the menstrual cycle.
- In males, the luteinizing hormone is called *interstitial cell-stimulating hormone (ICSH)* and stimulates the secretion of testosterone.
- Lactogenic hormone (prolactin) stimulates the secretion of milk and influences maternal behavior.
- Somatotropic hormone (STH), also called the *growth hormone (GH)*, accelerates the growth of the body.

The posterior pituitary (neurohypophysis) produces two hormones:

- Antidiuretic hormone (ADH), or vasopressin, maintains water balance by increasing the reabsorption of water by the kidneys.
- Oxytocin (pitocin) promotes the ejection of milk and stimulates uterine contractions during pregnancy.

Pineal Body

The pea-sized pineal body is a gland located deep within the brain. It produces the hormone melatonin. Melatonin regulates the release of substances in the hypothalamus of the brain that influence secretion of the pituitary **go-nadotropins** or sex hormones. It is believed that melatonin inhibits the activity of the ovaries and LH secretion. Thus it influences the menstrual cycle and onset of **pu-**

berty. Melatonin is also believed to be involved in the regulation of the "biological clock" or body's physiological reaction to changes in light and dark.

Thyroid

The thyroid, a butterfly-shaped gland with two lobes, is located in the neck. The thyroid produces hormones that regulate body metabolism. They are called *thyroxine* and *triiodothyronine*. Iodine is required for production of both of these hormones. Calcitonin, another hormone produced by the thyroid, decreases the amount of calcium in the blood.

Parathyroid

The parathyroid is actually four tiny glands attached to the back of the thyroid gland. They secrete parathyroid hormone, which also affects the amount of calcium in the blood. This hormone increases the blood's calcium level by breaking the bonds of calcium and phosphorus compounds in the bones. It also increases the rate of phosphorus excretion by the kidneys.

Thymus

The thymus is a butterfly-shaped gland located above the heart. It produces the hormone thymosin, which stimulates the lymphoid organs to produce T-lymphocytes or antibodies in newborns and young children. The thymus gland provides additional immunity until it disintegrates and is replaced with fatty tissue at the time of puberty.

Pancreas

The pancreas, located behind the stomach, produces the hormones insulin and glucagon. Insulin regulates transportation of sugar, fatty acids, and amino acids into the cells. It also participates in protein synthesis. The action of glucagon opposes that of insulin by increasing the blood sugar level. The pancreas is the only gland that has both endocrine and exocrine functions. Chapter 15 provides more information about the exocrine function of the pancreas.

Adrenal Glands

The adrenal glands are located above the kidneys. Each gland can actually be divided into two layers called the *adrenal cortex* and *adrenal medulla*. The adrenal cortex produces about 30 hormones including glucocorticoids, mineralocorticoids, and androgens. Three of the most important hormones of the cortex are cortisol, aldosterone, and androgen. Glucocorticoids produce an antiinflammatory response, metabolize food, and make new cells. Mineralocorticoids control the body's fluid level and electrolyte balance by influencing the rate of excretion of mineral salts (sodium and potassium) by the kidneys. Androgenic hormones stimulate development of male sexual characteristics, including increased body size, and affect the buildup of protein tissues (anabolism).

The adrenal medulla produces epinephrine (adrenalin) and norepinephrine. Epinephrine initiates the "fight or flight" reaction to stress. Epinephrine increases heart rate, blood pressure, and blood sugar, and it decreases the blood flow to the internal organs.

Gonads

The gonads are the primary sexual glands. In the female, the ovaries produce estrogen and progesterone. The ovaries are located in the lower abdomen beside the uterus. Estrogen and progesterone stimulate breast development, hair placement, and menstruation. Estrogen also initiates ovulation. Progesterone assists in the normal development of pregnancy.

In the male, the primary sexual organs are the testes, located in the external scrotal sac. The testes produce the hormone testosterone. Testosterone stimulates secondary characteristics of the male including a lowered voice, body hair growth, and muscular development.

Prostaglandins

Prostaglandins are fatty hormones that are produced by tissues throughout the body that influence the tissues surrounding the area. At least 16 types have been identified. Prostaglandins are known to decrease blood pressure, cause fever, increase hydrochloric acid secretion in the stomach, increase uterine contraction during pregnancy, and influence intestinal peristalsis. These "tissue hormones" are broken down quickly in the body.

Hormonal Changes of Puberty

Puberty is the time during which the body matures sexually. Hormones of the pituitary gland direct the changes that occur in puberty. These stimulate the gonads to secrete the hormones that cause the testes and ovaries to mature. In males, the testes enlarge. In females, the menstrual cycle (menarche) begins. Both acquire the ability to reproduce. Chapter 20 provides more information about the reproductive system.

The adrenal gland secretes the hormones that begin the development of secondary sexual characteristics, those body features different in males and females but not directly affecting reproduction. In the male, the voice deepens and facial hair begins to grow. In the female, the breasts enlarge and fatty tissue is deposited around the hips. In both males and females, height and weight increase. Emotional changes, which have been attributed to hormonal changes, may also occur during this growing time.

Hormonal Changes of Pregnancy

With the onset of pregnancy, many hormonal changes occur that influence the appearance and function of the woman's body. The placenta, or interfacing organ between the fetal and maternal circulation, produces a hormone called *human chorionic gonadotropin* (HCG). It stimulates the development and secretions of the ovaries to maintain the uterine lining. Human chorionic gonadotropin can be detected in the urine and is used for pregnancy testing.

The increased estrogen and progesterone from the ovaries is maintained until the placenta begins to produce these hormones for the duration of the pregnancy. Progesterone increases the mobility of the pelvic and lower back bones to allow the birthing process and may also result in backache. Dilation of the ureters and renal pelvis may lead to urinary frequency. Progesterone also decreases the mobility and tone of the gastrointestinal tract and causes relaxation of the pyloric sphincter and may cause heartburn and constipation.

During pregnancy, the pituitary and thyroid glands increase in size. This results in a higher metabolic rate. The adrenal gland's secretions increase, especially aldosterone. An increase in the plasma level of insulin may be due to an increase in lipids or fats in the blood. Additionally, the destruction of insulin is faster during pregnancy, which may lead to a condition called "gestational" diabetes in which the woman's pancreas cannot produce enough insulin. The changes in the hormonal levels during early pregnancy may also be responsible for the nausea and vomiting called "morning sickness."

Hormonal Changes of Menopause

Menopause, or climacteric, is the term used to describe the time during which the female stops menses. Menopause occurs after a decrease in secretion of the gonadotropins follicle-stimulating hormone (FSH) and luteinizing hormone (LH). This change leads to a decrease in the secretion of the hormone estrogen by the ovaries. Hot flashes, periods of feeling extreme heat, are the only universal symptoms of menopause. Estrogen replacement therapy may be given after menopause in some instances.

Assessment Techniques

Hormonal disorders except diabetes mellitus (type 1 and type 2) and thyroid disease are rare. Thyroid function may be assessed using the **basal metabolic rate** (BMR) and protein-bound iodine (PBI) studies. However, results of both of these tests can be affected by many other factors. Several newer methods now used for assessment of the endocrine disorders include **immunoassay,** radioiodine uptake (RAIU) studies, and glucose tolerance testing (GTT).

- Basal metabolic rate is the amount of energy needed to maintain the functions of a resting body, including circulation, respiration, digestion, and cell metabolism. The basal metabolic rate is measured by a test called *indirect calorimetry,* which measures the amount of oxygen consumed.
- Protein-bound iodine (PBI) is a blood test to measure the amount of proteins attached to thyroxine. Test re-

sults may be influenced by cough syrups, iodine used in tests, diuretics, steroids, and pregnancy.
- Immunoassay is a chemical test in which a blood specimen is mixed with a specific agent. The number of antigens formed indicates the presence of certain hormones.
- Radioiodine uptake (RAIU) involves drinking radioactive iodine and measuring the iodine absorbed by the thyroid with a Geiger counter. The rate that the thyroid removes the iodine from the blood indicates how well it is functioning.
- The glucose tolerance test (GTT) assesses the function of the pancreas, using urine and blood specimens.
- Glucose is given and specimens are compared over time. This measures the efficiency of the insulin production of the pancreas.

Disorders of the Endocrine System

Acromegaly (ak-ro-MEG-uh-lee) is an enlargement of the bones of the hands, feet, and jaws (Figure 17-3). It results from an increased secretion of somatotropic (so-mah-to-TROP-ik) hormone, usually caused by a pituitary tumor. Headache and lethargy also result. Treatment includes surgical removal of the tumor or radiation to destroy gland tissue.

Addison's (AD-ih-sunz) disease is caused by hyposecretion of the hormones produced by the cortex of the adrenal gland. The person experiences excessive skin pigmentation, decreased blood sugar, and decreased blood pressure,

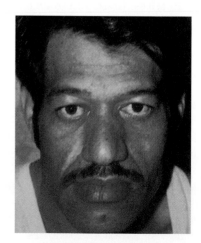

Figure 17-3 Acromegaly is characterized by enlargement of the bones of the hands, feet, and jaws with an increase in the soft-tissue covering them. *(Courtesy Henry M. Seidel, MD.)*

which result in muscle weakness, fatigue, gastrointestinal disturbances, and dehydration. Treatment includes administration of cortisone, a decrease in sodium intake, and monitoring the level of potassium and sodium in the blood.

Cretinism (KREE-tin-izm) is a condition resulting from a congenital deficiency of thyroid secretion or hypothyroidism (hi-per-THI-royd-izm). The basal metabolic rate, and mental and physical growth are decreased. Early indications of hypothyroidism include jaundice, excessive drowsiness, and a hoarse cry. Hypothyroidism can be treated by oral administration of thyroxine, and early treatment can minimize mental and physical damage.

Cushing's (KOOSH-ingz) syndrome is a disorder that causes hyperactivity of the adrenal glands, which has been triggered by oversecretion of the pituitary hormone ACTH. The person has a redistribution of fat, giving a distinctive "moon face" and "buffalo hump" appearance. Sexual dystrophy, increased blood pressure, unusual hair growth or hirsutism (HER-soot-izm), and easy bruising also result. Treatment depends on the cause of the hormone imbalance. If the cause is a tumor, it is surgically removed.

Diabetes insipidus (die-uh-BEE-tez in-SIP-i-dus) results from an acquired or inherited decrease in antidiuretic hormone secreted by the pituitary. The main sign is an increase in urine production (polyuria) that leads to an intense thirst (polydipsia), weakness, constipation, and dry skin. Treatment includes giving antidiuretic hormone by injection or nasal spray.

Diabetes mellitus (die-uh-BEE-tez mel-LIE-tus) is a complex disorder of carbohydrate, fat, and protein metabolism resulting from insufficient insulin production by the pancreas. Its cause is unknown. The person experiences unusual thirst, or **polydipsia,** increased urine output—**polyuria,** and unusual hunger—**polyphagia** (Table 17-2). **Hyperglycemia** may result, which is a greater-than-normal amount of glucose in the blood, causing nausea, headache, coma, and, if untreated, eventual death.

There are two main types of diabetes. Type 1 (formerly called insulin-dependent diabetes mellitus [IDDM]) can occur at any age and results when the pancreas does not produce insulin. Treatment includes injection of insulin to meet this need. Transplantation of a donor pancreas has been used with varied success. Type 2 diabetes (formerly non–insulin dependent diabetes mellitus [NIDDM]) is linked with obesity. The pancreas does not produce enough insulin to meet the need of the body. Treatment may include oral hypoglycemic medication and weight loss. In 2002 Florida became the first state to offer screening for diabetes mellitus to every newborn. The newborns will be monitored throughout their lifetime. The purpose of this program is to identify newborns with genetic risk for developing type 1 diabetes to refer them to clinical trials and research designed to end the disease.

Table 17-2 Signs and Symptoms of Diabetes Mellitus	
Hyperglycemia	**Hypoglycemia**
Increased thirst	Weakness
Increased urination	Trembling
Weight loss	Drowsiness
Increased appetite	Headache
Nausea	Confusion
Vomiting	Dizziness
Fatigue	Double vision
Ketoacidosis	Insulin shock

Dwarfism (DWARF-izm) usually is characterized by a normal trunk and head with shortened extremities. It results from hyposecretion of the growth hormone of the pituitary gland, which has been caused by a tumor, infection, genetic factors, or trauma (Figure 17-4). If discovered in the development years, dwarfism can be treated with injections of a somatotropic hormone (growth hormone) for 5 years or more. Dwarfism does not affect intelligence.

Gigantism (ji-GAN-tizm), or giantism, is an excessive growth of the long bones caused by hypersecretion of the somatotropic hormone. Treatment may include hormones to control growth and perhaps removal or destruction of the pituitary if diagnosed early.

Graves' (grayvz) *disease* is caused by hyperthyroidism (hi-per-THIE-royd-izm) or thyrotoxicosis (thie-ro-tok-sih-KO-sis). The person experiences nervousness, rapid pulse, weight loss, irritability, sensitivity to heat, increased basal metabolic rate and blood sugar, and sometimes **exophthalmos,** or protruding eyeballs. Treatment includes removal of part or all of the thyroid and drugs to decrease the thyroxine (thie-ROK-sin) level. Adults over 40 can be given radioactive iodine to destroy thyroid tissue.

Hyperparathyroidism (hi-per-pare-ah-THIE-roid-izm) causes hypercalcemia (hi-per-kal-SEE-mee-uh), an increased calcium blood level. It can cause kidney stone formation. The calcium is taken from the bones, which can lead to fractures and deformities. This condition is often caused by adenoma (ad-uh-NO-mah), a glandular tumor, and treatment requires its removal.

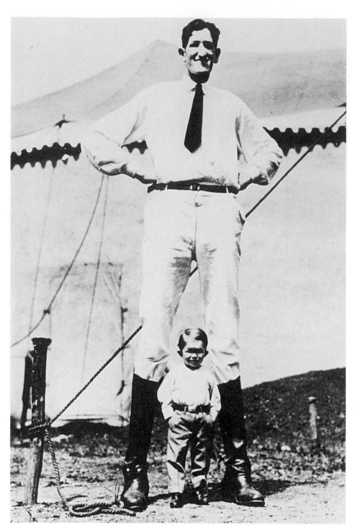

Figure 17-4 Dwarfism results from low levels of pituitary growth hormone during the early years and is the opposite of the condition of gigantism. *(From Seeley RR, Stephens TD, Tate P:* Anatomy & physiology, *ed 3, St Louis, 1995, Mosby.)*

Hypoglycemia results from increased insulin production by the pancreas. The low blood sugar causes fatigue, tremors, cold sweats, headache, and weight disturbances. Treatment includes a diet that is low in carbohydrates and high in protein.

Hypoparathyroidism (hi-po-par-uh-THIE-roid-izm) is a decreased secretion of parathyroid hormone that causes tetany. Blood calcium levels are decreased, interrupting function of the nerves. The person experiences a convulsive twitching. Death may result if the respiratory muscles are affected. Treatment is giving oral supplements of vitamin D, calcium, and parathormone.

Hypothyroidism (hi-po-THIE-royd-izm), also called *Hashimoto's disease,* results from an insufficient production of thyroxine. It may be caused by an autoimmune disorder

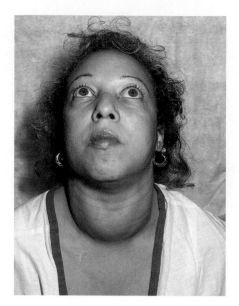

Figure 17-5 Simple goiter is a painless enlargement of the thyroid gland that may result from inadequate iodine intake in the diet. *(From Swartz MH:* Textbook of physical diagnosis, *ed 3, Philadelphia, 1998, WB Saunders.)*

of iodine deficiency. The thyroid enlarges to compensate for the deficiency, resulting in goiter (GOY-ter) (Figure 17-5). This leads to increase in fat tissue and sluggishness. Myxedema (mik-seh-DEE-muh) is the most severe form of hypothyroidism. The person experiences edema, obesity, lethargy, decreased heart rate, decreased intelligence, sensitivity to cold, and coarse skin. Treatment includes administration of oral thyroid extract.

Syndrome of inappropriate antidiuretic hormone (SIAD) involves water intoxication and the dilution of intracellular and extracellular body tissues, usually resulting from lung cancer. Antidiuretic hormone production is increased in the pituitary gland. The condition may lead to convulsions and death. Treatment is removal of the cancer, restriction of fluids, and drug therapy.

Virilism (VIR-i-lizm) results from increased secretion in the adrenal glands. The female may develop male sexual characteristics, including facial hair, broad shoulders, and small breasts. Treatment focuses on the cause of hypersecretion by the gland.

Issues and Innovations

Steroid Abuse

Abuse of hormones continues to be a problem, especially by athletes hoping for better performance. The Youth Risk and Behavior Surveillance System study of 1995 reported that 4.9% of adolescent boys and 2.4% of adolescent girls had used steroids at least one time in the last year.

Performance-enhancing or "ergogenic" steroids are commonly abused. These include somatotropic, or growth hormone, and androgenic anabolic steroids such as testosterone. The benefit, if any, from use of these hormones in sports training is far less than the health risk imposed. The effects of even a short use of these steroids can be long lasting or permanent.

Synthetic growth hormone was developed to treat children with a deficiency of this pituitary hormone. Some athletes believe that supplementing exercise with growth hormone will improve performance, but such improvement has not been shown scientifically. It is known that an oversupply of the hormone in adults leads to physical changes of acromegaly.

Androgenic anabolic steroids, including synthetic drugs similar to the hormone testosterone, have been banned by most major sports organizations. Muscle growth can be increased with use of anabolic steroids, but the risks and complications far exceed the benefits. Effects on men include early baldness, stunted growth, changes in liver structure, liver tumors, decreased sperm production, testicular atrophy, enlarged breasts, and increased risk of cardiovascular disease. Effects on women include menstrual irregularities, complete loss of menstrual cycle (amenorrhea), abnormal hair placement (hirsutism), baldness, and irreversible deepening of the voice. Among users of both sexes, bad breath, severe acne, headache, dizziness, hypertension, mood swings, and aggressiveness ("roid rages") are commonplace.

In 1988 anabolic steroids were classified as a controlled substance by federal law. Conviction for the selling of steroids results in a minimum sentence of 5 years in prison. The use of steroids may result in 1 to 6 years in prison.

Review Questions

1. Use the following terms in one or more sentences that correctly relate their meaning.

   Endocrine

   Hormone

   Hyperglycemia

   Polyphagia

   Polyuria

2. Describe the functions of the endocrine system.

3. Describe the location and function of each of the following parts of the endocrine system.

   Adrenal medulla

   Pineal body

   Pituitary

   Prostaglandin

4. Describe three tests used to assess the function of the endocrine system.

5. Describe three changes that occur during puberty as a result of hormonal changes.

6. Describe three changes that occur during pregnancy as a result of hormonal changes.

7. List five side effects and risks of using androgenic anabolic hormones.

Critical Thinking

1. Investigate and compare the cost of at least three tests used to diagnose disorders of the endocrine system.

2. Investigate the function of at least five common medications used in treatment of the endocrine system.

3. List at least five occupations involved in the health care of endocrine system disorders.

4. Compare the difference between the conditions of being a dwarf or midget.

5. Investigate and describe the function of the following exocrine glands.
   Lacrimal
   Mammary
   Salivary
   Sudoriferous

6. Investigate the incidence of steroid abuse in sports and the methods used to combat this problem.

7. Research and review an article regarding a recent development or treatment method relating to the endocrine system.

18
Nervous System

Learning Objectives

Define at least 10 terms relating to the nervous system.

Describe the function of the nervous system.

Identify at least 10 structures of the nervous system.

Describe at least five disorders of the nervous system.

Identify at least three methods used to assess the function of the nervous system.

Key Terms

Cerebrospinal Fluid
(ser-ee-bro-SPY-nal FLOO-id) Fluid contained in the brain's ventricles, intracranial spaces, and central canal of the spinal cord

Dementia
(de-MEN-shah) Organic loss of intellectual function

Epilepsy
(EP-ih-lep-see) Transient disturbances of brain function

Impulse
(IM-puls) Sudden pushing force; activity along nerve fibers

Intracranial
(in-tra-KRAY-nee-uhl) Situated within the cranium

Ischemia
(is-KEE-mee-uh) Insufficient blood to a body part caused by a functional constriction or actual obstruction of a blood vessel

Meninges
(me-NIN-jeez) Three membranes that surround and protect the brain and spinal cord

Myelography
(my-eh-LOG-rah-fee) X-rays of the spinal cord after injection of a contrast medium

Neurotransmitter
(noo-roe-TRANS-mitt-er) Chemical messenger, released from the axon of one neuron, that travels to another nearby neuron

Polyneuritis
(pol-ee-noo-RIE-tis) Inflammation of many nerves at once

Reflex
(REE-fleks) An involuntary action in response to a stimulus

Regenerate
(re-JEN-uh-rate) Natural renewal of a structure, as of lost tissue or part

Senile
(SEE-nile) Pertaining to or characteristic of old age; especially physical or mental deterioration accompanying aging

Nervous System Terminology*

TERM	DEFINITION	PREFIX	ROOT	SUFFIX
Anesthesia	Without sensation	an	esthes	ia
Cerebrospinal	Pertaining to the brain and spine	cerebro	spin	al
Craniotomy	Incision into the skull		crani	otomy
Encephalotomy	Incision into the brain		encephal	otomy
Hypnotic	Pertaining to sleep		hypnot	ic
Insomnia	Lack of sleep	in	somn	ia
Meningitis	Inflammation of the meninges		mening	itis
Microencephaly	Small brain	micro	encephal	y
Neuralgia	Nerve pain		neur	algia
Neurology	Study of the nerve		neur	ology

*A transition phrase or vowel may be added to or deleted from the word parts to make the combining form.

Abbreviations of the Nervous System

ABBREVIATION	MEANING
CAT	Computerized axial tomography
CNS	Central nervous system
CSF	Cerebrospinal fluid
CVA	Cardiovascular accident
H/A	Headache
MRI	Magnetic resonance imagery
NICU	Neurointensive care unit
PERLA	Pupils equally reactive to light
REM	Rapid eye movement
TIA	Transient ischemic attack

Structure and Function of the Nervous System

The nervous system is one of the most complex and interesting body systems. It is also one of the least understood. New discoveries are made almost daily about the capabilities of the nervous system.

The function of the nervous system is to sense, interpret, and respond to internal and external environmental changes to maintain a steady state in the body (homeostasis). The nervous system is divided into two major structures: the central nervous system (CNS) and the peripheral nervous system (PNS) (Figure 18-1).

The central nervous system is made up of the brain and spinal cord. It functions as the coordinator of the body's full nervous system and contains the nerves that control connections between **impulses** coming to and from the brain and the rest of the body. The central nervous system plays a crucial role in maintaining a healthy, normally functioning body. Because nervous tissues are delicate and easily damaged, tough membranes called **meninges** surround the tissues. The nervous tissue and meninges are further protected by bones (vertebrae and cranium).

The peripheral nervous system consists of 12 pairs of cranial nerves and 31 pairs of spinal nerves (Table 18-1) that reach all parts of the body. The cranial nerves originate in the brain, and the spinal nerves emerge from the spinal cord. The spinal cord nerves can act independently from the brain in some **reflex** reactions (Figure 18-2). Other reflex reactions of the nervous system may lead to the release of glandular secretions.

The organs of the peripheral nervous system contain sensory (afferent) and motor (efferent) neurons (Figure 18-3). Afferent neurons, or nerves, carry messages from the sensory cells of the body to the brain. Efferent, or motor, nerves carry messages from the brain to the body organs or parts. The connecting nerves (interneurons) of the central nervous system carry messages from afferent

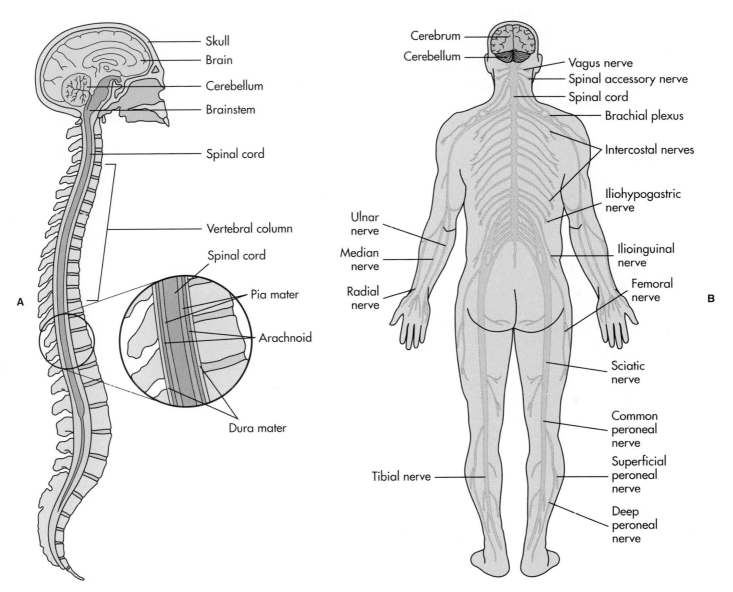

Figure 18-1   Divisions of the nervous system. **A,** The central nervous system. **B,** The peripheral nervous system. *(From Sorrentino S: Mosby's text for nursing assistants, ed 5, St Louis, 2000, Mosby.)*

Table 18-1 Functions of the Peripheral Nervous System

Nerve	Function
Cranial Nerves	
I Olfactory	Smell (S)
II Optic	Vision (S)
III Oculomotor	Raise eyelids, move eyes, focus lens, control pupil size (M)
IV Trochlear	Rotate eyes (M)
V Trigeminal	Facial and head sensation, control muscles in floor of mouth for chewing (B)
VI Abducens	Move eyes laterally (M)
VII Facial	Taste in anterior of mouth, control facial expression (B)
VIII Acoustic (auditory)	Hearing and balance (S)
IX Glossopharyngeal	Taste and swallowing (B)
X Vagus	Control muscles of speech, swallowing, and of thorax and abdomen; feeling from pharynx, larynx, and trachea (B)
XI Spinal accessory	Move neck and back muscles (M)
XII Hypoglossal	Move tongue (M)
Spinal Nerves	
C1-C8 Cervical (8 pair)	Neck and head movement; elevation of shoulders, movement of arms, hands and diaphragmatic breathing
T1-T12 Thoracic (12 pair)	Intercostal muscles of respiration and abdominal contractions
L1-L5 Lumbar (5 pair)	Leg movement
S1-S5 Sacral (5 pair)	Sphincter muscles of anus and urinary meatus; foot movement

S, Sensory; *M,* motor; *B,* both sensory and motor functions.

nerves to efferent nerves. Efferent nerves are classified as voluntary (somatic) or involuntary (autonomic).

The autonomic (involuntary) nervous system is a part of the peripheral nervous system. It has two parts: the sympathetic system and the parasympathetic system. The sympathetic nerves are stimulated in situations that require action such as the "fight or flight" reaction. The parasympathetic nervous system functions in response to normal, everyday situations. For example, the parasympathetic system would stimulate the digestion of food and slow the heart rate, whereas the sympathetic system would inhibit digestion and increase the heart rate.

Neuron

The basic structural unit of the nervous system is the nerve, which is a bundle of fibers that carries impulses.

Nerve fibers consist of neuron cells, which are the functional unit of the nervous system. There are three main types of neurons: afferent, efferent, and interneuron. Each carry messages, or impulses, to and from the body's organs.

The neuron has several important parts (Figure 18-4). The dendrites receive impulses and transmit them to the cell body. The cell body, which contains the nucleus of the neuron, transmits the impulse to the axon. The axon transmits the impulse away from the cell body to the dendrite of the next neuron. These impulse transmissions can travel more than 130 meters per second or 300 miles per hour.

Some neurons outside the central nervous system have a white, fatty substance covering the axon called *myelin*. Myelin, also called *white matter,* is arranged in bundles called *Schwann cells*. Layers of Schwann cells wrap around

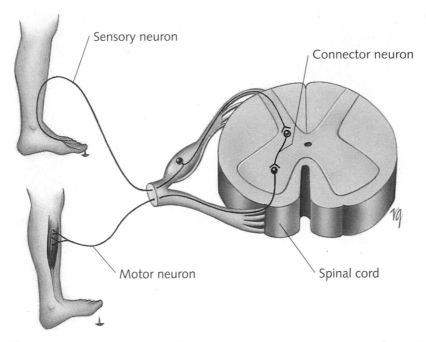

Figure 18-2   The spinal reflex arc. The motor response to injury is a reflex action controlled by the spinal nerves.

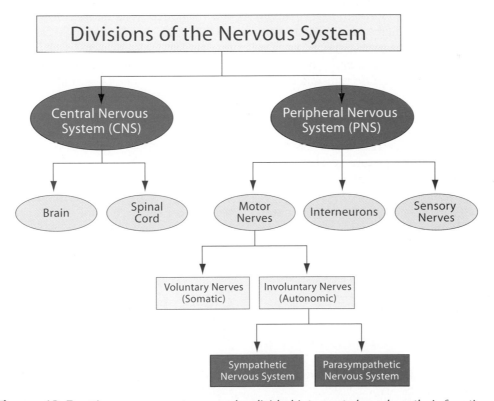

Figure 18-3   The nervous system may be divided into parts based on their functions.

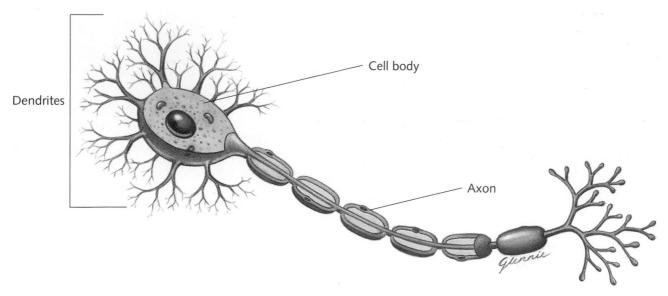

Figure 18-4   Neuron.

the axon forming the myelin sheath. The myelin sheath is covered with a membrane called the *neurilemma*. It is believed that neurilemma enables the axons to repair and **regenerate** themselves. Axons in the central nervous system, called *gray matter,* do not have neurilemma. Therefore they cannot repair or regenerate themselves. Another benefit of the myelin sheath is the microscopic spaces between the Schwann cells. These are called the *nodes of Ranvier* and greatly increase the speed of impulse transmission.

Neuroglia

Neuroglia are special nervous tissue cells that act as "glue" to support, bind, repair, and protect neurons. There are an estimated 900 billion neuroglia in the body. They can be divided into three major types.
- The astrocyte cells are believed to help transfer substances from the blood to the brain. They make up what is known as the "blood-brain barrier."
- The oligodendroglia in the central nervous system and Schwann cells in the peripheral nervous system help to develop the myelin sheath.
- The microglia destroy and engulf bacteria and fight infection.

The ependymal cells line cavities of the nervous system, producing and circulating fluid in the system.

Neuroglia divide to reproduce and may therefore become cancerous.

Synapse

A synapse is the space between two neurons. Neurons may be as close as one millionth of an inch to each other but still not touch. One neuron may send messages to up to 10,000 other neurons through the synapse. Impulses from one neuron are transmitted across the synapse to another neuron by a chemical called a **neurotransmitter.** The two most common neurotransmitters are acetylcholine and norepinephrine. One neurotransmitter may have different effects in varied synapses. More than 100 chemical messengers used by the nervous system have been identified.

Ganglia

Ganglia are groups of nerve tissue, principally nerve cell bodies, that are located outside the central nervous system. These cell bodies have some increased ability to transmit impulses as compared with nerve cells because they are clustered together in the ganglion.

Plexus and Dermatome

Four major networks of interwoven spinal nerves, called *plexuses*, provide impulses to specific regions of the body. They are called the *cervical, brachial, lumbar,* and *sacral* plexuses based on the spinal nerves that are involved in each group.

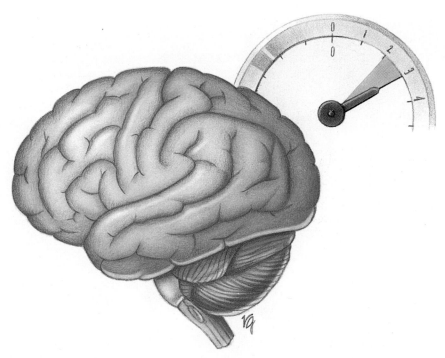

Figure 18-5   The brain weighs 2 to 3 pounds.

Sensations on the skin surface are controlled by specific spinal nerves. For example, the second cervical spinal nerve senses afferent messages on the top of the cranium. These areas are called *dermatomes*.

Brain

The brain is the largest structure of the nervous system and one of the largest organs of the body (Figure 18-5). It weighs about 2 to 3 pounds (0.9 to 1.4 kg). It uses about 20% of the blood flow from the heart. The brain's cells can survive only 4 to 6 minutes without oxygen and glucose from the blood.

The brain is covered by three layers of membranes called meninges: the dura mater, arachnoid, and pia mater. The pia mater is the innermost layer attached to the brain and spinal cord. The arachnoid is the middle layer and acts as a channel for **cerebrospinal fluid.** The dura mater is a leathery outer layer.

The brain has four lined cavities called ventricles. The inner layers of the brain, spinal cord, and ventricles are filled with a clear fluid called *cerebrospinal fluid.* This fluid acts as a cushion to protect the brain from injury and car-

ries nutrients to, and wastes from, the central nervous system cells.

The four major areas of the brain are the cerebrum, the diencephalon, the cerebellum, and the brain stem. The cerebrum is the largest area and is divided into two hemispheres. It is concerned with reasoning and the senses. Each of the hemispheres is further divided into lobes and sections based on function (Figure 18-6). The right hemisphere controls many of the functions of the left side of the body; the left hemisphere controls the right side. One side usually has more influence over the overall body functions.

The diencephalon contains the hypothalamus and the thalamus. The hypothalamus regulates and coordinates the activity of the autonomic nervous system. It also controls hormone secretion and appetite. The thalamus transfers sensory impulses to the sensory areas of the cerebral cortex.

The cerebellum directs coordination, muscle tone, and equilibrium. The brain stem includes the pons, medulla, and midbrain. It maintains the heartbeat, respiration, and blood pressure. Some areas of the brain have been identified with specific functions (Table 18-2).

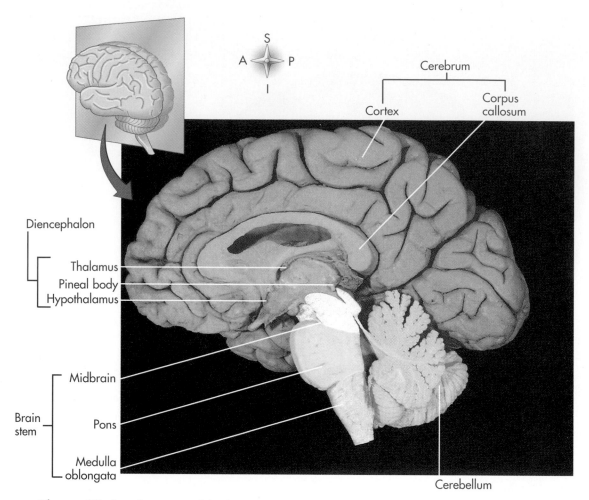

Figure 18-6 The parts of the brain. *(From Thibodeau GA, Patton KT:* Anatomy & physiology, *ed 5, St Louis, 2003, Mosby.)*

Assessment Techniques

Primary methods of assessing the nervous system include the following:

Electroencephalography (EEG) is a simple, painless test that measures the electrical activity of the brain and aids in location and treatment of disorders. Encephalography may be used in surgery by applying the electrodes directly to the brain tissue.

Lumbar puncture assesses cerebrospinal fluid for blood, foreign cells, infection, and chemical imbalances. Lumbar puncture is performed by a physician using strict sterile technique to avoid introduction of microorganisms into the spinal column.

Myelography is a type of x-ray of the interior of the spinal cord used to detect growths or displacement of the vertebral column.

Nerve conduction velocity tests the speed of impulses through nerves. This test stimulates nerves on a surface electrode placed on the skin and records the time needed to conduct the information to another electrode. This test may be used to diagnose nerve damage.

Computerized tomography (CT) is a special x-ray technique that uses scanning equipment to reconstruct sectional slices of the body at any angle to detect abnormalities.

Positron emission tomography (PET) is a type of CT using radioactive isotopes introduced into brain cells to detect disorders related to chemical functions.

Table 18-2 Functions of the Brain

Brain Part	Function
Cerebrum	
Frontal lobe	Personality, behavior, memory, reasoning, emotion
Broca's area	Speech
Sensory cortex	Sensations of heat and pain
Motor cortex	Controls movement
Angular gyrus	Written language
Wernicke's area	Understanding written or spoken language
Parietal lobe	Understanding speech or choosing words
Temporal lobe	Hearing and understanding speech and printed words, memory of music and visual scenes
Occipital lobe	Vision and its interpretation
Cerebellum	Coordination of voluntary movement, balance
Brainstem	
Pons	Breathing, relaying impulses between cerebellum and medulla
Medulla	Control of involuntary movements, heartbeat, blood pressure, respiration, and swallowing
Midbrain	Visual and auditory reflex

Magnetic resonance imagery (MRI) determines the movement of ions in tissue cells by measuring energy changes caused by radio waves (Figure 18-7). MRI is so sensitive that white matter and fluid in the brain can be seen.

Disorders of the Nervous System

Alzheimer's (AHLZ-hi-merz) disease is a form of **senile dementia,** but it also occurs in middle-aged adults. Although the specific cause is unknown, several forms of Alzheimer's have been identified, at least one of which is genetically linked. The person experiences a progressive loss of memory and intellectual impairment. There is no single diagnostic test for Alzheimer's disease. The Mini-Mental State Examination (MMSE) may be used to help with identifica-

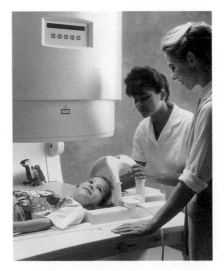

Figure 18-7   Magnetic resonance imagery allows the visualization of the body without use of radiation. *(Courtesy Siemens Medical Solutions USA.)*

tion of the condition. Lesions caused by deposit of plaque on brain cells can be seen on autopsy. Also, a PET scan may be used to identify it. Treatment helps the person control the symptoms, but no cure is known.

Cerebrovascular (se-ree-bro-VAS-kyoo-lar) accidents, commonly called *strokes* or *CVAs,* are cardiovascular disorders that directly affect the neurological system. Strokes affect about 4 of every 1000 people and are the third leading cause of death in the United States. A CVA is caused by loss of oxygen, or **ischemia,** to an area of the brain when a clot blocks a vessel or when a vessel breaks. The extent of damage depends on the area of the brain that is affected, and the person may experience mental or physical dysfunction. Prevention of a stroke includes controlling risk factors, such as hypertension, diabetes, and heart disease. Treatment helps the person recover from or cope with functional losses caused by tissue death such as the ability to walk or talk.

Down syndrome is one of the most common causes of mental retardation and the most common disorder of human chromosomes. The genetic disorder is caused by the presence of an extra chromosome. The resulting characteristics include short stature, short neck, broad hands with stubby fingers and toes, a large protruding tongue, and mental retardation. The degree of mental retardation varies greatly, but the average mental age that is reached is 8 years. Individuals with Down syndrome are also more likely to have respiratory infections, heart defects, and leukemia. There is no cure.

Encephalitis (en-sef-uh-LIE-tis) is inflammation of the brain caused by a virus, bacteria, or chemical agent. Encephalitis is usually an acute condition characterized by fever, headache, extreme irritability of the nervous system, and disorientation. Encephalitis may lead to convulsions and death. Treatment depends on the exact cause and may include antibiotics and precautions to reduce stimulation.

Guillain-Barré (ge-YANE bar-RAY) syndrome is also called infectious **polyneuritis.** The cause is unknown but it may appear shortly after a viral immunization or infection. The person experiences muscle weakness that rapidly moves from the legs to the face. Total paralysis of respiratory function may result. Treatment is supportive to maintain vital life functions. About 95% of the Guillain-Barré cases have complete recovery in a few weeks to several months.

Headache is a very common condition resulting from several different causes. However, headache can be the symptom of another, more serious disorder and should be investigated when occurring frequently. Tension headaches are directly related to stress. The muscles around the occipital area of the brain may constrict the blood flow to the area. Tension headaches are usually dull and steady in nature. They can be relieved with nonprescription analgesics.

Treatment includes relaxation techniques, massage of the neck and back muscles, and application of heat such as a hot shower.

Migraine headaches are vascular headaches of unknown cause. The pain results from the narrowing of blood vessels in the brain. Migraine headaches generally are throbbing, located in one area on one side of the brain, and involve gastrointestinal disturbances such as vomiting. They may last for several days. Treatment includes avoiding triggering factors such as certain foods. Relief from migraine headaches may require prescription medicine.

Sinus headaches result from the swelling of the membranes that line the sinus cavities. The pain is usually dull and shifts with head movement. Decongestants and nonprescription analgesics relieve this headache pain.

Head injury may occur when the brain impacts the skull as a result of a blow or rapid movement. Depending on the location of the injury, the person may experience nausea, confusion, increased blood pressure, and drowsiness. Treatment includes surgical relief of pressure on the brain if necessary. The person is assessed for neurological damage after a head injury for at least 24 hours.

Huntington's chorea is a degenerative neural disorder that affects brain tissues. The condition usually appears between the ages of 35 and 50. The person first experiences loss of balance and coordination, then progressively involuntary movements and dementia. Death occurs 10 to 20 years after the disease appears. An autosomal dominant gene causes the disease. If one parent has the gene for the disease, each child has a 50% chance of receiving it. The appearance of this gene can now be identified with gene mapping, allowing for counseling of families with a history of the disorder. There is no treatment.

Hydrocephalus (hi-dro-SEF-uh-lus) occurs when more cerebrospinal fluid is produced than is absorbed into the circulatory system. The excess fluid increases **intracranial** pressure and may enlarge the head. It may be caused by developmental defects, infection, trauma, or a tumor in the cranial space. Treatment includes removal of the excess fluid by a tube inserted into the intracranial space.

Intracranial (in-tra-KRAY-nee-al) tumors may be benign or malignant. Tumors of the nervous system usually involve neuroglia, blood vessels or membranes rather than neurons. A neuroma (noo-RO-ma) generally refers to a benign or noncancerous growth. A glioma would be more likely malignant or cancerous. It is also possible for a growth to be metastatic, originating from cells that have then been transported to the brain by the lymph vessels from another part of the body. Any type of growth can disrupt nervous system function with the symptoms depending on the portion of the brain or nerves that is compressed by the growth. The treatment may include surgical removal, radiation, or chemotherapy and varies with the location and type of growth.

Meningitis (men-in-JIE-tis) is a serious inflammation of the meninges caused by a bacterium, virus, or fungus. The person can experience a high fever, stiff neck, vomiting, severe headache, and convulsions. Damage to the nervous system may result in blindness, loss of hearing, paralysis, or retardation. Some cases of meningitis are self-limiting and require treatment only to relieve symptoms. In severe cases, treatment varies with the cause and usually includes antibiotics.

Meningocele (me-NING-go-seel) is a birth defect that occurs when the membranes covering the brain or spinal cord protrude through a congenital defect in the skull or spinal column. If treated rapidly with surgery to correct the defect, the damage done to the spinal cord and nerves can be minimized. The cause of meningocele is unknown. However, folic acid deficiency may play a part in neural tube defects. Environmental factors and a viral cause have also been theorized as a cause.

Multiple sclerosis (skle-RO-sis) results from a defect in electrical transmission of the neurons caused by degeneration of the myelin sheath. Multiple sclerosis usually appears in adults 20 to 40 years of age. The cause is unknown. Most scientists believe that the loss of myelin is caused by a virus or an autoimmune process. The person may first experience double vision or diplopia (di-PLO-pee-uh), loss of sensation, stiff extremities, or progressive loss of muscle control. Multiple sclerosis is treated with medication such as steroids and beta-interferon to help control the symptoms and disabilities. There is no cure.

Neural (noo-ral) *tube defect* is a defect in the formation of the skull and spinal column. It is caused primarily when the neural tube fails to close during the development of the embryo. Severe mental and physical disorders usually are present as well. Prenatal testing during the fourteenth to sixteenth week can determine whether a neural tube defect is present. Infection of the cerebrospinal fluid is the main concern after birth. In some cases, surgery may be performed to correct the deformity.

Neurofibromatosis (noo-ro-fi-bro-mah-TOE-sis), also called *Von Recklinghausen's* (REK-ling-how-zenz) *disease,* is caused by a defect in an autosomal dominant gene. It affects more than 100,000 people in the United States. The condition is believed to be caused by genetic mutation in half of the cases. The condition first causes large tan spots on the skin. Small benign tumors of nervous tissue develop with increased age. The tumors may cause loss of hearing or blindness if located in the ears and eyes. In many cases, the symptoms are mild and life expectancy is normal. There is no treatment, although unsightly tumors can be removed surgically.

Parkinson's (PAR-kin-sunz) disease commonly affects people over 50 years of age. It results from degeneration of certain brain cells and is sometimes called "shaking palsy." It results from a decrease in secretion of the neurotransmitter dopamine resulting from unknown causes. The person gradually feels stiffness and tremors, leading to uncontrolled muscular movement and rigidity. Treatment includes medication to decrease the symptoms. Drug therapy is usually successful but has many side effects. Surgery may be performed in some cases.

Poliomyelitis (po-lee-o-mi-uh-LIE-tis) is caused by a virus that spreads from the nose and throat to neural tissue. The virus destroys neural cell bodies and leads to temporary paralysis. Vaccination prevents the infection and has minimized the incidence of polio. Treatment of the disease includes measures to prevent deformity caused by loss of muscle function.

Sciatica (sie-AT-ih-ka) is characterized by constant pain radiating from the back and buttocks to the leg. Movement may also be limited in the affected leg. The cause is usually a rupture of an intervertebral disk and osteoarthritis (os-tee-o-ar-THRI-tis), producing pressure on the nerve or other nerve injury. Treatment of sciatica requires finding the cause of the pain and controlling it.

A *seizure* (SEE-zher) may result from injury, infection, or **epilepsy.** There are more than 40 types of seizure that may be classified into two groups. Partial seizures involve part of the brain, whereas generalized seizures involve the whole brain. Absence seizures, also called *petit mal* (PET-ee mahl) seizures, cause a lapse of consciousness for several seconds. Febrile and chemical seizures may result from drugs. Grand mal (grand mahl) seizures are a series of distinctive tonic and clonic spasms that last several minutes. In the tonic portion of the seizure, the muscles are contracted rigidly. The clonic phase involves involuntary muscle movements. Seizures may cause injury from uncontrolled movement. Seizures can often be controlled successfully with medication.

Spina bifida (SPI-nuh BIF-i-da) is a birth defect involving a malformed spinal column resulting from neural tube defects. In the United States, 1 of 1500 to 2000 babies is born with this defect each year. Spina bifida is partly hereditary but is also affected by the pregnant woman's diet and environment. At birth, the infant's spinal column is not closed completely over the spinal cord. The condition may cause problems with bowel and bladder control or paralysis. The opening can be closed surgically to minimize damage.

Spinal cord injuries (SCI) affect 7000 to 10,000 people in the United States each year. The majority, about 82%, are males between 15 and 25 years of age. About 47% of spinal cord injuries result from automobile accidents, whereas 21% result from falls and 15% from violence.

Most spinal injuries resulting from trauma occur in the cervical and lumbar area of the spinal column, which have the greatest mobility. Injuries to the cervical spine may cause quadriplegia (tetraplegia). In the lumbar region, paraplegia may result. The severity of the injury is diagnosed using x-ray, CT scans, and MRI. Treatment may include steroids to reduce the swelling in the cord and management to prevent complications resulting from lost sensory and motor function.

Transient ischemic attacks (TIAs) are often called "little strokes" and are caused by a decrease in blood to an area of the brain resulting from a small clot that temporarily lodges in a vessel. The person may experience slurred speech, numbness, or vision disturbances that usually disappear within a few days. Because the symptoms disappear, the condition may go unrecognized. Transient ischemic attacks may indicate an impending irreversible cerebrovascular accident. CVAs can be prevented with anticoagulants or vascular surgery to clear blocked blood vessels.

Trigeminal neuralgia (tri-JEM-in-al noo-RAL-jee-ah), also called *tic douloureux* (tik doo-loo-ROO), is characterized by sudden intense, unpredictable pain on one side of the face. The pain is caused by pressure on or deterioration of the trigeminal facial nerve. Treatment may include medication or surgery.

Issues and Innovations

Memory Research

The storage and recall of information is one of the most specialized functions of the nervous system. Three components of memory include sensory memory, short-term memory, and long-term memory. Sensory memory holds information for 20 to 30 seconds. Short-term memory is information retained for several minutes to several hours. The same information can be converted by repetition to long-term memory that may be retained for years. It is believed that information is stored in different areas of the brain according to whether the method of input is visual, auditory, or touch-related (kinesthetic). These areas are interconnected by chemical messengers for more efficient retrieval of information.

Researchers have also determined that memories are retained differently and in separate areas of the brain. For example, discursive or declarative information such as a multiplication table is stored in a different area than procedural information such as how to ride a bike or dance. And, an aphasic (without speech) injury might allow the person to remember the name of living things, but not non-living things. The temporal lobe is believed to store long-term memory. The hippocampus is the site for facts, events, novelties, and spatial relations.

The method that the brain uses to store and recall information is not clearly understood, but ribonucleic acid (RNA) may play a role. Most research on memory uses a marine slug named Aplysia or people who have sustained neurological changes resulting from injury or illness as subjects. The slugs are used for memory research because their ganglia are large and their behavior patterns are limited. The slugs do have the capacity to retain short-term memories of environmental changes. Researchers believe that the slug's memories result from a biochemical change in the synapse receptors. To create a new memory, the synapse reacts differently to the neurotransmitters it receives.

Neuroscientists believe that the 100 billion neurons of the brain communicate in a complicated network. Any single neuron may be connected to as many as 10,000 other neurons. Computer networks have been designed to try to simulate the action of the brain. Researchers hope to discover how the brain rearranges the connections to store new information and restore operations after damage to some neurons.

Parkinson's Correction

Parkinson's disease is a progressive neurological disorder characterized by three distinct functional changes. These three changes include slowness of movement (bradykinesia), tremor, and rigidity. More than 50,000 people in the United States are diagnosed with Parkinson's each year, with a total of up to 1 million affected. The usual treatment involves a series of drugs that alleviate symptoms and assist the body to make the neurotransmitter, dopamine, which is missing in Parkinson's.

The first transplant of adrenal gland cells to the brain in the United States was performed in 1987. Adrenal cells and fetal brain cells may be used to replace or stimulate the function of an area of the brain called the *substantia nigra* (sub-stan-shah NYE-grah) that normally produces dopamine. Researchers in Mexico who first performed the procedure reported a striking improvement in the condition. In the United States, implantation of fetal tissue has been limited because of a ban on fetal tissue research that was imposed in 1988. The federal government recently lifted the ban on fetal tissue research opening the way for more research in this area.

To date, the effectiveness of fetal tissue transplant to cure Parkinson's cannot be fully demonstrated. Only a few transplants have been completed and varied techniques were used in the procedure. Additionally, the supply of fetal tissue for transplant is very limited. Researchers at the University of California in San Diego are currently experimenting with genetically engineered skin cells to try to produce a larger supply of cells for transplant that have been "taught" to make dopamine. In 2002 Harvard researchers developed stem cells with all the characteristics of normal dopamine cells. This may lead to another treatment of the condition.

Review Questions

1. Use the following terms in one or more sentences that correctly relate their meaning.
   Epilepsy
   Impulse
   Myelography
   Reflex

2. Describe the function of the nervous system.

3. Identify the parts of the neuron.

4. Describe the location and function of each of the following parts of the nervous system.
   Autonomic nervous system
   Parasympathetic division
   Sympathetic division

5. Describe the function of each of the 12 cranial nerves.

6. List the function of the following parts of the brain.
   Frontal lobe
   Medulla
   Occipital lobe
   Parietal lobe
   Pons
   Temporal lobe

7. Describe three nervous system disorders that are caused by a pathogenic organism.

8. Describe three methods used to assess the function of the nervous system.

Critical Thinking

1. Investigate and compare the cost of at least three tests used in diagnosing disorders of the nervous system.

2. Investigate the function of at least five common medications used in treatment of the nervous system.

3. List at least five occupations involved in the health care of nervous system disorders.

4. Investigate the methods used to regain use of the brain following injury.

5. Research and review an article regarding a recent development or treatment method relating to the nervous system.

19
Sensory System

Learning Objectives

Define at least 10 terms relating to the sensory system.

Describe the function of the sensory system.

Identify at least 10 sensory system structures and the function of each.

Describe at least five disorders of the sensory system.

Identify at least three methods of assessment of the sensory system.

Key Terms

Accommodation
(uh-kom-uh-DAY-shun) Focusing of the eye for varied distances

Auditory
(AW-dih-tore-ee) Pertaining to the sense of hearing

Converge
(kon-VERJ) When two eyes move in a coordinated fashion toward fixation on the same near point

Cutaneous
(kyoo-TAY-nee-us) Pertaining to the skin

Equilibrium
(ee-kwih-LIB-ree-um) State of balance

Gustatory
(GUS-tuh-tore-ee) Pertaining to the sense of taste

Intraocular
(in-truh-OK-yoo-lar) Within the eye

Labyrinth
(LAB-ih-rinth) System of communicating canals in the inner ear

Olfactory
(OLE-fak-tore-ee) Pertaining to the sense of smell

Receptor
(ree-SEP-tor) Specific type of cell that responds to a specific stimulus

Refraction
(ree-FRAK-shun) Deviation of light when passing through a medium to another medium of a different density

Stimulus
(STIM-yoo-lus) Any agent that produces a reaction in a receptor

Vision
(VIZH-un) Act or faculty of seeing, sight

Sensory System Terminology*

TERM	DEFINITION	PREFIX	ROOT	SUFFIX
Gustatory	Pertaining to taste		gusta	tory
Intraocular	Within the eye	intra	ocul	ar
Kinesthetic	Pertaining to the sense of movement		kinesthet	ic
Nasal	Pertaining to the nose		nas	al
Ocular	Pertaining to the eye		ocul	ar
Olfactory	Pertaining to the sense of smell		olfac	tory
Ophthalmologist	Specialist in the eye and its disorders		opthalmal	ogist
Otoscope	Instrument used to view the eye	oto	scope	
Retinopathy	Disease of the retina		retin	opathy
Tympanitis	Inflammation of the eardrum		tympan	itis

*A transition phrase or vowel may be added to or deleted from the word parts to make the combining form.

Abbreviations of the Sensory System

ABBREVIATION	MEANING
aq	Aqueous
EENT	Ears, eyes, nose, throat
o.d.	Right eye
Oint	Ointment
Ophth	Ophthalmology
o.s.	Left eye
o.u.	Both eyes
PERLA	Pupils equally reactive to light
REM	Rapid eye movement
RK	Radial keratotomy

Structure and Function of the Sensory System

The sensory system consists of **receptors** in specialized cells and organs that perceive changes (stimuli) in the internal and external environment. The stimuli cause nerve impulses that are sent to the brain for interpretation. Environmental stimuli are perceived with the senses of **vision**, hearing, touch, taste, position, and balance. Specialized organs of the senses include the eye, ear, tongue, nose, and skin.

Eye

The eyes are considered the most important sensory organ because 90% of the information about the environment reaches the brain from the eyes.

The external structures of the eye are shown in Figure 19-1. The orbital cavity is composed of bones that protect and adipose tissue that cushions the eye. When the eyelids and eyelashes close or "blink," they protect the eye from injury. The conjunctiva is a mucous membrane that protects and lubricates the eyelids and part of the eye. The lacrimal apparatus forms tears that keep the eye moist and lubricated. Movement of the eye is controlled by the extrinsic muscles. Only one fifth of the eye is actually exposed to the environment.

The internal structures of the eye are shown in Figure 19-1. The sclera is a tough, white tissue that supports and gives structure to the eye. The sclera is covered with the clear, circular cornea that focuses images. The blood supply for the eye originates in the choroid, iris, and ciliary muscles. The iris and ciliary muscles are the intrinsic muscles of the eye.

The eyeball is not solid but is divided into sections, the anterior and posterior cavities. The anterior cavity is filled with a clear watery fluid called *aqueous humor*. The posterior cavity is filled with a semisoft gelatinlike substance

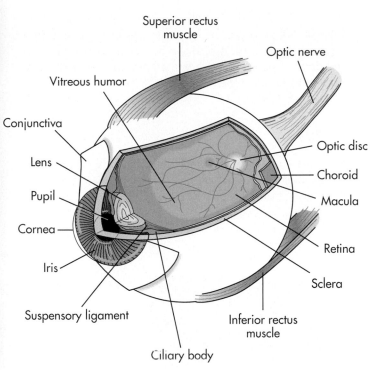

Figure 19-1   Structures of the eye. *(From Sorrentino S: Mosby's text for nursing assistants, ed 5, St Louis, 2000, Mosby.)*

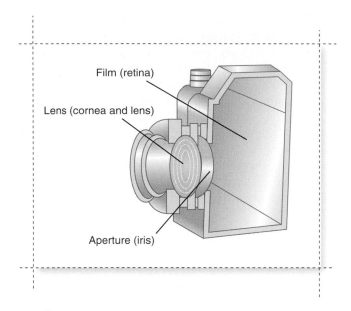

Figure 19-2   The eye functions like a camera.

called *vitreous humor.* Both the aqueous and vitreous humor help maintain the shape of the eye.

The opening called the *pupil* is in the choroid layer. The iris is a round, colored muscle that surrounds the pupil. The iris contracts and relaxes to adjust the amount of light entering the eye through the pupil. The lens is a convex, transparent tissue located directly behind the pupil that focuses and directs incoming light on the retina of the eye. The amount of light admitted into the eye is regulated by the movement of the iris.

Vision is similar to the action of a camera beginning with **refraction,** the process of the lens bending light rays as they enter the eye to focus on the retina (Figure 19-2). The eye changes the shape of the lens to focus near and far through the process of **accommodation.** The pupil constricts to focus the object on the retina and protect it from receiving too much light. The eyes **converge** on the object so that single binocular vision occurs and only one object is seen.

Specialized cells called *rods* and *cones* in the retina absorb the light. There are 100 million rods and 7 million cones in the retina of each eye. Rods are sensitive to dim light. Cones react to bright light and allow color distinction through three types of pigments that are sensitive to different wavelengths of light. The three photopigments recognize the primary colors: green, red, and blue. The impulses released by the pigments in the rods and cones are transmitted to the brain by the optic nerve.

Ear

The **auditory** or acoustic sense (hearing) is the primary function of the ear. A second function of the ear is to help maintain **equilibrium.** The ear has three parts called the *external, middle,* and *inner ear* (Figure 19-3).

The external ear channels the incoming sound waves or vibrations. The auricle or pinna is the flap of tissue on the side of the head that collects and transmits sound waves through the ear or auditory canal to the eardrum (tympanic membrane). Specialized glands in the ear canal produce earwax (cerumen) that protects the middle ear from entry of foreign particles.

The middle ear is an air-filled chamber that begins with the tympanic membrane, which changes sound waves into mechanical movements. Auditory bones (ossicles) transmit the sound vibrations. These three bones are called the *hammer (malleus), anvil (incus),* and *stirrup (stapes).* The ossicles amplify and transmit the sound to the inner ear. Two openings into the inner ear are the membrane covered round window and the oval window, which touches the stapes. Another opening exists between the middle ear and pharynx called the *eustachian tube.* The eustachian tube has two main functions. It allows the pressure of air in the middle ear to be equalized with the air pressure of the environment. Additionally, fluids and mucus from the middle ear are drained to the nasopharynx. Swallowing and yawning open the eustachian tube for these purposes.

The inner ear contains a series of canals called *bony labyrinth*, which includes the cochlea, semicircular canals, and vestibule with the membranous labyrinth inside of it. The movement of fluid and hair cells lining the cochlea converts the mechanical vibrations from the ossicles to neural impulses. There are 16,000 hair cells in each ear. Each hair cell has 100 stereocilia or bristles that transmit impulses to the auditory cranial nerves. The semicircular canals contain a clear fluid called *endolymph* that gives a sense of balance when the body is in motion. Two chambers called the *saccule* and *utricle* of the vestibule maintain static or resting equilibrium.

Hearing is a result of interpretation of sound waves. Sound waves are described by their amplitude (volume) and pitch (frequency). A sound is perceived when the tympanic membrane is vibrated or the hairs in the cochlea are stimulated. Sound waves may be transmitted through the air, bone, or fluid.

Tongue

Taste, or the **gustatory** sense, is perceived by specialized cells located in projections (papillae) on the tongue called "taste buds." Taste buds are chemoreceptors. The

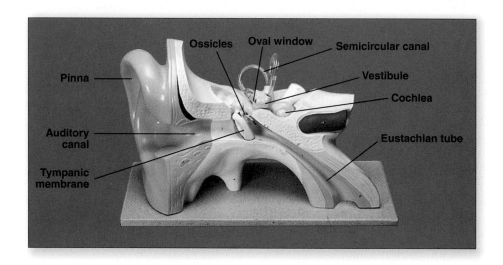

Figure 19-3 Structures of the ear.

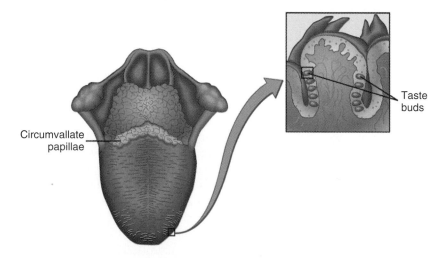

Figure 19-4 Taste buds are located on the tongue. *(From Thibodeau GA, Patton KT: Anatomy & Physiology, ed 5, St Louis, 2003, Mosby.)*

four tastes perceived by the tongue are sweet, sour, bitter, and salty (Figure 19-4). As more research is completed, new "tastes" may be identified. It is possible that "metallic" is also a primary taste. Before a taste can be sensed, the substance must be dissolved in fluid or saliva. The particular flavor of an item is identified by smell as well as taste.

Nose

The **olfactory** sense, or smell, originates in olfactory receptor cells in the nose that immediately transmit impulses to the brain through the olfactory cranial nerves (Figure 19-5). The nasal cavity is divided into two sections by the septum. Each side of the nose is further divided into three passageways by bony projections called *turbinates.* Specialized epithelial tissue near the roof of the nasal cavity contains the olfactory cells. Olfactory receptor neurons are stimulated by chemicals (gases) in the air. When the receptors reach a threshold, the olfactory bulb reacts and an impulse is transmitted to the brain. Air that is inhaled also circulates into the paranasal sinuses surrounding the nasal cavity.

The sense of smell is 10,000 times more sensitive than taste. More than 5000 distinct smells can be perceived. However, these smells result from a mixture of only 30 primary or "pure" odors. Some examples of primary odors include floral, putrid, and peppermint. Smells can reduce stress, affect blood pressure, recall memories, and aid in the sense of taste.

Skin

The **cutaneous** senses of the skin perceive touch, pressure, temperature, and pain through five specialized cells located in the skin (Figure 19-6). Touch, or the tactile sense, is the perception of textures such as smooth, rough, sharp, dull, soft, and hard. Light touch and motion near the skin is perceived by Meissner's corpuscles. Pacinian corpuscles, commonly found in deeper tissues of the tendons and ligaments, sense deep pressure. End-bulbs of Krause sense cold, low-frequency vibration and two-point discrimination. Corpuscles of Ruffini sense heat, deep pressure, and continuous touch. Pain receptors, also called *nociceptors,* are distributed throughout the skin, mucous membranes, skeletal muscles, and internal organs. Pain receptors are free nerve endings that respond to more than one type of **stimulus.** There are no pain receptors in the brain. Pain is the only type of nerve receptor found in visceral organs.

The sensation of stretching or knowing the position of muscles is determined by muscle spindles and Golgi tendon receptors. Muscle spindles in skeletal muscles sense the length of the muscles. Golgi tendon receptors, located in areas where muscles join to tendons, sense the tension of the muscle. These two proprioceptors help to maintain muscle tone and posture.

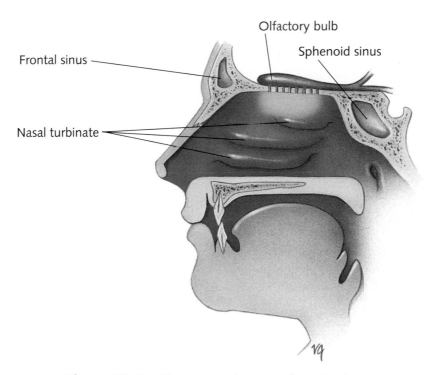

Figure 19-5   The nose and surrounding structures.

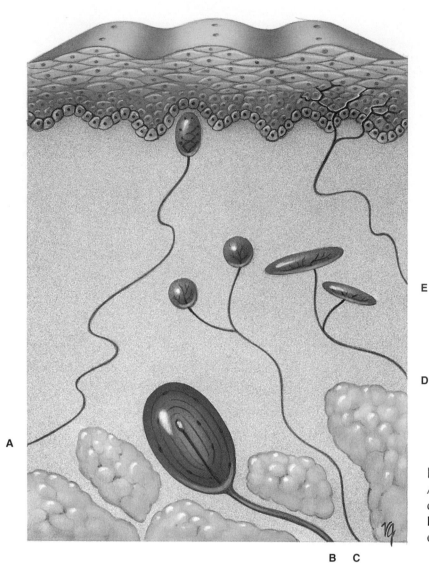

Figure 19-6 Nerve receptors of the skin. **A**, Meissner's corpuscle (touch). **B**, Pacinian corpuscle (pressure). **C**, Krause's end-bulb. **D**, Ruffini nerve endings (warmth). **E**, Free nerve endings (pain).

Assessment Techniques

Sight

Inner structures of the eye are examined by using an ophthalmoscope. The pupils are usually dilated to allow better visualization.

Visual acuity is assessed with a Snellen chart that shows letters or shapes identified from a distance. Normal vision (emmetropia) is 20/20 vision. This measurement indicates that a character of the designated size can be identified from a distance of 20 feet. A measurement of 20/100 would indicate that a person with normal vision would be able to identify the character at 100 feet but that the person being tested can identify it at 20 feet. A measurement of 20/200 is considered legal blindness.

Near vision may be tested with a Jaeger chart. Defective visual acuity can be corrected with eyeglasses or contact lenses.

Pressure of the inner eye, or **intraocular** pressure, is measured using a tonometer, which can detect glaucoma. It measures the force needed to indent the cornea with a plunger. The pressure is usually 13 to 19 mm mercury (Hg).

A "slit-lamp" is used to view the anterior eye for scratches or deformities. The eye is viewed through a binocular microscope, on which the patient rests the chin to prevent movement of the eyes.

The visual field, or space in which a person can see peripherally, is measured as the patient indicates that flashing pinpoints of light in the peripheral field are viewed while concentrating on a central point.

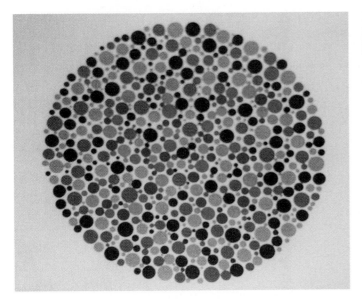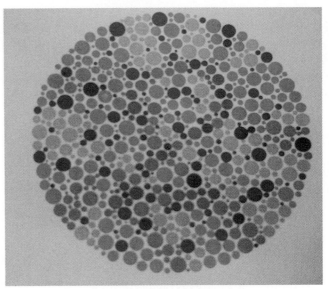

Figure 19-7   The most common type of color blindness is characterized by the inability to distinguish reds from greens. *(From Kinn ME, Woods M: The medical assistant, ed 8, Philadelphia, 1999, WB Saunders; modified from Ishihara S: Tests for colour-blindness, Tokyo, Japan.)*

Defects in color determination may be tested using a color blindness chart (Figure 19-7).

Hearing

The instrument used to view the structures of the ear is called an *otoscope*. Hearing ability can be measured using an audiometer that emits specific sounds of varied intensity and frequency through the air. Hearing ability may also be assessed using a vibrator on the mastoid process to measure bone conduction of sound waves. Normal hearing is in the range of 10 to 100 decibels (dB). Defective hearing can be corrected in some cases with a hearing aid that amplifies the sound. Impedance testing emits sound directly into the ear canal to measure the flexibility of the tympanic membrane. The Rinne test uses a tuning fork to assess transmission of sound through the ear structures. Weber's test uses a tuning fork to test for unilateral or one-sided hearing loss.

Disorders of the Sensory System

Achromatism (ah-KRO-mah-tizm), also called *color blindness*, is a common inherited defect. Monochromatism is complete color blindness in which only grays are seen.

Color blindness results from a recessive gene located on the X chromosome. It results when one or more of the three photopigments that assess color is defective. The person sees the color but cannot interpret it correctly. Green color blindness is most common; red is the second most common. Red-green color blindness is also possible. Blue color blindness is uncommon. There is no treatment for color blindness, although the person must learn to make adjustments for it. For example, the type of traffic signal at an intersection may be determined by placement of the lights rather than the color.

Amblyopia (am-blee-OH-pee-uh), also called "lazy eye," is poor vision in one eye often resulting from better vision in the other eye during infancy or early childhood. Exercises, corrective lenses, patching of the eye that has better vision, and surgery to shorten muscles around the eye may be used for treatment in young children. After 6 to 9 years of age, the development of the visual system is complete and the condition cannot be corrected.

Anacusis (an-ah-KYOO-sis), or hearing loss, can be either perceptive or conductive. Sensorineural (sen-so-ree-NOO-ral) hearing (perceptive) loss results from damage to neural tissues. Central nervous system tissue does not repair, so this type of hearing loss cannot be corrected. Transmission hearing loss (conductive) may result from otosclerosis (o-to-skle-RO-sis). Hearing loss may also result from infection or trauma to ear structures. Treatment of conductive hearing loss may *include surgery or use of hearing aids.*

Astigmatism (uh-STIG-muh-tizm) is a congenital defect of the eyeball that may increase with age. Imperfect curvature of the cornea results in blurred vision. Treatment is use of corrective lenses.

Cataract (KAT-uh-rakt) is a clouding of the lens that causes blurred or partial vision. The cause is unknown. Cataracts are not contagious and, if treated, do not cause permanent blindness. If untreated, cataracts may cause blindness. Some research indicates that antioxidants taken in food or supplements help to prevent cataracts from occurring. Cataracts can be corrected by surgical replacement of the cloudy lens.

Conjunctivitis (kon-junk-tih-VIE-tis), also called *pink eye,* is a bacterial or viral inflammation of the eyelid. Conjunctivitis is extremely contagious. The person has reddening of the eyelids and sclera with pus formation. The pus may lead to closure of the eye, especially in the morning. Conjunctivitis is treated with antibiotics.

Diabetic retinopathy (die-ah-BET-ik ret-in-OP-ah-thee) is a common condition of damaged blood vessels in the retina caused by uncontrolled diabetes mellitus. Visual loss results. Diabetes is the leading cause of blindness in people ages 25 to 74. The person may not notice the symptoms until the damage is so severe that it causes perceptible loss of vision. Treatment may not be necessary or may include laser surgery. The most important treatment is to control the diabetic condition to prevent damage.

Diplopia (dih-PLO-pee-uh), or double vision, results from muscle imbalance or paralysis of an extraocular muscle. It may also result from a problem with the sixth cranial nerve. Treatment of diplopia is to correct the cause.

Epistaxis (ep-ih-STAK-sis), or nosebleed, may result from disease, trauma, or other conditions such as hypertension, leukemia, or rheumatic fever. Most nosebleeds can be controlled easily with pressure at the base of the nose and application of cold. Application of heat (cautery) may be used to seal bleeding vessels.

Glaucoma (glaw-KO-muh) is a relatively common eye disorder in people over 35 years of age. Glaucoma results from an increase in the pressure inside the eye, caused by trauma or hereditary factors. The increased intraocular pressure can damage the optic disc and optic nerve and cause "tunnel" vision. The person may feel pain or no symptoms at all until damage occurs. Glaucoma can be controlled with medication that decreases the pressure.

Hyperopia (hi-per-O-pee-uh), or farsightedness, results from a congenital deformity in the eye. The condition is treated with corrective lenses.

Macular degeneration is the leading cause of blindness in people 65 and older. Macular degeneration results in a slow or sudden, painless loss of central vision. The first symptom may be visual distortion from one eye. Recent research indicates that high doses of antioxidant vitamins and zinc may slow vision loss. Treatment may include laser surgery.

Meniere's (men-ee-EERZ) disease is a collection of fluid in the labyrinth of the ear leading to dizziness (vertigo), ringing in the ear or tinnitus (TIN-ih-tus), pressure, and eventual deafness. The cause is unknown. Treatment includes medication, drainage of the fluid, or surgery.

Myopia (my-O-pee-uh), or nearsightedness, results from a congenital deformity in the eye. Treatment is corrective lenses or radial keratotomy (kare-uh-TOT-o-mee) in some cases.

Night blindness, or poor vision in dim light, results from a deficiency in the rods of the retina. This may be caused by insufficient vitamin A, cataracts, birth defect, or inflammation of the retina. Treatment may include supplementation of the diet with vitamin A.

Otitis media (o-TIE-tis MEE-dee-uh) is a middle ear bacterial or viral infection common in young children. It often appears in conjunction with a throat infection. The person feels pressure or pain in the ear. Otitis media may lead to hearing loss. Treatment includes antibiotics to cure the illness and may include myringotomy (meer-ing-GOT-o-me), the insertion of tubes to relieve pressure and fluid from the middle ear.

Presbyopia (pres-bee-O-pee-uh) is a type of farsightedness related to aging. The eye becomes less elastic and the fluid in the eye decreases. This can usually be treated effectively with corrective lenses. Other changes in the fluid may result in small clumps in the vitreous humor called *floaters* or flashes of light in the field of vision. These are not usually serious but should be monitored by periodic eye examination.

Retinal detachment may be due to injury or uncontrolled diabetes mellitus. It may occur gradually or be a medical emergency requiring immediate surgery. The person may experience a sudden appearance of light with eventual loss of visual field. Retinal detachment may be corrected with laser surgery that forms scar tissue that holds the retina in place.

Rhinitis (rie-NIE-tis) is inflammation of the lining of the nose caused by allergic reaction, viral infection, sinusitis, or chemical irritants. The person experiences drainage of nasal fluids, tears, and sneezing. Treatment depends on the cause and includes medication. Seasonal rhinitis (hay fever) may be caused by pollen in the air.

Ruptured eardrum may result from infection, an explosion, a blow to the head, or a sharp object inserted into the ear. The person experiences a slight pain and discharge from the ear. Healing usually occurs quickly. Scar tissue can form and result in hearing loss if the condition is chronic.

Sinusitis (sie-nus-I-tis) is a chronic or acute inflammation of the cavities of the cranium. Sinusitis is usually caused by spread of infection from the nasal passages to the sinuses or by nasal obstructions, which block the normal sinus drainage. The person experiences nasal discharge, sneezing, swelling below the eyes, and headache. Treatment may include medications or, in severe chronic cases, may require surgical correction of deformities.

Strabismus (strah-BIZ-mus) is a condition in which both eyes do not focus on the same point or direction. Strabismus may be caused by brain injury, a tumor, or infection, but is often the result of amblyopia. It may also be an inherited condition in which both eyes cannot be fixed on an object at the same time. Esotropia (es-o-TRO-pee-uh) or "crossed eyes" is the condition in which the muscles pull the eyes inward. Exotropia (ek-so-TRO-pee-uh) is the condition in which the muscles pull the eyes outward. Strabismus can be treated using eye exercises, patching, and corrective lenses. Surgery may be performed to correct the extraocular eye muscles.

A *sty* (stie) is caused by bacterial infection of the sebaceous glands of the eyelid. The sty contains pus and usually drains in 3 or 4 days. The person experiences pain, redness, and swelling. Treatment includes hot compresses, sometimes incision to drain the sty, and antibiotics.

Issues and Innovations

Vision Correction by Surgery

Radial keratotomy is a popular microscopic surgery that makes eight incisions into the cornea of the eye. These incisions cause a flattening of the cornea that corrects the refraction error causing myopia, or nearsightedness. The angle and depth of the cuts are calculated by computer and performed by an ophthalmologist. By 1994 more than 1 million people in the United States had undergone the procedure. A 10-year study by the U.S. National Eye Institute reports that the procedure was successful in two thirds of the cases. However, it also reports that 43% of those who had surgery later developed farsightedness.

Another surgical procedure in investigational stages is called *epikeratophakia.* This procedure involves freezing a donor cornea and then cutting it like a contact lens. A prescription correction can be provided with the cornea. The cornea is surgically implanted in the eye. In 4 to 6 months, the eye tissue attaches to the donor cornea and improved visual acuity results. The procedure has been used successfully to correct myopia, hyperopia, and cataract disorders.

In 1995 the FDA approved a computer-controlled laser surgery for vision repair called *photorefractive keratectomy* (PRK). PRK reshapes the cornea by shaving small pieces from the surface. It can be used to correct either near- or farsightedness. The cornea is reshaped as pieces of the cornea are removed by the laser. The main benefit of this procedure is that it does not weaken the cornea as might occur in radial keratotomy.

Noise Pollution

Noise in the environment can damage the nerve endings and cells in the inner ear. The ossicles of the ear amplify incoming sound 25 times before it reaches the inner ear. Hearing loss in industrial settings with strong noise pollution has been documented and has led to legislation to lower noise levels.

Loud music can also damage the cells in the inner ear. Once damaged, these cells cannot be repaired and the hearing loss is permanent. Environmental studies indicate that protection of the ears is needed with sound greater than 85 decibels (dB). Exposure to 2 hours of noise at 100 dB is known to cause some degree of permanent hearing loss. Even portable stereos with earphones can produce sound as loud as 115 dB.

Most people do not notice hearing loss until they cannot understand normal speech or they develop ringing in the ear (tinnitus). A sensation of fullness or buzzing in the ear after a concert or similar exposure to a loud noise indicates that damage has been done to the hair cells in the inner ear. This is called a "temporary threshold shift." In some cases, the hair cells may repair but repeated exposure leads to permanent hearing loss.

The volume of music is too high if it causes a ringing sensation or headache. It is too loud if a normal conversation cannot be heard. Because the ringer is in the earpiece, some cordless telephones have also been found to cause permanent damage to hearing when placed near the ear as it is ringing. Electronic noise canceling devices are used in headphones worn by airline pilots and may soon be available to the public. Chapter 33 provides more information regarding the environmental hazards of noise pollution.

Studies have confirmed that even casual use of cellular phones can damage the DNA in sensitive areas of the brain. Dr. Henry Lai of the University of Washington conducted a study that indicates that even low-level exposure to radio frequency electromagnetic fields and radio frequencies (EMF/RF) causes DNA damage to brain cells of rats, resulting in loss of short- and long-term memory and slower learning. He also concluded that the damage is cumulative. Research has provided extensive information on biological responses to power-frequency electric and magnetic fields (EMF). A strong link to development of cancer or other health problems due to EMF exposure has not been established.

Review Questions

1. Use the following terms in one or more sentences that correctly relate their meaning.
   Accommodation

   Intraocular

   Receptor

   Stimulus

   Vision

2. Describe the function of each of the five sensory organs.

3. Describe the location and function of each of the following parts of the sensory system.
   Corpuscles of Ruffini

   Iris

   Meissner's corpuscles

   Olfactory receptors

   Optic nerve

   Ossicle

   Pupil

4. Describe three methods of assessment of the sensory system function.

5. Describe the method by which radial keratotomy changes the vision of the eye.

6. Describe how hearing is damaged by noise.

Critical Thinking

1. Investigate and compare the cost of at least three tests used in diagnosing disorders of the sensory system.

2. Investigate the function of at least five common medications used in treatment of sensory system disorders.

3. List at least five occupations involved in the health care of sensory system disorders.

4. Investigate the current surgical techniques for correction of eye disorders with the use of laser technology.

5. Research the styles and cost of hearing aids.

6. Research and review an article regarding a recent development or treatment method relating to the sensory system.

20 Reproductive System

Learning Objectives

Define at least 10 terms relating to the reproductive system.

Describe the function of the reproductive system.

Identify at least 10 reproductive system structures and the function of each.

Describe at least five disorders of the reproductive system.

Identify at least three methods of assessment of the reproductive system.

Describe common patterns of growth and development of the neonate.

Key Terms

Conception
(kon-SEP-shun) Onset of pregnancy, union of sperm and egg (ovum)

Ectopic
(ek-TOP-ik) Located away from normal position

Erectile
(e-REK-til) Capable of becoming rigid and elevated when filled with blood

Fertility
(fer-TIL-ih-tee) Capacity to conceive or induce conception

Fibroid
(FIE-broyd) Tissue composed of threadlike, fibrous structure

Genital
(JEN-ih-tal) Reproductive organ

Gestation
(jes-TAY-shun) Development of young from conception to birth, pregnancy

Intercourse
(IN-ter-kors) Sexual union

Lactation
(lak-TAY-shun) Production and secretion of milk by the mammary glands (breasts)

Mammography
(ma-MOG-ruh-fee) Radiological view of breasts

Menses
(MEN-seez) Normal flow of blood and uterine lining that occurs in cycles in women

Menstrual cycle
(MEN-stroo-al) The recurring cycle of change of the reproductive organs induced by hormones in women

Ovulation
(o-vyoo-LAY-shun) Release of the egg (ovum) from the ovary

Sterility
(ster-IL-it-ee) Being unable to produce offspring

Reproductive System Terminology*

TERM	DEFINITION	PREFIX	ROOT	SUFFIX
Antenatal	Before birth	ante	nat	al
Colporrhaphy	Repair of the vagina		colpo	rrhaphy
Ectopic	Outside of the normal location		ectop	ic
Gynecology	Study of women		gyn/ec	ology
Hysterectomy	Removal of the uterus		hyster	ectomy
Mammography	Picture of the breast		mammo	graphy
Orchiectomy	Removal of the testes		orchi	ectomy
Prostatectomy	Removal of the prostate		prostat	ectomy
Uteropexy	Fixation of the uterus		uter/o	pexy
Vasectomy	Removal of a vessel		vas	ectomy

*A transition phrase or vowel may be added to or deleted from the word parts to make the combining form.

Abbreviations of the Reproductive System

ABBREVIATION	MEANING
circ	Circumcision
cx	Cervix
D&C	Dilation and curettage
del	Delivery
gyn	Gynecology
lap	Laparotomy
OB	Obstetrics
PEDS	Pediatrics
PMS	Premenstrual syndrome
TAH	Total abdominal hysterectomy

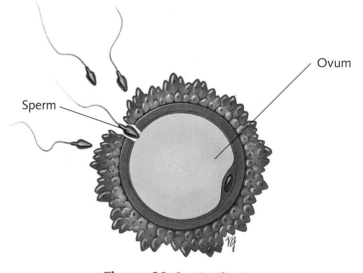

Figure 20-1 Fertilization.

Structure and Function of the Reproductive System

The function of the reproductive system is to produce offspring. The male and female reproductive organs (gonads) are different in structure to accomplish this function. Pu-berty is the age at which the reproductive organs mature sufficiently to allow reproduction.

The reproductive organs of both the male and female produce sex cells called *gametes*. The combination of genes of the female gamete (ova) and male gamete (sperm) is called *fertilization* (Figure 20-1). From the time of **conception** to 2 weeks, the fertilized ovum is called a *zygote*. From 2 to 8 weeks' **gestation,** the growing cells are called an *embryo*. From 8 weeks to birth, the unborn baby is called a *fetus*. During the first 30 days of life, the baby is considered to be a neonate.

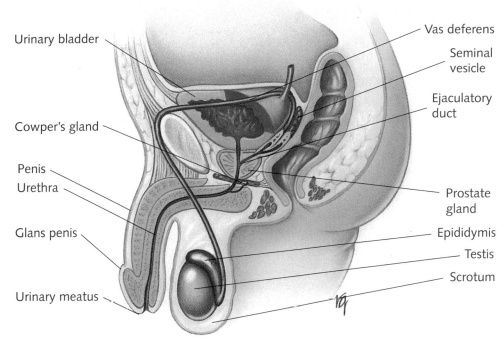

Urinary bladder

Cowper's gland

Penis

Urethra

Glans penis

Urinary meatus

Vas deferens

Seminal vesicle

Ejaculatory duct

Prostate gland

Epididymis

Testis

Scrotum

Figure 20-2   Male reproductive system.

Male Organs of Reproduction

The organs of reproduction of the male are shown in Figure 20-2. The testes, about 4 to 5 cm in length, produce the sperm. The testes also secrete an androgenic hormone (testosterone), causing the appearance of secondary sexual characteristics such as facial and body hair, deepened voice, increased muscle mass, and thickening of the bones.

The epididymis is a tube on the surface of each testis that stores the sperm while they mature. Sperm are transported by the vas deferens into the ejaculatory duct below the bladder. The seminal vesicle adds fluid that increases the volume and nourishes the sperm. The prostate gland, located below the bladder, secretes a fluid that protects the sperm.

The penis becomes rigid and elevated when filled with blood **(erectile)**. The penis encloses the urethra. The glans penis is covered with a loose-fitting, retractable casing called the *foreskin* (prepuce), which may be removed (circumcision). Both semen and urine are excreted through the urethra, but the systems operate separately. Semen is a thick, white secretion that contains the sperm and fluid. Expulsion of semen is called *ejaculation*. There are about 200 million sperm in each ejaculation.

The National Cancer Institute recommends a monthly self-examination of the testes (TSE) to detect testicular can-

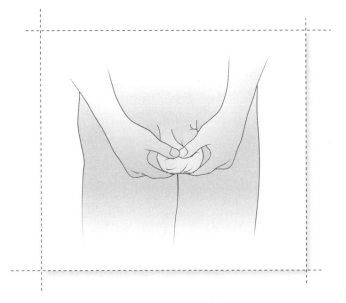

Figure 20-3   Testicular self-examination.

cer (Figure 20-3). Testicular cancer is the most common malignancy in young men between the ages of 20 and 34. There are about 7500 new cases and approximately 350 deaths each year in the United States. Testicular cancer represents about 1% of all cancers in men. However, it is the number one type of fatal cancer in men between 20 and 30 years of age.

Female Organs of Reproduction

The organs of reproduction in the female are shown in Figure 20-4. The ovaries are glands that produce eggs (ova) and the hormones estrogen and progesterone. The hormones prepare an egg (ovum) for fertilization, regulate the **menstrual cycle,** and help maintain pregnancy by promoting the growth of the placenta.

The fallopian tubes (oviducts) transport the mature ovum from the ovary to the uterus. Fertilization usually occurs in the fallopian tubes during the 5 days required for the ovum to move to the uterus. If the ovum is not fertilized, it degenerates and is excreted as part of the menstrual cycle.

The uterus is a muscular structure about the size of a small finger. The zygote is implanted in the uterus after conception. The cervix, or neck of the uterus, thins and opens for delivery of a fetus. The inner layer of the uterus, called the *endometrium,* is shed during each menstrual cycle.

The vagina is a muscular tube that extends from the cervix to the exterior of the body. It is the site of sexual **intercourse** and the passageway (birth canal) for delivery of the fetus.

The external structures of the female reproductive system are collectively called the *vulva* (Figure 20-5). The labia majora are folds of adipose tissue that protect the vaginal opening. The mons pubis is a pad of fat that joins the labia majora. The labia minora are pinkish folds of skin between the labia majora.

The clitoris is a small projection of erectile tissue located between the labia minora. Bartholin's glands secrete mucus and a lubricating fluid into the vaginal opening. The mammary glands (breasts) enlarge during puberty. The mammary glands have a system of ducts that secrete milk (**lactation**) after pregnancy.

Menstrual Cycle

The shedding of blood tissues of the uterus (menstruation) in the female signals the onset of puberty at about 10 to 16 years of age. The menstrual cycle, which lasts about 28 days, is a complex process of hormone secretion and tissue changes in the uterus (Table 20-1). A mature ovum is released from an ovary on about the fourteenth day of each cycle (Figure 20-6). Some women experience pain a few hours after **ovulation** called *Mittelschmerz.* This "middle pain" is believed to be caused by irritation of the peritoneum. If the released ovum is not fertilized, the lining of the uterus (endometrium) is released from the body along with the ovum. The sloughing of this bloody tissue, or **menses,** lasts from 3 to 7 days. The menstrual cycle continues until 45 to 50 years of age. The cessation of the cycle is called *menopause* (climacteric). Reduction in hormone production that occurs with menopause may cause a variety of symptoms, including "hot flashes," or transient periods of feeling warm. Reduced levels of both estrogen and

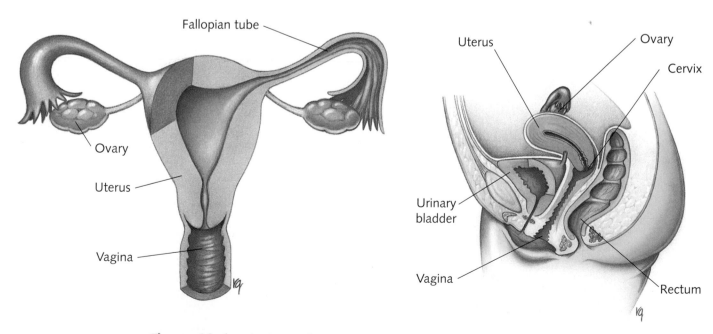

Figure 20-4 The internal structures of the female reproductive system.

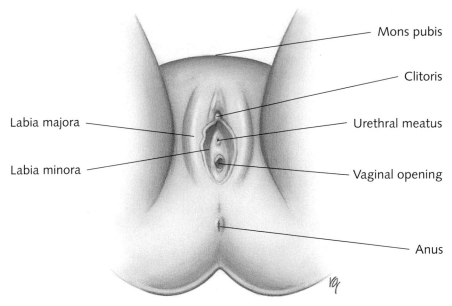

Figure 20-5   The external structures of the female reproductive system.

Table 20-1   Menstrual Cycle

Day(s)	Hormone Activity	Change in System
1	Pituitary secretes follicle-stimulating hormone (FSH)	Follicle cells mature and produce estrogen
	Pituitary secretes luteinizing hormone (LH)	Promotes estrogen production
2	Estrogen increases	Uterine lining begins to thicken; secondary sexual characteristics are maintained
3-13	No hormone activity	No change in system
14	Pituitary secretes FSH and LH	Mature follicle ruptures causing release of ovum* (ovulation); follicle of ovary becomes corpus luteum
15	Corpus luteum secretes progesterone and estrogen	Lining of uterus becomes more vascular; secretions of pituitary inhibited
16-23	No hormone activity	No changes in system
24	No hormone activity	Corpus luteum degenerates if ovum is not fertilized
25	Progesterone and estrogen secretion decreases	Blood vessels to uterine lining constrict; tissues disintegrate and slough
26-27	No hormone activity	No changes in system
28	No hormone activity	Menses begin and last approximately 5 days

*If the ovum is fertilized after leaving the ovary, it is implanted in the rich uterine wall. The corpus luteum continues to secrete progesterone throughout the pregnancy to maintain the uterine wall and inhibit the secretion of pituitary hormones.

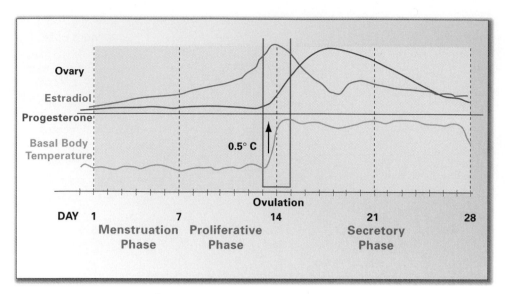

Figure 20-6   The menstrual cycle.

Pregnancy

Growth of an offspring in the uterus lasts about 280 days (9 months), or through the period of pregnancy. Pregnancy results from the union of the ovum and sperm, usually in the fallopian tube. The fertilized egg is known as a *zygote* for about 3 days. It is then considered to be the *morula* and enters the uterus. As a blastocyst, it implants in the uterine wall and is considered to be an *embryo* through the eighth week. From the eighth week until birth, it is considered to be a fetus.

Changes in the female reproductive system during pregnancy include an increase in muscle mass of the uterus and an elongation of the vagina. The uterus increases to 16 times normal size during pregnancy. The secretions, vascularity, and elasticity of the cervix and vagina also increase in preparation for the delivery of the fetus.

The amniotic sac is a membrane that surrounds the fetus in the uterus. The sac is filled with fluid to cushion and protect the fetus against infection and temperature changes. A portion of the uterus forms the placenta, which filters the blood of the mother to provide oxygen and nutrients for the fetus.

A baby born before the thirty-seventh week of pregnancy or weighing less than 2500 g (5 pounds ½ ounce) is considered to be premature. About 10% of babies in the United States fall in this category. Although there is no single cause for premature birth, some influencing factors

have been identified. These include social, environmental, economic, and nutritional deficits. The cost of care for a premature neonate ranges from $12,000 to $150,000.

Labor and Delivery

Labor is muscle contractions that signal the onset of delivery of the fetus. There are three stages of labor. In the first stage, muscle contractions of the uterus cause the amniotic sac to rupture and the cervix to open (dilate) to about 10 cm in diameter, allowing passage of the fetus. The second stage of labor is delivery of the baby, called *parturition*. Delivery of the afterbirth, or placenta, takes place about 15 minutes later and is the third stage of labor.

In the first 6 to 8 weeks after delivery of the baby, the mother is considered to be postpartum. During this time, the uterus shrinks back to normal size, and the hormonal balance of the body is reestablished.

Growth and Development

The physical and psychological stage of the newborn (neonate) changes rapidly from the moment of birth. *Growth* refers to the changes that can be measured by changes in height and weight as well as changes in body proportions. *Development* describes the stages of change in psychological and social functioning. These changes occur in spurts throughout the lifespan. At birth the baby, or neonate, is about 19 to 21 inches in length and weighs 7 to 8 pounds. The head is one fourth the length of the body compared with the adult ratio of one eighth. For the first 4 weeks, the baby is referred to as a neonate.

Assessment Techniques

Many disorders of the reproductive system can be assessed by palpation. Others are determined by blood tests, tissue culture, or by visual examination of the organs.

The most common methods of assessment of the male reproductive system are palpation and inspection of the organs (Box 20-1). Most disorders of the male reproductive system are treated by a physician specializing in urinary conditions (urologist). Cystoscopy can be used to view some of the reproductive structures. A blood test that measures a prostate-specific antigen (PSA) may be used to detect prostate cancer.

Disorders of the female reproductive system are treated by a specialist called a *gynecologist*. The vagina can be opened with an instrument called a *speculum* to allow inspection of the cervix. With a Pap smear, a few cells of the cervix are removed and studied microscopically to detect any potentially cancerous cells. Women over 35 years of age should have a Pap smear every 1 to 3 years.

Many abnormalities of the breast may be first discovered by self-examination (Box 20-2). **Mammography** is an x-ray technique used to visualize breast tissue to detect any possible cancerous changes early. Digital imaging software used in computerized mammograms can eliminate some errors in the reading. Although there is some disagreement regarding how frequently a mammogram should be performed, the American Cancer Society recommends that women have a mammogram every 2 years between the ages of 40 and 49 and on a yearly basis thereafter.

Several tests can be used to detect abnormalities of the fetus during gestation. These include amniocentesis, ultrasonography, and chorionic villus sampling (CVS). Amniocentesis is a procedure that removes a small amount of amniotic fluid between the sixteenth and twentieth week. This fluid can be used to detect fetal abnormalities (Figure 20-7). Ultrasonography uses high-frequency sound waves

---

Box 20-1   Testicular Self-Examination (TSE)*

1. While standing in front of a mirror, check for swelling on the scrotum.
2. Examine each testicle with both hands. Roll the testicle between the thumb and fingers. This should not be painful.
3. The epididymis may be confused with a lump but is located behind the testicle.
4. If you feel a lump, see a physician.

---

*TSE should be performed once a month after a warm bath or shower.

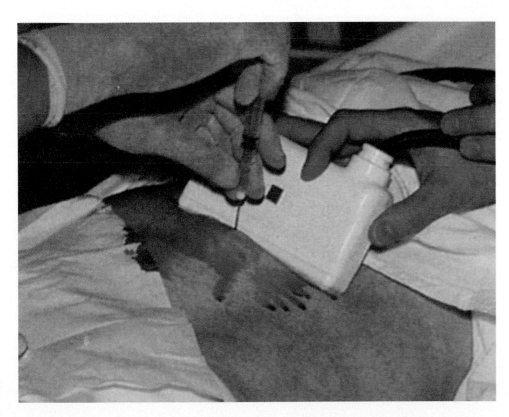

Figure 20-7   Laparoscopy allows the health care worker to see inside the abdomen through a very small incision.

to visualize structures deep in body cavities. Some evidence indicates that frequent sonograms (five or more) during pregnancy may lead to low birth weight. Chorionic villi are tiny vascular fibrils that help to form the placenta. Sampling of these fibrils using laparoscopy allows prenatal evaluation of the fetus. This procedure is often done in earlier stages of pregnancy than amniocentesis. CVS may cause birth defects such as missing fingers and toes in the unborn baby when performed early in the pregnancy.

Disorders of the Reproductive System

Benign prostatic hypertrophy (be-NINE pros-TAT-ik hi-PER-tro-fee) is an age-associated condition in men in which the prostate grows and may stiffen, causing blockage of the urethra (yoo-REE-thrah). The person may experience difficult and frequent urination and bloody urine, known as *hematuria* (hem-uh-TOO-ree-uh). Treatment may include surgical removal of part or all of the gland to remove the blockage.

Cancer of the female reproductive system occurs in several ways. Breast cancer is the most common cancer in women. According to *Science News* (June 1993), approximately one in eight women in the United States will be diagnosed with breast cancer in their lifetime. It can be painless and will spread, or metastasize (meh-TAS-tah-size), to other areas of the body if not detected early. Breast cancer can be detected by regular palpation for growths and with mammography (Figure 20-8 and Box 20-2). Less than 1% of breast cancers occur in men; however, the outcome for treatment is usually not as successful in men as in women.

Endometrial cancer is also common in women. Cervical cancer is associated with a history of sexually transmitted disease, smoking, and multiple sexual partners. Cervical

cancer can be detected early with a Pap smear. Treatment for cancer may include removal of the growth, radiation, and chemotherapy.

Cancer of the prostate is the second leading cause of death in men over 50 years of age. It is a slow-growing cancer that may show no symptoms for years. The person may experience a urinary disorder. Treatment may include removal of cancerous tissue and radiation.

Cancer of the testes, usually occurring in men 20 to 35 years of age, appears as a painless swelling of the scrotum. Rapid spread, or metastasis, is possible. Testicular cancer can be treated with surgery, radiation therapy, and chemotherapy. More than 90% of testicular cancer cases are cured by initial treatment.

Chancroid (SHANG-kroid) is a contagious bacterial infection characterized by painful sores (ulcers) on the **genital** area. The person may also have enlarged, painful lymph nodes, fever, and headaches. Chancroid is associated with poor hygiene and is transmitted by sexual contact. Treatment includes antibiotic medication and cleansing of the lesions.

Chlamydia (klah-MID-ee-uh), caused by the bacteria *Chlamydia trachomatis,* is the most common sexually transmitted disease according to the National Institute of Allergy and Infectious Diseases (NIAID). An estimated 4 million new cases occur each year. *Chlamydia* infection causes symptoms similar to those of gonorrhea, including painful urination and a discharge in both sexes. One of every two women infected has no symptoms. Pelvic inflammatory disease is a serious complication of chlamydial infection

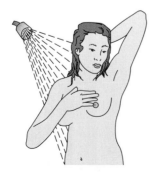

Figure 20-8   Breast self-examination. *(From Kinn ME, Woods M: The medical assistant, ed 8, Philadelphia, 1999, WB Saunders.)*

Box 20-2   Breast Self-Examination (BSE)*

1. In a supine position, flatten the right breast by placing a pillow under the right shoulder. Place the right arm behind the head.
2. Use the middle three fingers of the left hand to palpate for lumps using a circular rubbing motion from the center of the breast out.
3. Press firmly to feel through layers of the breast tissue.
4. Palpate the chest and axilla for lumps.
5. Repeat the procedure for the left breast.
6. Check the breasts while looking in a mirror for change in size, contour, dimpling, or discharge from the nipple.

---

*BSE should be completed once a month, 2 to 3 days after the menstrual cycle.

and may result in infertility in women. A pregnant woman may pass the infection to the newborn during delivery, leading to neonatal problems such as eye infections or pneumonia. *Chlamydia* can be treated successfully with antibiotics in 95% of the cases.

Cryptorchidism (kript-OR-kid-izm) is the failure of the testes to descend into the scrotal sac before birth. The undescended testes often descend later without intervention. If not descended by age 5, treatment may include hormone supplementation. Surgical correction, known as *orchiopexy* (OR-kee-o-pek-see), is possible but may result in reduced **fertility.**

An **ectopic** pregnancy is one that occurs in an abnormal location in the body. In ectopic pregnancies, the embryo or fetus does not usually survive, and the condition can be life-threatening to the woman if rupture results in internal bleeding. Ectopic pregnancies are now more common because of the greater incidence of sexually transmitted diseases, which damage the fallopian tubes. Ectopic pregnancies are associated with pelvic inflammatory disease and use of an intrauterine device (IUD) and some birth control pills. The person may experience lower abdominal pain, mild vaginal bleeding, and abdominal tenderness on palpation. Treatment is surgical removal of the embryo and, possibly, affected reproductive organs.

Endometriosis (en-do-mee-tree-O-sis) is growth of endometrial tissue in an area other than the uterus. The tissue continually grows and sheds, leading to abnormal bleeding and pain and sometimes to infertility. Treatment includes medication with pain relievers and steroids and possibly surgical removal of the affected organs.

Erythroblastosis fetalis (e-rith-ro-blas-TO-sis fet-AL-is) is a condition that may develop in an Rh+ fetus of an Rh- mother who has developed antibodies against the Rh blood protein in a prior pregnancy. Antibodies from the mother cross the placenta and attack the blood of the fetus. The condition leads to red cell destruction, jaundice, respiratory distress, and plaque formation in the brain of the fetus. Development of the Rh antibodies can be detected with a Coomb's test and blocked with an injection of RhoGAM. Treatment of the affected fetus can be done while the fetus is still in the uterus and at birth with transfusion.

Fetal alcohol syndrome (FAS) and *fetal alcohol effect* (FAE) include a group of physical and mental birth defects that result from damage to the fetus by alcohol consumed by the mother. The alcohol crosses the placenta and the fetus's liver is unable to remove it quickly. It is estimated that 1 in 750 births in the Unites States involves fetal alcohol syndrome with fetal alcohol effect five times as prevalent. The affected baby is often premature with smaller head and brain, low birth weight, and typical facial features of the disorder. In addition to learning and behavior problems, the baby may also suffer seizures and heart defects. There

is no safe level of alcohol consumption by the expectant mother to prevent this disorder. There is no cure for the affected child. Children affected with fetal alcohol effect and fetal alcohol syndrome are often placed in programs for children with special needs because of learning and behavioral problems and may need anticonvulsive medication or even brain surgery.

Fibroid tumors or *fibromyomas* are benign growths found in the uterus of 50% of women over 50 years of age. The person may experience bleeding or no symptoms. Treatment may include surgical removal if the tumors cause symptoms.

Genital warts, or *Condylomata cuinata,* are caused by one type of human papilloma virus. According to the NIAID, genital warts are very contagious with as many as 1 million new cases each year. Approximately two thirds of the people having sexual contact with people that have genital warts develop them. The presence of genital warts is commonly associated with genital cancers such as cervical, vulvar, and penile cancer. Warts on the external genitalia can be treated by surgical removal, freezing (cryotherapy), chemical or electrical burning, or injection of the warts with interferon. Although treatment removes the warts, it does not kill the virus, so they often reappear.

Gonorrhea (gon-or-REE-uh) is a bacterial infection and is one of the most prevalent sexually transmitted diseases. According to the NIAID, 1.5 million new cases occur each year. The most common symptom is painful urination and a white to yellowish-green discharge from the urethra. The female often experiences no symptoms but may have dysuria or pain in the abdomen. Gonorrhea can lead to **sterility** and arthritis if untreated. Gonorrhea may result in blindness in babies born to infected mothers. Treatment includes penicillin, but penicillin-resistant strains of gonorrhea are increasing.

Herpes simplex (HER-peez SIM-pleks) *virus* (HSV), or genital herpes, is one of the most common sexually transmitted diseases, affecting an estimated 30 million Americans. According to the NIAID, 500,000 new cases occur each year. Herpes is caused by a virus that results in blisters, which open into painful sores. Herpes lesions appear in episodes, triggered by factors such as sunlight, friction, emotional stress, and fever. Herpes is spread by sexual contact or secretions from open lesions. Women who have herpes lesions can transfer the virus to their babies during birth, causing mental retardation or death. There is no cure, but new treatment includes an antiviral medication that controls symptoms.

Human papilloma virus (HPV) affects an estimated 40 million Americans, according to the NIAID. More than 60 types of HPV have been identified. HPV infection often does not cause visible symptoms. It may appear as genital warts. HPV is associated with the development of cervical cancer in some cases. HPV may be treated by cryotherapy, burning (electrocautery), injection of interferon, or application of chemicals. Treatment removes the warts but does not eliminate the virus.

Klinefelter's (KLINE-fel-terz) *syndrome* is a defect appearing in males who carry an extra chromosome resulting in a karyotype of XXY. Males with this syndrome may develop breast tissue, tall stature, small testicles, below normal intelligence, and sterility. There is no treatment.

Leukorrhea (loo-ko-REE-uh) is a whitish vaginal discharge. A slight discharge is normal in the menstrual cycle when the ovum is released (ovulation) and just before menstruation. Any change in the color, odor, or character of the discharge may indicate a disorder. An excessive discharge may occur as a result of infection. Leukorrhea may be accompanied by redness, painful urination, or discomfort. Treatment of leukorrhea depends on the cause.

Menstrual (MEN-stroo-ul) *disorders* may result from endocrine, metabolic, and nutritional imbalances. Painful menstrual cramping, called *dysmenorrhea* (dis-men-o-REE-a), is often due to hormonal imbalance and faulty uterine structure. Excessive bleeding, or menorrhagia (men-o-RAY-jee-ah), or no bleeding, known as *amenorrhea* (a-men-o-REE-uh), may also occur. Menorrhagia may occur as a result of benign fibromas of the uterus. Amenorrhea may result from hormone imbalances, structural deformities, weight loss, and excessive exercise. Treatment depends on the severity and cause but may include surgical removal of the uterus in severe cases of menorrhagia.

Orchitis (or-KI-tis) is an inflammation of the testes usually resulting from sexually transmitted infection or mumps. The person may experience swelling, redness, and pain in the scrotum. Treatment may include elevation of the scrotum, ice packs, and pain-relieving medication.

Pelvic inflammatory (PEL-vik in-FLAM-ah-tore-ee) *disease* (PID) is relatively common, particularly in teenage women. Approximately 1 million women develop PID each year. Development of PID is usually associated with infection by gonorrhea or chlamydia and can become chronic. It affects all of the reproductive organs of the pelvis and causes scarring of the fallopian tubes. The woman experiences lower abdominal pain, fever, vaginal discharge, and menstrual disorders. According to the NIAID, an estimated 100,000 women become infertile each year as a result of PID. Ectopic pregnancy may result from damage to the fallopian tubes. Diagnosis can be done rapidly using a biotechnology technique called *polymerase chain reaction*. Treatment includes antibiotics and sometimes surgery.

Phimosis (fih-MO-sis) is a narrowing (stenosis) of the foreskin of the glans penis. Usually caused by infections, phimosis may interfere with urination and cause redness, swelling, pain, and pus formation. Treatment includes antibiotics, soaking, and surgical removal of the foreskin (circumcision).

Premenstrual (pre-MEN-stroo-al) *syndrome* (PMS) is a common collection of up to 150 symptoms occurring 3 to 14 days before the beginning of the bleeding part (menses) of the menstrual cycle. The woman may experience irritability, depression, impaired concentration, headache, and edema (eh-DEE-ma). The symptoms vary greatly and disappear with the menses. There are several theories to explain the symptoms of PMS, including hormonal or biochemical imbalance and poor nutrition. Treatment includes diet modification to eliminate sugar, caffeine, alcohol, nicotine, and processed foods. Vitamin B, calcium, magnesium, and chromium are prescribed in some cases. Exercise and stress reduction training may also be helpful.

Pubic (PYOO-bik) *lice* are yellow-gray parasites found in the pubic hair. They become dark in color when engorged with blood. They are usually transmitted sexually, but they can also be spread through clothes and bed linen. They cause itching. Treatment includes medicated shampoo, cream, or lotion to kill the parasite.

Sexually transmitted diseases (STDs) affect men and women of all social and economic backgrounds. More than 30 STDs have been identified by the NIAID and affect more than 13 million people each year. About two thirds of all STDs occur in people younger than 25, with nearly 2.5 million teenagers infected each year. Some common sexually transmitted diseases are chlamydia, herpes simplex, human papilloma virus, gonorrhea, and syphilis. Other STDs include trichomoniasis, hepatitis B, scabies, AIDS, and pubic lice.

Syphilis (SIF-ih-lis), currently at its highest rate in 40 years, is caused by a spirochete (SPY-ro-keet) bacteria, *Treponema pallidum* (trep-o-NEE-mah PAL-ih-dum), and occurs in three stages. Painless sores, or chancres, first appear 10 to 90 days after infection and disappear in a few weeks in the second stage. The infection spreads into the blood stream and causes fever, swollen glands, and rash that then disappear in 10 to 14 days. Third-stage syphilis may appear years later as the nervous system tissue is damaged, leading to death in one third of untreated cases. Syphilis may cause birth defects in babies of mothers with syphilis. Syphilis can be successfully treated with antibiotics.

Trichomonas vaginalis (trik-o-MO-nas VAJ-ih-nal-es) is a parasitic protozoa. The person may have no symptoms or may experience a foul-smelling, yellowish-green discharge and redness of the vulva, urinary frequency, or painful urination (dysuria). Treatment includes oral medication.

Vaginitis (vaj-ih-NIE-tis) is a nonspecific infection that may cause a scant, gray, foul-smelling discharge. Treatment includes antibiotics such as ampicillin.

Yeast infection is an overgrowth of yeast in the vagina that appears as a curdy, cheeselike discharge. This infection commonly occurs in women who are diabetic or are taking medication such as antibiotics, steroids, or commercial douches that alter the pH of the vagina. Treatment includes antifungal, or mycostatic (MY-ko-stat-ik), medication or potassium hydroxide.

Issues and Innovations

Alternatives in Conception

Technological advances have given people many choices regarding reproduction. Effective birth control methods have been developed to prevent pregnancy, although teenage and unwanted pregnancy remains a major problem. In a February 2002 release, the CDC reported that the United States had the highest rate of pregnancy, abortion, and childbirth of all the industrialized nations. This was true even though the rate of sexual activity in other countries is considered to be similar. The *Encyclopedia Britannica* reports that 1 million, or one in every nine, girls between the ages of 15 to 19 become pregnant each year. About one half of the pregnancies of teenagers are terminated by abortion. The effectiveness of contraceptive methods varies a great deal (Table 20-2). Abstinence is the only birth control method that successfully prevents pregnancy and sexually

Table 20-2   Contraceptive Methods

Method	Effectiveness	Description
RU486	100%	Abortifacient drug (mifepristone) taken orally up to 9 weeks of pregnancy along with prostaglandin, resulting in abortion of fetus 1 to 1.5 weeks later; ban against use lifted in United States in 1993; also used for treatment of breast cancer, endometriosis, glaucoma, and brain tumors
Abstinence	100%	Refraining from sexual activities that could result in pregnancy
Norplant	99.8%	Capsules implanted under the skin of the upper arm containing levonorgestrel, a synthetic progesterone that stops ovulation; effective for 5 years
Vasectomy	99.8%	Surgical cutting of the vas deferens of the man so that sperm does not leave the testes; may be reversed in approximately 50% of cases
Tubal ligation	99.6%	Surgical cutting of the fallopian tubes of the woman so that the ovum does not reach the uterus; may be reversed in 25% of cases
Birth control pills	94%-97%	Contains estrogen and progesterone hormones to prevent ovulation or progesterone only to prevent implantation of the ovum; not recommended in some women because of health risk; Depo-Provera (DMPA) developed in 1992 as a synthetic form of progesterone
Intrauterine device (IUD)	94%	Inserted into uterus by doctor; IUD scrapes lining of uterus to prevent implantation of ovum
Barrier methods	88%	Condoms cover the erect penis to collect sperm entry into uterus
	84%	Diaphragms cover the entrance to the cervix with a soft cap that prevents the sperm from entering; best used with spermicidal jelly; must be individually fitted and checked yearly
	79%	Spermicidal agents are chemicals in creams, jellies, suppositories, or foams inserted into the vagina before intercourse to kill sperm cells
	73%-92%	Cervical cap inserted 1 hour before intercourse to block entry of sperm
"Natural" methods	60%-75%	Rhythm method, or fertility awareness, requires abstention during ovulation by counting days or checking body temperature
	81%-96%	Withdrawal is the removal of the penis before ejaculation

transmitted diseases. Abortion remains a controversial moral and legal issue.

In vitro (from the Latin *vitrum,* "glass") fertilization is a technique of conception for those who are otherwise infertile. The first "test tube" baby was born in England in 1978, with hundreds more now living throughout the world. The procedure involves removal of eggs from the ovary with a surgical needle. The egg is incubated and then joined with sperm cells. Some of the fertilized eggs are then implanted by laparoscopy into the uterus of the female who will carry the pregnancy. An ethical concern of this method relates to the status of the unused embryos, which can be frozen and implanted later or discarded. In 1993, a procedure called *intracytoplasmic sperm injection* (ICSI) was performed for the first time in the United States. In this procedure, a single sperm cell is injected into an egg, which is then implanted into the uterus. This procedure is used for infertility problems that result from low sperm count or misshaped or immotile sperm. Fertility drugs provide another method to increase the chances of pregnancy by stimulating the ovaries to secrete eggs. Fertility drugs may lead to multiple or premature births.

The issue of surrogacy has become an ethical and legal concern. In surrogacy, the sperm and ovum are artificially fertilized and implanted in a woman who agrees to give the baby to the couple after birth. A fee is usually given to the woman for bearing the child. Surrogate mothering is an alternative for women for whom pregnancy is a health risk or impossibility. In some cases, the woman bearing the child has been reluctant to give the baby to the couple as agreed. Some states have passed laws to make surrogacy illegal.

More than 10% of live births or more than 4 million infants in the United States are born before 37 weeks of gestation or prematurely. With innovations such as the drugs used to replace pulmonary surfactant in the care of premature infants, a fetus can now survive outside the uterus (called *viability*) at a much younger age, even at less than 20 weeks' gestation.

Surgery has also been successful to correct a defect in a fetus as early as the twenty-fifth week of gestation. Approximately 50 "open" fetal surgeries have been performed. The fetus is partially removed from the uterus in a procedure similar to a cesarean section and replaced after the surgical correction is completed. Open fetal surgery was used successfully to remove a lung tumor on a 26-week-old fetus in Georgia. Two children have survived *in utero* abdominal surgery. "Closed" fetal procedures are more common and use ultrasound to place a needle in the uterus or umbilical cord to treat the fetus. Some closed fetal procedures include transfusion in cases of Rh blood incompatibility, removal of excess lung fluid, administration of heart medication, and clearing urinary system obstructions.

Infertility

Infertility is an inability to conceive. About one of every six couples are infertile because of abnormalities in the reproductive system or problems with production of gametes. The National Center for Health statistics reports an overall consistent rate in the number of infertile couples with a total of more than 2 million. Approximately 40% of infertility problems can be traced to low sperm count. Another common cause is damage to the fallopian tubes that occurs with sexually transmitted diseases, especially pelvic inflammatory disease. Infertility is also associated with prolonged use of birth control methods. The intrauterine device is known to damage uterine tissue and birth control pills alter the hormonal balance of the body to prevent ovulations. Repetitive elective abortion by scraping the uterus (dilation and curettage) also may hinder successful pregnancy. Hormonal changes resulting from stress and excessive exercise may also cause infertility. The tendency of couples to delay childbearing until their late twenties or early thirties may also be a factor.

Redefining the Sexes

Changes in family structure and sexual orientation have become a major national concern. Alternative sexual lifestyles remain a controversial issue, such as relations between members of the same gender (homosexual) or both genders (bisexual). Transvestites dress in the clothes of the opposite gender.

Some people have also undergone surgeries to change their sexual appearance (transsexual). The person who seeks transsexual treatment is given hormones to produce secondary sexual characteristics such as voice and hair changes and breast tissue growth. Plastic surgery cosmetically changes genital structure. Internal reproductive organs and the genetic makeup of the cells are not changed. Sexual intercourse is possible for the transsexual, but conception is not.

Review Questions

1. Use the following terms in one or more sentences that correctly relate their meaning.
   Conception
   Fertility
   Gestation
   Intercourse

2. Describe the function of the reproductive system.

3. Describe the location and function of each of the following parts of the reproductive system.
   Cervix
   Fallopian tube
   Ovary
   Penis
   Uterus
   Vagina

4. Describe three reproductive system disorders that are caused by a pathogen.

5. Describe three methods used to assess the reproductive system.

6. Differentiate between the effectiveness of three methods of contraception.

7. Describe three methods of artificial insemination and the circumstances that might lead to the choice of each method.

8. Describe the development of the newborn from conception to neonate.

Critical Thinking

1. Investigate and compare the cost of at least three tests used in diagnosing disorders of the reproductive system.

2. Investigate the function of at least five common medications used in treatment of the reproductive system.

3. List at least five occupations involved in the health care for reproductive system disorders.

4. Investigate the cost of *in vitro* fertilization.

5. Investigate the current legal issues regarding surrogate mothering contracts.

6. Investigate the postpartum disorder sometimes called the "blues."

7. Investigate the frequency of occurrence and cause of sudden infant death syndrome (SIDS).

8. Research and review an article regarding a recent development or treatment method relating to the reproductive system.

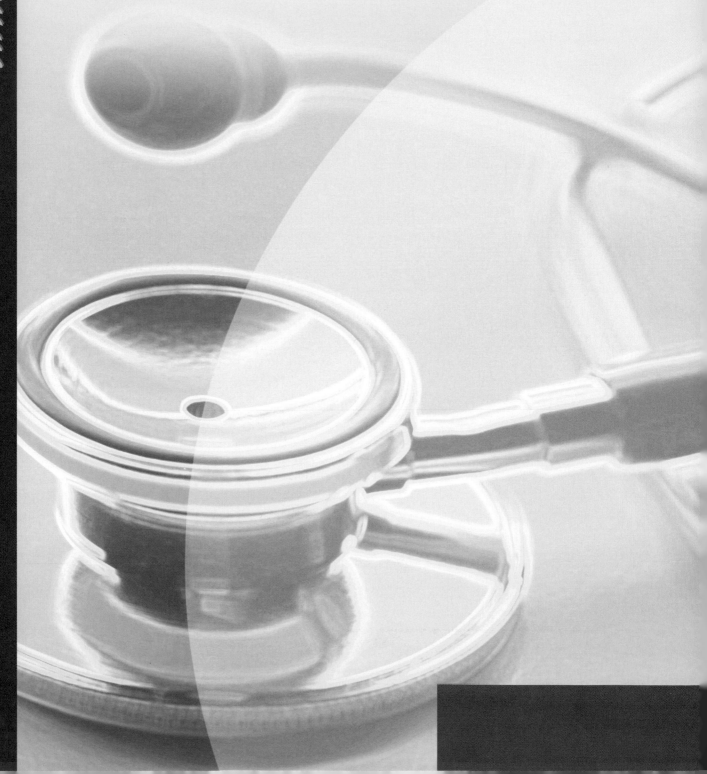

Career Clusters

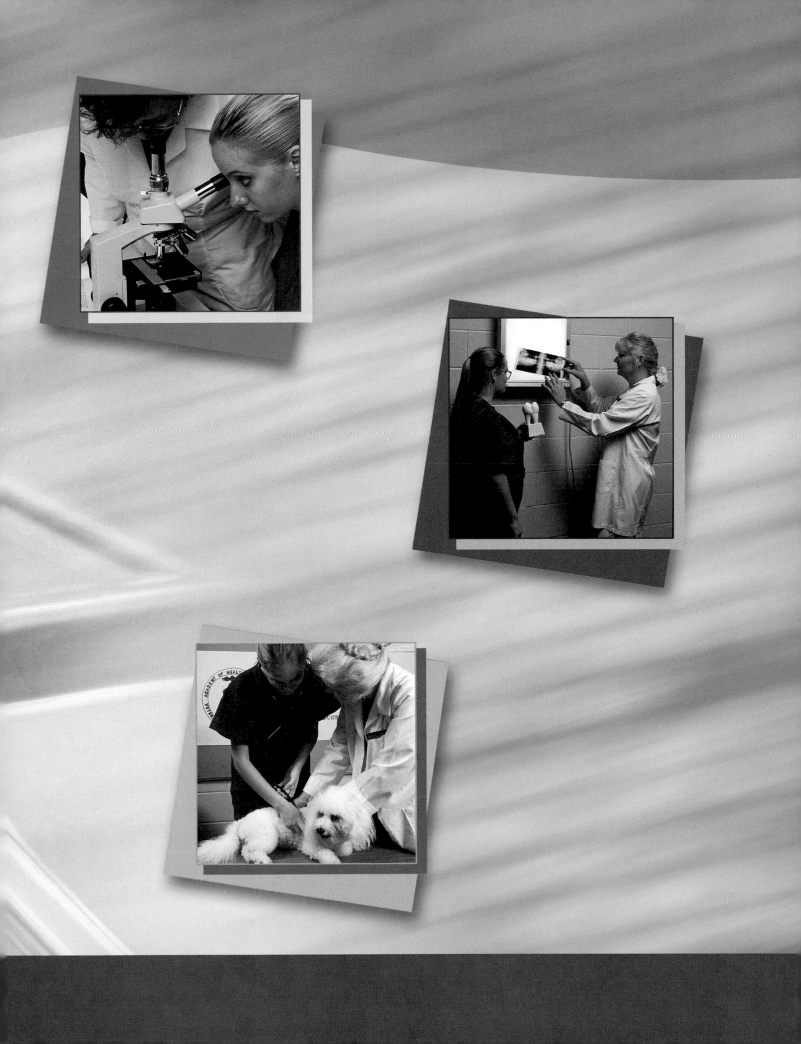

21
Laboratory Careers

Learning Objectives

Define at least 10 terms relating to laboratory careers.

Specify the role of selected laboratory health care workers including personal characteristics, levels of education, and credentialing requirements.

Differentiate between pathogenic and nonpathogenic microorganisms.

Identify six groups of microorganisms that may be pathogenic in humans.

Describe the conditions that are favorable for growth of microorganisms.

Identify three ways in which the skin serves as a defense against infection.

Key Terms

Donor
(DOE-ner) Person who supplies living tissue or who furnishes blood or blood products for transfusion to another person

Fomite
(FOE-mite) Inanimate object capable of carrying germs

Immunity
(im-YOO-nih-tee) High level of resistance to certain microorganisms or diseases

Infection
(in-FEK-shun) Invasion and multiplication of pathogenic microorganisms in the body tissues

Microorganism
(mie-cro-ORG-un-izm) Microscopic living organism, microbe

Nonpathogenic
(non-path-o-JEN-ik) Microorganism that does not produce disease

Pathogen
(PATH-o-jen) Microorganism that produces disease

Phagocyte
(FAY-go-site) Cell that surrounds and destroys microorganisms and foreign particles

Phlebotomy
(fle-BOT-uh-mee) Incision into a vein to withdraw blood

Recipient
(re-SIP-ee-int) One who receives tissue from another, such as in a blood transfusion

Sterile
(STARE-ul) Free from all living microorganisms

Laboratory Careers Terminology*

TERM	DEFINITION	PREFIX	ROOT	SUFFIX
Aerobic	Pertaining to air		aerob	ic
Antitoxin	Against poisoning	anti	toxin	
Microbiology	Study of life on the microscopic level	micro	bio	ology
Microorganism	Small living thing	micro	organism	
Nonpathogen	Does not originate (cause) disease	non	path/o	gen
Pathogen	Originates (causes) disease		path/o	gen
Pathologist	One who studies disease		path	ologist
Phagocyte	Cell that eats	phag/o	cyte	
Urinalysis	Test to study urine		urin	alysis
Zoologist	One who studies animals		zoo	o/logist

*A transition phrase or vowel may be added to or deleted from the word parts to make the combining form.

Abbreviations for Laboratory Careers

ABBREVIATION	MEANING
ABC	Aspiration, biopsy, cytology
AFB	Acid-fast bacillus
bl wk	Blood work
BUN	Blood, urea, nitrogen
CPK	Creatine phosphokinase
ESR	Erythrocyte sedimentation rate
H & H	Hemoglobin and hematocrit
SMAC	Sequential multiple analysis computer
spG	Specific gravity
UA	Urinalysis

Careers

Laboratory careers include workers with a broad range of interests and abilities (Box 21-1). Opportunities in this area include clinical laboratory, blood banking, research, and related fields in life science.

Clinical Laboratory Science

Laboratory personnel do not usually have contact with the patient. The laboratory provides a clean, well-lighted, and controlled working environment with regular hours. Most of the laboratory work is done while sitting. Excellent vision and manual dexterity are needed to perform laboratory work.

The pathologist is a medical doctor who examines specimens of body tissue, fluids, and secretions to diagnose disease. Other medical practitioners rely on the pathologist as a consultant who determines the effectiveness of treatments and the cause of death. The pathologist must first complete medical school and then obtain specialized education and training in this area. Hospitals, medical schools, all levels of government, and private industry employ pathologists. In many hospitals, the pathologist supervises the laboratory.

The laboratory technologist, also called the *clinical laboratory scientist* (CLS), performs clinical laboratory testing and analyzes the results using independent judgment. For example, the technologist cross-matches blood to be used for transfusion. The technologist calibrates the equipment and assists in determining the accuracy and utility of new tests and procedures under the supervision of the pathologist or laboratory supervisor. Technologists usually complete a bachelor's degree followed by a training program of up to 1 year in length. The Board of Registry for Laboratory Technologists requires a baccalaureate degree and an examination to become a certified technologist (CT). Licensure of technologists is required in some states.

Box 21-1 Laboratory Careers

Blood donor unit assistant
Chemistry technologist
Cleaner, laboratory equipment
Cytologist
Cytotechnologist
Dairy technologist
Feed research aide
Histologic technician
Histopathologist
Immunohematologist
Laboratory assistant, culture media
Laboratory sample carrier
Medical laboratory assistant
Medical laboratory technician
Medical technologist
Medical technologist, chief
Microbiology technologist
Pathologist
Phlebotomist
Poultry scientist
Zoologist

Laboratory health care workers perform tests to monitor and provide support for the functions of other health care providers.

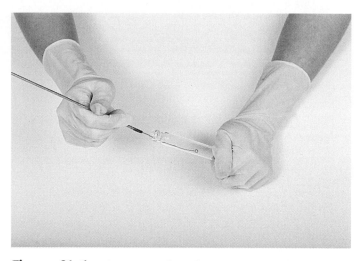

Figure 21-1 Care must be taken not to touch the loop to the sides of the test tube during transfer of microorganisms.

Several areas of specialization are possible for the laboratory technologist. The microbiology technologist may collect the specimen directly from the patient or receive materials from an autopsy. The technologist then grows and isolates the **microorganisms** to assist with their identification (Figure 21-1; Skill 21-1). Cytotechnologists specialize in preparation and screening of cells for diagnosis after collection by scraping, brushing, or aspirating body cells from an organ or site (Figure 21-2). These microscopic cells may be used to diagnose cancer, infectious agents, or inflammation. Chemistry technologists analyze body fluids and wastes. Other areas of specialization are the study of blood (hematology) and the study of resistance to **pathogens** (immunology).

Medical laboratory technicians (MLT), also called *clinical laboratory technicians* (CLT), perform daily tasks under the supervision of the laboratory technologist or pathologist. The responsibilities include preparation of tissue slides and performance of simple blood tests. The technician obtains blood samples, prepares tissue slides, analyzes body specimens, and performs cell counts and urinalysis. Technicians complete at least 2 years of training.

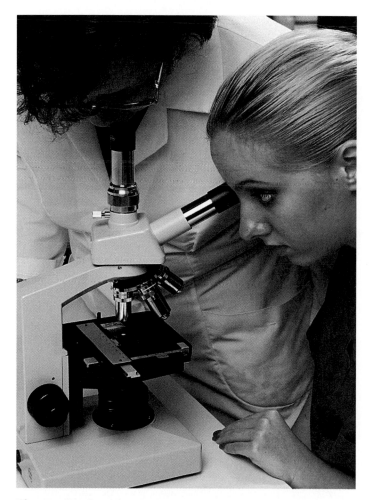

Figure 21-2 The microscope allows the health care worker to study many microorganisms.

Skill 21-1

Transferring Bacteria

1. Maintain medical asepsis by using the guidelines provided in the Standard and Transmission-Based Precautions, including good handwashing technique and use of gloves as needed.

2. Microorganisms may be nonpathogenic in certain areas of the body, but pathogenic in others.

3. Hold the test tube so that the opening is not straight up, to prevent dust from entering it while the cap is off.

4. Flame a wire loop by holding the wire in the center of the flame until red hot. Flaming the loop kills any microorganisms that may be present on it.

5. Remove the cap or lid. Hold the cap so that the inside edges do not touch anything. If the inside surface or edges of the lid touch anything that is not sterile, the specimen is contaminated.

6. Pass the opening of the test tube through the flame. Heat will kill any bacteria that might be present on the edges of the test tube.

7. Insert the wire loop into the test tube or onto the plate without touching any edges. Edges are considered to be contaminated.

8. Run the loop or applicator on the surface of the agar to remove or add bacteria to the surface. Do not break the surface of the agar. If the surface of the agar is broken, the microorganism will grow down and under the media.

9. Reflame and recap the tube or replace the lid on the agar plate. Immediately recapping the tube avoids contamination.

10. Flame the loop to kill all bacteria before putting it on any surface.

11. Label all containers with the date and type of bacteria.

12. Incubate bacterial cultures for growth. The best temperature for most bacteria is 35° to 36° C.

To qualify for the medical laboratory technician certification examination through the American Society for Certified Pathologists (ASCP), an associate degree from an accredited college or university program or 5 years of full-time acceptable clinical laboratory experience is needed. Some states require certification or licensure for technicians.

Medical laboratory technicians may specialize in one area, such as histology. This involves the preparation of tissues for diagnosis, research, and teaching purposes. Histology technicians may work in many different settings including the hospital, forensics labs, immunopathology research, veterinary practice, or marine biology. Histology technicians (HT) may be certified and must be licensed in some states. The certified histological technician must complete an associate degree and 1 year of acceptable experience in histopathology or 3 years of experience under the supervision of a certified pathologist.

Medical laboratory assistants perform routine tests under the supervision of the technologist or other qualified personnel. Areas of testing that are performed by the assistant may include urinalysis, hematology, serology, and bacteriology. Laboratory assistants complete 1 year of training in a hospital or 2 years in college or vocational programs. Certification is possible after successful completion of an accredited program and a registry exam. Phlebotomists obtain and process blood specimens to aid in the diagnosis and treatment of disease (Figure 21-3). Phlebotomists may be trained on the job or in community college or vocational programs.

Blood Banking

Careers in blood banking include **donor** recruitment, collection and processing of donor blood, testing and typing of blood, laboratory supervision, and teaching. Specialists in blood bank technology (SBB) select donors, draw blood, classify (type) blood, and run pretransfusion tests to ensure the safety of the **recipient.** Blood bank specialists act as a resource in solving blood-related problems. Applicants as blood bank specialists must have a baccalaureate degree and certification as a medical technologist. The blood bank specialist program of study is 12 months long. After successful completion of the program and examination, the blood bank specialist may be qualified for certification.

Life Science

Life scientists or researchers study living organisms and life processes including growth and reproduction. Many areas of specialization are possible in research and development in the health care industry. The educational requirements for research are a master's degree or doctoral-

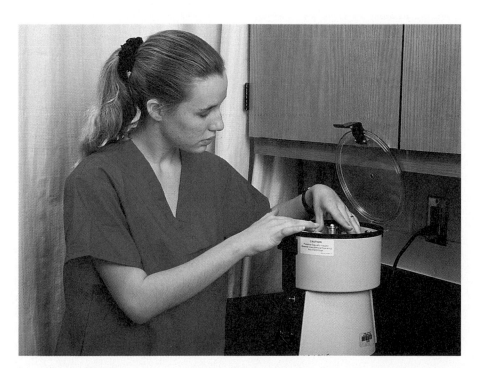

Figure 21-3   The phlebotomist uses a centrifuge to process blood.

level preparation. Medical research is conducted in the areas of biology, anatomy, biochemistry, genetics, physics, physiology, and microbiology. Life scientists are responsible for the development of new drugs, plant varieties, methods of treatment, and methods of environmental protection. Biotechnologists or genetic engineers explore the genetic design of plants and animals. Chapter 34 provides more information regarding career opportunities in biotechnology. Approximately one fourth of life scientists work for the federal government. One third of the life scientists work in private industry. Universities and similar agencies employ others.

Microbiologists study bacteria, algae, viruses and other microorganisms that cause disease or may be used to prevent it. Some accomplishments of microbiological research include the development of vaccines for polio and other diseases. Microbiologists also help to determine the method of transmission of diseases. Clinical microbiologists work in a medical, veterinary, or laboratory setting to identify microorganisms in specimens. This may include the development of new drugs. Microbiologists usually work in a laboratory of a hospital or private industry such as pharmaceuticals. Microbiologists may begin work with a 4-year university degree. Higher salary offers are given to employees with a master's or doctoral degree. Most researchers and supervisors in microbiology hold a doctoral degree. Licensure is not required of microbiologists. There are several specialty areas of microbiology, including virology, mycology, and immunology.

Virologists specialize in researching the method by which viruses infect cells and cause disease. More recently, virologists have helped develop viruses that are used to transport and manipulate genetic material. Mycologists study fungal organisms such as molds and yeast.

Immunologists use the body's defense mechanisms (antibodies) to fight disease. Biotechnology techniques used by the immunologist include cell typing and tissue culturing to produce transplant skin or tumor grafts. Recombined or genetically manipulated cells can be implanted directly into the body in a process called *cell fusion.* Commercially produced tissue cultures can be used for grafts. Cell cultures that are being developed include liver, connective tissue, bone marrow, and blood vessels. An artificial pancreas tissue has been developed and is currently being tested.

Biochemists study the chemical nature of living things. In cells, the work involves the methods of reproduction, growth, and metabolism. Biochemists analyze and research the effect of hormones, enzymes, serums, and foods on the tissues and organs of animals. Some areas of study for biochemists include processes such as aging, tooth decay, and viral infection. Clinical biochemists may work in medical laboratories or private industry such as

pharmaceuticals. A master's or doctoral degree is preferred for positions in biochemistry. Licensure for biochemists is not required. Certification may be required for jobs in hospitals.

Biochemistry technologists use specimens such as urine, spinal fluid, blood, and gastric juices to study the hormonal and chemical composition that might cause disease. Technologists work under the supervision of a biochemist. Education and training may include a 2-year associate degree or vocational program. A position as a research or laboratory assistant may be available for individuals with a bachelor's degree.

Content Instruction

Laboratory health care workers provide a picture of the patient's health status at one point in time. This may be done with a variety of laboratory tests. Many of the complex processes of the body are possible because a constant balance is maintained in chemical and electrical components of the cells. When an imbalance occurs, laboratory tests may indicate the cause. Because the normal values of many laboratory tests vary from one person to another, they are given in ranges. The result of a test may be affected by age, gender, pregnancy, medication, diet, exercise, and other differences in lifestyle. Chapter 11 provides more information about the normal values of laboratory tests dealing with blood. Information about urinalysis testing is found in Chapter 16.

Microbiology

Microbiology is the study of life forms that can be seen only with powerful magnification. Microorganisms (microbes) are present in the air and on the surfaces of all objects. Many microorganisms live on the surface of or inside the body without causing harm **(nonpathogenic).** When an animal harbors or hosts a microorganism without self-injury, it is called a *carrier.* Microorganisms that usually live in a certain location of the body are considered normal flora (Table 21-1). Microorganisms may be nonpathogenic in certain circumstances but cause disease (pathogenic) in others. For example, *Escherichia coli* is normally found in the intestines but is pathogenic if it enters the urinary tract.

Some microorganisms are always present (resident) and some are found temporarily (transient). Microorganisms that damage the host organism on or in which they live are called *parasites.* Microorganisms can be further separated into groups that can live in the presence of oxygen (aerobic) and those that cannot (anaerobic).

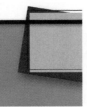

Table 21-1   Microorganisms Normally Found in the Body*

Location	Microorganism	Action
Skin	*Corynebacterium* spp. *Propionibacterium* spp. *Staphylococcus epidermis* *Streptococcus aureus*	Underarm odor
Mouth and throat	*Actinomyces* spp. *Bacillus* spp. *Candida albicans* *Fusobacterium* spp. *Lactobacillus* spp. *Staphylococcus viridans* *Streptococcus* spp.	Tooth decay and plaque formation
Upper respiratory tract	*Corynebacterium* spp. *Hemophilus* spp. *Neisseria* spp. *Staphylococcus* spp. *Streptococcus* spp.	
Intestines	*Bacterioides* spp. *Bifidobacterium* spp. *Clostridium* spp. *Escherichia coli*	
Genital tract	*Corynebacterium* spp. *Lactobacillus* spp. *Staphylococcus* spp. *Streptococcus* spp.	Maintains acidic environment

*Blood, urine, and the internal body systems are normally sterile, or free from all microorganisms.

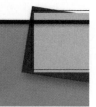

Table 21-2   Relative Size of Organisms and Structures

Organism or Structure	Size in Microns*
Virus	0.01-0.05
Rickettsia	0.2-0.5
Bacteria	0.5-1.5
Red blood cell	5
Lymphocyte	5-8
Human sperm (without tail)	60
Human egg	100
Human hair (width)	100
Paramecium (protozoan)	200

*1 Micron = 1 micrometer = 0.001 mm = 10^{-6} meter.

Most microorganisms survive well in conditions for growth such as warmth, darkness, moisture, and a source of food. The size of microorganisms is an important factor in determining a method of prevention of illness (Table 21-2).

Infection is a state of disease caused by the presence of pathogenic microorganisms in the body. For a microorganism to cause disease, several factors must be present (Figure 21-4). There must be a portal of entry for the organism, and the microorganism must have a mode of transmission or method of transfer. Infectious microorganisms may be transferred by direct contact or in droplets of air. They may be transferred by other animals, plants (vectors), and **fomites.** Fomites include countertops, eating utensils, linens, and other inanimate objects. There is a period of time before the infection shows its effects (incubation) and a period of time during which the microorganism is able to cause an infection in another (communicability).

There are four major groups of microorganisms that cause disease in humans. They are bacteria, fungi, protozoans, and viruses (Table 21-3). Bacteria are the most common cause of human disease and infection. Bacteria are single-celled organisms that are neither animals nor plants (Figure 21-5). Bacteria are placed into smaller groups according to their shape. Bacilli are rod-shaped microorganisms. Cocci are round and spirilla are spiral in shape. Bacteria may grow as single cells or clump together in colonies. Cultures or samples of bacteria are grown on a variety of media such as nutrient agar or broth. Clinical laboratory personnel may also identify metazoans. Metazoans are microscopic animals that may be parasites in humans.

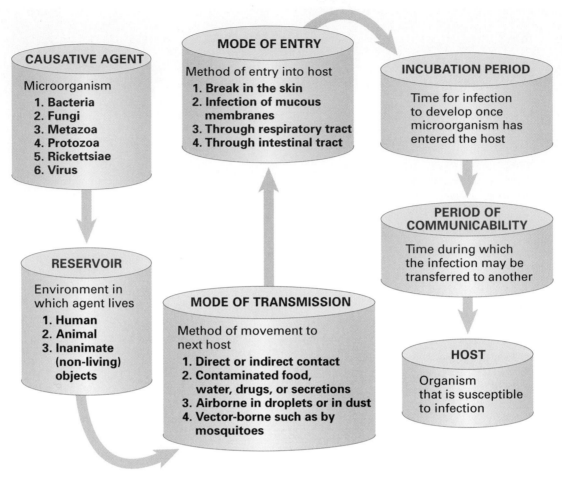

Figure 21-4 Infectious process.

The fungi group contains yeast and molds. Fungi grow in groups or colonies on other organisms, so they are parasitic. Protozoans, which are protists, are animal-like, unicellular organisms that cause a variety of disorders. Viruses are not really cells, but they contain bits of genetic information that can reproduce and cause illness inside a cell of the body. Rickettsiae are very small, bacteria-like organisms that cannot live outside living tissue.

Epidemiology

Epidemiology is the study of diseases occurring in human populations. The field of epidemiology has expanded from this original goal to the study of contagious (communicable) diseases. Epidemiology now includes study of the distribution, causative factors, and prevalence of infectious, chronic, and degenerative diseases. This includes cardiovascular disorders, cancer, arthritis, mental illness, congenital defects, nutritional disorders, and accidents. Some diseases known to result from contaminated environmental resources include cholera, typhoid, malaria, and typhus. With modern advancements in the control of the environment, these diseases are unusual in developed countries such as the United States.

Epidemiological studies use demographic data, such as the number of times a condition occurs (prevalence), in relation to the total number of people in the community. Information from epidemiological studies is provided to health care workers to help control and prevent the spread of disease. The ratio of sick (morbidity) to well individuals and death rate (mortality) are considered. These figures are based on census information gathered by departments of vital statistics. More than 40 diseases must be reported to the Center for Disease Control (CDC) so that measures may be taken to control their spread. Methods of control may include sanitation measures to destroy the host or pas-

Table 21-3   Pathogenic Microorganisms and Their Associated Diseases

Type of Microorganism		Examples of Diseases
Bacteria		Anthrax, boils, botulism, bronchitis, carbuncles, cholera, diphtheria, dysentery, gangrene, gonorrhea, leprosy, meningitis, osteomyelitis, pertussis, pink eye, pneumonia, scarlet fever, sinus infection, sore throat, syphilis, tetanus, tonsillitis, trench mouth, tuberculosis, typhoid fever, urinary tract infection

Fungi
   Mold
   Yeast
		Athlete's foot, histoplasmosis, ringworm, thrush, vaginitis

Protozoans		African sleeping sickness, amebic dysentery, malaria
Metazoans		Hookworm, intestinal diarrhea, pinworm, tapeworm, trichinosis
Viruses		AIDS, chickenpox, cold sores, genital herpes, hepatitis, measles, mumps, poliomyelitis, rabies, warts
Rickettsiae		Rocky Mountain spotted fever

sive carrier of the pathogen (reservoir), immunization, or limiting exposure by quarantine. Immunization against some childhood diseases is a legal requirement for admission to school.

Communicable diseases are those caused by specific organisms that are capable of producing a contagious disease. Infectious disease is the concern of the entire community. An epidemic is an outbreak of disease that affects a large number of people in one area. Infectious diseases can be caught by direct contact with another person, by indirect contact or through the air. Other infectious diseases are transmitted by vectors, or carriers, such as animals or insects (Table 21-4).

Organisms causing infectious disease adapt and evolve at a rapid rate. New diseases are discovered or rediscovered

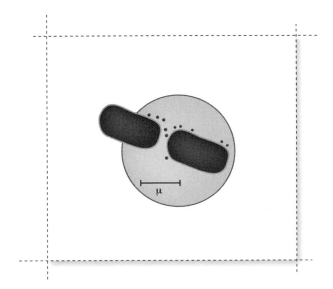

Figure 21-5   Bacteria surrounded by different viruses.

Table 21-4 Causes, Reservoirs, and Modes of Transportation of Communicable Diseases

Disease	Causative Agent	Reservoir	Mode of Transmission
Botulism	Bacteria	Soil, water, intestinal tract of animals, fish	Ingestion of contaminated canned foods
Cholera	Bacteria	People	Ingestion of contaminated water, feces, vomitus, food
Coccidioidomycosis (valley fever)	Fungus	Soil	Inhalation of spores
Conjunctivitis	Bacteria	People	Contact with discharge from infected area or from respirations
Dermatophytosis (ringworm)	Fungus	People, animals	Direct or indirect contact, especially with toilet articles
Diphtheria	Bacteria	People	Direct or indirect contact with lesions or contaminated articles; raw milk
Gastroenteritis	Virus	People	Probably feces to mouth, air droplets, food contamination
Giardiasis	Protozoa	People, domestic animals	Fecal contamination of water; hand-to-mouth transfer of feces
Gonorrhea	Bacteria	People	Direct contact
Hepatitis A	Virus	People	Direct contact; food or water contaminated with fecal matter
Hepatitis B	Virus	People	Blood to blood, parenteral
Hepatitis non-A, non-B, C	Virus	People	Blood to blood, parenteral
Herpes simplex I (cold sores)	Virus	People	Direct contact with saliva
Herpes simplex II	Virus	People	Direct contact
Herpes zoster (chickenpox)	Virus	People	Direct contact, airborne droplets
Influenza	Virus	People, swine, horses, birds	Direct contact, nasal droplets, soiled articles
Leprosy (Hansen's disease)	Bacteria	People	Not established; nasal droplets
Malaria	Protist	People	Mosquito bite
Measles (rubeola)	Virus	People	Droplets, direct contact, urine
Mononucleosis (Epstein-Barr virus)	Virus	People	Person-to-person contact with saliva, nasal secretions
Mumps	Virus	People	Droplet spread; direct contact with saliva

Table 21-4　Causes, Reservoirs, and Modes of Transportation of Communicable Diseases—cont'd

Disease	Causative Agent	Reservoir	Mode of Transmission
Pediculosis	Lice	People, hair	Direct contact, contact with infested materials
Plague (bubonic)	Bacteria	Wild rodents	Flea bite; contact with infected tissues
Poliomyelitis	Virus	People	Direct contact, transfer of feces to mouth
Rabies	Virus	Wild and domestic animals	Saliva, airborne rarely
Rocky Mountain spotted fever	Rickettsia	Ticks	Tick bite
Rubella (German measles)	Virus	People	Nasopharyngeal secretions, blood, urine, feces, droplets, direct contact
Salmonellosis	Bacteria	Animals, turtles	Ingestion of organism in contaminated food, feces
Syphilis	Bacteria	People	Direct contact
Tetanus (lockjaw)	Bacteria	Soil, intestinal canals, people	Puncture wounds
Trichomoniasis	Protozoa	People	Direct contact
Typhoid fever	Bacteria	People	Feces-contaminated food or water
Typhus	Rickettsia	People	Body louse
Whooping cough (pertussis)	Bacteria	People	Direct contact with respiratory secretions, droplets, contaminated articles
Yellow fever	Virus	People, mosquitoes	Mosquito bite

each year. The emergence of the HIV virus identified in 1959 is one example. The Lyme disease disorder was first documented in 1975 and the Hanta virus in 1976. In 1993 the parasite *Cryptosporidium* was found in the water supply in Milwaukee, Wisconsin. Approximately 400,000 people became ill from it. Another 300 people in the Northwest have become ill with a strain of *E. coli* in undercooked meat. Two microorganisms that have evolved to form more harmful strains are the tuberculosis and streptococcus bacteria. In 1995 the Ebola virus reappeared in Africa for the first time since 1976. The host and cure for this deadly virus that causes massive hemorrhaging in its victims remain unknown.

Secretions Analysis

One of the most common methods of studying secretions is through separation of the liquid and solid portions of a specimen using centrifugal force (Figure 21-6). The speci-

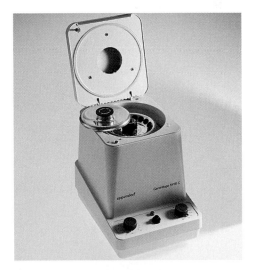

Figure 21-6　Blood and other body fluids may be separated using the centrifuge. *(Courtesy Ward's Natural Science Establishment, Rochester, NY.)*

men is spun at a high speed to cause the formed, or solid, part to settle as sediment on the bottom of the tube. Either portion can then be visualized with a microscope or used for testing to identify cells and microorganisms.

Clinical chemistry deals with the analysis of the serum portion of blood, urine, spinal fluid, and other body fluids. Many tests can be done on these types of specimens including tests for the presence of drugs, microorganisms, electrolytes, and enzymes.

Hematology is the study of the components of formed, or solid, elements of blood and blood-forming tissues.

Whole blood (formed elements) includes the red and white blood cells and platelets. Chapter 11 provides more information regarding the structure and function of blood. Blood can be collected in small amounts using a finger puncture (Figure 21-7). Larger specimens are obtained using venipuncture, or **phlebotomy.** Serology is the study of antibody reactions in serum, whole blood, or urine.

Immunology is the study of how the blood cells prevent disease caused by microorganisms. The work of the blood bank portion of the laboratory is also known as *immunohematology.* This is a specialized branch of immunology that

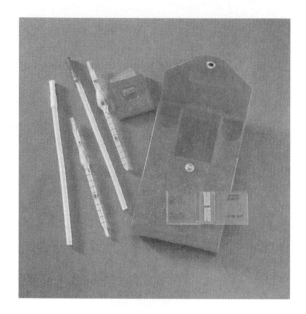

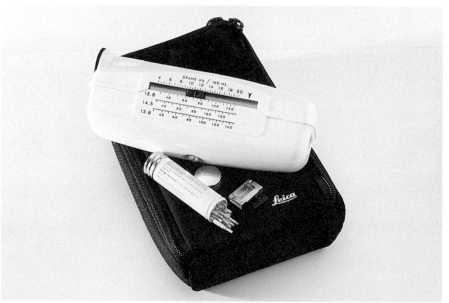

Figure 21-7 The hemacytometer is used to count red and white blood cells. *(Courtesy Ward's Natural Science Establishment, Rochester, NY.)*

studies and identifies blood groups. More than 300 blood factors are used to cross-match blood before it is used for transfusion. Blood component therapy separates blood into parts that can be used for specific conditions. For example, plasma, platelets, and the proteins serum albumin and gamma globulin can be separated from red blood cells. New technology includes intrauterine transfusion of blood to unborn babies to treat blood disorders. Stored or refrigerated blood is good for only 35 days, but frozen blood can be kept up to 3 years. Blood banks store and provide blood for replacement in surgery or illness. Chapter 11 provides further information regarding tests performed by the blood bank.

Defense Systems of the Body

Humans have several methods of defense against pathogenic microorganisms. The first line of defense is the skin. The skin surface is acidic and dry and acts as a barrier to prevent microorganisms from entering the body. A second defense mechanism is the action of phagocytic cells of the immune system. **Phagocytes** react to a microorganism as a foreign body. They surround and digest it, if possible. The immune system also prevents infection by producing antibodies and antitoxins to combat the action of pathogens that enter the body. **Immunity** is the ability to resist or overcome infection caused by microbes. Immunity can be either inborn or acquired. An individual is born with an innate (inborn) immunity to some organisms. Acquired immunity results when the body produces cells or antibodies to combat a specific organism once exposure occurs. Laboratory tests can determine the type of microorganism causing an infection, whether antibodies have been formed, and the most effective treatment when the body's defenses fail. Immunity to some microorganisms results from administering a vaccine. A vaccine contains a form of the organism that has been treated so that it will increase immunity but not cause the illness.

Performance Instruction

One of the skills used by the laboratory personnel is the preparation of bacterial cultures. This includes using **sterile** technique to prepare growth media and transfer microorganisms. Agar is a growth medium on which bacteria can grow and may be made of nutrients from seaweed, potato, or blood. Agar plates are prepared using sterile technique to prevent contamination by undesired microorganisms (Figure 21-8). The microorganism to be cultured or grown may be transferred to the agar plate using a sterilized loop or culture swab (Figure 21-9). After the transfer of bacteria or inoculation of the plate is completed, it is labeled with the name of the patient, date, and time of collection and placed in an incubator. After the microorganism has grown on the plate, the colonies may be counted or sampled for identification (Figure 21-10; Skills 21-2 and 21-3).

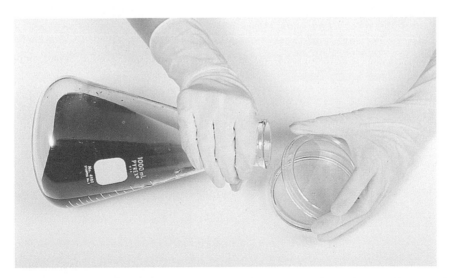

Figure 21-8 The agar media may be sterilized separately from the sterile petri dish if sterile technique is used during transfer.

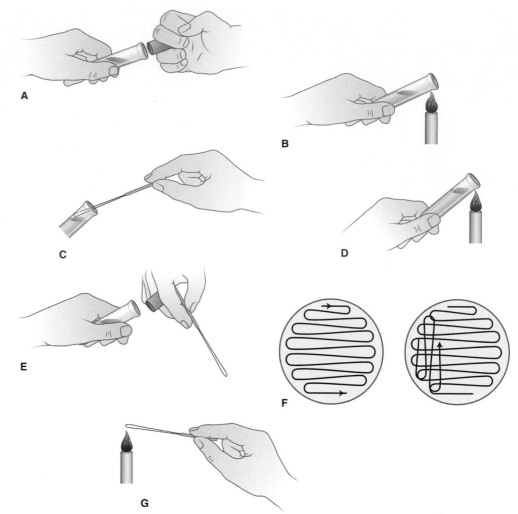

Figure 21-9 **A,** The cap is removed so that it can be held during the procedure to prevent contamination from a counter-top. **B,** The lip of the test tube is flamed to kill any microorgan-isms that may be present on the outside of the test tube. **C,** The inoculating loop is inserted into the test tube to remove a specimen. **D,** The lip of the test tube is flamed again to kill any contaminants. **E,** The cap is re-placed on the test tube without touching it to any surface. **F,** The plate is streaked in a pat-tern to promote even growth of the microorganism. **G,** The in-oculating loop is flamed to kill all microorganisms before it is touched to any surface.

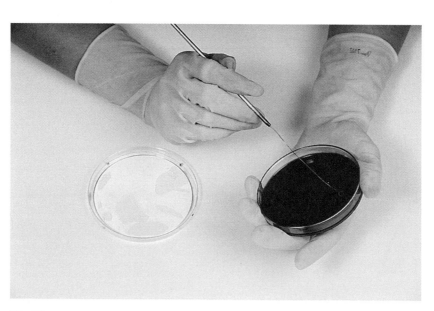

Figure 21-10 The microorganism is spread evenly over the surface of the agar with-out breaking it.

Skill 21-2

Preparing an Agar Plate

1. Maintain medical asepsis by using the guidelines provided in the Standard and Transmission-Based Precautions, including good handwashing technique and use of gloves as needed.

2. Prepare the agar mixture according to the manufacturer's instructions.

3. Using a funnel, pour warm agar into the clean test tubes or petri dishes until they are half full. Agar will harden when cooled. If the tube is too full, the tube cannot be slanted and contamination may occur at the edge.

4. Allow the agar to cool and cap the tubes with cotton balls. Tubes may be cooled in a slanted position to provide more surface area for bacterial growth.

5. Sterilize the tubes or agar plates in an autoclave. Tubes and petri dishes may be sterilized before adding sterile agar if sterile technique is used for the transfer.

6. Refrigerate the sterilized, hardened agar with the container closed until used. Petri dishes must be stored in an inverted position. Once sterilized, the container must remain sealed to ensure sterility. Storing petri dishes in an inverted position prevents condensation from forming on the inner surface of the lid.

Skill 21-3

Making a Streak Plate

1. Maintain medical asepsis by using the guidelines provided in the Standard and Transmission-Based Precautions, including good handwashing technique and use of gloves as needed.

2. Follow the procedure given to remove bacteria from an agar plate or slant or to collect a culture swab.

3. Open sterile agar plate slightly. The less the plate is opened, the less chance for contamination by microorganisms carried on air droplets.

4. Touch the loop or swab carrying the inoculate microorganism (inoculum) on one spot of the petri dish and spread it across the plate. Do not break the surface of the agar. Colonies will grow under the agar if the surface is broken.

5. Reflame the loop and allow it to cool. The swab is not resterilized. The loop must cool before retouching it to the agar because excessive heat may kill the microorganism.

6. Touch the loop to the area that has been streaked and carry the inoculum across the plate in right angles to the first streak area.

7. Remove the loop and reflame it before placing it on any surface. Discard the swab in the designated location for biological waste. Flaming the loop prevents the undesired contamination of any surface.

8. Cover, label, and incubate the petri dish. Store in inverted position. Label the dish on the bottom side. Labeling the dish on the top may prevent the viewing of the microorganisms when they grow.

9. Incubate the dish for 2 or 3 days before observing growth.

Clinical laboratory workers may also use a microscope to identify bacteria. Microscopes are delicate instruments that require special handling and care (Figure 21-11; Skill 21-4). Care must be taken to prepare slides so that no air bubbles are formed and they are not contaminated by debris (Figure 21-12; Skill 21-5). They also use microscopes to identify urine particles. The specimen is placed in a centrifuge before viewing to separate solid particles from the liquid portion. The laboratory worker may also be asked to perform venipuncture or draw blood after specialized training. This blood collected may then be used to determine the hematocrit, hemoglobin, erythrocyte sedimentation rate, or blood cell count.

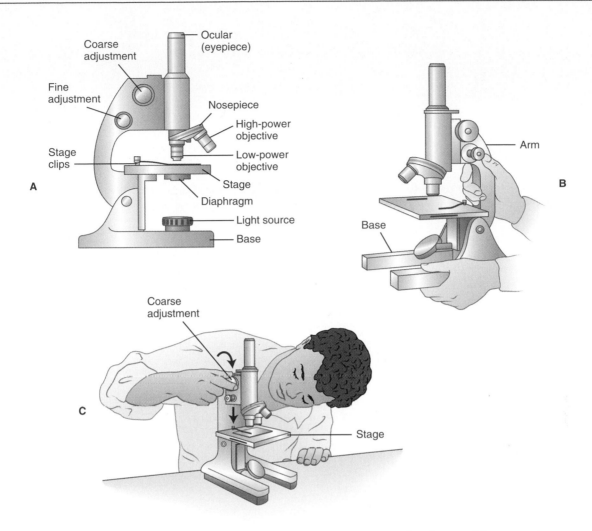

A

B

C

Figure 21-11   **A,** The microscope is a precise instrument made of several lenses to in-crease magnification. **B,** Care must be taken in moving a microscope to prevent breakage. **C,** The image is never viewed through the eyepiece of a microscope when the stage is being moved toward the objective lens.

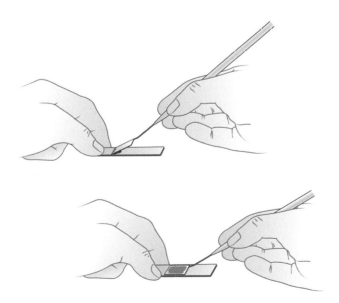

Figure 21-12   Air bubbles on a wet mount microscope slide can be prevented by placing the cover slip on it from one side to the other.

Skill 21-4

Using a Microscope

1. Maintain medical asepsis by using the guidelines provided in the Standard and Transmission-Based Precautions, including good handwashing technique and use of gloves as needed.

2. Place the microscope at least "thumb's length" from the edge of the table. Plug the cord in so that it is coiled away from the edge of the table. Fold and place the dust cover away from the working area. Microscopes are very expensive and may be easily damaged if dropped.

3. Turn on the light. Adjust the diaphragm to the desired opening. The diaphragm allows different light intensities to better clarify objects.

4. Revolve or turn the nosepiece until the low or shortest objective is in place.

5. Use the coarse adjustment to move the objective away from the platform.

6. Center the slide on the stage carefully, touching only the edges of the slide and corner label if one is present. Carefully adjust the stage clips to hold the slide in place and avoid chipping on the slide.

7. While looking at the slide from the side, lower the objective to the stage. The slide is viewed from the side at any time the stage and objective are being moved together, to avoid cracking the slide or contaminating the objective by touching them together.

8. Focus the slide by moving the objective away from the stage.

9. While looking at the slide from the side, move the high-power lens into place.

10. Use the fine adjustment only to focus the object. If the microscope is "parfocal," it is designed to maintain the focus from one objective to the next.

11. Before removing the slide from the stage, move the objective away from it by raising the nosepiece.

12. Turn off the light, coil the cord, and replace the dust cover before returning the microscope to its designated location.

13. Clean and return the slides and materials to their designated location.

Skill 21–5

Preparing a Wet Mount Slide

1. Maintain medical asepsis by using the guidelines provided in the Standard and Transmission-Based Precautions, including good handwashing technique and use of gloves as needed.

2. Rinse a microscope slide and cover slip with water.

3. Use a soft cloth to dry the slide and cover slip.

4. Use a medicine dropper to place a drop of water on the center of the slide.

5. Place the specimen to be viewed in the drop of water.

6. Lower the cover slip from one side of the drop of water to the other to prevent air bubbles from forming on the slide.

7. Place the wet mount slide on the stage of the microscope and position it so that the specimen is centered over the light source.

8. Using the coarse adjustment, lower the low-power objective as far as it will go without touching the slide. (Never lower an objective while looking through the eyepiece.)

9. While looking through the eyepiece, move the objective up until the specimen is in focus.

10. Using the fine adjustment knob, complete the focusing of the specimen.

Review Questions

1. Use the following terms in one or more sentences that correctly relate their meaning.
   Immunity
   Infection
   Microorganism
   Pathogen
   Phagocyte

2. Describe the duties, educational preparation, lines of authority, and credentialing of five laboratory personnel.

3. Describe the difference between pathogenic and nonpathogenic organisms.

4. List four types of pathogenic microorganisms. Give an example of each.

5. List five environmental conditions that are favorable to the growth of microorganisms.

6. Describe the three methods of defense of the body against infection.

Critical Thinking

1. Compare the size of pathogenic organisms with methods used to prevent their spread.

2. Convert the measurements in Table 21-2 to make a model demonstrating the relative size of listed items using a scale of 100 meters equals 0.1 mm.

3. Investigate the cost of education for two laboratory health care providers.

4. Investigate the types of contrast media and reagents used in laboratory health care. Explain why different reagents are needed to process different specimens.

5. Compare the temperature at which bacteria prefer to grow and the normal temperature range of humans.

6. Research and describe five of the diseases that are reportable to the CDC. Explain why it is important for these disease statistics to be gathered by a central agency.

22

Imaging Careers

Learning Objectives

Define at least seven terms relating to careers in medical imaging.

Specify the role of selected diagnostic medical health care workers including personal characteristics, levels of education, and credentialing requirements.

Discuss three important developments in the field of diagnostic imaging.

Identify one imaging technique that does not use radiation.

Key Terms

Echocardiography

(ek-o-kar-dee-OG-ruf-ee) Recording the position and motion of the heart walls or its internal structures using ultrasonic waves

Fluoroscopy

(floor-OS-kuh-pee) Immediate visualization of part of the body on a screen using radiography

Isotope

(ISE-uh-tope) One or more forms of an atom with a difference in the number of neutrons

Polarity

(po-LARE-it-ee) Distinction between positive and negative charges of particles

Radiographic Contrast Media

(ray-dee-uh-GRAF-ik KON-trast MEE-dee-uh) A chemical that does not permit passage of x-rays

Radiography

(ray-dee-OG-ruf-ee) Making film records of internal structures by passing radiographs or gamma rays through the body to make images on specially sensitized film; roentgenography

Tomography

(tom-OG-ruf-ee) Radiograph producing a detailed cross section of tissue at a predetermined depth

Ultrasound

(ul-truh-sound) Visualization of deep structures of the body by recording reflections of sound waves directed into the tissues

Imaging Careers Terminology*

TERM	DEFINITION	PREFIX	ROOT	SUFFIX
Angiogram	Record or image of a vessel		angi/o	gram
Echocardiograph	Record or image of the heart using sound	echo	cardi/o	graph
Fluoroscopy	Look with a fluorescent screen		fluor/o	scopy
Hemogram	Record or image of blood		hem/o	gram
Mammography	Making a record or image of a breast		mamm/o	graphy
Myelogram	Record or image of bone marrow		myel/o	gram
Radiologist	One who studies radiation (interprets radiographs)		radi/o	logist
Radiology	Study of radiation		radi/o	logy
Sonogram	Record or image made using sound waves		son/o	gram
Tomography	Making a record or image of a plane of the body		tom/o	graphy

*A transition phrase or vowel may be added to or deleted from the word parts to make the combining form.

Abbreviations for Imaging Careers

ABBREVIATION	MEANING
BE	Barium enema
CAT	Computerized axial tomography
CT	Computer tomography
CXR	Chest x-ray
EEG	Electroencephalogram
EKG	Electrocardiogram
IVP	Intravenous pyelogram
MRI	Magnetic resonance imagery
NMT	Nuclear medical technician
PET	Positron emission tomography

Careers

The careers in diagnostic imaging include workers with a broad range of interests, abilities, and training (Box 22-1). The career opportunities in this area include **radiography** and related occupations. The radiology department of most health care facilities provides techniques in addition to radiography, such as monitoring of the heart (electrocardiography) and the brain (electroencephalography).

Medical Imaging

Operators of radiographic machinery are called *radiographers* or *radiologic technologists*. Radiologic technologists work under the direction of a physician (radiologist) and may specialize in one area of diagnosis or treatment (Figure 22-1). Responsibilities of the medical radiographer include transferring and positioning the patient and selecting the proper technical factors to ensure the quality of the radiographs. They also use safety equipment and administer opaque media (dye) to make the internal body parts visible. Radio-opaque materials may be administered by mouth, rectum, or by the intravenous route. Radiographers may take portable films at the bedside or in the emergency or operating room. The radiographer must use sterile technique, maintain records, and assist with special procedures such as arteriograms.

Job opportunities in radiology are found in hospitals, privately owned facilities, and physician offices that provide radiological services. The job involves some hazard of radiation exposure. Each worker wears a film badge that records the level of exposure to radiological materials. The federal government regulates the levels that are considered to be safe. Programs of study for radiographers range from 1 to 4 years; 2 years is the most common length. Radiographers need a strong background in human anatomy because identification of anatomical landmarks is important to obtain the best possible radiographs. To work as a technologist, a college or university degree may also be required. At least 33 states require licensure for radiographers.

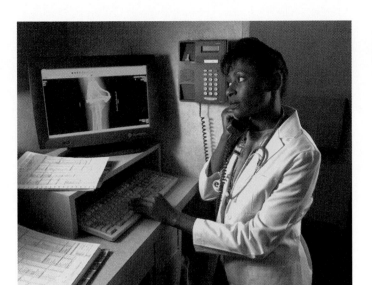

Figure 22-1   The radiologist is a physician who specializes in tests and treatments using radiographic materials. *(Courtesy Swissray International Inc., Elmsford, NY.)*

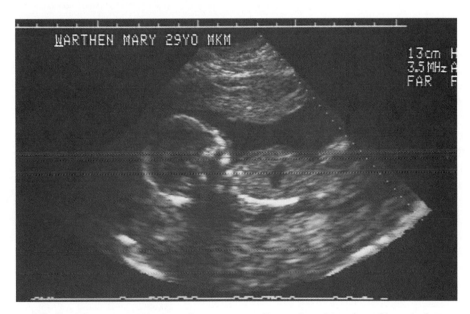

Figure 22-2   The sonogram produces a two-dimensional image of internal structures.

One area of specialty for radiographers uses the properties of radioactive materials to make diagnostic evaluations and provide therapy. Along with other imaging technologists, the nuclear medicine, or radioisotope, technologist (NMT) provides basic and emergency care, prepares and administers radioactive compounds, and participates in research activities. Radioactive compounds (radiopharmaceuticals) may be injected into the blood stream, swallowed, or inhaled. The gamma ray emissions are traced through the body, and the length of time they remain in the body provides important diagnostic information. Some of the tests possible using nuclear medicine are blood volume, red blood cell survival, and fat absorption analysis. Brain, thyroid, lung, bone, and heart scans are also part of diagnostic nuclear medicine.

The diagnostic medical sonographer, or **ultrasound** technologist, produces two-dimensional images of internal organs, utilizing sound waves at high frequency (Figure 22-2). The technologist positions the patient, explains the procedure, and adjusts the equipment to produce the images. The technologist also labels the images for identification. Certification, after completion of a 2-year community college program, is the minimum training requirement for an ultrasound technician.

Related Imaging Personnel

Radiological physics is concerned with the application of ionizing radiation to medical diagnosis and therapy. Physicists assist a physician with the care of patients, equipment selection, quality control, teaching, and radiation safety. Physicists may assist with selection of imaging or therapy equipment from technical and financial viewpoints and are responsible for developing and directing quality control programs for equipment and procedures. They may be responsible for establishing and supervising radiation safety programs including monitoring personnel, handling radioactive materials, and advising radiation safety committees. Physicists may provide required in-service education to staff that work with radiation. The preparation for becoming a radiological physicist involves earning a master's degree (M.S.) or doctorate (Ph.D.) in medical physics or a related discipline. Practical experience in a hospital is also required as part of a 2- to 3-year postgraduate program or clinical medical physics residency program. Physicists must pass a certification examination given by the American Board of Radiology.

Medical dosimetrists work under the supervision of the medical physicist. They calculate and plan radiation doses to treat cancer. Educational backgrounds of the medical dosimetrist vary but include mathematics and physics.

Electrocardiograph (EKG) technicians, although not imaging personnel, may work in the radiology department or area. Electrocardiograph technicians attach electrode leads or pads on the patient to monitor or test the action of the heart. The results of the tests are edited and mounted for study by the cardiologist. The electrical impulse of the heart activity is monitored and recorded by the equipment. The patient may be asked to sit, lie down, or walk during the test. Technicians may learn on the job or in community college or vocational programs. Specialized training qualifies the electrocardiograph technician to work in the areas of cardiac catheterization, **echocardiography**, continuous monitoring, and blood flow studies. Certification and registration is possible for the cardiology technologist with additional training. More information regarding electrocardiography may be found in Chapter 24.

Electroencephalographic (EEG) technologists measure the electrical activity of the brain to aid in diagnosis of disorders. Although not using radiographic materials, they may be included in the radiology department of the health care facility. The responsibilities of the EEG technologist include placing the electrode instrument on the patient, adjusting the machine, and monitoring the patient during testing. The electroencephalogram technologist training may range from 1 to 2 years. Electroencephalogram technologists may seek registration after completion of an accredited program.

Content Instruction

Medical imaging became a reality when Wilhelm Conrad Roentgen discovered "x-rays" in 1895. He called the electromagnetic energy "X" because it was unknown. Contrast agents were developed by pharmacists to allow better visualization of the inside of the body using this technique. By the 1950s, several other radioactive **isotopes** and other energy forms, such as sound waves, were being used for diagnosing disorders.

Most medical imaging of today continues to be diagnostic radiology using conventional radiographs. There are more than 100 tests that use radiographs (Figure 22-3). They include everything from examination of a simple fracture to angiography to visualize blood vessels. **Fluoroscopy** is a type of radiography that shows the internal organs in real time. Mammography is the fastest growing diagnostic procedure.

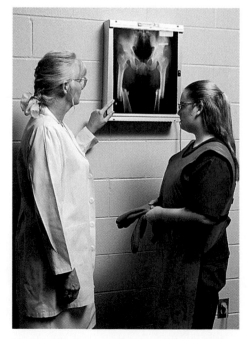

Figure 22-3 Radiographs are viewed using a light box to illuminate the film.

Radiographers may receive advance certification to perform mammography. A mammogram is a radiograph of the breast used to detect breast cancer. Using a mammogram, it is possible to detect a tumor that cannot be felt. The Mammography Quality Standards Act (MQSA) is a federal law designed to ensure that mammograms are safe and reliable. The Food and Drug Administration (FDA) must accredit all mammography facilities in the United States. The radiograph may be taken by a technologist and is read or interpreted by a radiologist. Digital mammography, approved in January 2000, is a technique for recording radiograph images in computer code instead of on radiograph film. Digital technology reduces radiation exposures, allows correction of the image for under- or overexposure of the radiograph, and allows examination of all areas of a breast with varying tissue densities.

The field of radiography has expanded greatly as modern methods of imaging have combined the use of computers with radiographic procedures. Computerized **tomography** revolutionized the field by linking the use of computers to radiographs. The images produced by "CT scans" provide cross-sectional views of the whole body instead of just one region.

Positron emission tomography (PET) uses computers and radiographic technique to visualize the metabolic activities of the body as well as its structure. In this procedure, gamma rays are produced in the body when a radioactive biochemical such as glucose or nitrogen is inhaled or ingested. A computer produces colored images that are dependent on the amount of gamma rays produced. Because the radioactive materials used have a very short period of activity, the patient is not exposed to much radiation. The biochemical activity of the brain in addition to blood flow in the heart and vessels are studied using this technique. The location of higher brain functions such as speech, memory, and emotion have been demonstrated using this technique.

Magnetic Resonance Imaging (MRI) is a process that creates superb image resolution and tissue contrast (Figure 22-4). It is particularly useful in diagnosing problems of the brain and spine. Magnetic resonance imagery forms pictures by measuring the magnetic field produced by ions in body cells. Radio frequencies are used to change the electronic pulses of the hydrogen nucleus in cells to one **polarity**. The speed of realignment when the radio frequencies are changed determines the type of image that is produced to represent the tissue. There is no exposure to radiation. As in many innovative health care practices, most technologists in this field began in another area of radiography and were trained for the new technology on the job.

Near infrared spectroscopy (NIRS) is a new technique that allows noninvasive measuring of cerebral functions. Because near infrared light passes through the human body easily, the light that penetrates the skull and brain can be detected by the spectrograph. In this region, oxyhemoglobin (oxyHb) and deoxyhemoglobin (deoxyHb) have differing spectrums that can be individually measured. Blood flow change in the cerebral cortex and the change in the amount of oxygen saturation that accompany neural activity can be measured.

Digital radiography is an emerging technique that is being used to reduce the time needed for and the expense of processing film (Figure 22-5). Although the time and expense of this procedure is reduced and the contrast is better than images taken with film, the amount of exposure to radiation is increased with this method.

Interventional radiology is another development in the imaging field. With this technique, small tubes or catheters are inserted into the blood vessels to correct abnormalities. An example of interventional radiology is the balloon angioplasty used to enlarge a vascular constriction by inflating a balloon in a narrowed portion of the vessel. Injecting small amounts of **radiographic contrast media** into diseased arteries to see vascular structures and narrowing determines the location for placement of the balloon. Although rare, interventional techniques have also been used to correct malformations of the brain's blood vessels.

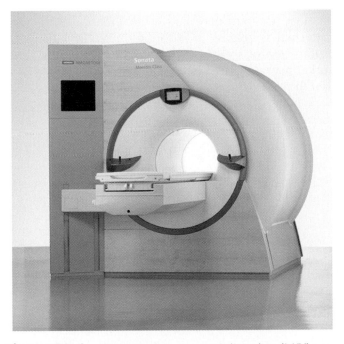

Figure 22-4   A magnetic resonance imaging (MRI) machine. *(Courtesy Siemens Medical Solutions USA.)*

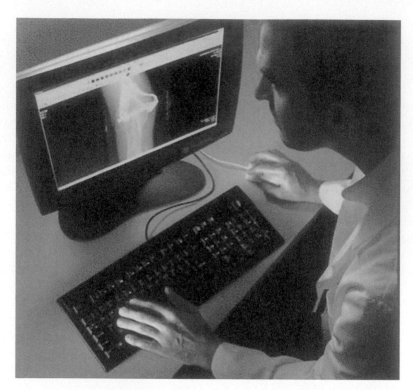

Figure 22-5 Digital radiography produces images that show better contrast than images produced by conventional methods. *(Courtesy Swissray International Inc., Elmsford, NY.)*

Performance Instruction

Because imaging involves the use of radiation, exposure is monitored and regulated by the federal government. The entry-level worker does not usually participate directly in procedures that require radiation. However, the radiology assistant may assist with procedures in many ways such as helping to move and position patients for examination or treatment (Figure 22-6). An entry-level worker may also perform loading and processing of films used in radiology (Skills 22-1 and 22-2).

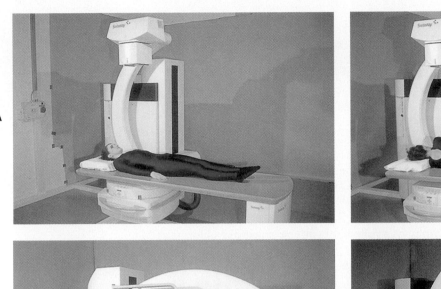
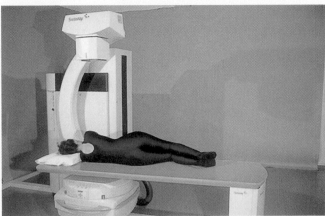
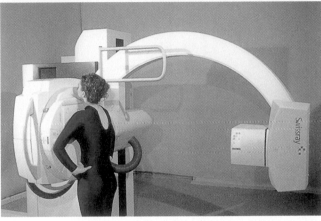
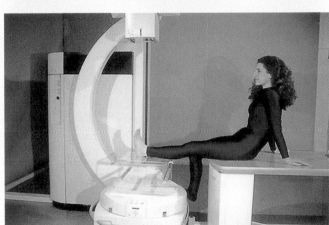

Figure 22-6   Correct positioning is important to ensure that radiographs provide the best image possible. **A**, Chest. **B**, Spine. **C**, Chest. **D**, Ankle. *(Courtesy Swissray International Inc., Elmsford, NY.)*

Skill 22-1

Loading and Unloading Film

1. Maintain medical asepsis by using the guidelines provided in the Standard and Transmission-Based Precautions, including good handwashing technique and use of gloves as needed.

2. Gather all supplies in a dark room environment. White light will fog unexposed film.

3. Close the darkroom door and turn off the white light. Check for white light leaks.

4. Turn on safe light. Safe light illuminators will not fog unexposed film.

5. Use the fingertips to open the back panel of the film holder with the front side down placed on the work surface.

6. Open the unexposed film storage bin and select a film.

7. Touch the film on the edges with only the fingertips to place the unexposed film into the film holder.

8. Close the film holder. The film holder protects the unexposed film from exposure until used.

9. Turn off the safe light. Turn on the white light.

10. Place the film holder in the proper storage area.

Skill 22-2

Processing Film

1. Maintain medical asepsis by using the guidelines provided in the Standard and Transmission–Based Precautions, including good handwashing technique and use of gloves as needed.

2. Gather all supplies in a darkroom environment. White light will fog exposed film.

3. Close the darkroom door and turn off the white light. Check for white light leaks.

4. Turn on the safe light. Safe light illuminators will not fog unexposed film.

5. Open the film holder (cassette or magazine).

6. Open the unexposed film storage bin and select film.

7. Touch only the edges to remove processed film. Touching the film will alter the image.

8. Place the film on the feed tray of an automatic processor.

9. Hold the edges of the film firmly and push it forward until caught on rollers. A bell will ring to indicate that the film has entered the processor completely.

10. Place unexposed film into the cassette.

11. Remove processed film when it is released by the processor.

12. Turn off the safe light. Turn on the white light.

13. Place the film in the proper storage area.

Review Questions

1. Use each of the following terms in one or more sentences that correctly relate their meaning.

   Fluoroscopy

   Radiography

   Tomography

   Ultrasonography

2. Describe the duties, educational preparation, and credentialing of five careers in medical imaging.

3. Describe the history of developments in radiography.

4. Compare the uses of conventional radiograph and magnetic resonance imagery.

Critical Thinking

1. Research and compare the cost of various types of imaging tests.

2. Explore and describe three common contrast media used in imaging.

3. Investigate and compare the cost of education and available programs for two health care careers in medical imaging.

23 Nursing Careers

Learning Objectives

Define at least eight terms relating to nursing careers.

Specify the role of nurses and related providers, including personal qualities, levels of education, and required credentialing.

Differentiate between the role of the registered nurse, licensed practical nurse, and nurse assistant.

Identify three items considered to be intake and three to be output.

Identify three conditions that indicate the need to measure intake and output.

Describe methods of maintaining a clean and safe facility or unit.

Key Terms

Apical
(AY-pik-ul) Pertaining to, or located at, the apex of the heart

Asepsis
(ay-SEP-sis) Process of removing pathogenic microorganisms or protecting against infection by such organisms

Emesis
(EM-e-sis) Vomit

Intravenous
(in-truh-VENE-us) Within a vein or veins

Perinatal
(pare-ih-NAY-tul) Pertaining to the period shortly before and after birth

Pulse
(puls) Heartbeat that can be felt, or palpated, on surface arteries as the artery walls expand with blood

Unit
(YOO-nit) Part of a facility, including equipment and supplies, organized to provide specific care

Vital
(VIE-tul) Necessary to life

Nursing Careers Terminology*

TERM	DEFINITION	PREFIX	ROOT	SUFFIX
Abduction	Move away from the center	ab	duction	
Atrophy	Without nutrition (waste away)	a	troph	y
Bradypnea	Slow breathing	brady	pnea	
Cyanoderm	Blue skin	cyan/o	derm	
Dypsnea	Painful breathing	dys	pnea	
Hematemesis	Vomiting blood	hem/at	emesis	
Hemiplegia	Pertaining to being half paralysed (one side of the body)	hemi	pleg	ia
Insomnia	Pertaining to being without sleep	in	somn	ia
Intravenous	Inside a vein	intra	venous	
Sublingual	Below the tongue	sub	lingual	

*A transition phrase or vowel may be added to or deleted from the word parts to make the combining form.

Abbreviations for Nursing Careers

ABBREVIATION	MEANING
AP	Apical
BSN	Bachelor of science in nursing
HCA	Home care assistant
I & O	Intake and output
LPN	Licensed practical nurse
NA	Nurse assistant
RN	Registered nurse
PCA	Personal care attendant
PO	By mouth
ROM	Range of motion

Careers

Nurses make up the largest group of health care workers, with more than 2 million jobs (Box 23-1). Nursing is also one of the 10 occupations that are projected to have the largest number of new jobs in the future. In fact, the American Nurses Association and Bureau of Labor Statistics project a shortage of more than 1 million nurses by 2010. Levels of workers classified as the registered nurse, licensed practical nurse, and nursing assistant give nursing care. Nurses and related caregivers work with their patients in a close or primary relationship. The function of the nurse is to promote optimal health and provide care during illness. The duties of the nurse focus on the patient's physical and mental needs.

Nurses must have the ability to get along with other people and communicate well. They must provide, without prejudice, the best care possible for every patient. Especially during critical moments, the nurse must be self-controlled, efficient, and show problem-solving ability.

Registered Nurse

The registered nurse (RN) may complete a 2-year community college program, 3-year hospital diploma program, or 4-year college or university program to qualify to take the licensing examination. However, the 3-year programs are being phased out in many locations. Registered nurses may hold a bachelor's (B.S.N.), master's (M.S.N.), or doctorate (Ph.D.) degree. Registered nurses supervise the nursing care of patients. Most nurses work under the supervision of a physician in a hospital, a long-term care facility, home health, or other health care agencies.

Community health nursing is concerned with the care of the family and community. The primary focus of community or public health nursing is the prevention of disease and promotion of the highest possible level of health and well-being. The public health nurse identifies needs, determines the plan for care, mobilizes appropriate re-

Box 23-1   Nursing Careers

Birth attendant
Child care attendant, school
Community health nurse
Counselor
Geriatric nurse assistant
Licensed practical nurse
Nurse aide
Nurse anesthetist
Nurse midwife
Nurse, office
Nurse practitioner
Nurse, private duty
Nurse, school
Occupational health nurse
Orderly
Practical nurse
Registered nurse

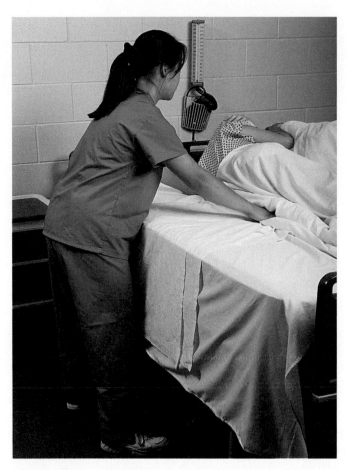

Figure 23-1   Making beds is just one way a nurse provides for a patient's comfort.

sources, and evaluates the services given to the patients. Professional public health nursing did not evolve until the twentieth century. Most public health nurses work for government health agencies. They visit people in their homes to provide care and evaluate the environmental conditions that may affect that care. A bachelor's degree in nursing is required for public health nursing.

Advanced preparation by the registered nurse may lead to work as a nurse practitioner, clinical nurse specialist, nurse anesthetist, or nurse midwife. Nurse practitioners perform physical exams, order and interpret tests, and may recommend or prescribe medication in some states. Nurse practitioners emerged as a profession to meet the needs of rural communities. They function independently from the physician in these settings and assume primary responsibility for care. Nurse practitioners commonly specialize in the areas of adult, pediatric, family, or geriatric practice. Nurse practitioners are certified by the state in which they practice. Nurse midwives provide perinatal care and deliver babies under the supervision of an obstetrician. Nurse anesthetists provide anesthesia during obstetrical and surgical procedures under the supervision of an anesthesiologist.

Areas of specialization for the registered nurse include units, such as the operating room, recovery room (postanesthesia), critical care, and emergency room, as well as practices, such as oncology, cardiovascular, and many others. Nursing opportunities are available all days of the week and all hours of the day.

Licensed Practical Nurse

Licensed practical or vocational nurses (LPN or LVN) complete a 1- to 2-year program and provide personal care under the direction of a physician, dentist, or registered nurse. Many licensed practical nurses work in a hospital assisting by making beds, taking vital signs, and providing personal hygiene for patients (Figure 23-1). Other practical nurses provide care in long-term care facilities. Licensed practical nurses may legally administer certain medications, insert catheters, and dress wounds. In some states, they may also take orders from the physician and input the orders in a computer for implementation. They may also assist physicians with procedures and train students at some levels.

Nurse Assistant

The nurse assistant (NA) works under the direction of the registered nurse or licensed practical nurse to provide basic care. Nurse assistants may be called *orderlies* (if male), *per-*

sonal care assistants (PCA), *personal care attendants,* or *patient care technicians* (PCT). In most states, nurse assistants must complete a certification program of at least 75 hours in length and complete a nationally approved written and skill examination.

Nurse assistants may provide care in the patient's home and are called *home care assistants* (HCA). Their role includes assistance with personal care, such as bathing, bed-making, and meal preparation, as well as general maintenance of the home. Home care assistants usually work with a patient over an extended period of time. The home care assistant may be trained to perform all the functions of the nurse assistant.

Content Instruction

Fluid Balance

Within a 24-hour period, the fluid that is taken into the body and eliminated from the body should be approximately equal in volume to maintain the balance of the electrolytes and fluid needed to perform body processes. When an individual is unable to eat, has severe diarrhea, or high fever, the output may be greater than intake. In some instances, the patient may be unable to ingest adequate liquids because of physical limitations. The order may be given to "force fluids." Forcing fluids means to offer at least 100 mL (cc) of liquid each hour.

Oral intake is considered to be anything that is liquid at room temperature and taken by mouth (Figure 23-2). This includes foods such as ice cream and Jell-O. The average

adult takes in 32 qt (3.3 L) of fluid daily in food and beverages. Intravenous (IV) fluids and tube feeding are considered to be intake.

Administration and measurement of intravenous fluids is a function of the registered nurse. All members of the nursing staff observe the site of insertion for any redness, swelling, and complaint of pain that may indicate problems with the treatment. When the fluid is nearly gone, this is reported to the registered nurse or, in some cases, the licensed practical nurse that changes the fluid.

Output includes urine, vomit (emesis), drainage from wounds, and liquid stool. The body also loses fluid that cannot be measured in the form of perspiration on the skin and through lungs during respiration.

Personal Care

Personal or direct care is usually needed for the hospitalized patient. Assistance with activities of daily living (ADLs) as well as treatments may be needed if the patient is weak or ill (Figure 23-3; Skill 23-1). The manner in which the health care worker provides personal care often determines the patient's reaction to having someone assist with these activities or treatments. The health care worker should approach direct contact with the patient in a professional, calm, and caring manner.

Personal hygiene on a daily basis includes morning (am), afternoon (pm) and evening (hs) care. Before eating in the morning, the patient is assisted to the bathroom or to use a bedpan or urinal. The patient is assisted to wash hands and face and to brush the teeth before or after eating breakfast as desired. The bed linens and unit are

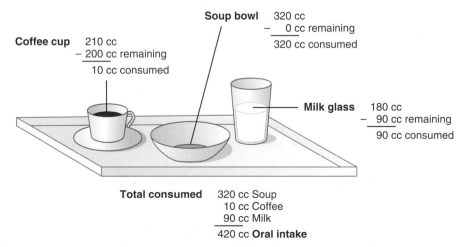

Figure 23-2 Oral intake is determined by estimating the amount of liquid that is not consumed when the meal is finished. To estimate the amount consumed, the amount remaining is subtracted from the total amount held by the container.

Skill 23-1

Assisting the Patient to Eat

1. Maintain medical asepsis by using the guidelines provided in the Standard and Transmission-Based Precautions, including good handwashing technique and use of gloves as needed.

2. Gather all necessary supplies and equipment, including the patient's tray, a chair for the assistant, washcloth, and hand towel.

3. Prepare the tray according to the nutritional requirements. Dietary requirements may be limited by the patient's condition or ability to eat.

4. Assist the patient to assume an upright position. The upright position helps encourage eating and promotes digestion.

5. Assist the patient to use the restroom if desired.

6. Assist the patient to wash his or her face and hands.

7. Place the tray in front of the patient. Open containers and remove food covers.

8. Sit next to the patient during the meal. The assistant should be seated, relaxed, and not appear hurried to encourage the patient to eat.

9. Assist the patient with eating as needed. The patient should be allowed to do as much as possible without assistance to preserve independence and dignity. A hand towel may be used as a napkin under the chin to catch any food that is dropped.

10. Talk with the patient during the meal. Maintaining a conversation with the patient helps make the meal a pleasant experience and encourages eating.

11. Pause at times to allow the patient to rest. The patient needing assistance with the meal also needs time to rest during the meal.

12. Assist the patient to clean his or her face, hands, and teeth after eating.

straightened and the patient positioned for comfort in a sitting position when possible. After eating, the patient is assisted to bathe and shave as desired. The linens and gown are changed. The hair is combed or brushed. A bed bath, backrub, and range-of-motion (ROM) exercises may be provided if the patient has limited movement (Figure 23-4).

Range-of-motion exercises are designed to move the muscles and tendons of the joints for patients that are not able to move independently or have limited abilities. Movement of the joints may prevent contracture or reduction in the amount of movement possible. Range of motion exercises should be performed once every 8 hours when the patient is not mobile (Skill 23-2).

Throughout the day, the patient is assisted with hygiene needs of elimination such as using the bathroom or bedpan. Also, assistance is given with washing of the hands and face as needed. The unit is straightened including pro-

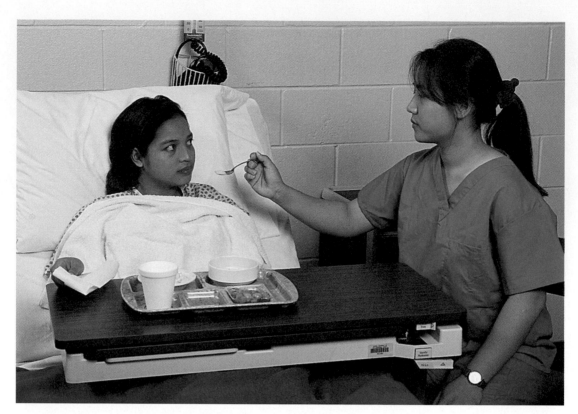

Figure 23-3 Creating an atmosphere of being unhurried and interested in assisting with the patient's daily activities is important.

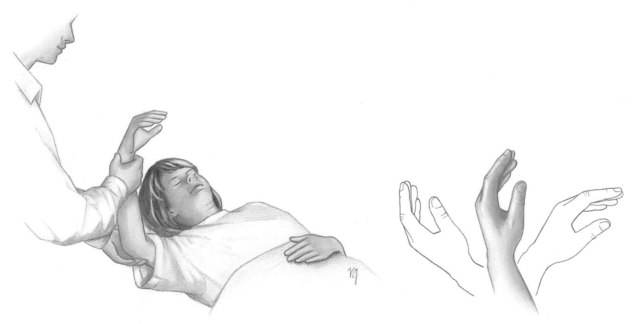

Figure 23-4 Range-of-motion exercises may be performed as part of the bed bath.

Skill 23-2

Performing Range-of-Motion Exercises

1. Maintain medical asepsis by using the guidelines provided in the Standard and Transmission-Based Precautions, including good handwashing technique and use of gloves as needed.

2. Identify the patient and explain the procedure. Range-of-motion exercises may be performed during the bed bath or at another time. The type of exercises that can be accomplished by the patient is determined by his or her condition. The patient should perform as much of the exercise as possible. If the patient cannot perform the movements, the health care worker can provide the same benefits by moving the parts of the body.

3. Provide for privacy. Position the patient comfortably in the supine position. The supine position allows movement of all body parts.

4. Ensure safety by keeping all unattended side rails in an upright position.

5. Exercise the neck five to 10 times. The neck can be hyperextended, rotated, flexed, and moved in a lateral flexion.

6. Exercise the shoulder five to 10 times. The shoulder can be flexed, extended, abducted, adducted, and rotated by grasping the hand and elbow to keep the arm straight.

7. Exercise the elbow five to 10 times. The elbow can be flexed and extended by grasping the hand and upper arm.

Continued

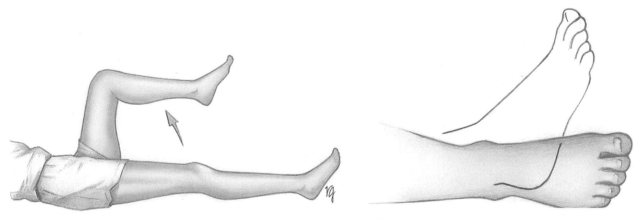

Figure 23-4, cont'd

Skill 23-2—cont'd

Performing Range-of-Motion Exercises—cont'd

8. Exercise the forearm five to 10 times. The arm can be turned downward, or pronated, and turned upward, or supinated.

9. Exercise the wrist five to 10 times. The wrist can be flexed and extended by bending the wrist with the fingers.

10. Exercise the thumb and fingers. The fingers can be abducted, adducted, extended, and flexed. The thumb can also be rotated.

11. Exercise the hip five to 10 times. The hip can be flexed, extended, abducted, adducted, and rotated by grasping the knee and ankle to keep the leg straight.

12. Exercise the knee five to 10 times. The knee can be flexed and extended by supporting the upper leg and foot.

13. Exercise the ankle five to 10 times by flexing and extending it.

14. Exercise the toes five to 10 times. The toes can be flexed, extended, abducted, and adducted.

15. Repeat the exercises on the other side of the body.

16. Position the patient for comfort and safety.

17. Record the treatment. Any observations about the skin, complaint of pain, muscle spasm, and degree of assistance with the exercises should be recorded. The time of treatment and joints exercised are also recorded.

viding fresh water at the bedside periodically throughout the day (Skill 23-3).

At bedtime, the patient is assisted to use the bathroom, bedpan, or urinal as needed. Oral hygiene is provided as well as changing damp or soiled linens and gown. The patient is given a backrub to promote sleep.

Unit Maintenance

Maintaining an orderly and safe environment for care of the patient is the responsibility of all health care practitioners. Clean sheets and a tidy unit benefit the patient and the health care team. Sheets may be changed with the patient out of the bed (unoccupied) or in bed (occupied). Special bed-making skills may be needed in the case of postsurgical patients. Sheets should be changed regularly and when soiled. When changing linens, rules of medical asepsis are followed to keep the environment as clean as possible and prevent the spread of microorganisms. Sheets that are free of wrinkles are more comfortable and help prevent the formation of bedsores (decubitus ulcers), which are caused by pressure.

Performance Instruction

One of the duties that may be provided by nurses is the bed bath (Figure 23-5). Patients who are unable to perform this task alone may need assistance with bathing.

Skill 23-3

Maintaining the Unit

1. Maintain medical asepsis by using the guidelines provided in the Standard and Transmission–Based Precautions, including good handwashing technique and use of gloves as needed.

2. Change the sheets daily and when soiled. Remove soiled linens from the room frequently.

3. Replace equipment, supplies, and the patient's possessions to the designated location after each use.

4. Throw trash in the appropriate location and empty frequently.

5. Supply the patient with fresh water once a shift and as needed.

6. Clean surfaces of tables regularly and as soiled.

7. Keep the call bell within reach of the patient at all times.

The assistant uses standard isolation precautions such as wearing gloves to avoid the spread of microorganisms throughout this procedure. Patients are encouraged to perform as much of the care as possible independently. A routine is established for assisting with the bed bath moving from the cleanest areas such as the eyes to dirtier areas such as the face, hands, back, and so forth. A backrub may be given at the same time as the bed bath to increase circulation and provide comfort (Figure 23-6; Skills 23-4 and 23-5).

Some conditions of the heart and peripheral arteries may lead to a difference or deficit in the pulse rate at the heart and at the radial artery. In this instance, the assistant must use the apical-radial method to assess the pulse. The procedure requires two people. One person counts the pulse rate using a stethoscope over the heart while at the same time another counts it over the radial artery.

Oral intake may be recorded by estimating the amount of fluids consumed after a meal is finished (Skill 23-6). Additionally, all of the liquid taken at other times of the day is counted. Some patients may not be able to move to the restroom to use the toilet. The patient may then use a urinal, bedpan, or catheter for elimination (Figure 23-7). Privacy is provided for the patient as the bedpan is placed under the patient in a position that collects the waste material as it is eliminated (Skill 23-7). Urine output may be collected and measured using a catheter, bedpan, or urinal (Skill 23-8). The amount of fluid intake and output should be fairly close over a 24-hour period.

Assistants also assist the patient by making beds (Figure 23-8). Bed linens are usually changed daily in hospitals but may need to be changed more frequently when a person is ill as a result of body secretions. Linens may be changed with the patient out of the bed (unoccupied) or in the bed (occupied). The assistant must use good body mechanics and safety guidelines to prevent injury to himself or the patient during the procedure. This includes raising the bed to a comfortable working height to maintain good body mechanics and keeping the bed rails raised if the assistant is not directly at the bedside. The patient is made comfortable and the bed lowered to the lowest level when the bed is completed (Skills 23-9 and 23-10).

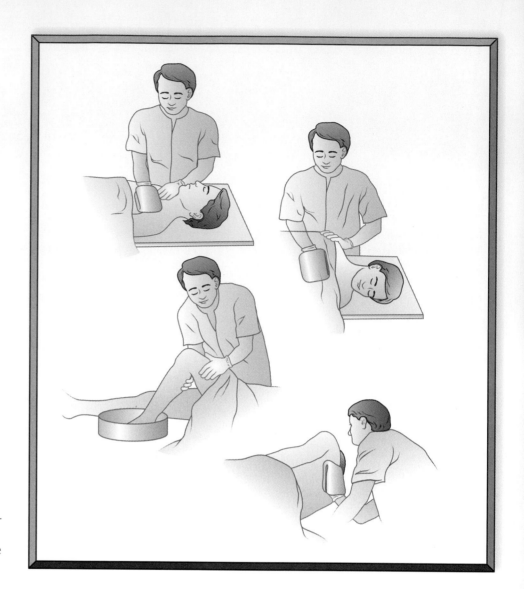

Figure 23-5 The bed bath provides comfort and cleanliness for the patient confined to a bed while protecting his or her dignity.

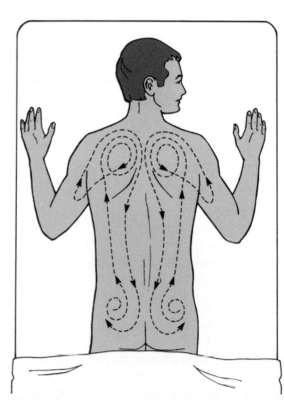

Figure 23-6 The backrub stimulates circulation to the tissues of the back and provides comfort. *(From Sorrentino SA:* Mosby's textbook for nursing assistants, *ed 4, St Louis, 1996, Mosby.)*

Skill 23-4

Giving a Backrub

1. Maintain medical asepsis by using the guidelines provided in the Standard and Transmission-Based Precautions, including good handwashing technique and use of gloves as needed.

2. Identify the patient and explain the procedure. The backrub may be performed during the bed bath. Patients who are unable to leave their beds should have a massage at least every 8 hours. Bedsores may occur if circulation to an area has been decreased because of immobility. Backrubs increase circulation to the back area as well as promoting comfort.

3. Provide for privacy by drawing curtains or closing the door.

4. Ensure safety by keeping all unattended bed rails in an upright position.

5. Assist the patient to turn to the far side.

6. Apply lotion to the hands and rub from the neck to the buttocks in circular motions. The strokes should be firm and smooth. To loosen muscles, knead them with the fingers. The patient may prefer a specific type of lotion or that no lotion be used.

7. Observe for reddened pressure areas on the bony prominences. Pressure areas that are noted and treated promptly may prevent bedsores.

8. Reposition the patient for safety.

9. Report any unusual findings immediately and record observations.

Skill 23-5

Giving a Bed Bath

1. Maintain medical asepsis by using the guidelines provided in the Standard and Transmission–Based Precautions, including good handwashing technique and use of gloves as needed.

2. Collect all necessary equipment including clean bath towels, washcloths, bath blanket, gown, soap, and warm water. Water for bathing should be about 110° F (43° C).

3. Ensure safety throughout the procedure by keeping all unattended bed rails raised.

4. Identify the patient and explain the procedure. The type of bath given is determined by the patient's mobility and condition.

5. Provide for privacy. A bath blanket is used to cover the patient before removing the gown and top bed linens. The patient should be covered at all times during the procedure to preserve his or her dignity.

6. Assist the patient to use the restroom or bedpan if necessary. Exposure to water stimulates the need for urination.

7. Assist the patient with oral hygiene. The male patient may need assistance with shaving.

8. Wash the eyes without using soap, which may irritate the eyes. The eyes should be wiped from the inner to the outer aspect, each with a separate part of the washcloth. A mitt can be made with the washcloth to provide better control.

9. Wash the face, ears, and neck with soap. Rinse and dry. Establishing a routine of washing head to toe and far side to near side ensures speed and complete coverage.

10. Place a towel under each area of the body as it is cleaned. The towel prevents water and soap from collecting in the bed linens under the patient.

11. Wash, rinse, and dry the patient in sections of the arms, chest, abdomen, legs, and feet. The body is washed and dried in parts to promote comfort. The skin should be washed with firm but gentle strokes. Patting the skin dry prevents damage to sensitive areas.

12. Change the water. The water becomes progressively soapy, dirty, and cool with use.

13. Turn the patient to the far side to wash, rinse, and dry the back from neck to buttocks. A back massage or rub may be done at this time to increase circulation and provide comfort.

14. Allow the patient to wash, rinse, and dry the genital area, unless he or she needs assistance. The genital area should be washed thoroughly to prevent infection and odor.

15. Wash, rinse, and dry the perineal area from front to back. Microorganisms that normally live in the intestinal tract can cause infection when transmitted to the urinary tract.

16. Depending on patient preference, apply lotion and antiperspirants during the bath.

17. Assist the patient to dress. The patient may need assistance to comb, brush, or arrange the hair.

18. Reposition the patient for comfort and safety.

19. Clean and replace equipment in the storage area. Place the soiled bath linens in the designated area.

20. Change the bed linens if necessary.

21. Record observations. Report any unusual findings to the supervisor immediately. The bed bath provides a time for the patient to voice opinions about care that is being given and for the health care worker to observe any problems with the patient's skin.

Measuring Oral Intake

1. Maintain medical asepsis by using the guidelines provided in the Standard and Transmission–Based Precautions, including good handwashing technique and use of gloves as needed.

2. Collect the food tray after the patient has finished eating. Compare the remains with the list of food and liquid served. Be alert to families and visitors who may eat what the patient does not want.

3. Estimate the amount of liquids consumed during the meal. Anything that is a liquid at room temperature is considered to be oral intake. Examples include ice, ice cream, and Jell-O. Oral intake is measured in cubic centimeters (cc).

4. Record oral intake in designated area.

5. Replace the tray on the cart.

Skill 23-7

Assisting with the Bedpan

1. Maintain medical asepsis by using the guidelines provided in the Standard and Transmission-Based Precautions, including good handwashing technique and use of gloves as needed.

2. Collect the necessary equipment and supplies including a bedpan, washcloth, hand towel, toilet tissue, and disposable gloves. Urine and feces are body secretions, and care should be taken to prevent exposure to them.

3. Explain the procedure to the patient and provide for privacy.

4. Raise the bed to a comfortable working height, making sure that all unattended side rails are up. Side rails should be up when the bed is raised to prevent injury if the patient should attempt to move around or leave the bed.

5. Position the patient in the supine position with the head slightly raised.

6. Fold the top linens to the foot of the bed. Keep the lower body lightly covered with a gown or top sheet. Linens and other materials are moved to prevent contamination with urine or feces.

7. Assist the patient to flex the knees and raise the hips.

8. Place the bedpan under the patient's buttocks. The patient may be turned to the side and rolled onto the bedpan if unable to raise the buttocks.

9. Cover the patient with the top sheet.

10. Raise the head of the bed to a sitting position.

11. Check the positioning of the bedpan.

12. Raise the side rail and lower the bed. Place toilet paper and call bell within reach. Instruct the patient to call when finished using the bedpan.

13. If the patient is strong enough to sit unassisted, he or she may be left alone to provide some privacy. It may be difficult for a person to feel free to eliminate waste with someone present.

14. Knock or call to the patient before entering the curtained area.

15. Raise the bed and lower the side rail and head of the bed.

16. Put on gloves to assist the patient to raise off the bedpan in the same manner in which the bedpan was placed.

Continued

Skill 23-7—cont'd

Assisting with the Bedpan—cont'd

17. Cover the bedpan and place it aside.

18. Clean the perineal area if the patient is unable to do so.

19. Assist the patient to wash his or her hands.

20. Lower the bed and reposition the patient for comfort and safety. Clean the call bell with disinfectant and place it within reach of the patient.

21. Take the bedpan to the bathroom or dirty utility room to empty. Measure the urine if the patient is on intake and output.

22. Rinse the bedpan and empty it into a toilet or proper receptacle. Clean it with disinfectant.

23. Discard gloves in appropriate container.

24. Return with a clean cover to the patient's bedside.

Skill 23-8

Measuring Urine Output

1. Maintain medical asepsis by using the guidelines provided in the Standard and Transmission-Based Precautions, including good handwashing technique and use of gloves as needed.

2. Gather all necessary equipment and supplies, including paper towel, alcohol pledget, graduated cylinder, paper, and pen.

3. Identify the patient and explain the procedure.

4. Empty the catheter bag, urinal, or bedpan into a graduated cylinder. Paper tissue should not be placed in the bedpan because the tissue displaces the urine and makes the reading too high.

5. Clean the draining tube of the catheter bag with an alcohol pledget before reinserting it into the bag.

6. Place the graduated cylinder on a flat surface out of the patient's vision. Read it at eye level. The angle of the container will change the reading.

7. Record the amount, color, and consistency of the specimen. Report any unusual findings to the supervisor.

8. Rinse the graduated cylinder, urinal, or bedpan with cool water and empty the contaminated water into the toilet. Return the urinal or bedpan to a convenient location for the patient.

9. Dispose of the used paper toweling, disposable gloves, and alcohol pledget in the appropriate container.

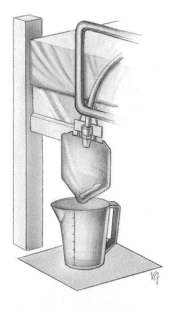

Figure 23-7 When a catheter is used, a paper towel is placed under the graduated cylinder to prevent any urine from contaminating the floor during emptying of the catheter bag.

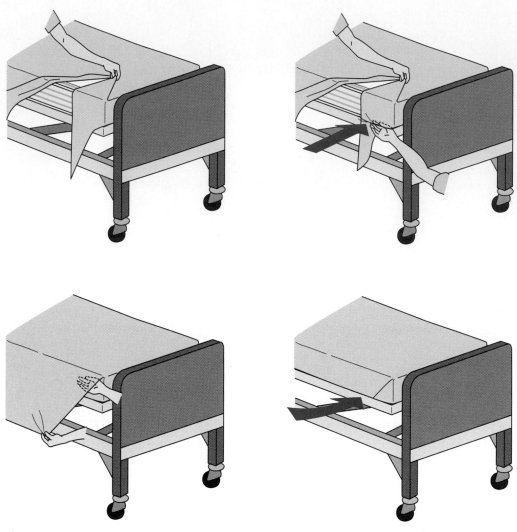

Figure 23-8 The unoccupied bed is made with mitered corners. *(From Sorrentino SA: Mosby's textbook for nursing assistants, ed 5, St Louis, 2000, Mosby.)*

Skill 23-9

Making an Unoccupied and Surgical Bed

1. Maintain medical asepsis by using the guidelines provided in the Standard and Transmission-Based Precautions, including good handwashing technique and use of gloves as needed.

2. Collect clean linens in order of use: mattress pad, bottom sheet, draw sheet, top sheet, blanket, bedspread, and pillowcases. Do not allow the linens to touch the uniform. The linens are considered to be cleaner than the uniform and should be held away from it.

3. Place the linens on a clean surface in their order of use so the mattress pad is on top. Once brought into a room, linens may not be returned to the linen cart. If not soiled, some linens may be reused on the same bed, depending on agency policy.

4. Raise the bed to a comfortable working height.

5. Remove dirty linens to an appropriate receptacle. To prevent the spread of microorganisms in the unit, dirty linens should be placed directly into the linen basket or bag, not on the other furniture or the floor.

6. Push the empty mattress to the head of the bed. The mattress slides to the foot of the bed when the head of the bed is raised.

7. Place the mattress pad on the mattress, extending it from the area of the shoulders to the knees.

8. Without shaking it, place the bottom sheet on the bed with the center fold in the middle of the bed and with the hem seams down. Place the sheet so that the bottom edge is even with the mattress at the foot of the bed. Shaking the sheets in the air increases the number of microorganisms on the linens.

9. Tuck in the top edge of one side of the bed to make a mitered corner. Tuck the sheet on the one side from the head to the foot of the bed.

10. Miter the other corners and tuck the sheet tightly on the opposite side of the bed. Wrinkles are uncomfortable and may lead to skin irritation and bedsores, or decubitus ulcers.

11. Place the draw sheet on the bed so that it covers the area from the shoulders to the knees. Tuck each side tightly. The draw sheet may be used to move the patient because most of the weight of the patient is located in the trunk of the body.

12. Place the top sheet and blanket on the bed with the blanket 4 to 6 inches lower than the sheet to make a cuff.

Continued

Making an Unoccupied and Surgical Bed—cont'd

13. Place the bedspread on the bed. A closed bed is made when the bedspread, blanket, and top sheet cover the bottom sheet completely. The top sheet, blanket, and bedspread may be folded back to the foot of the bed to make an open bed. In a surgical bed, the top linens are not tucked under the mattress to provide easy access to the bed and to make postsurgical assessment easier.

14. Place the pillowcase on the bed next to the pillow. Using the center of the closed end of the pillowcase, grasp the center of the pillow and pull the cover on. Place the pillow so the open edge is away from the door. To prevent the spread of microorganisms, do not hold the pillow under the chin to assist in putting on the pillowcase.

15. Return the bed to its lowest level.

Skill 23-10

Making an Occupied Bed

1. Maintain medical asepsis by using the guidelines provided in the Standard and Transmission-Based Precautions, including good handwashing technique and use of gloves as needed.

2. Collect clean linens, following the same procedure as for the unoccupied bed.

3. Identify the patient and explain the procedure.

4. Provide for the privacy and safety of the patient. Place side rails in the upright position.

5. Raise the bed to a comfortable working height and lower the head of the bed. Remove the pillows to make moving the patient easier. One pillow may be left under the patient's head for comfort.

6. Lower the side rail. Without exposing the patient, assist him or her to turn to one side.

7. Roll the soiled sheets toward the patient. The sheets are wrapped as tight as possible because the patient will later be asked to roll over these linens to the clean side.

8. Make the unoccupied side of the bed, placing the clean sheets for the occupied half of the bed under the roll of soiled sheets. The bottom side of the soiled sheets is cleaner than the top.

9. Raise the side rail and assist the patient to roll across the sheets to the cleaner side.

10. Lower the side rail and make the unoccupied side of the bed. Remove the soiled linens and immediately place them in an appropriate container.

11. Assist the patient to return to the center of the bed.

12. Place the clean top sheet over the soiled top sheet and remove the soiled sheet. Do not expose the patient at any time during this procedure. Add the blanket to the top sheet.

13. Make the top sheet and blanket corners. Raise the side rail.

14. Change and replace the pillowcases.

15. Lower the bed to its lowest level.

16. Reposition the patient for comfort, privacy, and safety.

Review Questions

1. Use each of the following terms in one or more sentences that correctly relate their meaning.
   Apical
   Pulse
   Vital

2. Describe four nursing specialties.

3. Describe the education, role, and credentialing of three levels of nursing.

4. Describe the importance of assessing fluid balance in the body.

5. Describe the importance of a clean unit and bed.

6. List three types of intake and output.

7. List five conditions that indicate assessment of intake and output.

8. Describe the process of forcing fluids and indications for its use.

Critical Thinking

1. Investigate the requirements and cost of education programs for three types of nurses.

2. Write a narrative paragraph describing to a patient the procedure for and importance of monitoring intake and output.

3. While nurses give direct care to patients, it is common for the patient to share information with the nurse. For each of the following situations, write one or more sentences that describe the action the nurse should take. Justify the action chosen for each of the situations. Chapter 4 provides additional information regarding ethical and legal responsibilities of health care workers.

   a. The nurse notices several old scars that are small and circular on the patient's back and chest while giving a bed bath.

   b. The nurse hears a patient arguing with someone on the phone indicating that no one is coming to give the patient a ride on discharge from the facility.

   c. The patient tells the nurse that he or she will never follow the physician's orders once discharged from the facility because the orders are too impractical.

4. Research and describe the factors that have led to the projected nursing shortage. Describe three actions that might be taken by educational and health facilities to recruit and keep more nurses in the profession.

24
Medical Careers

Learning Objectives

Define at least 10 terms relating to careers in medicine and related fields.

Specify the role of selected medical care providers, including personal qualities, levels of education, and credentialing requirements.

Define visual acuity and describe at least two methods used to determine it.

Describe two types of electrocardiography used by medical personnel.

Key Terms

Acuity
(uh-KYOO-it-ee) Clearness or sharpness of perception

Allopathic
(al-o-PATH-ik) Treatment of disease and injury with active intervention

Anesthesiology
(an-es-thee-zee-AHL-uh-jee) Study of medicine to relieve pain during surgery

Biomechanics
(by-o-meh-KAN-iks) Study of the mechanical laws and their application to living organisms, especially locomotion

Internship
(IN-tern-ship) Period of initial training under the supervision of a qualified practitioner

Osteopathic
(os-tee-o-PATH-ik) Treatment of disease and injury with an emphasis on the relationship between the body organs and musculoskeletal system

Residency
(REZ-ih-dent-see) Period of training in a specific area under the supervision of a qualified health care practitioner

Vision
(VIZH-un) Capacity for sight

Medical Careers Terminology*

TERM	DEFINITION	PREFIX	ROOT	SUFFIX
Chiropractic	Pertaining to manipulation of the spine by hand (literally, done by hand)	chiro/pract	ic	
Electrocardiogram	Record of the electrical activity of the heart	electro	cardio	gram
Gynecology	Study of women		gyne/c	ology
Ophthalmic	Pertaining to vision		ophthalm	ic
Orthoptics	Science of vision using both eyes	orth	opt	ics
Osteopathy	Therapeutic approach to medicine (literally, disease of bone)	osteo	path	y
Phlebotomy	Incision into a vessel		phleb	otomy
Podiatrist	One who treats the feet		pod/ia	trist
Psychiatry	Medicine dealing with mental, emotional, and behavioral disorders		psych/ia	try
Psychology	Study of the mind		psych	ology

*A transition phrase or vowel may be added to or deleted from the word parts to make the combining form.

Abbreviations for Medical Careers

ABBREVIATION	MEANING
AMA	American Medical Association
DC	Doctor of chiropractry
DO	Doctor of osteopathy
DPM	Doctor of podiatry
EKG	Electrocardiogram
MA	Medical assistant
MD	Medical doctor
PA	Physician assistant
RMA	Registered medical assistant
CST	Certified surgical technologist

Careers

Physicians and other medical care providers work with their patients in a close or primary relationship (Box 24-1). The function of medical care providers is to promote optimal health and provide care during illness.

Physicians

There are two types of medical doctors, the MD (Doctor of Medicine) and DO (Doctor of Osteopathic Medicine). Although **osteopathic** doctors are also physicians, the largest group of physicians providing direct care is the medical doctors (MDs), or **allopathic** physicians. The education for the medical doctor includes 4 years of medical school after completion of a college or university degree. Additional training under the supervision of a practicing doctor is needed for specialization. The additional training may be a 1-year **internship** that includes general training. Most physicians complete a **residency,** or training of several years in length, in an area of specialty.

Medical doctors provide care through all phases of life. About one third of medical doctors and one half of osteopathic doctors are primary care physicians. They are usually the first doctor to see the patient, and they see patients on a regular basis. Some of the many areas of specialization in medicine include **anesthesiology,** surgery, pediatrics, obstetrics, and urology (Figure 24-1). Information regarding the specialty of psychiatry is provided in Chapter 29. Information regarding careers in pathology is provided in Chapter 21. Most medical doctors work in private practice, although an increasing number work for health maintenance organizations or as hospital staff. Medical doctors are licensed by the state after

Box 24-1   Medical Careers

Allergist-immunologist
Anesthesiologist
Cardiologist
Chiropractor
Chiropractor assistant
Dermatologist
Dispensing optician
Family practitioner
General practitioner
Gynecologist
Intern
Internist
Medical assistant
Medical officer
Neurologist
Obstetrician

Ophthalmologist
Optical engineer
Optometric assistant
Optometrist
Osteopathic physician
Otolaryngologist
Pediatrician
Physiatrist
Physician
Physician assistant
Podiatric assistant
Podiatrist
Proctologist
Surgeon
Urologist

Physicians and other medical care providers work with patients in a variety of care settings.

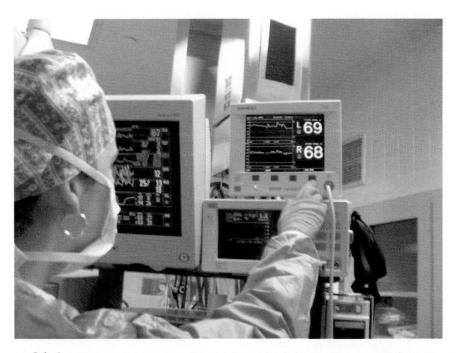

Figure 24-1   Surgery is one area in which medical doctors can specialize. *(Courtesy Somantics Corporation, Troy, Mich.)*

successful completion of medical school and passing a comprehensive board examination. There are 24 specialty boards in medicine.

Ophthalmologists are medical doctors who diagnose and treat diseases and injuries to the eyes. The ophthal-mologist may prescribe medication and perform surgery. Ophthalmologists write prescriptions for glasses and give instruction for corrective eye exercise. Ophthalmology re-quires a medical degree and license to practice medicine as well as specialty education and experience.

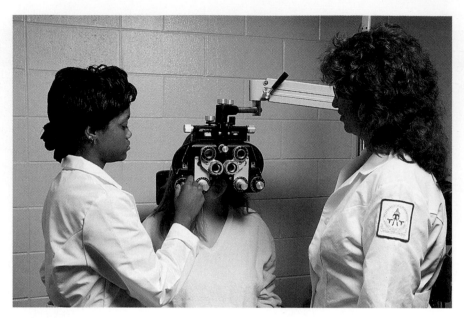

Figure 24-2 The optometrist uses an ophthalmoscope to view the interior eye and detect ocular diseases.

Education for the doctor of osteopathy (DO) emphasizes the overall body and the physiology of movement. The philosophy of osteopathic medicine is based on the belief that the human body is an integrated organism with a natural ability to resist disease and to heal itself. In addition to using the modern tools of medicine, osteopaths are trained to perform manipulation. The moving or manipulation of muscles and bones is called **biomechanics.** The education for osteopathic physicians is very similar in length to the medical doctor. After successful completion of an accredited program and a national examination, osteopathic physicians are licensed by the state in which they practice. There are more than 14,000 osteopathic physicians in the United States. To continue practice in many states, osteopathic physicians must complete at least 150 hours of continuing education every 3 years.

Other Medical Care Providers

Podiatrists (DPM) treat common foot disorders by using corrective devices, orthopedic shoes, surgery, and medication. Podiatry school includes 4 years of classroom and clinical instruction following completion of at least 2 years of college. Podiatrists are licensed by the state and may be required to complete an internship to qualify. There are more than 10,000 podiatrists in the United States.

The role of the physician assistant (PA) is different from other health care professions in that it was not developed to meet the needs of advanced medical technology. It was developed to relieve some of the tasks performed by the medical doctor to extend the availability of care. Physician assistants, working under the direction of a physician, perform about 70% of the duties of the medical doctor, including taking the patient history, conducting the physical exam, performing minor surgical procedures, and ordering diagnostic tests. In some states, physician assistants may write prescriptions. New roles for the physician assistant include serving as house staff in hospitals, emergency settings, and occupational health clinics. Most PA programs accept students with 2 years of college and prior experience in the health care industry. Education for the physician assistant includes 2 years of classroom and clinical training. Three physician assistant programs train surgeon assistants. Completion of the program may result in a certificate or academic degree. Physician assistants may be registered or licensed by the state in which they practice. Every 6 years, they must be recertified, based on completion of at least 100 hours of continuing education.

Orthoptics is the clinical science of **vision** using both eyes (binocular). Orthoptists are eye muscle specialists who work under the direction of an ophthalmologist and who help the patient develop the ability to use both eyes together. Exercises may be used to improve vision. Most orthoptists complete 2 years of college and 24 months of specialized training. Certification is recommended for most employment opportunities.

Opticians (also called *ophthalmic dispensers*) design, fit, and adapt lenses and frames based on an optical prescription. The optician grinds lenses to fit the patient's needs. Training for opticians is available on the job, in vocational schools, and in 2-year colleges. Licensing of opticians is required in at least 26 states.

Optometrists examine and test eyes to evaluate vision and detect diseases of the eye for referral to a medical doctor (Figure 24-2). The optometrist may use lenses or therapy to improve vision. Optometry requires at least 2 years of college work followed by 4 years of professional study at an accredited optometric school. The degree earned is Doctor of Optometry (OD). Optometrists are licensed by the state.

Support Personnel

Surgical technologists (ST), also called *surgical* and *operating room technicians,* assist during surgical operations under the supervision of the surgeon and registered nurse (Figure 24-3). Surgical technologists help prepare the operating room. They assemble and sterilize the instruments, drapes, and solutions. Technologists may also prepare the patient by shaving and cleaning the incision site. Surgical technologists assist the rest of the team to put on sterile gowns and gloves. During the surgery, surgical technologists pass the instruments and materials needed for the procedure to the surgeon. Surgical technologists receive training in community college, university, military, and vocational school programs. In 2001 there were 350 accredited programs, which last 9 to 24 months in length. Technologists may achieve voluntary certification after completing an accredited program and a national examination.

Medical assistant (MA) is expected to be one of the fastest growing occupations through the year 2010. The medical assistant performs both clerical and clinical functions under the supervision of a physician. Clerical duties that may be performed by the medical assistant include answering the telephone, filling out insurance forms, handling correspondence, and scheduling appointments, hospital admissions, and laboratory services (Skill 24-1). The medical assistant prepares the treatment room, drapes and positions patients, sterilizes equipment, and maintains and inventories supplies and equipment (Figure 24-4; Skill 24-2). Medical assistants who have a specialty may make casts or take radiographs and electrocardiographs. The medical assistant may also greet and interview patients and assess vital signs. Training for the medical assistant ranges from 1 to 2 years in a vocational or community college program. Some medical assistants are trained on the job by the employing physician. Certification of medical assistants is possible through the American Association of Medical Assistants. The American Medical Technologists organization grants a certification called *Registered Medical Assistant* (RMA) to those who have 5 years of service and have completed an approved course. The American Registry of Med-

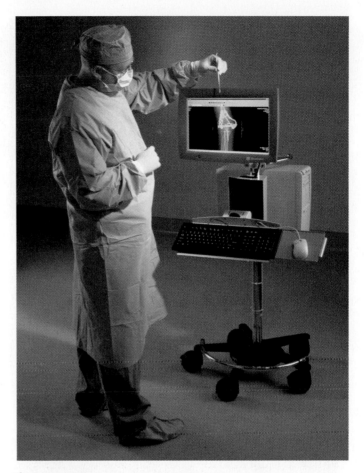

Figure 24-3   Radiographs allow the surgery team to prepare for procedures. *(Courtesy Swissray International, Inc, Elmsfed, NY.)*

ical Assistants also awards the RMA to those who have completed an approved course, have 1 year of experience, and have a letter of recommendation from an employer.

The podiatric assistant performs routine procedures such as patient preparation, equipment sterilization, development of radiographs, and general office duties. Podiatric assistants may be trained on the job or attend vocational school.

Ophthalmic assistants and technicians provide care to the patient of the ophthalmologist by measuring vision, changing dressings, administering eye and oral medications, applying contact lenses, and assisting with specialized ocular tests. Ophthalmic assistants maintain equipment and supplies. Assistants may learn on the job or complete a home-study course offered by the American Association of Ophthalmology. Technicians perform all of the tasks of the assistant and may be trained to prepare specimens for examination and to assist with ocular surgery. Ophthalmic technicians complete a 2-year certificate program.

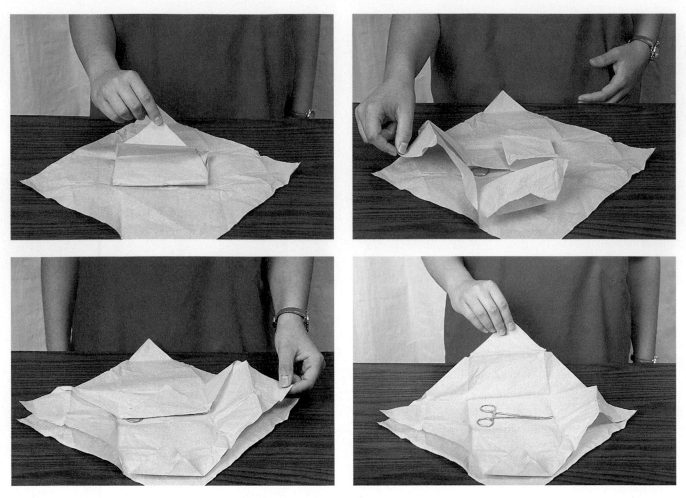

Figure 24-4   Opening a sterile package.

Content Instruction

Paraoptometric personnel extend the optometrist's capability by performing the routine tasks of vision care. Paraoptometric personnel work under the supervision of a doctor of optometry. Optometric technicians complete an associate or 2-year degree. They perform tests such as vision screening, measuring pressure on the cornea (tonometry), and recording patient histories. Technicians may also determine the power of existing lenses and assist with frame selection and fitting. Technicians instruct patients on the care and proper method of contact wear. They assist the optometrist during examinations and may work with children who have disabilities such as wandering eyes (amblyopia). Optometric assistants may be trained on the job or in 1-year programs.

Vision

Visual **acuity** is the ability to differentiate shapes and color to interpret their meaning. The ophthalmoscope is used to view the interior of the eye to examine its structures. Another assessment method is the field vision test that measures how wide the field of vision reaches around each eye.

Comprehensive eye examination includes testing for visual acuity for distance and near objects. It also measures focusing, tracking, and fixation skills. The ability to use both eyes together at the same time (binocular vision) is assessed as well as depth perception (stereopsis) (Skill 24-3).

Skill 24-1

Answering the Telephone

1. Maintain medical asepsis by using the guidelines provided in the Standard and Transmission-Based Precautions, including good handwashing technique and use of gloves as needed.

2. Answer the telephone promptly.

3. Speak in a polite, clear, and well-modulated voice.

4. Determine who is calling, the person for whom the call is intended, and the nature of the business.

5. Do not give out any information about patients or other personnel unless directed to do so by the supervising personnel.

6. In a designated location, write the name of the caller, to whom the message is directed, the time and date of the call, the telephone number of the caller, and any information that is given by the caller.

7. Repeat the name of the caller, the telephone number, and information to verify its accuracy with the caller.

8. Deliver the message to the person for whom it is intended as directed by supervising personnel.

Skill 24-2

Opening Sterile Packages

1. Maintain medical asepsis by using the guidelines provided in the Standard and Transmission-Based Precautions, including good handwashing technique and use of gloves as needed. The hands are never sterile. If a clean hand touches a sterile object or surface, the object or surface is contaminated.

2. Place the sterile package on a clean, dry surface or hold the package above the level of the waist. The edges and parts of sterile packaging that fall below the level of the waist are considered to be contaminated. The surface must be dry because moisture allows microorganisms to move through the wrapping material by capillary action, called the *wicking effect*.

3. Check the color of the sterilization tape. The tape changes color when the temperature and pressure of the autoclave reach sufficient levels to destroy all microorganisms and endospores. Remove the tape if the color has changed.

4. Open the far side of the package first. If any part of the arm or hand passes over the sterile area, the item is considered contaminated because particles of dead skin and microorganisms may fall into the sterile area.

5. Open one side and carefully avoid crossing over the sterile field. When holding the package, the free hand is passed under it to avoid contamination.

6. Open the near corner last. If the sterile object is being held, secure the ends of the package before passing the contents to the sterile field. If the unsterile parts of the draping cross over the edge of the sterile field, the area is contaminated.

Skill 24-3

Measuring Visual Acuity

1. Maintain medical asepsis by using the guidelines provided in the Standard and Transmission-Based Precautions, including good handwashing technique and use of gloves as needed.

2. Identify the patient and explain the procedure.

3. Hang the Snellen chart on a light-colored wall at eye level 20 feet from the location of the patient. Make sure there is no glare and the chart is completely illuminated. The patient might not be able to read the chart accurately if the light is placed incorrectly.

4. Place the patient's heels on a line 20 feet from the chart. If the patient is sitting, the back of the chair should be 20 feet from the chart. The chart is designed to measure the height of the letters that can be read correctly from a distance of 20 feet.

5. Cover the patient's left eye when testing the right eye. Have the patient read the letters on each line, beginning with the 100 line and descending to the smallest line that can be read. If the patient wears glasses, have the patient complete the test first with the glasses on, then repeat the procedure with the glasses removed for comparison. The comparison of vision with and without the glasses indicates the effectiveness of the corrective lenses.

6. Repeat the procedure to test the left eye and then both eyes together.

7. Record the visual acuity as a proportional value. The numerator is the distance from the chart (20 feet). The denominator is the height of the letters of the smallest line that is read accurately. Normal vision is considered to be 20/20.

Electrocardiogram

Electrical currents in the heart are measured using an electrocardiogram. This may be done with 3 to 12 leads (or electrodes) or more attached to the person being tested (Figure 24-5). The electrocardiograph is a strip of graph paper that is produced as the heart's electrical activity is recorded. More information regarding electrocardiographs and the function of the heart may be found in Chapter 10.

Performance Instruction

Physical Examination and Treatment

The medical assistant may assist with a physical examination or simple medical procedure. Preparation of the examination room includes providing the needed equipment, supplies, and linens for the procedure to be completed (Figure 24-6). The assistant greets the patient,

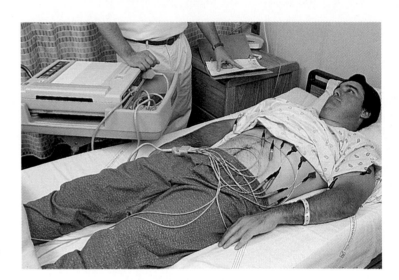

Figure 24-5 Cables are connected from the EKG machine to the electrodes. *(From Sorrentino S:* Mosby's text for nursing assistants, *ed 5, St Louis, 2000, Mosby.)*

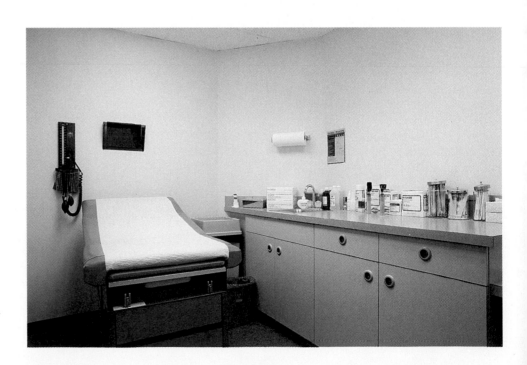

Figure 24-6 Preparing the examination room is an important duty of the medical assistant.

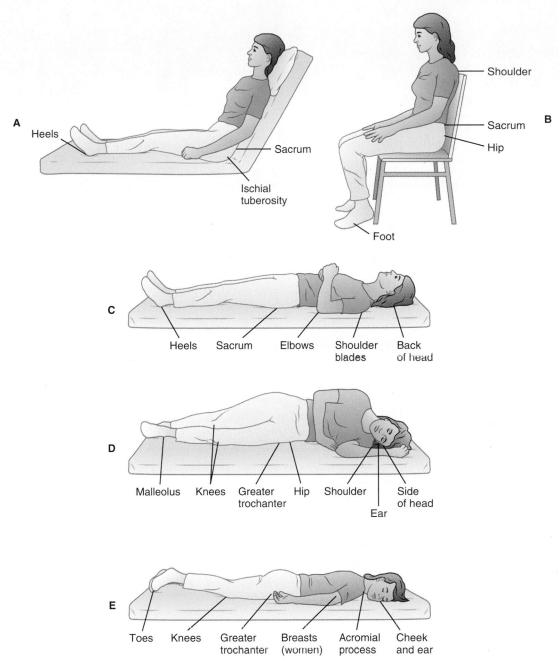

Figure 24-7   The best position is determined by the health care worker or ordered by the physician. **A,** Modified semi-Fowler's position. **B,** Sitting position. **C,** Horizontal or supine position. **D,** Left Sims' position. **E,** Prone position.

takes him or her to the examination room, and takes vital signs. If necessary for the procedure, the assistant explains the use of an examination gown and provides the patient with privacy to change into it. The assistant then assists the physician in positioning and giving treatment to the patient (Figure 24-7). All specimens are labeled at the time that they are collected with the patient's name, identification number, date and time of collection, and the name of the physician. The patient is provided with privacy to redress when the procedure is completed. The assistant then cleans and prepares the room for the next procedure (Skills 24-4 and 24-5).

Skill 24-4

Assisting with the Physical Examination

1. Maintain medical asepsis by using the guidelines provided in the Standard and Transmission–Based Precautions, including good handwashing technique and use of gloves as needed.

2. Prepare the examination room with necessary linens, equipment, and supplies for the procedures to be completed.

3. Assist the patient to the room and take vital signs.

4. Instruct the patient to undress and put on an examination gown.

5. Leave the room briefly to provide the patient with privacy.

6. Knock before reentering the room.

7. Position and drape the patient for examination.

8. Hand supplies and equipment to the examiner as they are needed.

9. Label all specimen containers with appropriate information including date, time, type of specimen, the patient's name, and name of person collecting the sample. Place specimens in designated areas for examination.

10. Instruct the patient regarding procedures to follow before leaving the office.

11. Provide the patient with privacy to dress when the examination is completed.

12. Clean and restock the examination room.

Skill 24-5

Assisting with Suture Removal

1. Sutures may be removed by trained personnel under the supervision of the physician.

2. Maintain medical asepsis by using the guidelines provided in the Standard and Transmission-Based Precautions, including good handwashing technique and use of gloves as needed.

3. Position the patient and remove clothing as necessary to expose the sutured area. Provide privacy as needed.

4. Put on examination or nonsterile gloves to remove dressings. Gloves prevent the spread of microorganisms from body fluids contained in the dressing to the health care worker.

5. Remove the dressing gently, and retain it or dispose of it in the appropriate container. The tape may be loosened using hydrogen peroxide to prevent reopening of the wound.

6. Clean the suture line and skin around it with an antiseptic.

7. Use aseptic technique to open a sterile suture removal kit. The opened tray is considered the sterile field for this procedure. Only the handles of the forceps and suture scissors are touched by the health care worker so that the tips that touch the patient remain sterile.

8. Grasp the knot of the suture and pull it away from the skin.

9. Slip the curved cutting edge of the scissors under the short end of the suture and cut as close to the skin as possible. Cutting the suture close to the skin decreases the chance of infection because less of the exposed suture is pulled through the tissue.

10. Slowly and steadily pull the knot of the suture straight up from the skin. A slow, steady pull prevents tissue damage and pain.

11. Remove every other suture first to assess healing of the suture line. If gaps in the wound occur, the physician may want to resuture the wound.

12. If no gaps occur, remove all remaining sutures.

13. Clean the site again with antiseptic. Leave the wound area exposed unless directed to use a dressing.

14. Inform the patient of any restrictions in movement that might be necessary.

15. Dispose of used items appropriately in the biohazard waste receptacle.

Vision Assessment

Vision may be tested by the medical or optometric assistant using a Snellen chart that measures the ability to see symbols from a specified distance (Figure 24-8). The patient is asked to sit or stand 20 feet from the chart and identify the characters on the chart with each eye separately and then together. The height of the characters on the chart that can be seen is used to describe the patient's vision. For example, a measurement of 20/30 means that the patient can see characters that are 30 mm high when the patient is 20 feet from the chart. A reading of 20/20 is considered normal vision.

Electrocardiogram

The electrical activity of the heart may be measured using an electrocardiogram (EKG). If the heart muscle is damaged, changes in the EKG may be used to locate the damaged area. The supine position is usually used for taking an EKG. To get a clear reading, the contact pads of the electrodes should have good contact with the person. This may require shaving of the area as well as removal of oils and perspiration. Rubbing alcohol may be used to clean the skin before application of the electrodes (Skill 24-6).

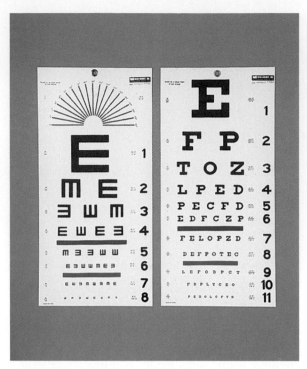

Figure 24-8   Snellen and Jaeger charts are used to measure visual acuity.

Skill 24–6

Obtaining an EKG*

1. Maintain medical asepsis by using the guidelines provided in the Standard and Transmission-Based Precautions, including good handwashing technique and use of gloves as needed.

2. Review the procedure with the supervising personnel and patient.

3. Provide for privacy. Assist the patient with elimination needs.

4. Raise the bed to a comfortable working height.

5. Measure and record vital signs.

6. Expose the chest, arms, and/or legs as needed for electrode placement.

7. Wear gloves to wash and shave designated electrode sites.

8. Clean electrode sites with alcohol.

9. Apply electrodes to chest, arms, and legs.

10. Connect cables from the EKG machine to the electrodes.

11. Plug in EKG machine.

12. Instruct the patient to lie still without talking during the test.

13. Obtain 8 to 12 inches of heart tracing for each lead. Notify the supervising personnel if any unusual patterns are seen.

14. Turn off the EKG machine.

15. Remove the tracing from the machine.

16. Return the patient to a comfortable bed level and position.

17. Return all equipment to the designated location.

* Medical assistants may perform this procedure when specially trained, if it is allowed by the state, and if the medical assistant is supervised by licensed personnel.

Review Questions

1. Use each of the following terms in one or more sentences that correctly relate their meaning.
   Allopathic
   Biomechanics
   Osteopathic

2. Describe the function of the medical health care providers.

3. Describe the education, role, and credentialing of three medical health care providers.

4. Describe two methods of assessment of vision.

Critical Thinking

1. Investigate the requirements and cost of education programs for five types of medical health care providers.

2. Describe a normal and abnormal pattern for an electrocardiogram. (Chapter 10 provides more information regarding cardiovascular assessments.)

3. Use Figure 24-7 and the information learned from the anatomy and physiology chapters to determine what position would be used for the following procedures: chest radiograph, electrocardiograph, injection, lumbar puncture, phlebotomy, suture of hand wound.

25
Dental Careers

Learning Objectives

Define at least 10 terms relating to dental health care.

Specify the role of the dentist, dental hygienist, dental assistant, and dental laboratory technician, including personal qualities, levels of education, and credentialing requirements.

Identify the difference between the dentition of the child and adult.

Identify at least five structures of the oral cavity.

Describe the location, structure, and function of four types of teeth.

Chart at least three types of dental variations using a selected method of charting.

Describe methods of prevention and detection of caries and periodontal disease.

Describe techniques of brushing and flossing to promote dental health.

Key Terms

Abscess
(AB-ses) Localized collection of pus in a cavity formed by destruction of tissue

Alloy
(AL-oy) Solid mixture of two or more metals

Alveoli
(al-VEE-o-lie) Bony cavities in maxilla and mandible in which the roots of the teeth are attached

Calculus
(KAL-kyoo-lus) Calcium phosphate and carbonate with organic matter, deposited on the surfaces of teeth; tartar

Caries
(KARE-eez) Decalcification of the surface of the tooth followed by disintegration of the inner part of the tooth; cavity

Deciduous
(de-SID-yoo-us) The teeth that erupt first and are replaced by permanent dentition; primary teeth

Dentition
(den-TISH-un) Used to designate natural teeth in the mouth

Gingiva
(JIN-jiv-uh) Gum of the mouth, mucous membrane with supporting fibrous tissue

Halitosis
(hal-ih-TOE-sis) Offensive or bad breath

Hygiene
(HI-jeen) Proper care of the mouth and teeth for maintenance of health and the prevention of disease

Mandible
(MAN-dih-bul) Bone of the lower jaw

Maxilla
(mak-SIL-uh) Irregularly shaped bone that forms the upper jaw

Periodontal
(pare-ee-o-DON-tul) Situated or occurring around a tooth

Permanent
(PER-muh-nent) The teeth that erupt and take the place of deciduous dentition; secondary teeth

Plaque
(plak) Mass adhering to the enamel surface of a tooth, composed of mixed bacterial colonies and organic material

Restoration
(res-tore-AY-shun) Replacement of part of a tooth, usually with silver alloy, gold, or esthetic composite material

Dental Careers Terminology*

TERM	DEFINITION	PREFIX	ROOT	SUFFIX
Buccal	Pertaining to the cheek		bucc	al
Endodontics	Pertaining to treatment of disease of the inside of the tooth	endo	dont	ics
Gingivitis	Inflammation of the gums		gingiv	itis
Mandibular	Pertaining to the lower jaw		mandibul	ar
Maxillofacial	Pertaining to the upper jaw and face	maxillo	faci	al
Mesial	Pertaining to the middle		mesi	al
Odontology	Study of the tooth		odont	ology
Orthodontics	Pertaining to correcting tooth placement	ortho	dont	ics
Pedodontics	Pertaining to teeth of children	ped/o	dont	ics
Prosthodontist	One who places artificial appliances on teeth	prosth/o	dont	ist

*A transition phrase or vowel may be added to or deleted from the word parts to make the combining form.

Abbreviations for Dental Careers

ABBREVIATION	MEANING
ADA	American Dental Association
amal	Amalgam
ant	Anterior
DA	Dental assistant
DDS	Doctor of dental surgery
DH	Dental hygienist
DLT	Dental laboratory technician
DMD	Doctor of medical dentistry
ext	Extract, extraction
post	Posterior

Box 25-1   Dental Careers*

Dental assistant
Dental health director
Dental hygienist
Dental laboratory technician
Dentist
Endodontist
Oral pathologist
Oral surgeon
Orthodontic technician
Orthodontist
Pedodontist
Periodontist
Prosthodontist

*The dental health care team promotes prevention of dental diseases and provides restorative care of structures of the oral cavity.

Careers

The dental team includes the dentist, dental hygienist, dental assistant, and dental laboratory technician (Box 25-1). The goal of the dental team is to provide optimal care of the oral cavity for all patients. Dental team members work in a variety of settings including group practice, specialty practice, schools, government or community clinics, and in dental insurance and supply companies.

Dentist

The role of the dentist has changed greatly because improved methods of dental care and nutrition have reduced the number of **caries.** Dentists now perform a variety of services including public education directed to prevent tooth decay, detection of disease such as cancer, cosmetic improvement of appearance, and correction of oral problems such as misaligned teeth and jaws (Figure 25-1). Some

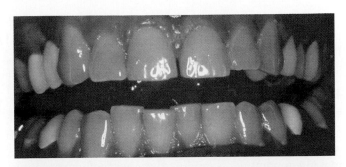

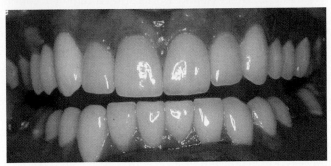

Figure 25-1 Bonded veneers improve the appearance, change the shape, and restore the function of teeth. *(Courtesy Joyce Bassett, DDS, FAGD, Scottsdale, Ariz.)*

dentists perform surgery to correct facial and dental deformities caused by accidents or birth defects. Pain control and anesthesia in dentistry has become two of the roles of the professional because many people become anxious and even phobic when needing dental care. Types of anesthesia that may be administered include local, sedation, and general anesthesia. Some sedation may even cause retrograde amnesia or the inability to remember the treatment.

Dentists are highly respected professionals. Dentistry offers a great deal of flexibility and independence. Private practitioners can choose to work either full or part time. Many dentists now choose to work in a group practice to share the cost of maintaining an office. Dentists are needed in all types of communities.

Dentistry offers eight specialties that allow practice in specific areas:

1. Endodontics: treatment of disease of the dental pulp, usually with root canal
2. Oral and maxillofacial surgery: extraction and treatment of injury, disease, and deformity of the mouth, such as cleft palate
3. Oral pathology: laboratory testing and biopsy to diagnose oral conditions
4. Orthodontics: prescription and fitting of braces to correct misaligned teeth or jaws
5. Pedodontics: prevention of disease and decay and therapeutic care of children's teeth from birth through adolescence
6. Periodontics: treatment of gum disease and education for prevention

7. Prosthodontics: design and fitting of bridgework and dentures as well as substitutes for missing teeth or tissue
8. Public health dentistry: promotion of prevention and treatment of dental disease

Dentists work with people of all ages and personalities. They must possess leadership ability and good interpersonal skills. The work requires creativity and decision-making ability. Much of dentistry involves precise work by hand, so manual dexterity is needed.

The educational requirement for a dentist includes at least 2 years of college classes before entering dental school. More than 90% of students entering dental school have completed a 4-year degree at a college or university. Dental school training ranges from 3 to 4 years and offers either a doctor of dental surgery (DDS) or a doctor of medical dentistry (DMD) degree. Two additional years of training are needed to practice in one of the eight areas of specialization. After successful completion of an accredited dental program and a national examination, dentists are licensed by the state.

Dental Hygienist

With the purpose of providing preventive oral health, dentists developed dental **hygiene** as a career in the early 1900s. As of 2000, dental hygiene was projected to be one of the 30 fastest growing occupations. Dental hygienists work in a variety of settings that range from private practice to corporate clinics located in foreign countries. Some areas in which the dental hygienist may specialize include clinical work, education, administration, research, consumer advocacy, or veterinary dental practice. Hygienists may work flexible hours depending on the type of practice.

The scope of practice of the dental hygienist varies from state to state. It is influenced by the level of education and type of practice in which the hygienist works. The role of the hygienist includes recording the patient's health history, removing **calculus** and **plaque** from above and below the gum line, examining the teeth and oral structures, and screening for oral cancer and blood pressure abnormalities. Hygienists expose, process, and may interpret dental radiographs (Figure 25-2). In addition to removing plaque from the teeth surfaces, dental hygienists also polish and floss the teeth as part of the cleaning procedure. In some practices, the hygienist applies a fluoride treatment to the teeth. Dental hygienists instruct patients on the procedures for home care including making dietary recommendations. The hygienist may be responsible for the recall system to alert patients of the next appointment. They may also place temporary fillings and apply cavity-preventive agents such as fluoride and sealants. Expanded functions of the dental hygienist may include administration of local anesthesia.

The practice of hygiene requires manual dexterity to use dental instruments in the small area of a mouth. Good health and personal cleanliness are also important characteristics of the hygienist. The education for a hygienist ranges from a 2-year community college to a 4-year college or university program. The community college program usually includes 2 years of prerequisite work in addition to dental training.

Dental hygienists are licensed by the state in which they practice after they have successfully completed an accred-

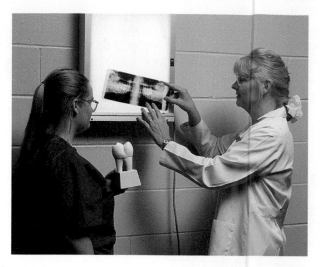

Figure 25-2 The use of dental radiographs is regulated by law to protect the patient and caregiver from unnecessary exposure to radiation.

ited program and a national examination. Hygienists are registered with the National Board of Registered Dental Hygienists.

Dental Assistant

The role of the dental assistant varies greatly with the size and type of practice in which the assistant works. The job responsibilities may include answering the telephone, making appointments, and working with billing accounts. Assistants are responsible for maintaining infection control. They clean and sterilize instruments, prepare the treatment room and dental materials, and assist with procedures (Figure 25-3). Exposing radiographs, taking and recording dental histories, and assessing vital signs are also responsibilities of the dental assistant. The dental assistant must work under the supervision of a dentist.

Personal qualities that are important for a dental assistant include the ability to work well with others. Good physical and psychosocial health is also needed. There are no educational standards required by all states for a dental assistant, and some tasks can be learned with on-the-job training. Accredited programs for dental assistants run 1 to 2 years. Certification is available through the Dental Assisting National Board. Some states require licensure or registration.

Dental Laboratory Technician

Dental laboratory technicians are the only members of the dental health care team who do not work directly with pa-

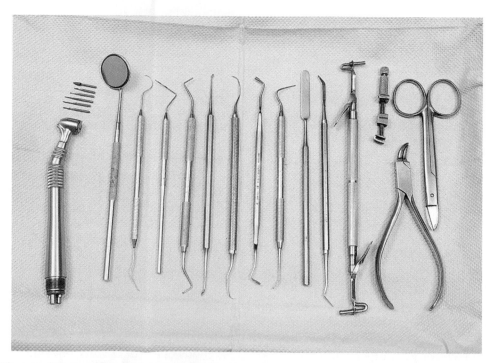

Figure 25-3 Cleaning and sterilizing dental instruments are part of the dental assistant's role.

tients. Technicians make prostheses following the orders of a dentist. These prostheses include bridges, dentures, crowns, inlays, space maintainers, and corrective orthodontic appliances. Dental lab technicians work with a variety of materials including gold **alloy**, nonprecious metal, porcelain, wax, acrylic, and wires. Most dental technicians work in commercial laboratories and receive a salary for a standard 40-hour week.

The work of the dental laboratory technician involves minute detail and requires excellent manual dexterity. An awareness of detail, accuracy, and patience are necessary as well as artistic ability. Most dental laboratory technicians learn their work on the job. However, 30 programs in dental laboratory technology were approved by the Commission on Dental Accreditation in 2000. Certification for dental laboratory technicians is available through the National Association of Dental Laboratories.

Content Instruction

Maintaining Dental Health

Neglect or improper care of the teeth can lead to formation of cavities (caries) or **periodontal** disease (pyorrhea) with resulting tooth loss. Cavities, or caries, are inflammation or disease of the inner tooth. They result from the destruction of the enamel that protects the tooth.

Periodontal disease is caused by infection in the supporting structures of teeth such as the **gingiva** and bones. Periodontal disease affects one out of every two people in the United States. It can be acute or chronic. Most periodontal disease begins in the mouth by age 13. It may be asymptomatic for 20 to 30 years. Eventually, bleeding gums may result. The major cause of periodontal disease is formation of bacterial plaque. Plaque is composed of 75% bacterial colonies and 20% organic material that sticks to the surface of the tooth. Plaque is usually colorless and forms in 12 to 24 hours. Bacteria normally found in the mouth produce lactic and formic acids, which irritate the gum and cause tenderness and inflammation. The gingiva then pulls away from the irritant, allowing more plaque to form. Acids also dissolve the protective enamel on the surface of the tooth. Plaque may harden and discolor and become tartar (calculus). Plaque can reach the root of the tooth and the bone supporting the tooth (Figure 25-4). The tooth eventually falls out. The most common types of periodontal disease are gingivitis and periodontitis. Gingivitis is the early stage of the disease. Periodontitis may result in formation of pockets of pus called **abscesses.**

Only 60% of people in the United States brush and 25% floss their teeth regularly. Brushing removes plaque and

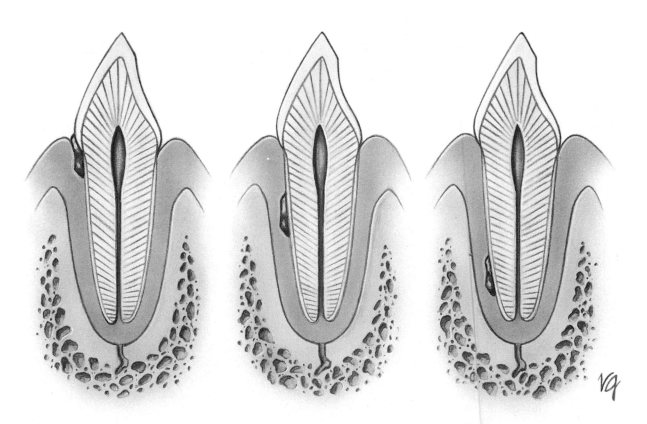

Figure 25-4   Dental caries and gingivitis develop as plaque is pushed into the soft tissues that support the mouth.

Skill 25-1

Assisting with Oral Hygiene Instruction

1. Maintain medical asepsis by using the guidelines provided in the Standard and Transmission-Based Precautions, including good handwashing technique and use of gloves as needed.

2. The teeth should be brushed for at least 5 minutes, twice daily. Regular brushing removes organic material and prevents bad breath (halitosis).

3. Use a soft brush with rounded bristles and a small head. Soft bristles prevent injury to the gum tissues, and a small head allows all areas of the mouth to be reached. Replacing worn brushes ensures effectiveness.

4. Use a toothpaste of individual choice. Toothpastes contain a foaming agent and mild abrasive. Some toothpastes contain fluoride, which helps to strengthen teeth. Tartar-softening agents have been added to some varieties.

5. With the brush held at a 45-degree angle to the gumline, move the brush in the direction of the tooth growth. Thoroughness in brushing is more important than technique to remove debris.

6. The back side of the front teeth is cleaned by tilting the brush upward.

7. Brush the gums and the tongue. Brushing the soft tissues of the mouth removes debris and increases circulation to the area.

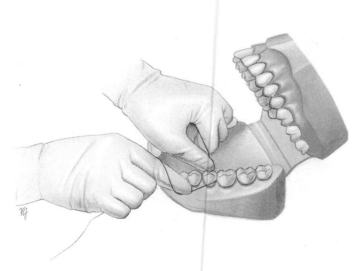

Figure 25-5 Flossing instruction is made easier with an enlarged model of teeth.

prevents bad breath (**halitosis**) (Skill 25-1). Flossing removes plaque from areas the toothbrush cannot reach (Figure 25-5; Skill 25-2). Sugar and sticky foods increase the chance of plaque formation. Local irritants that inflame the gums include smoking and chewing tobacco products. Poorly aligned teeth (malocclusion) and grinding of the teeth (bruxism) also increase the chance of periodontal disease. Medications, such as oral contraceptives, steroids, and chemotherapeutic agents, affect the gingiva by making it more susceptible to gingivitis and periodontitis. Systemic conditions also contribute to formation of caries and periodontal disease. They include hormonal imbalances such as in pregnancy, diabetes, and immunological deficiency. A balanced diet provides the proper nutrients needed to maintain dental health.

More than 23 million people in the United States are toothless (edentulous). Dentures are replacement prosthe-

Skill 25-2

Teaching Patients to Floss Teeth

1. Maintain medical asepsis by using the guidelines provided in the Standard and Transmission-Based Precautions, including good handwashing technique and use of gloves as needed.

2. Floss at least once daily. Plaque forms within 24 hours on teeth. Flossing reaches areas of the teeth that are missed by a toothbrush.

3. Use a 12- to 18-inch length of waxed or unwaxed floss supported between two fingers. Used properly, waxed and unwaxed floss are both effective. Supporting the floss between the fingers prevents cutting injury to the gums.

4. Move floss back and forth in a C-shape motion on the side of each tooth. The floss should reach below the gum line without cutting the tissue.

ses for total tooth loss. Dentures function to chew food, present a normal facial appearance, and allow clear speech. Dentures wear out and must be replaced. It is important that denture wearers continue to maintain dental health routines to prevent destruction of gum tissues. The gums should be brushed daily. Dentures should be cleaned daily by brushing, soaking in cleaning solution, or placing in an ultrasonic cleaner.

Structures of the Oral Cavity

Functions of the teeth include the mechanical portion of digestion, shape of the face, and aid in the production of speech. **Dentition** is the natural teeth in their normal position in the mouth.

The teeth are located in sockets **(alveoli)** of the **mandible** and **maxilla.** The areas of the mandible and maxilla in which the teeth are located are called the *mandibulary* and *maxillary arches.* The mandible is the longest and strongest bone of the face. It is the only movable bone of the skull. The sinuses are air cavities, lined with mucous membrane, that decrease the weight of the skull and also warm air during respiration. The frontal and maxillary sinuses connect with the maxillary bicuspid teeth.

The mouth, or oral cavity, is covered with mucous membrane (Figure 25-6). The roof of the mouth is divided into two portions. The anterior portion, or hard palate, is attached to the bones of the skull by the membranous tissue that covers it. The membrane of the posterior portion hangs loosely and is called the *soft palate.* The mandible and maxilla are surrounded by the inner surface of the lips. The lips are connected to the midline of the mandible and maxilla by a fold of mucous membrane called the *frenulum.* The tongue (lingua) lies on the floor of the mouth.

Tooth Formation

Tooth formation begins during the second month of gestation. At birth, the neonate has 44 teeth buds at various stages of development in the gums (gingiva). Twenty primary or **deciduous** teeth begin to erupt at about 6 months of age. The majority of deciduous teeth erupt by the age of 2 to 3 years, although the rate of tooth development varies greatly between individuals. Twenty-four of the buds are permanent teeth. The **permanent** teeth replace the deciduous teeth by about the twelfth year, but they may not completely appear until age 20 (Figure 25-7).

Structures of the Tooth

The tooth is divided into two sections called the *crown* and *root* (Figure 25-8). The crown is covered with shiny, white

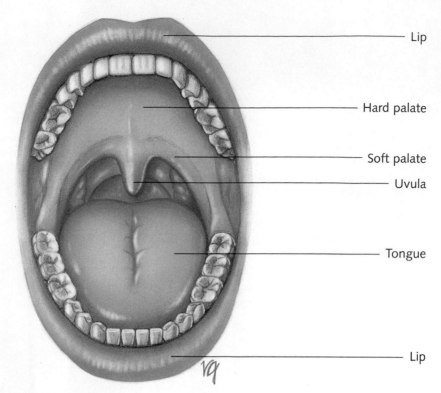

Lip

Hard palate

Soft palate

Uvula

Tongue

Lip

Figure 25-6 Structures of the oral cavity (the frenulum cannot be seen below the tongue).

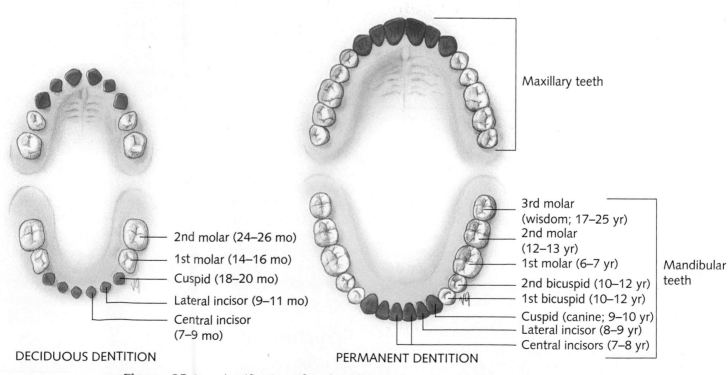

Maxillary teeth

2nd molar (24–26 mo)

1st molar (14–16 mo)

Cuspid (18–20 mo)

Lateral incisor (9–11 mo)

Central incisor (7–9 mo)

3rd molar (wisdom; 17–25 yr)

2nd molar (12–13 yr)

1st molar (6–7 yr)

2nd bicuspid (10–12 yr)

1st bicuspid (10–12 yr)

Cuspid (canine; 9–10 yr)

Lateral incisor (8–9 yr)

Central incisors (7–8 yr)

Mandibular teeth

DECIDUOUS DENTITION

PERMANENT DENTITION

Figure 25-7 Identification of teeth with eruption times (anterior teeth are shaded).

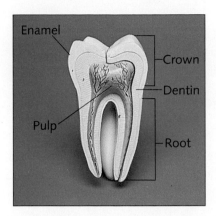

Figure 25-8   Structure of a molar tooth.

enamel, which is the hardest substance in the body. Enamel is composed mostly of calcium and phosphorus. The middle layer of the crown is composed of dentin. It forms the bulk of the tooth. Dentin is harder than bone but softer than enamel. Although it does not have nerves, dentin reacts to tactile (touch), thermal (temperature), and chemical stimulation. The inside layer of the crown and root is made of soft tissue called *pulp*. Pulp contains the nerves and blood vessels of the tooth. It forms and nourishes the dentin of the tooth.

Cementum, a hard, bonelike substance on the outside surface of the root, anchors the tooth. The neck (cervix) of the tooth is the narrowed area where the enamel of the crown and the cementum of the root join. The periodontal ligament is located between the alveolar bone and cementum. It holds the tooth in place. The gum tissue around the root of the tooth is the gingiva.

Types of Teeth

Descriptive anatomy of the tooth is called *odontology*. Teeth can be divided into four main types. They are the incisors (8), cuspids (4), bicuspids (8), and molars (12). The incisors, located in the front of the mouth, help to cut food. The cuspids, also called *canines* or *eyeteeth,* are the longest teeth in the mouth and they tear food. Bicuspids, or premolar teeth, are not present in the deciduous teeth. Bicuspid teeth tear and crush food. The molars are located in the back of the mouth. The largest and strongest teeth, molars, grind the food. The third molars are commonly called *wisdom teeth,* but they do not appear in every person. They may be removed if the space in the jaw is insufficient for the new teeth.

Identification of Teeth

Teeth in the upper jaw are called *maxillary teeth.* Those in the lower jaw are referred to as *mandibular.* The teeth in the front of the mouth (incisors and cuspids) are identified as being anterior. The bicuspids and molars are considered to be located posteriorly.

Each tooth can be named individually by its type and location. Location of a defect or structure of the crown of the tooth can also be identified using five surfaces of the crown (Figure 25-9). The Universal System for numbering teeth was adopted by the American Dental Association in 1968. It numbers the adult teeth from 1 to 16 beginning with the right maxillary third molar to the left maxillary third molar. Numbering the mandibulary teeth begins with the left third molar as 17 to the right third molar as number 32. Primary teeth are lettered in the same manner from A to T (Figure 25-10). Other systems used for charting include the Federation Dentaire International System and the Palmer system. The type of cavity (caries) or **restoration** can be charted using the five classes developed by G.V. Black.

Performance Instruction

Dental health care personnel use radiographs or x-rays to visualize the teeth in the gums. Both intraoral and extraoral films may be used. The standards for safety and limits of exposure to radiation are regulated by the U.S. National Council on Radiation Protection (NCRP). Dental care workers wear a film badge that records the amount of exposure to radiation.

New technology has changed dental practice. Computerized probes measure and record the depth of a pocket or recession of the gum. Lasers are used to soften calculus and seal some applications. Intraoral camera systems enlarge and visualize the inside of the mouth for the patient and dentist (Figure 25-11). Digital images have reduced the use of radiation for some images. Another innovation is the use of electronic dental anesthesia, which blocks the pain caused by dental work with electronic impulses.

One of the duties performed by the dental assistant is charting of dental conditions at the direction of the dentist (Figure 25-12). The assistant must be familiar with the structures of the individual teeth and their location in the mouth. The assistant also prepares the dental operatory and equipment for procedures (Figure 25-13). This includes adjusting the height of the chairs and placement of the lights, disinfecting surface areas, and sterilizing dental instruments after use (Skill 25-3). When needed, the assistant prepares restorative materials such as amalgam or cement (Figure 25-14). Amalgam is an alloy of silver and mercury that may be used to fill teeth. The assistant also prepares gels or alginate materials to make impressions of the teeth in the mouth. These models are then filled with plaster to make molds.

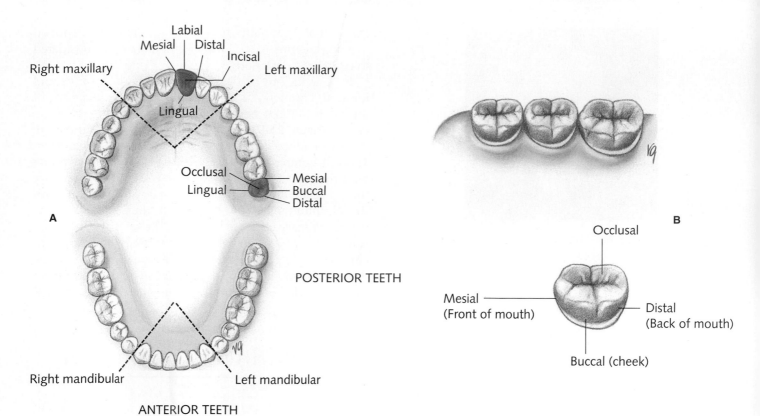

Figure 25-9 **A**, Five surfaces of the crown. **B**, Surface of a posterior crown (lingual side is not visible).

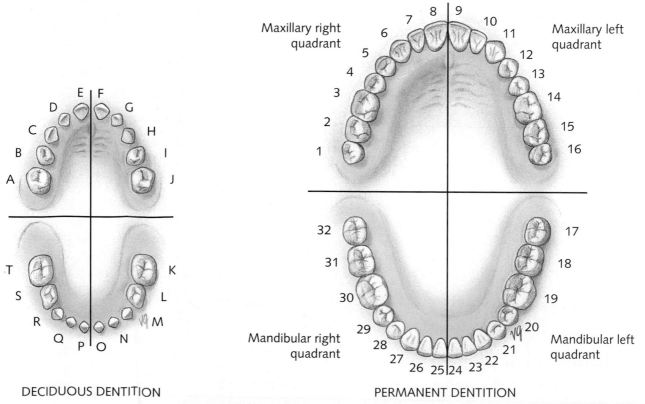

DECIDUOUS DENTITION

PERMANENT DENTITION

Figure 25-10 Universal system of tooth identification.

Skill 25-3

Maintaining and Preparing the Dental Operatory

1. Maintain medical asepsis by using the guidelines provided in the Standard and Transmission-Based Precautions, including good handwashing technique and use of gloves as needed.

2. Remove all evidence of prior visits, and position the dental chair in an upright position before escorting the patient to the treatment room. Make sure the light is out of the way while entering and exiting the room. Height of the chair and armrests can be adjusted to fit any size person comfortably.

3. Make sure the chair is in an upright position when escorting the patient from the operatory.

4. Clean the operatory surfaces and chair with disinfectant daily, according to the manufacturer's directions. Cleanliness of equipment and supplies reduces the spread of microorganisms that may cause infection.

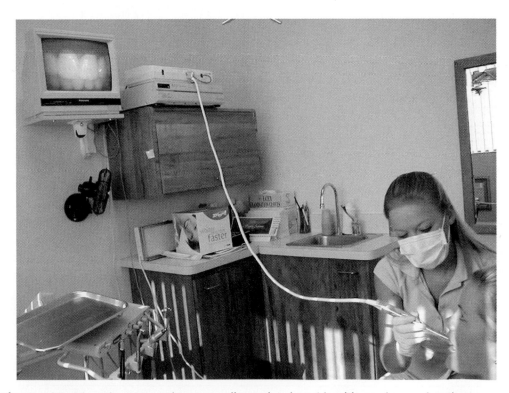

Figure 25-11 The intraoral camera allows the dental health worker and patient to see the tooth structure on a larger scale. (*Courtesy Joyce Bassett, DDS, FAGD, Scottsdale, Ariz.*)

Initial Clinical Examination ▬▬▬▬▬▬▬

(Use this form on initial visit only)

Date_____

Patient Name_____ Patient #_____

Chief Dental Complaint
Oral Habits
Existing Illnesses/Current Drugs Used
Allergies
History Verification - A health (medical and dental) history has been completed and reviewed by:
Dr._____
Initials_____Date_____

Blood Pressure		Pulse	
Date Last Dental Exam			
General Physical Condition			
Under Physician's Care Now?			
History of Bleeding?			
Reaction to Anesthetic?			
Existing Xrays		Date	Xrays Required

Existing Prosthesis

Max.	Date Placed:	Condition:
Min.	Date Placed:	Condition:

A

Oral, Soft Tissue Examination and TMJ Evaluation

Area	Description of Any Problem
Pharynx	
Tonsils	
Soft Palate	
Hard Palate	
Tongue	
Floor of Mouth	
Buccal Mucosa	
Lips	
Skin	
Lymph Nodes	
Occlusion	

TMJ Evaluation

Right	☐ Crepitus	☐ Snapping/Popping
Left	☐ Crepitus	☐ Snapping/Popping

Tenderness to Palpation:

TMJ	☐ Right	☐ Left

Muscles _____

Deviation on Closing _____ Rmm _____ Lmm

Needs further TMJ evaluation ☐ Yes ☐ No
If Yes, use TMJ evaluation form

Oral Hygiene	☐ Excellent	☐ Good	☐ Fair	☐ Poor
Calculus	☐ None	☐ Little	☐ Moderate	☐ Heavy
Plaque	☐ None	☐ Little	☐ Moderate	☐ Heavy
Gingival Bleeding		☐ Localized	☐ General	☐ None
Perio Exam	☐ Yes	☐ No		

Additional Comments: _____
_____
_____
_____
_____

Figure 25-12 Clinical examination form. **A**, front. (*Courtesy Colwell, a Division of Patterson Dental Supply Inc, St Paul, Minn.*)

Missing Teeth and Restorations

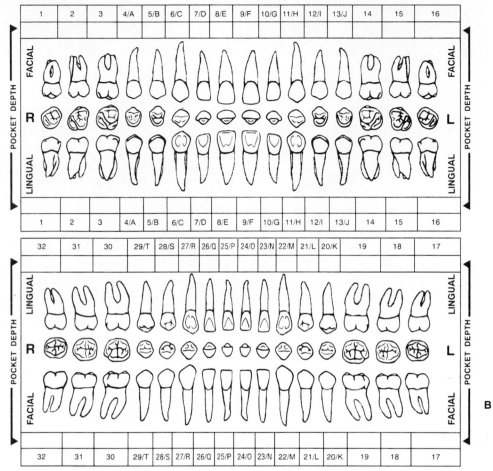

Diagnosis and Treatment Plan

Date	Tooth	Surface	Service Planned	

Consent to treatment plan obtained: Date_____   Dr._____

Figure 25-12, cont'd   Clinical examination form. **B**, back. *(Courtesy Colwell, a Division of Patterson Dental Supply Inc, St Paul, Minn.)*

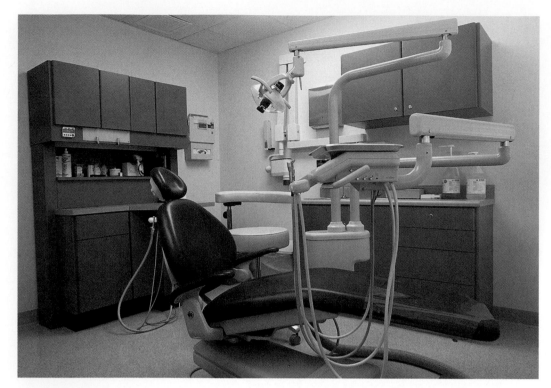

Figure 25-13 The dental operatory is arranged for convenience and comfort.

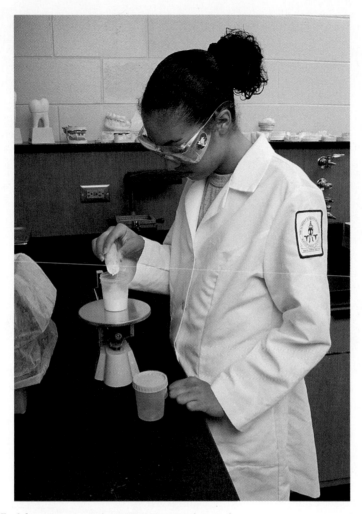

Figure 25-14   The dental assistant must know how to prepare a variety of dental materials.

Review Questions

1. Use each of the following terms in one or more sentences that correctly relate their meaning.
   Calculus
   Gingival
   Halitosis
   Hygiene
   Plaque

2. List the four members of the dental health care team.

3. Describe the purpose of the dental health care team.

4. Describe the role of four dental specialties.

5. List each of the four types of teeth and the purpose and number of each in the adult mouth.

6. Draw and label the five surfaces of a molar tooth.

7. Describe the formation of plaque and calculus.

8. List three factors that contribute to the formation of plaque.

9. Describe the correct technique for brushing and flossing teeth.

Critical Thinking

1. Investigate and compare the cost of various types of dental treatments and procedures.

2. Investigate five common medications used in dental health care.

3. Investigate and compare the cost of education for the dental assistant, dental hygienist, and dentist.

4. Investigate the relative number of private and corporate practices for dentists.

26

Complementary and Alternative Careers

Learning Objectives

Define at least 10 terms relating to careers in complementary and alternative medicine.

Specify the role of selected complementary and alternative care providers, including personal qualities, levels of education, and credentialing requirements.

Describe the methods used in allopathic, holistic, and homeopathic health care.

List five domains of complementary and alternative health care as described by the National Institutes of Health.

Key Terms

Allopathic
(al-o-PATH-ik) System of medical practice that uses remedies designed to produce effects that are different than those caused by the disease being treated

Biofeedback
(bie-o-FEED-bak) Conscious control of biological functions normally controlled involuntarily

Chiropractic
(kie-ro-PRAK-tik) System of therapy based on the theory that health is determined by the condition of the nervous system

Holistic
(ho-LIS-tik) Practice of medicine that considers the person as a whole unit, not as individual parts

Homeopathic
(ho-me-o-PATH-ik) System of medical practice that uses remedies designed to produce similar effects to those caused by the disease being treated

Hydrotherapy
(hie-dro-THER-uh-pee) External use of water to treat disease

Subluxation
(sub-luk-SAY-shun) Incomplete dislocation of a joint

Complementary and Alternative Terminology*

TERM	DEFINITION	PREFIX	ROOT	SUFFIX
Aromatherapy	Treatment with odors	aroma	therapy	
Chiropractic	Pertaining to manipulation of the spine by hand		chiro/pract	ic
Homeopathic	Treatment with similar disease	homeo	path	ic
Hydrotherapy	Treatment with water	hydro	therapy	
Hypnotherapy	Treatment using hypnosis	hypno	therapy	
Neuromuscular	Pertaining to the nerves and muscles	neuro	muscul	ar
Orthopedic	Pertaining to correction of bones		orthoped	ic
Osteoarthritis	Inflammation of the bones and joints	osteo	arthr	itis
Radiography	Picture taken using radiation	radi/o	graph	y
Thermography	Picture taken showing heat	therm/o	graph	y

*A transition phrase or vowel may be added to or deleted from the word parts to make the combining form.

Abbreviations for Complementary and Alternative Medicine

ABBREVIATION	MEANING
ADHD	Attention deficit hyperactivity disorder
BCIA	Biofeedback Certification Institute of America
CAM	Complementary and alternative medicine
DC	Doctor of chiropractic
EEG	Electroencephalogram
EMG	Electromyogram
GSR	Galvanic skin response
ND	Doctor of naturopathy
NIH	National Institutes of Health
TMJ	Temporomandibular joint dysfunction

Careers

Complementary medicine, alternative medicine, and **holistic** health are therapies based on wellness and natural treatment. Complementary and holistic health practices are used at the same time as conventional medical techniques. Alternative health care is used in place of conventional methods. Integrative medicine is nonallopathic practices that have been shown to be effective by research.

Based on information gathered in a 1997 survey, the *Journal of the American Medical Association* reported that more than 42% of Americans use therapies outside of mainstream medicine. The Reuters Health Information published a study in 1999 that found that 69% of Americans had used some form of alternative medicine in the previous year.

Some hospitals have opened alternative health clinics and are conducting studies to determine the effectiveness of their treatments (Table 26-1). More than 20 states have laws that allow the practice of complementary and alternative medicine (CAM). Some of the conditions that draw consumers to complementary health care include chronic pain, arthritis, addiction, headache, anxiety, chronic fatigue, sprains, and muscle strains.

Table 26-1   Alternative Therapies Studies*

Therapy or Treatment	Indication
Acupuncture	Depression, attention deficit hyperactivity disorder (ADHD), osteoarthritis, postoperative dental pain
Hypnosis	Chronic low back pain, accelerated fracture healing
Ayurvedic herbal	Parkinson's disease
Biofeedback	Diabetes, low back pain, painful jaw disorders
Electric current	Tumor
Imagery	Asthma, breast cancer

*The National Institutes of Health (NIH) has provided grants for study of the effectiveness of these alternative therapies.

Box 26-1   Complementary and Alternative Methods*

Alternative Medical Systems

Acupuncture
Ayurveda
Counseling
Herbal medicine
Homeopathy
Hydrotherapy
Naturopathy
Oriental massage

Mind-Body Interventions

Aromatherapy
Art therapy
Counseling
Hypnotherapy
Meditation
Mental healing
Music therapy

Biological-Based Therapies

Biological therapies
Dietary therapy
Herbal therapy
Orthomolecular therapy

Manipulative and Body-Based Methods

Alexander technique
Chiropractic
Massage therapy
Osteopathy
Reflexology

Energy Therapies

Crystal therapy
Electrical therapy
Magnet therapy
Qi gong
Reiki
Therapeutic touch

*Most of the complementary and alternative health care practitioners received education and credentials in another health care practice.

The National Institutes of Health (NIH) groups CAM practices into five domains (Box 26-1). These five domains include alternative medical systems, mind-body interventions, biological-based treatments, manipulative and body-based methods, and energy therapies.

Many of the health care workers specializing in CAM have education and training in other health careers. For example, holistic practitioners include nurses, physicians, veterinarians, pharmacists, and many other professionals. Two CAM professions that have specific educational requirements include the chiropractor and naturopath.

Chiropractor

Chiropractors or doctors of **chiropractic** (DC) treat health problems associated with the muscular, skeletal, and nervous system. Chiropractic physicians adjust the spinal column and other body joints to correct subluxations. **Subluxations** are incomplete or partial dislocations of the spine.

The chiropractor uses radiography and other tests to diagnose and assess progress in the adjustment. Chiropractors use a holistic approach to treatment emphasizing health and wellness. Treatments are drugless and nonsurgical. When appropriate, the chiropractor may refer a patient to an **allopathic** practitioner.

Education for the chiropractor includes a minimum of 2 years of college and completion of a 4- or 5-year chiropractic program. There are 16 programs accredited by the Council on Chiropractic Education in the United States. Licensure by the state is required for chiropractic practice.

Box 26-2	Areas of "Diplomate" Certification for Chiropractors

Diagnostic imaging
Internal disorders
Neurology
Nutrition
Occupational and industrial health
Orthopedics
Sports injuries
Thermography

Box 26-3	Applications for Biofeedback

Anxiety and panic disorders
Asthma
Attention deficit hyperactivity disorder (ADHD)
Epilepsy
Headache
Hypertension
Irritable bowel syndrome
Neck and shoulder pain
Neuromuscular disorders
Raynaud's syndrome
Rheumatoid arthritis
Temporomandibular joint dysfunction (TMJ)
Urinary and fecal incontinence

Certification (diplomate) for clinical specialties in orthopedics, neurology, sports injury, and other areas may be granted by professional associations (Box 26-2).

Naturopath

Licensed naturopathic doctors (NDs) are primary care physicians that focus on treatment of the whole person with emphasis on wellness and disease prevention. They perform all of the routine medical exams, laboratory tests, and office procedures, such as minor surgery used by the allopathic doctor. They do not use synthetic medication nor do they perform major surgeries. Naturopathic doctors may refer patients to allopathic practitioners for specialized treatment or major surgery.

Naturopathic physicians attend a 4-year graduate medical school. In addition to the standard curriculum of medical school, naturopathic doctors study nutrition, homeopathy, botanical medicine, and **hydrotherapy.** The degree earned is called a *doctor of naturopathy*. There are three accredited schools of naturopathic medicine in the United States. At least 11 states license naturopathic doctors.

Other Complementary and Alternative Practitioners

Massage therapists (also known as *masseuses* or *masseurs*) use skillful touch to loosen muscles and relieve pain (Figure 26-1). In addition to working with the manipulation of muscle, skin, tendon, and ligaments, massage therapists may also apply light, water, or vibration devices. Forms of massage include Swedish, polarity, sports, infant, facial, and scalp. Education and training for massage therapists vary from state to state. The American Massage Therapy

Association has approved 55 schools. Thirteen states require licensure.

Hypnotherapists help clients to overcome bad habits and treat emotional problems using hypnosis. The method of hypnosis may differ greatly from one practitioner to another. Many hypnotherapists are licensed in a related field such as medicine, nursing, or psychology. Licensure is not required, although a permit to practice may be needed.

Acupuncturists insert needles into peripheral or surface nerves to control pain, provide anesthesia, relieve symptoms, and modify psychosomatic (mind-caused) disorders. Acupuncture has been in use for 5000 years. It originated with the Chinese. The practitioners of today usually hold credentials in another health care field and are trained in the application of needles. Acupuncture is believed to release endorphins and other mood-elevators when the appropriate meridian points, or "mens," are stimulated. The training for acupuncture varies greatly and may include up to 2 or 3 years of study after completion of a minimum of 2 years of college. There are 10 schools approved by the National Accreditation Commission for Schools and Colleges of Acupuncture and Oriental Medicine in the United States. Only 20 states regulate the practice of acupuncture. A national board examination for acupuncturists is available on a voluntary basis. Acupressure is a similar treatment that applies pressure, instead of needles, to the points.

Biofeedback is a technique used to change normally involuntary reactions of the body using conscious control, such as lowering heart rate or changing the size of blood vessels (Box 26-3). For example, a person may raise the

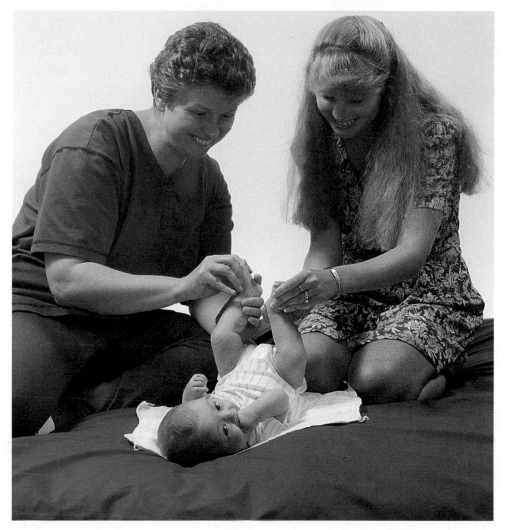

Figure 26-1   A massage therapist teaches a new mother how to massage her infant. *(From Fritz S:* Mosby's fundamentals of therapeutic massage, *ed 2, St Louis, 2000, Mosby.)*

temperature of one hand higher than the other. Raising the temperature of both hands using biofeedback has been demonstrated to reduce the blood flow to the brain and relieve headache symptoms. Biofeedback practitioners may practice other areas of health care, such as nursing or medicine. Certification for biofeedback is possible through the Biofeedback Certification Institute of America (BCIA), which requires that the applicant is licensed or working under the supervision of a licensed health care practitioner.

Content Instruction

Alternative Medical Systems

Many of the alternative medical systems were developed before the conventional biomedical approach. Some are still practiced by cultures throughout the world. For example, traditional oriental medicine emphasizes proper balance of a person's *qi* (pronounced "chee") or vital energy.

Table 26-2 Relaxation Response

Technique	Oxygen Consumption	Respiratory Rate	Heart Rate	Alpha Waves	Blood Pressure	Muscle Tension
Transcendental meditation	Decreases	Decreases	Decreases	Increases	Decreases*	Not measured
Zen and yoga	Decreases	Decreases	Decreases	Increases	Decreases	Not measured
Autogenic training	Not measured	Decreases	Decreases	Increases	Inconclusive	Decreases
Progressive relaxation	Not measured	Not measured	Not measured	Not measured	Inconclusive	Decreases
Hypnosis with suggested deep relaxation	Decreases	Decreases	Decreases	Not measured	Inconclusive	Not measured

*In patients with elevated blood pressure.

Some of the practices that are part of the alternative medical systems domain include acupuncture, herbal medicine, and oriental massage.

India's traditional system of medicine is called *Ayurveda* and places equal emphasis on the body, mind, and spirit. The treatments are designed to restore harmony and include such things as diet, exercise, meditation, massage, sun exposure, herbs, and controlled breathing. Other systems have been developed by the Native Americans, Africans, and Central and South Americans.

Homeopathic medicine is a Western system based on the concept that "like cures like." Practitioners believe that small dosages of plant extracts and minerals that produce the same symptoms of a disease cure it by stimulating the body's defense and health mechanisms.

Naturopathic medicine emphasizes restoration of health and sees disease as a change in the body's natural process. It is based on the medical philosophy called *vitalism* that sees a person as a combination of body, spirit, and mind. Some examples of techniques used by naturopaths include nutrition, acupuncture, herbal medicine, hydrotherapy, spinal manipulation, electrical therapy, ultrasound and light therapy, counseling, and pharmacology.

Mind–Body Intervention

Mind-body interventions are not all recognized by the NIH to be complementary and alternative medicine. The NIH recognizes interventions such as hypnosis, meditation, prayer, dance, music, art therapy, and mental healing. The mind-body interventions that are considered to be part of mainstream medicine are educational or behavioral in nature. All of these techniques are designed to help the mind treat the body.

Biological–Based Therapy

Many of the biologically based therapies that are considered to be CAM overlap with conventional medicine and involve special dietary supplements or programs. Herbal therapy uses plants that act on the body. Special diet programs that are considered to be CAM include those proposed by Drs. Atkins, Pritikin, and Weil. Use of chemicals such as magnesium, melatonin, and vitamins in megadoses is called *orthomolecular therapy*. Biological therapies that are used to treat cancer include laetrile and shark cartilage. Bee pollen is used to treat autoimmune and inflammatory diseases.

Energy Therapy

Electromagnetic fields originating from an external source and energy originating in the body (biofields) are used in energy therapies. Biofields have not been experimentally proven to exist. Energy therapies involving pressure and manipulation of the body include Qi gong, Reiki, and therapeutic touch. External sources of therapy include magnets and electrical devices.

Performance Instruction

Biofeedback techniques are designed to change blood pressure, muscle tension, heart rate, and other bodily functions that are not normally under voluntary control. The technique allows people to use signals from their own bodies to change their health (Table 26-2). Biofeedback machines or techniques include electromyogram (EMG) to measure

Skill 26-1

Using Biofeedback*

1. Maintain medical asepsis by using the guidelines provided in the Standard and Transmission–Based Precautions, including good handwashing technique and use of gloves as needed.

2. Apply a stress dot to the back of the hand between the thumb and index finger.

3. Match the color of the dot to the stress dot color chart.

4. Increase the level of relaxation by breathing evenly and deeply.

5. Relax the muscles of the hand by holding a fist for 5 seconds and then releasing it. Repeat with the other hand.

6. Compare the color of the stress dot with the chart.

*Procedures vary with the type of device used to measure physiological changes.

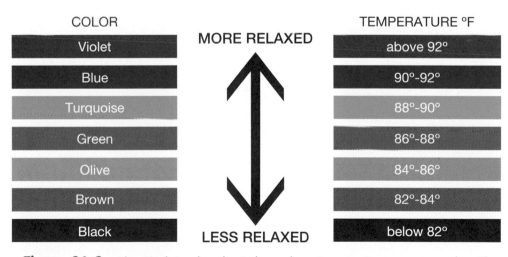

Figure 26-2 The Biodot color chart shows how temperature corresponds with relaxation.

muscle tension, Galvanic skin response (GSR) monitors to measure sweat production, skin temperature sensors, and electroencephalograms (EEG) to measure brain wave activity. Other techniques include measuring vital signs. Stress dots made of liquid crystal were developed as a way to measure the change in temperature of the skin (Skill 26-1). When the temperature of the hand becomes warmer, that indicates a more relaxed state (Figure 26-2). Through conscious thought, a person may learn to adjust to a more relaxed state.

Review Questions

1. Use the following terms in one or more sentences that correctly relate their meaning.
   Allopathic
   Holistic
   Homeopathic

2. List three health professions that might practice allopathic and alternative therapies.

3. Describe two differences between the practice of medical and naturopathic doctors.

4. Describe each of the five domains into which the National Institutes of Health places complementary and alternative therapies.

Critical Thinking

1. There are a group of practitioners in the United States that call themselves *certified naturopaths*. They have not completed the training and education of the licensed naturopathic physician. Explain how this situation has occurred, how a consumer can be confident about the training of a practitioner, and what could be done to remedy the confusion.

2. Research one of the complementary and alternative methods listed in Box 26-1 including its use, effectiveness, and credentialing of practitioners.

27
Veterinary Careers

Learning Objectives

Define at least 10 terms relating to veterinary care.

Specify the role of selected veterinary workers, including personal qualities, levels of education, and credentialing requirements.

Describe the function of the veterinary team.

Identify the functions that animals serve in the daily life of humans.

Identify at least three characteristics of a healthy animal.

Identify at least five signs of disorders in animals.

Identify at least five methods of restraint for care or examination of animals.

Describe at least five disorders affecting animals.

Identify at least three methods of assessment of disorders in animals.

Key Terms

Bovine
(BOH-vine) Pertaining to cattle

Canine
(KAY-nine) Pertaining to dogs

Carcass
(KAR-kus) Dead body of an animal

Equine
(EE-kwine) Pertaining to horses

Feline
(FEE-line) Pertaining to cats

Immunize
(IM-yoo-nize) Secure against a particular disease

Parasite
(PARE-uh-site) Plant or animal that lives on or within another living organism at the expense of the host organism

Quarantine
(KWAR-an-teen) Period of detention or isolation as a result of a disease suspected to be communicable

Theriogenology
(theer-ee-o-gen-OL-o-gee) Branch of veterinary medicine dealing with reproduction

Vaccination
(vak-sin-AY-shun) Introduction of a microorganism that has been made harmless into a human or animal for the purpose of developing immunity

Veterinary
(VET-er-in-air-ee) Pertaining to animals and their diseases

Veterinary Careers Terminology*

TERM	DEFINITION	PREFIX	ROOT	SUFFIX
Cutaneous	Pertaining to the skin		cut/an	eous
Encephalitis	Inflammation on the inside of the brain	en	ceph/al	itis
Hepatitis	Inflammation of the liver		hepat	itis
Intravenous	Inside the vessel	intra	ven	ous
Pathology	Study of disease		path	ology
Rhinotracheitis	Inflammation of the nose and windpipe	rhino	trache	itis
Toxicology	Study of poison		toxic	ology
Tracheobronchitis	Inflammation of the windpipe and bronchus	tracheo	bronch	itis
Urologic	Pertaining to urine		urolog	ic
Zoology	Study of animals		zoo	ology

*A transition phrase or vowel may be added to or deleted from the word parts to make the combining form.

Abbreviations for Veterinary Careers

ABBREVIATION	MEANING
CENSHARE	Center for the Study of Human-Animal Relationships
CPV	Canine parvovirus
CVT	Certified veterinary technician
DVM	Doctor of veterinary medicine
EE	Equine encephalomyelitis
FP	Feline panleukopenia
FUS	Feline urologic syndrome
FVR	Feline viral rhinotracheitis
RVT	Registered veterinary technician
VMD	Veterinary medical doctor

Careers

Veterinary care personnel work in a variety of settings including private practice, public health, research, zoos, circuses, and racetracks (Box 27-1). Those interested in aquatic animals may work in the area of marine biology. The purpose of animal health care is to prevent illness and provide care for sick and injured animals. Animal health care providers also prevent the spread of disease carried by animals to humans (zoonosis).

Good physical health is needed for those who work with animals. The work may involve lifting and manipulating heavy animals and supplies for their care. Veterinary personnel may be exposed to disease and injury by unrestrained animals. They must work well with others and with the animals receiving care.

Veterinarian

Veterinarians make up the largest group of animal health care providers. Their professional oath describes the use of their knowledge and skills "for the benefit of society, for the protection of animal health, the relief of animal suffering, the conservation of livestock resources, the promotion of public health, and the advancement of medical knowledge."

It is estimated that veterinarians in the United States treat more than 99 million cattle (**bovine**), 54 million hogs (swine), and 10 million sheep in the livestock industry. More than 8 million horses (**equine**), 52 million cats (**feline**), and 55 million dogs (**canine**) are kept as domestic pets. More than 171 million turkeys, 374 million egg-producing chickens, and 4,282 million broiler-production chickens are raised annually in the United States. Veterinarians are instrumental in artificial insemination procedures to produce selected types of stock. Methods used for this selective breeding include embryo transplants and freezing.

Box 27-1   Veterinary Careers*

Animal breeder
Animal health technician
Animal keeper
Animal maintenance supervisor
Animal-nursery worker
Dog groomer
Feed-research aide
Horseshoer (farrier)
Marine biologist
Stable attendant
Veterinarian
Veterinarian, lab animal care
Veterinarian, poultry
Veterinary hospital attendant
Veterinary laboratory technician
Veterinary livestock inspector
Veterinary meat inspector
Veterinary pharmacologist
Veterinary virus serum inspector
Zoo laboratory assistant
Zoo veterinarian

*Animal health care workers provide care, regulation, and treatment for large and small animals in urban and rural areas.

Veterinarians are licensed by the state in which they practice. The veterinarian must first obtain a college or university degree followed by the completion of study at a 4-year accredited veterinary college. The degree earned is a doctor of veterinary medicine (DVM). One college awards a degree called a *veterinarian medical degree* (VMD). Passing a written and oral examination is necessary for licensure. There are 27 schools of veterinary medicine in the United States. Veterinarians who work in research may have an additional doctoral degree in pathology, toxicology, or laboratory animal medicine.

There are 16 recognized specialty boards in veterinarian medicine. These are anesthesiology, cardiology, dermatology, internal medicine, laboratory animal medicine, microbiology, neurology, ophthalmology, pathology, preventive medicine, radiology, surgery, reproduction (**theriogenology**), toxicology, veterinary practice, and zoo medicine.

Veterinarians must work well with people and with animals. The profession requires good hearing, vision, and manual dexterity. Veterinarians may work long hours, and in rural areas a great deal of travel may be required. Care of animals may result in injury or exposure to disease.

Three out of four veterinarians work in private practice. Many veterinarians work exclusively with either large or small animals although some, especially those in rural areas, work in a mixed practice. Animal care veterinarians diagnose, perform surgery, and provide treatments and medication for sick and injured animals. They also **immunize** animals against disease and advise owners on ways to keep pets healthy. Veterinarians who care for companion animals usually work in hospitals or clinics. In rural areas large animal care may be provided through a traveling van equipped as a clinic.

Veterinarians may also specialize in fields such as wildlife and international economics. Wildlife veterinarians may travel to treat animals affected by oil spills and natural disasters. Economic veterinarians may travel throughout the world to help set policies and procedures to deal with international food and agriculture.

Research veterinarians work to find better methods to prevent and cure animal disorders. Many of these methods have been a direct benefit to treatment of human disorders. Veterinary research has led to the development of many modern drugs and treatments. Some animals commonly used for research include dogs, cats, guinea pigs, mice, rats, rabbits, gerbils, and monkeys. Laboratory animals are usually bred specifically for the purpose of research to have healthy and similar specimens. Small animals are preferable to larger animals because the generations and life cycles are shorter.

Veterinarians specializing in toxicology and pathology protect humans from diseases transmitted by animals. They also work to control and eliminate disease in livestock. The federal government employs veterinarians in the Department of Agriculture and in the Public Health Service. In public health, a veterinarian may work as an epidemiologist to prevent the spread of disease transmitted by animals.

Veterinary Technician

Veterinary technicians (VTs) may work in research settings, private clinics, food inspection, and laboratories or perform research under the supervision of a veterinarian, scientist, or senior technologist. The research technician prepares and tests serums (**vaccinations**) used to prevent animal diseases. Meat and dairy products are inspected for quality and purity by animal technicians. Veterinary technicians in private practice assist the veterinarian by performing a variety of duties including obtaining information, preparing animals and equipment, collecting specimens, and assisting with procedures. Technicians may also administer medications, prepare lab samples, and apply bandages or dressings to wounds (Box 27-2).

Technicians may be trained to perform extended duties such as teeth cleaning, removal of sutures, and administra-

Box 27-2	Duties of the Certified or Licensed Veterinary Technician

Obtain and record animal case histories from and communicate with owner

Maintain the examination and kenneling facilities

Prepare animals for examination, treatment, or surgery

Assist with examination, treatment, or surgery

Monitor animal's condition after examination, treatment, or surgery

Collect specimens

Perform laboratory tests

Expose and develop radiographs

Train and supervise animal or kennel caretakers

Clean teeth, administer medication, and perform other extended duties after advance training

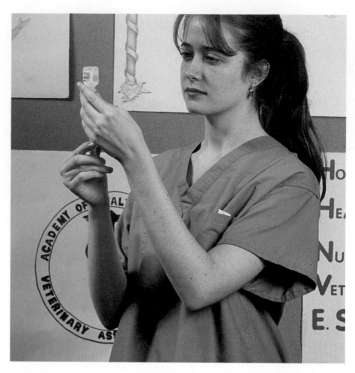

Figure 27-1 Injections are given only by trained personnel under the supervision of a licensed health care worker.

tion of intravenous fluids. One method that the technician may use to administer medications is injection (Figure 27-1). Medical asepsis is maintained throughout the procedure to prevent the spread of microorganisms. The correct dosage, medication, and route must be determined before giving an injection. The injection sites for animals are determined by the route of administration and type of animal.

The technician completes a minimum of 2 years of college-level vocational training for this occupation. Some colleges offer an associate degree in veterinary technology. There are more than 75 programs accredited by the American Veterinary Medical Association. Continuing education is necessary as the role of the technician expands. Animal technologists work in a more expanded role and must complete a 4-year baccalaureate degree program. In most states, the animal health technician and technologist must be certified (CVT), registered (RVT), or licensed (LVT).

Veterinary Assistant

Veterinary assistants provide a variety of services for animals as part of the care given in a clinic or animal hospital. The duties of the assistant include maintaining a clean and safe environment, observing behavior, preparing animals for examination or treatment, and maintaining daily records. Many animals show unusual behavior in an unfamiliar setting, so the assistant must show understanding and patience. Assistants may learn their training on the job or in a vocational program.

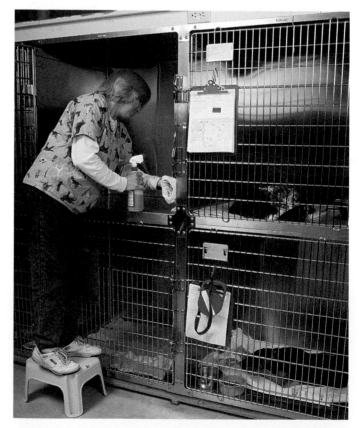

Figure 27-2 Kennel cleanliness prevents the spread of disease.

One of the duties of the veterinary assistant is to maintain the kennel or cage (Figure 27-2). Living quarters for animals such as dogs and cats are cleaned and disinfected at least once daily to prevent the spread of microorganisms from one animal to another. The living area should be well ventilated and kept at a comfortable temperature. Animals need fresh food, water, and exercise on a daily basis (Skill 27-1). When needed, the assistant may bathe and groom the animals (Figure 27-3). Restraint may be necessary during bathing and grooming if the animal is uncooperative. The skin and coat is observed during bathing and any unusual findings are reported to the veterinarian. The animal is wetted thoroughly with lukewarm water before the soap is applied. Care is taken to prevent the soap from entering the animal's eyes. The animal is rinsed thoroughly and dried before returning it to the cage or kennel. The nails may be clipped during the procedure if necessary (Skill 27-2).

Animal Caretaker

Animal caretakers may be called by a variety of titles depending on the job responsibilities. Some examples of animal caretakers include kennel, stable, shelter, pet shop, wildlife, and grooming attendants, such as a farrier (one who shoes horses) assistant. The animal caretaker performs routine tasks of daily care and assessment for domestic and exotic animals under the supervision of the facility supervisor or a veterinarian. The animal caretaker may be trained on the job or complete a home study program for kennel technicians offered by the American Boarding Kennel Association. There are no special educational or experience requirements for many entry-level jobs in animal care.

Animal Breeder

Animal breeders raise animals using selective breeding to maintain or improve the traits of existing breeds as well as to develop new breeds. Breeders use genetic traits to meet the needs of the owners. For example, they breed cows to produce better and more milk. Some breeders produce small animals for ownership as pets or use in research. They provide all care for the animals until a buyer takes them. In addition to on-the-job training, many breeders have a 4-year university degree in animal science because knowledge of the animal and genetics is important.

Marine Biologist

Aquatic or marine biologists study plant and animal life in saltwater environments. Marine biology is also known as *marine ecology* or *biological oceanography*. The environmental conditions that affect marine life include the water salinity, temperature, acidity, light, and oxygen content. An

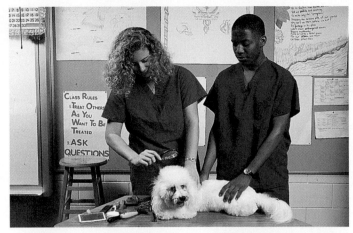
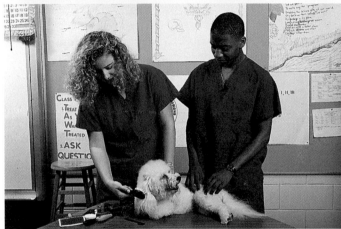
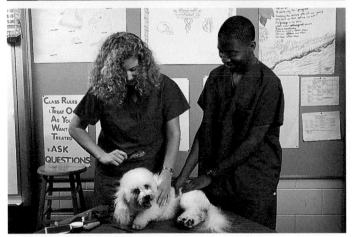

Figure 27-3 Grooming requires patience and confidence in handling methods.

example of the work completed by a marine biologist might include using research data to make a mathematical model to demonstrate changes in numbers of marine creatures. Marine biologists may study one species or the effect of environmental influences on a specific ecological area. Education for the marine biologist includes a master's or doctoral degree from a university. Employment may be

Skill 27-1

Maintaining the Cage or Kennel

1. Maintain medical asepsis by using the guidelines provided in the Standard and Transmission-Based Precautions, including good handwashing technique and use of gloves as needed.

2. Clean and disinfect the animal's living quarters daily. Microorganisms, present in the waste of infected animals, must be removed to prevent the spread to other animals.

3. Remove waste material on a regular basis during the day. Waste that is left may be spread to other cages by the movement of the animal.

4. Check the area for appropriate ventilation, proper temperature, and shaded areas. A restrained animal cannot move to a more comfortable area in the cage or kennel. Dogs and cats cannot sweat to lower the body temperature, and they may become ill if left in an environment that is too hot.

5. Supply fresh food and water daily. The amount of food and number of feedings required depends on the breed. Nutritional requirements vary for different species and breeds of animals. Like humans, animals need all of the nutrient groups each day.

6. Exercise kenneled animals at least twice daily for 30 to 45 minutes. Animals that are kept as pets need human companionship and exercise to remain emotionally and physically healthy.

available for those with a 4-year college or university degree in botany or zoology as a marine biology technician. Other professionals working as marine biologists include physiologists and ecologists. Marine biologists are employed in colleges or universities, by private industry, and by the federal government. Most marine biologists work in large marine laboratories.

Content Instruction

Animals as Pets

Animals serve many functions for humans. They provide a source of food in meat and milk products. The skins and coats of animals are used to make clothing and jewelry. Some animals are kept for observation and enjoyment in zoos. Animals can also be trained to live with people (domesticated) for companionship, service, and protection.

Animals kept for companionship are called *pets*. About 80 million people in the United States have at least one pet. Common pets include dogs, cats, turtles, birds, fish, small rodents, horses, and snakes (Figure 27-4). Cats are more common than dogs as pets. Several research studies have indicated that people with pets have reduced stress and lower blood pressure during interaction with their companions. Some animals such as guide dogs for the visually impaired are used for service. Watchdogs are used for protection.

Skill 27-2

Bathing and Grooming

1. Maintain medical asepsis by using the guidelines provided in the Standard and Transmission-Based Precautions, including good handwashing technique and use of gloves as needed.

2. Observe the condition of the skin and coat. Report any unusual findings to the veterinarian.

3. Select the proper shampoo or dip. Shampoos may be specific for the type of animal and type of condition. Shampoos may be designed for animals that are being bathed to remove parasites or debris or for those being prepared for sale or show.

4. Dilute the shampoo or dip according to the manufacturer's instructions.

5. Prepare the water or solution at a lukewarm temperature (100° to 115° F).

6. Place the animal into a half-full tub. Restrain the animal if necessary. Protect the animal's ears with cotton and the eyes with a lubricating ointment made for that purpose.

7. Wet the animal thoroughly. Rub the soap into the skin, and avoid getting soap in the eyes.

8. The soap or solution may have directions that specify the length of time of application to be effective. Rinse the soap off completely, and remove the animal from the tub. Soap that is left on the animal may cause skin irritation.

9. Dry the animal completely. Brush and comb hair as needed. Loose and matted hair should be removed.

10. Clean the ears and teeth. Clip nails if needed. Some animals may need to be anesthetized to clean their teeth and clip their nails.

11. Reward the animal with affection before returning it to the cage or pen. The animal may not like to be bathed, so the procedure should be made as pleasant as possible to avoid behavior problems at the next bath.

12. Record observations. Immediately report any unusual findings to the veterinarian or owner.

13. Clean any used equipment and return it to the designated area.

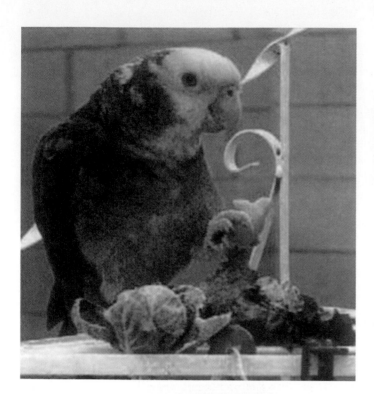

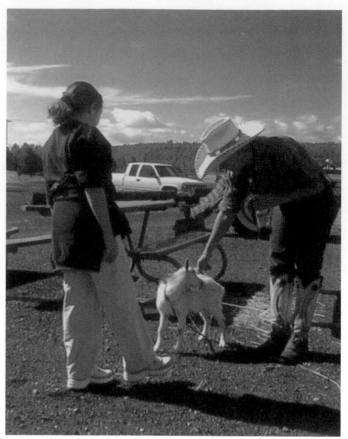

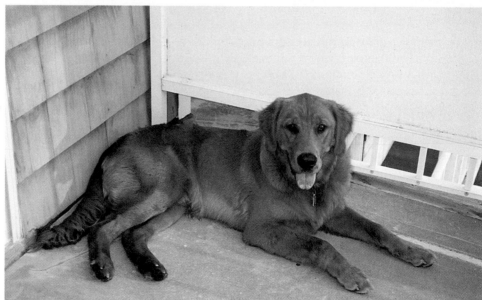

Figure 27-4   Pets come in all shapes and sizes.

The birthrate of domestic animals is a serious problem in the United States. *Neutering* is the process of surgical sterilization to prevent unwanted births. In female animals, the procedure is called *spaying*. In males, the procedure involves the removal of the testes (orchiectomy). Each year more than 18 million unwanted or homeless domestic animals are destroyed.

Induction of death in a sick, severely injured, or unwanted animal is called *euthanasia*. The decision to end the life of a pet rests with the owner who has assumed the responsibility for the care and accepted the companionship of the animal. Often the decision is very difficult and is based on the owner's understanding of the quality of life. Euthanasia may also be necessary if an animal becomes vicious, dangerous, or unmanageable. Euthanasia is usually accomplished by injection of an anesthetic drug. The death is quick and painless. The owner and family of an animal that dies face the same process of grief felt with the death of a person. In addition, the person who chooses euthanasia for a pet may feel a sense of responsibility for the death. The dead animal is disposed of in a sanitary manner to prevent infestation of the **carcass** with microorganisms. The animal is placed in a plastic bag and disposed of in a city disposal, buried, or incinerated. If the animal carcass must be kept for any length of time, it is refrigerated or frozen until disposal is possible.

Animals in Health Care

Pet therapy for physically and mentally ill people is rapidly becoming an accepted treatment method in many health care settings. Involvement with pets has been shown to improve both physical and psychological health. For example, stroking the coat of a pet has been demonstrated to lower blood pressure and heart rate. At least 30 colleges and universities have research programs in the area of human and companion-animal bonding. The Center for the Study of Human-Animal Relationships (CENSHARE) is located at the University of Minnesota.

Most scientists agree that using animals for research is essential. Animal advocates believe that animal research is overused and could be replaced with other methods. Animals are used to test cosmetics and other products before human use is approved. One example of a controversial test is the Draize test in which chemicals are sprayed into an animal's eyes to determine any possible damage that might occur.

Surgical transplant of animal organs or tissues has also been attempted. In 1984 a baboon heart was transplanted into a human baby whose heart was underdeveloped. Baby Fae lived 20 days with the baboon heart. Transplant into an adult was attempted in 1993. Other species have been used for heart valves and tissue grafts. More than 20 million animals are in use by research laboratories throughout the country. Many of these laboratories are regulated by the National Institutes of Health, which finances their research. The U.S. Department of Agriculture supervises the standard of care in other locations for animals, such as zoos and places where animals are sold.

Animal Disorders

More than 150 diseases (zoonoses) can be transmitted from animals to humans. Some of these include anthrax, rabies, leptospirosis, cat scratch fever, ringworm, tapeworm, toxoplasmosis, and Rocky Mountain spotted fever. Most disorders that affect animals harm only their own species and do not harm humans (Table 27-1). Animals, like humans, are affected by both infectious and noninfectious diseases. Animal parasites are one of the most common and deadly of infections. **Parasites** are small organisms that live in or on a host, causing it harm (Table 27-2). The infested animal may need to be isolated or **quarantined** to prevent the spread of infectious organisms.

Some indications that an animal is sick include abnormal behavior, especially sudden viciousness or listlessness (lethargy), abnormal discharge from any body opening, lumps, limping, or difficulty moving. Loss of appetite, large weight gain or loss, and excessive water consumption are also indications of illness. Difficult, abnormal, or uncontrolled waste elimination are other signs. Redness, swelling or discharge from the eyes or ears, abnormal stance, foul odor, loss of hair, and twitching or scratching may also indicate a problem.

Performance Instruction

Daily Care and Assessment

The procedures for the daily care of animals provide for the basic needs of the animal. Every animal should be fed regularly with the correct amount and type of food for the species. Fresh water should be available to animals at all times. The living space of a pet should be clean and dry. Bedding, appropriate for the climate, should be provided. Animals that are pets also need human companionship and exercise. The animal caretaker must observe the behavior of an animal to determine any change indicating illness. Observation is made about the intake of food, level of activity, attitude, and pattern of waste elimination (urination and defecation). The healthy animal should be alert and responsive. The animal should eat regularly and have a full, glossy coat. The nose is moist and cool in most animals with normal temperature. Vital signs may be assessed to determine more specific observations.

The method used to assess an animal's health is determined by the species. Medical asepsis is maintained while

Table 27-1   Animal Disorders

Class	Condition or Disease	Cause	Method of Transfer	Signs and Symptoms	Prevention, Treatment, and Outcome
Bovine (cattle)	Brucellosis	Unknown	Unknown	May be asymptomatic; reproductive problems	Unknown
	Scours (calf enteritis)	Bacteria	Soiled environment	Diarrhea, dehydration, weight loss, depression, death	Replace fluids, electrolytes; quarantine; antibiotics
	Mastitis	Microorganisms	Dairy equipment	Loss of milk production; swelling of udder; milk clotted or watery; fever, death	Prevent injury to udders; antibiotics
	Bovine leptospirosis	Bacteria	Urine shed in water, soil or splashed in eyes, feed; rats, rodents	Decreased milk production; milk contaminated; fever	Vaccination*; antibiotics
Canine (dogs)	Canine heartworm (dirofilariasis)	Worm	Mosquitoes	Worms in heart 14 in (35 cm) long; impaired circulation, difficulty breathing, cough, listlessness, weight loss	Drugs to prevent infections, kill worms
	Canine parvovirus (CPV)	Virus	Fecal waste	Depression, loss of appetite, fever, diarrhea, feces light or yellow-gray with blood	Vaccination*; replace lost body fluids; antibiotics for secondary infections
	Rabies	Virus	Saliva	Irritability, viciousness, drowsiness, paralysis of lower jaw	Vaccination†; supportive treatment, usually fatal
	Canine distemper	Virus	Secretions of nose and eyes, urine and feces; air droplets; inanimate objects	Damage to nervous system; discharge from eyes, nose; intestinal upset, weight loss, paralysis, convulsions	Vaccination*; supportive treatment; death in 50% of dogs affected
	Infectious canine hepatitis	Virus	Unknown	Fever, depression, loss of appetite, vomiting, abnormal thirst, diarrhea, death	Unknown
	Kennel cough (infectious tracheobronchitis)	Unknown	Unknown	Fever, cough, gagging, loss of appetite	Usually self-limiting; may become bronchopneumonia and be treated with antibiotics

*Can prevent the disease.
†Required by law for most domestic pets.

Table 27-1   Animal Disorders—cont'd

Class	Condition or Disease	Cause	Method of Transfer	Signs and Symptoms	Prevention, Treatment, and Outcome
Equine (horses)	Colic	Feeding, mis-management, worms	Unknown	Severe abdominal pain, distension; frequent urination	Walking, preventing horse from rolling
	Distemper (strangles)	Bacteria	Direct contact, air droplets, contact with contaminated objects	Fever, loss of appetite, cough, enlarged lymph glands, yellow nasal discharge	Vaccination (reduces severity); quarantine; antibiotics; hot compresses on lymph glands; rest
	Sleeping sickness (equine encephalomyelitis) (EE)	Virus	Birds, as carriers, reservoir; mosquitoes	Fever, difficulty swallowing, teeth grinding, staggering, paralysis	Vaccination*; 80% to 90% die; those that recover have neural damage
	Swamp fever (equine infectious anemia)	Unknown	Unknown	Fever, depression, weight loss, weakness, leg swelling, death	Unknown
	Internal parasites	Bots-flies, strongyli, ascarides, pinworms	Licked from hair, grass blades, contaminated water	Diarrhea, weight loss, anemia	Dewormers/unknown
Feline (cats)	Feline panleukopenia (FP)	Virus	Direct contact with blood, urine, fecal material, fleas	Vary greatly; decrease in WBC, depression, loss of appetite, dehydration, vomiting	Vaccination*; supportive measures to counteract signs, symptoms; quarantine; death in hours or days if untreated
	Feline viral rhinotracheitis (FVR)	Virus	Unknown	Fever, conjunctivitis, nasal discharge, sneezing, death	Unknown
	Feline infectious peritonitis (FIP)	Unknown	Unknown	Fever, loss of appetite, depression fluid accumulation, death	Unknown
	Feline leukemia	Unknown	Unknown	Weight loss, anemia, depression, death	Unknown
	Feline urologic syndrome (FUS)	Unknown	Unknown	Painful, frequent urination; blood in urine; depression, death	Antibiotics, surgery
Porcine (swine)	Clostridial diarrhea	Bacteria	Unknown	Listlessness, diarrhea, bloody stool, death	Unknown

Table 27-2 External Parasites

Parasite	Description	Effects	Treatment
Ear mite	Ear mites are crablike parasites commonly found in dogs and cats.	Severe itching; scratching may lead to bacterial infection; bacterial infection in the ear may penetrate the brain and cause convulsions or death; scratching may lead to bleeding sores	Includes medication
Flea	Fleas have eggs that lie dormant during the winter and emerge in warm weather. They hatch into wormlike larvae, which eventually become fleas. Fleas may jump from one location to another. They can live in carpeting and on clothing.	Itching	Includes sprays, dips, powders, specially treated collars, and tablets
Louse	Lice are very small and may penetrate the animal's skin to suck blood.	Itching; dangerous to small animals because of bacterial infection	Includes medication
Mite	Mange, caused by the mite, can be present at any time of the year. With some types of mange, dogs do not scratch. Mange may be contagious to people as well as to other animals.	Patches of hairlessness and red, irritated skin	Includes shaving the hair, medicated baths, and oral or injected medication
Tick	The tick looks like a small wart or seed. Ticks embed themselves into the skin of the animal. Ticks can live in carpeting and on household items.	Possibly itching; may carry disease to animals and humans	Includes medicated shampoo and removal

handling animals because some diseases in animals can be transmitted to humans. For dogs and cats, the animal's alertness, appetite, and condition of the coat are some indicators of health. The eyes and ears should be clear and clean in appearance. The nose, membranes of the mouth, posture, and vital signs are also indicators of the animal's health (Skill 27-3).

Animal caretakers may need to help with delivery of the young, called *whelping* in dogs. Signs of the beginning of labor in animals may appear as restlessness, panting, scratching, or tearing 4 to 24 hours before delivery. In dogs, the first puppy should appear within 3 hours of the onset of true labor. Each puppy is born in a separate amniotic sac, which should be removed after birth. This may be done with a clean towel if the mother does not do it. The nose and mouth of the newborn must be kept clear of mucus, and the umbilicus tied. Respiration must be stimulated and cardiac massage performed if the heartbeat is absent. Abnormal labor (dystocia) should be reported to a veterinarian immediately. The newborn should nurse or drink milk from the mother within the first 12 hours of life.

When an animal becomes ill, one of the duties of the veterinary care worker is to prepare the room for examinations and treatments (Figure 27-5). This includes cleaning and disinfecting the room and equipment to prevent the spread of microorganisms. Supplies are gathered before the procedure to minimize the stress for the animal and owner. After completion of surgical procedures, the veterinary care worker may clean and sterilize instruments. Medical asepsis is maintained during handling of all specimens and contaminated instruments. Gloves may be worn during these procedures. Instruments are rinsed in cold water and scrubbed with a soapy brush before autoclaving for sterilization. Some may need to be oiled or sharpened according to the manufacturer's directions. Instruments may be

Skill 27-3

Assisting with Assessment of a Dog or Cat

1. Maintain medical asepsis by using the guidelines provided in the Standard and Transmission–Based Precautions, including good handwashing technique and use of gloves as needed. Some animal disease may cause illness in humans. Also, the hands of the assistant may transfer many pathogens from one animal to another.

2. Restrain the animal if necessary.

3. Observe the animal's alertness and appetite for water and food.

4. Observe the condition of the animal's coat. The coat should be glossy and full. A dull or shedding coat may indicate inadequate nutrition or the presence of parasites.

5. Observe and describe the condition of the eyes and ears. Swelling, redness, or discharge may indicate infection or the presence of a parasite.

6. Observe and describe the condition of the nose. The nose should be cool and moist.

7. Observe and describe the condition of the mucous membranes of the mouth. The membranes should be pink and moist.

8. Observe and describe the condition of the stool and urine. The color, amount, odor, and consistency should be noted.

9. Observe the animal's stance and posture for normalcy.

10. Assess the vital signs. The pulse can be counted using the femoral artery in many animals. In the horse, the submaxillary artery can be felt under the jaw bone. Temperature is taken rectally for 3 minutes. Normal values for vital signs differ according to the species. The vital signs provide a specific determination of the animal's condition. Abnormal vital signs indicate illness or infection.

11. Release and reward the animal with affection. The animal may feel more positive about the assessment procedure when rewarded.

arranged in advance in prepared sets for surgical procedures (Skill 27-4).

Treatment Techniques

Restraint may be needed to examine or treat an animal. Each animal responds differently to being handled by a stranger and should be observed before approach. The handler should always have a means to exit the area if necessary. The work area should be clean, quiet, and free from clutter to avoid accidents. If use of restraint is necessary, it should not impair the animal's circulation or respiration. Some methods of restraint include the use of gloves, boxes, nets, bags, muzzles, snares, and leashes (Figure 27-6). Horses can be restrained using a nose twitch, stanchion, halter, rope, or hobble. Cattle are restrained in a similar method with nose tongs, headgates, squeeze chutes, halters, hobbles, nose rings, bull staffs, or electric stock prods. Swine can be restrained using hog snares, hog hurdles, ropes, and headgates.

Collection of blood samples may be accomplished in a variety of locations on animals. The site that is used depends on the amount of blood needed and type of animal. Some veins that might be used to collect blood from domestic animals, such as the dog and cat, include the jugular, cephalic, saphenous, sublingual, anterior vena cava, and the ear (Figure 27-7).

Fecal specimens may be collected to look for internal parasite infestation. Flotation, which is the mixing of fecal material with solutions, may be used to find the eggs (ova) of parasites. Viewing feces by microscope (direct smear) provides another method. Fecal solutions can also be centrifuged, or separated by spinning, to reveal parasites.

Urine samples may be collected from some animals by placing a collecting receptacle under the animal as it voids. Catheterization may be necessary to collect the specimen.

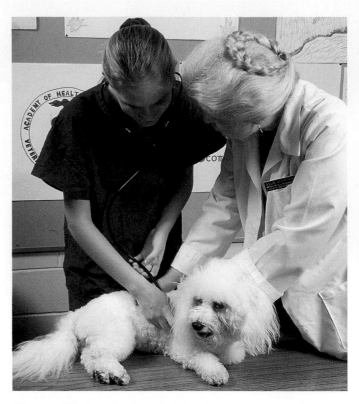

Figure 27-5 The examination room is arranged to provide easy access to materials and to limit the animal's movement.

Urine may also be obtained by surgical puncture of the urinary bladder with a sterile needle (cystocentesis). Urine can be obtained from an unconscious animal by continuous, gentle pressure on the bladder. Bacterial or fungal cultures may be obtained using a variety of collection methods and supplies such as culture tubes and tissue samples.

Skill 27-4

Preparing the Examination Room

1. Maintain medical asepsis by using the guidelines provided in the Standard and Transmission-Based Precautions, including good handwashing technique and use of gloves as needed.

2. Check the records to determine the necessary equipment and supplies for the visit. Advance preparation for anticipated needs make the treatment procedures more efficient and less traumatic for the animal.

3. Clean and disinfect the room and equipment. Many disease-causing organisms live outside the animal's body for long periods of time. Organisms on inanimate objects can be transmitted from one animal to another.

4. Restock the disposable items. Supplies should be available during a procedure to prevent delay.

5. Escort the animal to the examination room. Some veterinarians prefer that the animal owner not be present. The pet may sense and react to the owner's anxiety about the treatment.

6. Assist with examination or treatment as needed. The animal may need to be restrained, or supplies may need to be opened for the veterinarian.

7. When the procedure is completed, return the animal to the cage or kennel as directed by the veterinarian. The animal may need observation or monitoring of vital signs after some procedures.

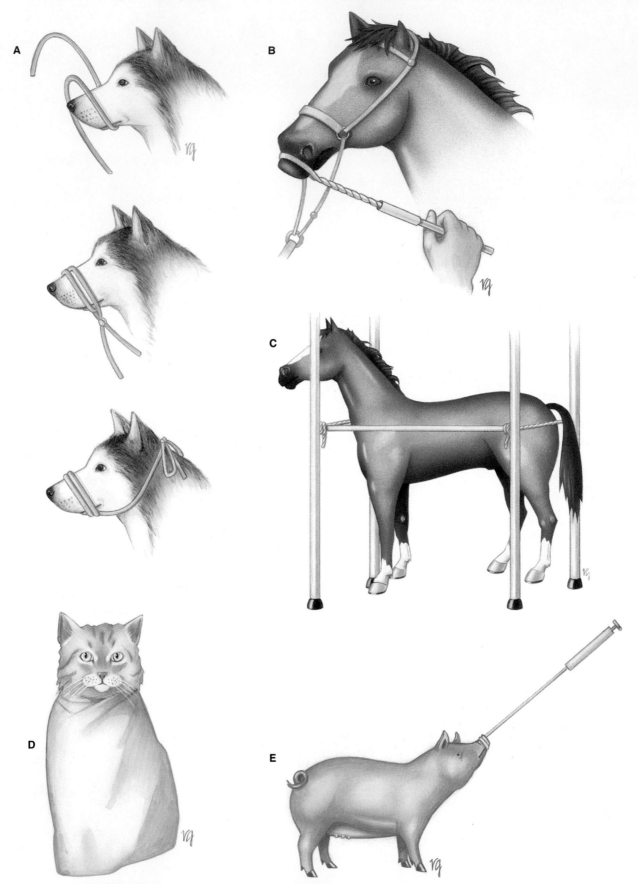

Figure 27-6   Methods of restraint. **A,** Muzzle. **B,** Twitch. **C,** Chute. **D,** Bag. **E,** Snare.

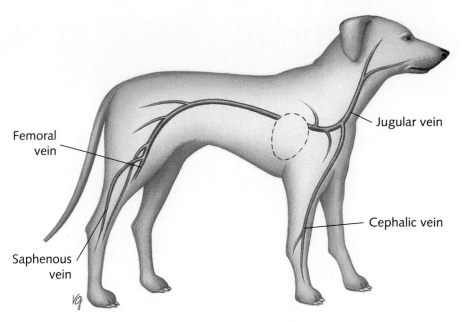

Figure 27-7   Venous blood collection sites.

Review Questions

1. Use each of the following terms in one or more sentences that correctly relate their meaning.
   Canine
   Feline
   Quarantine
   Vaccination
   Veterinary

2. Describe the function of the veterinary team.

3. Describe the function of the veterinary technician.

4. Describe the functions that animals serve in the daily life of humans.

5. Describe five methods of restraint used for animal treatment and care.

6. Identify six signs of illness in animals.

7. Describe six common disorders that affect animals.

8. Describe five methods of assessment of disorders in animals.

Critical Thinking

1. Investigate and compare the cost of various types of treatments related to veterinary care.

2. Investigate five common medications used in veterinary care.

3. Investigate the use of pets as therapeutic members of the health care team.

28

Community and Social Careers

Learning Objectives

Define at least eight terms relating to community and social health care.

Describe the function of the community and social health care team.

Specify the role of the community and social health care team members, including personal qualities, educational requirements, responsibilities, and credentialing requirements.

Identify at least six services provided by community health care agencies.

Specify the difference between physical and psychological drug dependency.

Identify at least four signs and symptoms of withdrawal from an addictive substance.

Key Terms

Communicable
(kum-YOO-nik-uh-bul) Capable of being transmitted from one person or animal to another

Demographic
(dem-o-GRAF-ik) Pertaining to the study of people as a group, especially of statistical groupings according to age, gender, and environmental factors

Dependence
(dee-PEN-dents) Addiction to drugs or alcohol

Hallucination
(huh-loo-sin-AY-shun) Sensory perception that occurs in waking state but does not have external stimulus

Immunization
(im-yoo-niz-AY-shun) Process of becoming secure against a particular disease or pathogen

Pollution
(puh-LOO-shun) Condition of being defiled or impure

Vector
(VEK-tur) Carrier that transfers an infective agent from one host to another

Withdrawal
(with-DRAW-ul) Unpleasant symptoms resulting with stoppage of drugs or substances on which a person is dependent; symptoms include anxiety, insomnia, irritability, impaired attention, and physical illness

Community and Social Careers Terminology*

TERM	DEFINITION	PREFIX	ROOT	SUFFIX
Anesthetic	Pertaining to a lack of feeling	an	esthet	ic
Arthritis	Inflammation of the joints		arthr	itis
Chronic	Pertaining to time		chron	ic
Disable	Opposite of fitness	dis	able	
Euphoria	State of feeling well	eu	phor	ia
Gerontology	Study of aging		geront	ology
Hypertrophy	Increase in nourishment (size)	hyper	troph	y
Hypnotic	Pertaining to a state of sleep		hypnot	ic
Narcolepsy	Condition to uncontrolled sleep		narco	lepsy
Sociologist	One who works with society		sociol	ogist

*A transition phrase or vowel may be added to or deleted from the word parts to make the combining form.

Abbreviations for Community and Social Careers

ABBREVIATION	MEANING
ACSW	Academy of Certified Social Workers
DHHS	Department of Health and Human Services
DSW	Doctorate of social work
FDA	Food and Drug Administration
GHB	Gamma hydroxybutyrate
MSW	Master of social work
NIH	National Institutes of Health
PhD	Doctor of philosophy
THC	Tetrahydrocannabinol
WHO	World Health Organization

Careers

Community and social health care has broad goals and focuses on the health needs of a population (Figure 28-1). The primary goal of community and social health care

workers is prevention of illness and injury and provision of care to a population. The community and social health care worker is involved in the search for the source of disease and the use of technical and regulatory means to protect the population from environmental, social, and behavioral hazards. Health problems addressed by community and social health care workers are often related to environmental hazards, sanitation, and work and living conditions. Other health problems may originate because of population growth and social and behavioral aspects of life.

Employees in community and social health careers may be trained as physicians, social workers, dentists, nurses, and counselors as well as other health care providers (Box 28-1). These health care providers usually work for the government or volunteer agencies. They must develop the ability to consider many aspects of a problem or condition and analyze the many options that are provided by, or limited by, public health agencies. Community and social health care workers must also be able to function well in an environment that involves many regulations and agencies.

Community Health Providers

Community nutrition workers provide food and nutrition education through public health clinics and programs (Figure 28-2). They screen patients to determine eligibility, based on health risk and income, for the program. Other job duties may include testing blood, taking dietary histories, assessing vital signs, and counseling on basic nutri-

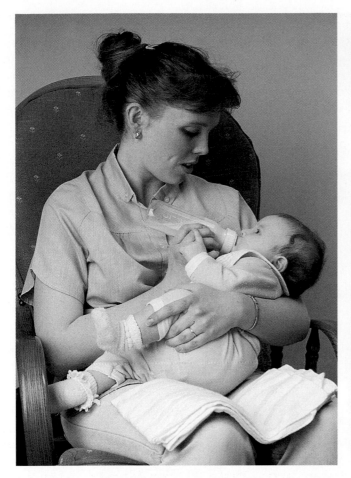
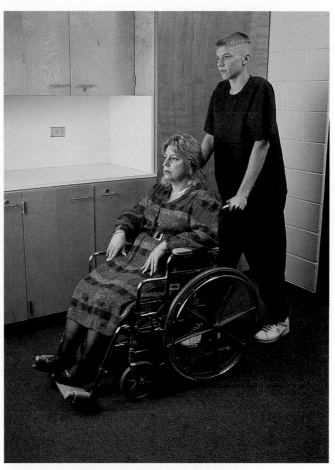

Figure 28-1 Community and health care workers may work in many areas, ranging from maternal and child care to advocacy for people with physical challenges.

Box 28-1 Community and Social Health Careers

Child life specialist
Child welfare caseworker
Community dietician
Community health nurse
Community organization director
Community service and health education director
Counselor
Counselor, residence
Counselor, vocational-rehabilitation
Director of counseling

Geriatric social worker
Mental health aide
Occupational health nurse
Red Cross executive director
Sheltered works director
Social group worker
Social services aide
Social worker, delinquency
Social worker, medical
Sociologist, clinical

tion. The minimum qualification is a high school education and experience working with the public or training in nutrition education.

Caseworker supervisors direct and coordinate the activities of agency staff, volunteers, and students working in child welfare. The supervisor assigns the cases and assists with services. Graduate-level preparation plus social work experience is usually required. Caseworkers may investigate physical and psychological home conditions to determine the need for intervention of the agency workers.

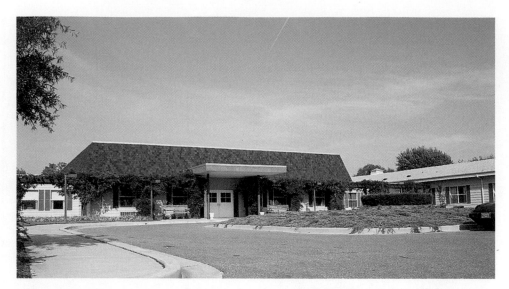

Figure 28-2   Community nutrition workers often present programs in public health clinics.

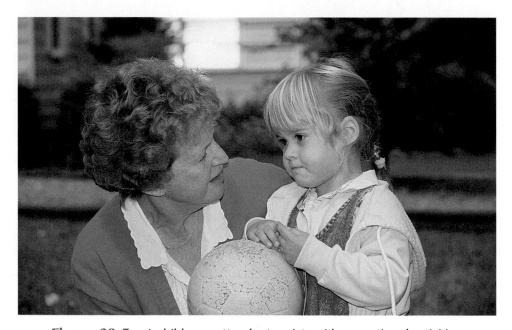

Figure 28-3   A child care attendant assists with recreational activities.

Caseworkers provide counseling for children, parents, and foster parents. The caseworker determines the suitability of foster homes and adoption applicants and places children in appropriate settings. Bachelor's preparation in social work is the minimal level for employment, but a master's degree is preferred.

Under the supervision of the caseworker, case assistants perform such tasks as completing forms and explaining the services of the agency. Duties may include assisting patients to complete applications for unemployment compensation, food stamps, medical care, and other services.

On-the-job or vocational school training for case assistants may be adequate for employment.

Under the supervision of the director, attendants for children's institutions provide care for children who are housed in city, county, private, or other institutions such as orphanages, child care homes, and day-care centers. The duties include waking and assisting the children who need help in dressing. The responsibilities may also include assistance with feeding, schooling, and recreational activities. The attendant may be responsible for discipline when children misbehave. Attendants with high school diplomas are

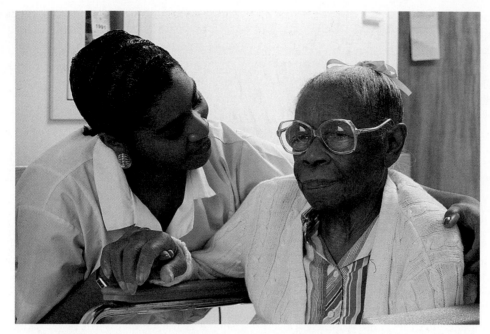

Figure 28-4   Geriatric social workers help to improve quality of life for the elderly.

preferred. There is little advancement possible without additional education and training.

Disabled children may be assigned to a child care attendant while attending school. The attendant helps the student perform tasks needed to attend classes. Duties may include transporting the child, replacing braces or slings, and helping with participation in activities (Figure 28-3). Most school attendants are employed by the school system, and a high school diploma is required for employment.

Social Care Providers

Health sociologists identify and explain the social factors affecting the care of patients. They specialize in the study of the effect of social factors on the incidence and course of disease. By gathering and interpreting data about the community, the health sociologist can advise the community and health care workers about the response to a new technology or service that may be expected. Health sociologists (medical sociologists) work in universities or for the government. Most health sociologists have a doctoral (PhD) degree. Neither certification nor licensure is required for the health sociologist.

Geriatric social workers specialize in providing assistance to the elderly (Figure 28-4). Some examples of positions for geriatric social workers include evaluation of patients for social services, working in a hospital to provide treatment for the elderly, working in group homes or senior centers, hospices, and working in long-term care facilities. Most states require geriatric social workers to be licensed or registered. A master's degree in social work

Box 28-2	**Areas of Specialization for Social Workers**

Administration
Child welfare and family services
Clinical practice (psychotherapy)
Criminal justice
Gerontology
Health care
Mental health practice
Occupational
Plan and policy making
School
Substance abuse

allows geriatric social workers to advance beyond entry level positions.

There are three levels of education for professional social workers. These are the bachelor's degree (BSW), the master's degree (MSW), and the doctoral degree (DSW). Certification is available through the Academy of Certified Social Workers (ACSW). A master's or doctoral degree is usually required for social workers employed in mental health and medical environments. Most social workers specialize in one area of practice (Box 28-2). Professional social workers use counseling, referral, and advocacy to help patients to deal with their problems. Areas of specialization include child welfare, family counseling, corrections, aging, medical, and psychiatric care.

Counselors help their patients to solve problems of personal, social, career, and educational development. They work in a variety of settings, such as schools, rehabilitation agencies, mental health or correctional facilities, and colleges, or they may have a private practice. They may specialize in marriage, family, career selection, grief, or other types of guidance practice.

Most counseling positions require a master's degree for entry-level work. An internship or supervised field experience is needed for certification or licensure by the state. Most states require counselors to be licensed, certified, or registered.

Vocational and rehabilitation counselors assist disabled individuals and students to identify career opportunities and to learn a trade. They help the disabled individual to adjust during training and to find employment when the program is completed. Vocational counselors must complete a bachelor's degree for entry-level employment, but a master's degree may be required. Most vocational counselors work for state or local rehabilitation agencies and schools.

Some counselors specialize in treatment of drug or substance abuse. Duties of the substance abuse counselor include providing help for abusers and implementing preventive programs. Substance abuse counselors may be educated as psychologists, nurses, social workers, or in related occupational fields as well as counseling.

The child life specialist works in health care settings and focuses on the emotional and developmental needs of children. These specialists use play therapy, activities, and communication to reduce the stress of illness and improve the child's understanding of health care treatments and the environment. Children do not have the emotional maturity to understand confinement, the lack of privacy, separation from family, and pain resulting from tests and treatments during treatment for illness.

Educational programs in child life care are available at the baccalaureate and graduate level. Supervised field training in a hospital or clinic may be part of the program. Individuals with training in education, recreation, and child development may also qualify for this occupation. Voluntary certification for child life professionals is available through the Child Life Certifying Commission. Child life specialists may have assistants who hold a 2-year community college degree. Presently, child life specialists are not required to be licensed or certified.

The social and human service assistant field includes workers in many areas, including social work assistant, case management aide, and community outreach worker. This position is projected to be one of the fastest growing occupations between 2000 and 2010. The social and human service assistant may give care directly to the patient or indirectly by helping a professional responsible for the care. Job duties of the social and human service assistant vary with the type of employment. Examples may include assessing patient needs for benefits, arranging transportation, organizing group activities, and keeping records of care given. There are no specific educational or certification requirements for the social and human service assistant.

Content Instruction

Substance Abuse

Drug **dependence** or addiction is the physical or psychological need to continue taking a drug or other substance. Psychological dependence is a state of mind that needs the substance to achieve a desired feeling. Physical dependence results when the body develops a need for the substance to function. **Withdrawal** occurs when the substance is not taken. Withdrawal causes extreme nervousness, uncontrollable trembling, excessive sweating, and painful cramps. Other symptoms may include nausea and imaginary visions (**hallucination**). A person may develop tolerance to the substance and require a larger dose of the drug to achieve the same effect.

The reasons that people use or abuse mind-altering substances vary greatly. These include the desire to experience new sensations, relax, gain acceptance from others, or escape boredom. Some users state these substances provide a temporary sense of control over the body or relieve a bad feeling or personal problem. As with any mind-altering substance, the problem or feeling remains when the effects of the drug wear off. Substance abuse is the misuse of drugs including alcohol. Abuse may result from use of legal or illegal drugs (Table 28-1). Stimulants may be used to increase the activity of the central nervous system. Depressants have the opposite effect. Narcotics depress the central nervous system, but they also result in a "pleasurable" feeling followed by drowsiness, sleep, or unconsciousness. Some household cleaning and paint products are used to produce a change in mental status. There is an increasing trend of the abuse of inhalants by teenagers (Box 28-3). It is estimated that 17% of high school seniors have used inhalants. These are very dangerous and have been the cause of death in many young people.

Alcohol is the most commonly abused substance in the United States, and alcoholism is a major medical problem. Treatment of alcoholism includes detoxification and therapy to prevent drinking. Most drug programs teach that not drinking (abstinence) is the only reasonable goal for the addicted individual.

Treatment of the symptoms of substance abuse is usually the first step after diagnosis. Once the person's addiction is controlled, treatment of the mental disorder can be started. Although many factors such as age, values, culture,

Table 28-1   Commonly Abused Chemicals

Category	Chemical	Commercial and Street Names	Intoxicating Effects	Potential Harmful Effects
Cannabinoids	Hashish	Boom, chronic, gangster, hash, hash oil, hemp	Euphoria, slowed thinking and reaction time, confusion, impaired balance and coordination	Cough, frequent respiratory infections; impaired memory and learning; increased heart rate
	Marijuana	Blunt, dope, ganja, grass, herb, joints, Mary Jane, pot, reefer, sinsemilla, skunk, weed	Euphoria, slowed thinking and reaction time, confusion, impaired balance and coordination	Cough, frequent respiratory infections; impaired memory and learning; increased heart rate
Depressants	Barbiturates	Amytal, Nembutal, Seconal, phenobarbital, barbs, reds, red birds, phennies, tooies, yellows, yellow jackets	Reduced pain and anxiety; feeling of well-being; lowered inhibitions; slowed pulse and breathing; lowered blood pressure; poor concentration, sedation, drowsiness	Confusion, fatigue; impaired coordination, memory, judgment; respiratory depression and arrest, addiction, depression, unusual excitement, fever, irritability, poor judgment, slurred speech, dizziness
	Benzodiazepines (other than flunitrazepam)	Ativan, Halcion, Librium, Valium, Xanax; candy, downers, sleeping pills, tranks	Reduced pain and anxiety; feeling of well-being; lowered inhibitions; slowed pulse and breathing; lowered blood pressure; poor concentration	Confusion, fatigue; impaired coordination, memory, judgment; respiratory depression and arrest, addiction
	Flunitrazepam*	Rohypnol; forget-me pill, Mexican Valium, R2, Roche, roofies, roofinol, rope, rophies	Reduced pain and anxiety; feeling of well-being; lowered inhibitions; slowed pulse and breathing; lowered blood pressure; poor concentration, visual and gastrointestinal disturbances, urinary retention, memory loss for the time under the drug's effects	Confusion, fatigue; impaired coordination, memory, judgment; respiratory depression and arrest, addiction
	GHB*	Gammahydroxybutyrate; G, Georgia home boy, grievous bodily harm, liquid ecstasy	Reduced pain and anxiety; feeling of well-being; lowered inhibitions; slowed pulse and breathing; lowered blood pressure; poor concentration, drowsiness, nausea/vomiting, headache, loss of consciousness, loss of reflexes, seizures, coma, death	Confusion, fatigue; impaired coordination, memory, judgment; respiratory depression and arrest, addiction
	Methaqualone	Quaalude, Sopor, Parest; ludes, mandrex, quad, quay	Reduced pain and anxiety; feeling of well-being; lowered inhibitions; slowed pulse and breathing; lowered blood pressure; poor concentration, euphoria	Confusion, fatigue; impaired coordination, memory, judgment; respiratory depression and arrest, addiction, depression, poor reflexes, slurred speech, coma

Adapted from the National Institutes of Health "Commonly Abused Drugs."
*Associated with sexual assaults.

Continued

Table 28-1 Commonly Abused Chemicals—cont'd

Category	Chemical	Commercial and Street Names	Intoxicating Effects	Potential Harmful Effects
Dissociative anesthetics	Ketamine	Ketalar SV; cat Valiums, K, Special K, vitamin K	Increased heart rate and blood pressure, impaired motor function, at high doses, delirium, depression, respiratory depression and arrest	Memory loss; numbness; nausea/vomiting
	PCP and analogs	Phencyclidine; angel dust, boat, hog, love boat, peace pill	Increased heart rate and blood pressure, impaired motor function, possible decrease in blood pressure and heart rate, panic, aggression, violence	Memory loss; numbness; nausea/vomiting, loss of appetite, depression
Hallucinogens	LSD	Lysergic acid diethylamide; acid, blotter, boomers, cubes, microdot, yellow sunshines	Altered states of perception and feeling; nausea, increased body temperature, heart rate, blood pressure; loss of appetite, sleeplessness, numbness, weakness, tremors	Chronic mental disorders, persisting perception disorder (flashbacks)
	Mescaline	Buttons, cactus, mesc, peyote	Altered states of perception and feeling; nausea, increased body temperature, heart rate, blood pressure; loss of appetite, sleeplessness, numbness, weakness, tremors	Chronic mental disorders, persisting perception disorder (flashbacks)
	Psilocybin	Magic mushroom, purple passion, shrooms	Altered states of perception and feeling; nausea	Chronic mental disorders, persisting perception disorder (flashbacks), nervousness, paranoia
Opioids and morphine derivatives	Codeine	Empirin with Codeine, Fiorinal with Codeine, Robitussin A-C, Tylenol with Codeine; Captain Cody, Cody, schoolboy; (with glutethimide) doors & fours, loads, pancakes and syrup	Pain relief, euphoria, drowsiness; less analgesia, sedation, and respiratory depression than morphine	Respiratory depression and arrest, nausea, confusion, constipation, sedation, unconsciousness, coma, tolerance, addiction
	Fentanyl	Actiq, Duragesic, Sublimaze; Apache, China girl, China white, dance fever, friend, goodfella, jackpot, murder 8, TNT, Tango and Cash	Pain relief, euphoria, drowsiness	Respiratory depression and arrest, nausea, confusion, constipation, sedation, unconsciousness, coma, tolerance, addiction
	Heroin	Diacetylmorphine; brown sugar, dope, H, horse, junk, skag, skunk, smack, white horse	Pain relief, euphoria, drowsiness, staggering gait	Respiratory depression and arrest, nausea, confusion, constipation, sedation, unconsciousness, coma, tolerance, addiction

Adapted from the National Institutes of Health "Commonly Abused Drugs."

Table 28-1   Commonly Abused Chemicals—cont'd

Category	Chemical	Commercial and Street Names	Intoxicating Effects	Potential Harmful Effects
	Morphine	Roxanol, Duramorph; M, Miss Emma, monkey, white stuff	Pain relief, euphoria, drowsiness	Respiratory depression and arrest, nausea, confusion, constipation, sedation, unconsciousness, coma, tolerance, addiction
	Opium	Laudanum, paregoric; big O, black stuff, block, gum, hop	Pain relief, euphoria, drowsiness	Respiratory depression and arrest, nausea, confusion, constipation, sedation, unconsciousness, coma, tolerance, addiction
Stimulants	Amphetamine	Adderall, Biphetamine, Dexedrine; bennies, black beauties, crosses, hearts, LA turnaround, speed, truck drivers, uppers	Increased heart rate, blood pressure, metabolism; feelings of exhilaration, energy, increased mental alertness, rapid breathing; hallucinations	Rapid or irregular heartbeat; reduced appetite, weight loss, heart failure, tremor, loss of coordination; irritability, anxiousness, restlessness, delirium, panic, paranoia, impulsive behavior, aggressiveness, tolerance, addiction
	Cocaine	Cocaine hydrochloride; blow, bump, C, candy, Charlie, coke, crack, flake, rock, snow, toot	Increased heart rate, blood pressure, metabolism; feelings of exhilaration, energy, increased mental alertness, increased temperature	Rapid or irregular heartbeat; reduced appetite, weight loss, heart failure, chest pain, respiratory failure, nausea, abdominal pain, strokes, seizures, headaches, malnutrition
	MDMA (methylenedioxy-methamphetamine)	DOB, DOM, MDA; Adam, clarity, ecstasy, Eve, lover's speed, peace, STP, X, XTC	Increased heart rate, blood pressure, metabolism; feelings of exhilaration, energy, increased mental alertness, mild hallucinogenic effects, increased tactile sensitivity, empathic feelings, hyperthermia	Rapid or irregular heartbeat; reduced appetite, weight loss, heart failure, impaired memory and learning
	Methamphetamine	Desoxyn; chalk, crank, crystal, fire, glass, go fast, ice, meth, speed	Increased heart rate, blood pressure, metabolism; feelings of exhilaration, energy, increased mental alertness, aggression, violence, psychotic behavior	Rapid or irregular heartbeat; reduced appetite, weight loss, heart failure, memory loss, cardiac and neurological damage; impaired memory and learning, tolerance, addiction
	Methylphenidate	Ritalin; JIF, MPH, R-ball, Skippy, the smart drug, vitamin R	Increased heart rate, blood pressure, metabolism; feelings of exhilaration, energy, increased mental alertness, increase or decrease in blood pressure, psychotic episode	Rapid or irregular heartbeat; reduced appetite, weight loss, heart failure, digestive problems, loss of appetite, weight loss

Continued

Table 28-1 Commonly Abused Chemicals—cont'd

Category	Chemical	Commercial and Street Names	Intoxicating Effects	Potential Harmful Effects
	Nicotine	Bidis, chew, cigars, cigarettes, smokeless tobacco, snuff, spit tobacco	Increased heart rate, blood pressure, metabolism; feelings of exhilaration, energy, increased mental alertness	Rapid or irregular heartbeat; reduced appetite, weight loss, heart failure; additional effects attributable to tobacco exposure: adverse pregnancy outcomes, chronic lung disease, cardiovascular disease, stroke, cancer, tolerance, addiction
Other compounds	Anabolic steroids	Anadrol, Oxandrin, Durabolin, Depo-Testosterone, Equipoise; roids, juice	No intoxication effects	Hypertension, blood clotting and cholesterol changes, liver cysts and cancer, kidney cancer, hostility and aggression, acne; adolescents, premature stoppage of growth; in males, prostate cancer, reduced sperm production, shrunken testicles, breast enlargement; in females, menstrual irregularities, development of beard and other masculine characteristics
	Inhalants	Solvents (paint thinners, gasoline, glues), gases (butane, propane, aerosol propellants, nitrous oxide), nitrites (isoamyl, isobutyl, cyclohexyl); laughing gas, poppers, snappers, whippets	Stimulation, loss of inhibition; headache; nausea or vomiting; slurred speech, loss of motor coordination; wheezing	Unconsciousness, cramps, weight loss, muscle weakness, depression, memory impairment, damage to cardiovascular and nervous systems, sudden death

Adapted from the National Institutes of Health "Commonly Abused Drugs."

Box 28-3   Warning Signs of Inhalant Abuse

Empty lighters
Empty plastic bags
Fingernails painted with inhalants such as Liquid
    Paper
Hair bands wrapped around wrists or upper arm
    (soaked in inhalant)

Loss of appetite
Nausea
Persistent cough
Runny nose or nosebleed
Sores or rashes around the mouth
Stains on skin or clothing

---

gender, family relationships, and other disorders influence the type of treatment, most treatments have similar components. Medication may be used to control mood and behavior. Psychotherapy, group therapy, behavior modification, and cognitive therapy may also be used.

Public Health Resources

Public health care agencies are concerned with maternal and child health, dental care, tuberculosis control, sexually transmitted disease control, mental illness, care of the aged, addiction, and chronic and **communicable** diseases. State services include **immunization,** sanitation, animal control, vital statistics, public health nursing services, referral services, air and water **pollution** control, **vector** control, food and drug control, and community-sponsored blood testing (Figure 28-5). Health needs are determined by surveying the community needs.

Every country in the world has a department that determines the health policies and protection plans for the citizens. The World Health Organization (WHO) is a nongovernmental agency that is organized to protect the health of the world community. In the United States, health agencies are organized on local, state, and federal levels.

The federal health agencies provide regulation of and protection against hazards that affect all of the states. They collect and distribute **demographic** health statistics, support local and state agencies, and organize and support disaster relief programs. The Department of Health and Human Services (DHHS) is the main organization for public health care at the federal level.

The Centers for Disease Control (CDC) is an agency of the Public Health Service. It provides programs that prevent and control communicable, vector-borne, and chronic illnesses. The Food and Drug Administration (FDA) regulates foods, drugs, medical devices, and cosmetics. The National Institutes of Health (NIH) deal with research in determining the cause, treatment, and methods of prevention

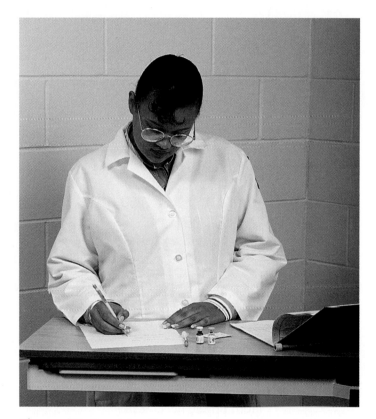

Figure 28-5   A health care worker prepares for immunizations.

of diseases. Other departments of the Public Health Service include the Health Resources Administration and Health Services Administration.

State and local agencies enforce state health laws and provide care for residents. These agencies are involved in preventive, environmental, and community health care services. Community health care provides services for individuals who do not use private health care because of

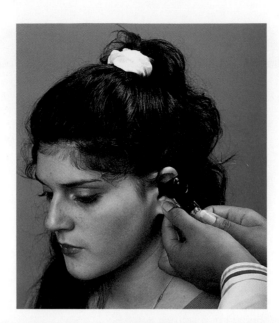

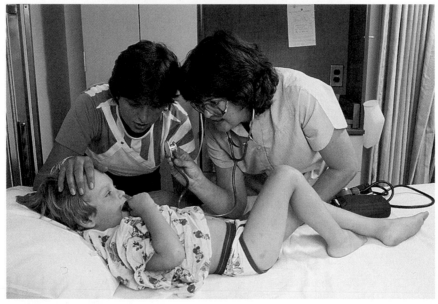

Figure 28-6 Community health care centers often provide care for those who cannot afford private health care.

economic, cultural, or similar reasons (Figure 28-6). Immunization and education programs of the community health services are directed to provide care for the entire community. Eligibility for community health services is determined by state and federal regulations.

Performance Instruction

Most of the duties that are performed as part of the health care treatment in mental and community settings are performed by licensed personnel. This is due to the legal and privacy rights of the people seeking care in this setting. The entry-level worker may provide assistance in these duties when supervised by licensed personnel.

Research has shown that hospital and medical experiences can be upsetting to children and their families. The child life specialist and related personnel help to meet the social and mental needs of the hospitalized child. Some examples of activities that may reduce anxiety for the child are tours of surgery, radiology, and other departments that may be visited during the hospital stay. Explanation and demonstration of equipment and supplies to be used are also helpful.

Review Questions

1. Use the following terms in one or more sentences that correctly relate their meaning.
   Dependence
   Hallucination
   Withdrawal

2. Describe the role of each member of the community and social health care team.

3. List six services provided by community and social health care agencies.

4. Differentiate between physical and psychological dependence.

5. List four signs and symptoms of withdrawal.

Critical Thinking

1. Investigate and compare the cost of various types of community and social health care services.

2. Research and identify the types of immunizations required for school attendance.

3. Discuss situations that might lead to substance abuse and alternative coping mechanisms.

4. Plan a health fair based on study of the needs of the community. Investigate the community resources, publicity, and other factors needed to produce the fair.

29
Mental Health Careers

Learning Objectives

Define at least eight terms relating to mental health care.

Describe the function of the mental health care team.

Specify the role of selected members of the mental health care team, including the personal qualities, levels of education, and credentialing requirements.

Define mental health and mental hygiene.

Describe at least four psychoneurotic disorders.

Describe at least two types of psychosis.

Describe procedures for use of physical restraint.

Identify at least three techniques of reality orientation.

Key Terms

Behavior
(bee-HAYV-yur) Conduct, actions that can be observed

Phobia
(FOE-bee-uh) Persistent abnormal dread or fear

Psychology
(sie-KOL-uh-jee) Study of human and animal behavior, normal and abnormal

Psychoneurosis
(sie-ko-noo-RO-sis) Functional disturbance of the mind in which the individual is aware that reactions are not normal

Psychosis
(sie-KO-sis) Major mental disorder in which the individual loses contact with reality

Psychotherapy
(sie-ko-THARE-uh-pee) Treatment of discomfort, dysfunction, or diseases by methods designed to understand and cope with problems

Reality Orientation
(ree-AL-it-ee o-ree-en-TAY-shun) Awareness of position in relation to time, space, and person

Restraint
(reh-STRAYNT) Physical confinement

Mental Health Careers Terminology*

TERM	DEFINITION	PREFIX	ROOT	SUFFIX
Anorexia	Condition of being without appetite	an	orex	ia
Bipolar	Having two extremes	bi	polar	
Hydrophobia	Condition of being afraid of water	hydro	phob	ia
Insomnia	Condition of lacking sleep	in	somn	ia
Neurotic	Pertaining to a functional disorder or disease of the nerves		neuro/t	ic
Phobia	Pertaining to fear		phob	ia
Photophobia	Fear of light	photo	phob	ia
Psychology	Study of the mind		psych	ology
Psychopathology	Study of disease of the mind	psych/o	path	ology
Psychosis	Condition of the mind		psych/o	sis

*A transition phrase or vowel may be added to or deleted from the word parts to make the combining form.

Abbreviations for Mental Health Careers

ABBREVIATION	MEANING
ECT	Electroconvulsive therapy
EdD	Doctor of education
EEG	Electroencephalogram
LOC	Level of consciousness
NCHSW	National Commission for Human Services Workers
Neuro	Neurology
NIMH	National Institute of Mental Health
PhD	Doctor of philosophy
PsyD	Doctor of psychology
RO	Reality orientation

Box 29-1   Mental Health Careers*

Psychiatric aide
Psychiatric technician
Psychiatrist
Psychologist, chief
Psychologist, clinical
Psychologist, counseling
Psychologist, developmental
Psychologist, educational
Psychologist, engineering
Psychologist, experimental
Psychologist, industrial
Psychologist, school
Psychologist, social

*The function of the mental health care team is to provide care and treatment for patients with disorders of the mind, emotion, or behavior.

Careers

The function of the mental health care team is to provide care and treatment for individuals with disorders of the mind, emotion, or behavior (Box 29-1). Mental health care workers must have an interest in **behavior** and the ability to communicate well. The work is challenging and requires the worker to be creative in finding unusual solutions to problems. Mental health care workers must be emotionally stable and mature. They must be able to lead and inspire others while demonstrating patience and perseverance.

The field of mental health care is constantly growing. With the increasing age of the population in general and

Box 29-2   Areas of Specialty for Psychologists

Childcare counseling
Clinical psychology
Community psychology
Consumer psychology
Counseling psychology
Developmental psychology
Educational psychology
Engineering psychology
Family therapy
Forensic psychology
Health psychology
Hospital practice
Human relations
Industrial or organizational psychology
Marriage therapy
Military practice
Neuropsychology
Private practice
Quantitative and measurement psychology
Rehabilitation psychology
Research psychology
School psychology
Social psychology
Sports psychology
Substance abuse therapy

Psychiatrists determine the type and severity of the disorder and plan the necessary therapy, which may include medication to treat the problem. Psychiatrists must complete at least a 4-year residency after earning a medical degree. Specialties in psychiatry include **psychotherapy,** child practice, psychoanalysis, behavior therapy, forensics, and industrial or organizational practice. About half of all psychiatrists work in private practice with the remainder working in hospitals, clinics, research, and educational centers.

Psychologist

Psychologists are professionals who specialize in treatment of mental and emotional disorders. They study human behavior and mental processes to understand and explain human actions. Methods of treatment include personal interviews, intelligence and aptitude testing, and observation. Most psychologists earn a doctoral (PhD, EdD, or PsyD) degree and complete an internship before the licensure or certification required to practice independently. The doctor of **psychology** degree is offered by professional schools that emphasize training for clinical practice. Psychologists may specialize in the area of educational, social, clinical, cross-cultural, quantitative, consumer, environmental, developmental, rehabilitative, or organizational behavior (Box 29-2). More than 40% of psychologists are self-employed.

Master's degree preparation in psychology allows an individual to work in a limited variety of settings including schools, businesses, and mental health centers. Many individuals with master's degrees work under the supervision of a doctor of psychology. Certification or licensing is required in all states.

Support Personnel

Psychiatric technicians take an active part in the treatment of patients. They may interview, lead group sessions, give daily care, or make home visits. In some cases, they may administer medications. Education for the psychiatric technician includes a 2-year associate degree. Many states require the psychiatric technician to be licensed. Psychiatric technicians may also be known as *mental health technicians, human service workers,* or *mental health associates.* Certification for mental health technicians is available from the National Commission for Human Service Workers (NCHSW).

Psychiatric assistants help patients with problems of mental health under the direction of nurses and physicians. The responsibilities of the psychiatric assistant include helping the patient with activities of daily living such as dressing and eating. The assistant also socializes with the patients and may play games or lead recreational activ-

the higher cost of care, many of the mental health care services have moved into the homes of the patients, residential facilities, and neighborhood clinics. Additionally, more allied and support staff personnel are providing care and treatments that were done by professionals in the past.

It is now commonly accepted that a person's emotional and mental state may cause or have some effect on all physical disorders. According to testimony given by physicians to the Congress of the United States, more than half of all physician office visits do not result from physical illness. Disorders of the mind (psyche) may be caused by mental illness, loss of contact with reality, the inability to understand the environment, isolation, depression, or destructive life events.

Psychiatrist

Psychiatrists are licensed physicians specializing in the treatment of mental, emotional, and behavioral disorders.

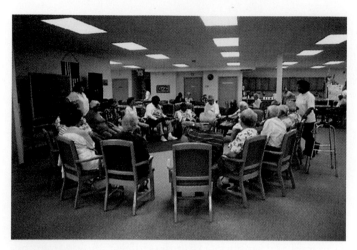

Figure 29-1   An adult day-care center for patients with Alzheimer's disease is an alternative to a long-term care environment.

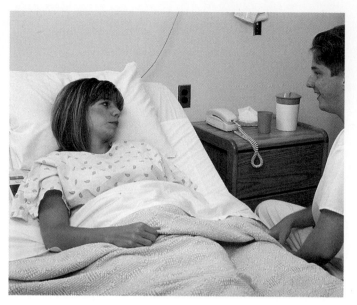

Figure 29-2   Anxiety and depression may affect anyone at any time of life.

ities. The psychiatric assistant observes patients for unusual behavior and reports the observations to the professional staff. Some psychiatric hospitals and community colleges offer on-the-job training programs to prepare psychiatric assistants. These training programs usually last 4 to 6 months.

Content Instruction

Mental Health

In the past, people with mental or developmental problems were placed in institutions called *asylums* or *sanatoriums*. The majority of people with mental illness in the United States now live in the community, not in institutions. Society believes that people with mental illness and developmental disabilities have the potential to improve and the right to try to live an independent life. The living environment for those with mental impairments must provide protection, opportunities for development, and support for daily tasks. Most experts feel that living at home is the optimal arrangement for individuals with mental or developmental disabilities. Other alternatives include foster care, day-care centers, halfway houses, and small group homes that provide supervised assistance (Figure 29-1).

Mental health is a state of mind in which a person can cope with problems and maintain emotional balance and satisfaction in living. Mental disorders may be classified as organic or functional. Organic disorders are caused by injury to the brain such as by high fever, tumor, or toxic substances such as drugs. Functional disorders have no known brain injury. Functional disorders include psy-

choneuroses, psychoses, and personality disorders. The severity of mental illness ranges from minor anxiety to a condition that prevents an individual from relating with other people. More than 16 million Americans seek some form of mental health care each year.

Psychoneuroses are functional disturbances of the mind. The individual with neuroses does not lose touch with reality and often knows that the reactions experienced are not appropriate. Anxiety and depression are two emotions experienced by everyone (Figure 29-2). Anxiety is a feeling of fear or apprehension. Depression is a feeling of sadness. In some people, these emotions may be experienced without cause or in an overwhelming manner. Panic disorder is a condition of feeling an unreasonable fear with no known cause. **Phobias** are specific unrealistic fears. For example, agoraphobia is fear of being in a place where escape may not be possible, and it may lead to a reluctance to leave the home. Another neurosis is hypochondria, or the belief in imaginary illness.

Psychoses are severe or major mental disorders in which the individual is not in contact with reality. The individual with a psychosis does not know that the behavior and thoughts are abnormal. There are several types of schizophrenia that result in a separation from the real world and in fixed ideas or obsessions. Manic-depressive or bipolar **psychosis** is a condition of repeating cycles in which severe depression is followed by extremely elated or excited behavior. In a condition of paranoia, the person feels persecuted and plotted against by others.

Deprivation syndrome is a condition in children resulting from inadequate nutrition and an environment un-

Table 29-1   Forms of Therapy

Type of Therapy	Description
Behavioral	Focus is on symptoms and managing specific complaints, such as phobias
Cognitive	Focus is on patient's thinking and logic regarding dysfunctional behavior
Desensitization	Form of behavioral therapy that removes phobias by progressively exposing the patient to the source of fear
Family	Focus is on unhealthy patterns of interaction and inappropriate demands and expectations between family members
Gestalt	Focus is on challenging patient's defenses to strive for wholeness
Group	Focus is on interaction with others in a controlled setting
Humanistic	Focus is on helping the patient remove emotional barriers; nondirective
Interpersonal	Focus is on improving social skills
Play	Focus is on the patient's (child's) expression of problems through the use of play
Psychoanalytic	Focus is on continued, intensive treatment with one practitioner
Psychodynamic	Focus is on personal relationships
Short-term	Focus is on specific problems

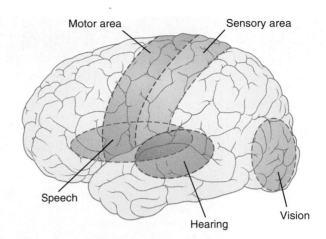

Figure 29-3   Functional areas of the brain. *(From Milliken ME, Campbell G:* Essential competencies for patient care, *St Louis, 1995, Mosby.)*

suited for normal growth and development. These children develop an intellectual slowing (retardation) and difficulty fitting into society. Other mental disorders may result from the abuse of drugs and alcohol. Dissociative disorders are those in which the person loses or changes identity. An example of a dissociative disorder is an individual with multiple personalities.

Mental disorders are treated in many ways (Table 29-1). Psychotherapy is discussion to help understand and cope with problems. Some disorders may be treated or con-

trolled with medication. Treatment may include group therapy, in which people share their thoughts and feelings with others who have the same problem. Electroconvulsive therapy may be used to treat depression by using electric shock to interrupt temporarily the normal function of the brain. Some disorders may be treated with behavioral modification to change the individual's lifestyle.

Research is being conducted on the relationship of the function of the brain to psychological behavior. This field is called *neurobiology*. One example of the result of neurobiological research is the demonstration of "right-brain" and "left-brain" control. It is now known that the right hemisphere of the brain controls creative and nonverbal thinking, whereas the left hemisphere controls logical and verbal thought (Figure 29-3). One new concept that is being researched by neurobiologists hypothesizes that there are periods of "neuroplasticity" or specific developmental times during which the brain needs certain experiences for optimal development to occur.

Other research has lead to the theory that genes influence a person's personality and mental behavior. Studies conducted by the Minnesota Center for Twin and Adoption Research using identical twins that were separated at birth often reveal that the twins display the same mannerisms, pursue the same interests and careers, and even marry the same type (in appearance and personality) of individual. This field of study is often called *sociobiology*.

Mental Hygiene

Mental hygiene includes the methods used to preserve and promote mental health. Mentally healthy people can learn stress reduction techniques and adopt changes in lifestyle.

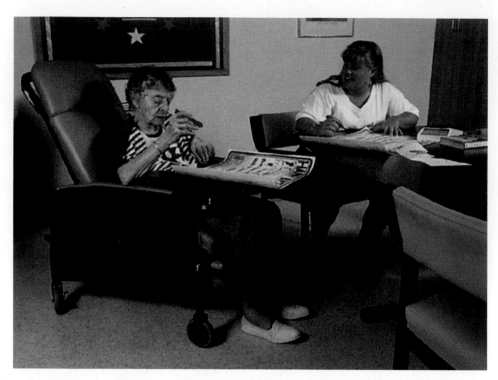

Figure 29-4   The geriatric chair is also a physical restraint. Restraints are used only with a physician's order so that the patient is protected from injury. *(From Sorrentino S: Mosby's textbook for long-term care assistants, ed 3, 1999, St Louis, Mosby.)*

The individual with mental disorders may need special treatment techniques to live safely and in the best manner possible. Examples of these techniques include the use of protective restraints and **reality orientation.**

Restraints, or protective devices, are used to protect patients from harming themselves or others (Figure 29-4). Confinement may be to a bed or chair. Restraints may be made of cloth or leather. In many states, a written order from a physician is required for use of restraints. Without a doctor's order, the use of restraints is considered to be false imprisonment. Restraints must be applied correctly to avoid injury to the patient and are used for as short a time as possible. As well as meeting the physical needs of the restrained patient, the health care worker must also make sure that the patient's mental needs are met. Anxiety resulting from confinement may be reduced by visiting with the patient frequently and providing other distractions such as activities.

Loss of orientation (confusion) may result in many situations. Loss of hearing, sight, or confinement may lead to temporary confusion. Confusion may result from a reduced blood supply to the brain. Confusion is frightening and frustrating for the person. Reality orientation (RO) is a form of rehabilitation that promotes or maintains awareness of person, place, and time by reinforcing the correct information (Skill 29-1).

One of the methods used to help patients maintain their sense of reality is a systematic approach to orientation. Calendars, clocks, and a routine for daily activities helps keep the patient oriented to place and time. Several times daily, the health care workers talk with and address the patient by name to help maintain the patient's orientation to person.

Performance Instruction

Restraint

Use of restraints must be ordered by a physician and only after proper instruction is given for its use. The least restrictive type of **restraint** is preferred. Safe restraints should not have tears, frayed edges, or other damage. Towels, bedsheets, tape, and other improvised restraints are not safe for use. The restraint should be applied according to manufacturer's instruction. They should be snug but allow some movement and blood circulation in the restrained area. Circulation in the restrained area should be checked every 15 minutes. Restraints should not be secured to moving parts of the bed or chair that might change the movement in the restrained area. Proper body alignment should be observed and maintained during restraint.

Skill 29-1

Reality Orientation

1. Maintain medical asepsis by using the guidelines provided in the Standard and Transmission-Based Precautions, including good handwashing technique and use of gloves as needed.

2. Identify the patient and explain the procedure.

3. Face the individual and speak clearly and slowly. Speaking in this manner helps the patient to process the information.

4. Call the individual by name or title (Mr., Mrs., Ms., or Miss) according to his or her preference. It is not appropriate to call adults by their first name without permission.

5. Identify yourself to the patient by name and role.

6. Tell the individual the date and time of day.

7. Give simple and clear instructions or answers to any questions.

8. Allow enough time for a response. Older people require more time to process new information.

9. Keep calendars and clocks with large numbers in clear view.

10. Assist the patient to use glasses and hearing aids if needed.

11. Provide items of current information, such as newspapers, and place familiar objects and pictures in view. Remind the patient of special events such as holidays.

12. Maintain a cycle of day and night activities. Street clothes should be worn during the day and pajamas or nightgowns at night.

13. Be consistent with the procedure. Routine helps the patient to retain information.

Reality Orientation

Confusion may result from many disorders or displacement to a health care facility. Care for a confused person should include stating of the caregiver's name and role with each visit to the room as well as clarifying and repeating procedures as often as needed for the person to understand. The patient should also be called by name with every contact. Speaking slowly and clearly is one method to improve understanding. Instructions should be short and simple. A calm, relaxed environment and a routine may help reduce anxiety caused by confusion. Clocks, calendars, newspapers, and other articles may help the person remain oriented to the present.

Review Questions

1. Use each of the following terms in one or more sentences that correctly relate their meaning.
   Behavior
   Phobia
   Psychology
   Psychoneurosis

2. Describe the function of the mental health care team.

3. Specify the role of the members of the mental health care team.

4. Define mental health and mental hygiene.

5. Define *psychoneurosis*. Describe four types of psychoneuroses.

6. Define *psychosis*. Describe two types of psychoses.

7. Specify the need for physical restraint and two precautions that may be used to avoid injury.

8. Describe three techniques that can be used to promote orientation to reality in a confused patient.

Critical Thinking

1. Investigate and compare the cost of various types of mental health care treatments and tests.

2. Investigate five common medications used in mental health care treatments.

3. Investigate the local availability of mental health care facilities and services in the area.

30
Rehabilitative Careers

Learning Objectives

Define at least 10 terms relating to rehabilitative health care.

Identify the function of the rehabilitative health care team.

Describe the role of at least five of the rehabilitative health care team members, including personal qualities, levels of education, and credentialing requirements.

Identify at least five methods or devices used to improve activities of daily living for the disabled.

Describe two types of hearing loss and two methods of assessing defects in hearing.

Identify at least five common drug types including the expected action of each.

Identify the necessary components of a legal drug prescription including the personnel qualified to write one.

Describe three other types of rehabilitative treatments.

Key Terms

Articulation
(ar-tik-yoo-LAY-shun) Enunciation of words and syllables, how sounds are spoken

Audiology
(aw-dee-OL-uh-jee) Science of hearing

Disability
(dis-uh-BIL-uh-tee) Lack of ability to function in the manner that most people function physically or mentally

Dispense
(dis-PENTS) Prepare, package, compound, or label for delivery according to a lawful order of a qualified practitioner

Dosage
(DOSE-age) Regulation of size, frequency, and amount of medication

Frequency
(FREE-kwen-see) Number of times an event occurs in a given period; measured in cycles per second (hertz [Hz]) in hearing

Hydrotherapy
(hie-dro-THAIR-uh-pee) Application of water

Nebulizer
(NEB-yoo-lie-zer) Device used to deliver a spray or mist of medication into the lungs

Orthotics
(or-THOT-iks) Art or science of custom designing, fabrication, and fitting of braces

Pharmacology
(farm-uh-KOL-uh-jee) Study of the actions and uses of drugs

Prosthesis
(pros-THEE-sis) Artificial device applied to replace a partially or totally missing body part

Prosthetics
(pros-THET-iks) Art or science of custom design, fabrication, and fitting of artificial limbs

Rehabilitation
(re-huh-bil-i-TAY-shun) Restoration of normal form and function after injury or illness

Therapy
(THEIR-uh-pee) Treatment of disease; science and art of healing

Rehabilitative Careers Terminology*

TERM	DEFINITION	PREFIX	ROOT	SUFFIX
Aphasia	Without speaking	a	phas	ia
Audiogram	Record of hearing	audio	gram	
Audiology	Study of hearing		audi	ology
Dysarthria	Difficulty articulating	dys	arthr	ia
Extracorporeal	Pertaining to outside of the body	extra	corpore	al
Hydrotherapy	Water therapy	hydro	therapy	
Myoelectronics	Pertaining to electric and muscles	myo	electron	ics
Pedorthist	One who corrects child (bones)	ped	orth	ist
Pharmacology	Study of drugs		pharmac	ology
Tracheotomy	Hole in the windpipe		trache	otomy

*A transition phrase or vowel may be added to or deleted from the word parts to make the combining form.

Abbreviations for Rehabilitative Careers

ABBREVIATION	MEANING
ADLs	Activities of daily living
CCC	Certificate of Clinical Competence
COTA	Certification of Occupational Therapy Assistants
CPT	Chest physical therapy
DEA	Drug enforcement agency
DTR	Registered dance therapists
FDA	Food and Drug Administration
OTC	Over the counter
PDR	*Physician's Desk Reference*
Rx	Prescription

Careers

Rehabilitative careers provide a variety of working opportunities (Box 30-1). The **rehabilitation** team includes physicians, surgeons, physical therapists, occupational therapists, social workers, counselors, pharmacists, orthotists, and prosthetists who provide services designed to overcome physical, developmental, behavioral, or emotional disabilities. The disabilities include impaired muscle strength, physical endurance, sensory or muscle coordination, concentration, and spatial discrimination.

The rehabilitation team works closely with the patient and family members to restore these functions. These occupations require optimism, creativity, persistence, and the ability to work with a variety of people. Additionally, the health care worker in rehabilitation must have strong listening and verbal skills, analytical ability, and patience to meet challenges and solve problems.

Physical Therapist

Physical therapists work to restore function, relieve pain, and prevent **disability** after disease, injury, or loss of a body part. Physical therapists may specialize in many areas of practice including rehabilitation, community health, sports, industry, research, education, and administration (Figure 30-1). Additionally, physical therapists may work for a hospital or other health care facility or practice privately. Admission to the less than 30 college programs in physical therapy is competitive. Entry-level practice with a bachelor's degree in physical **therapy** or a related area and completion of certification is being phased out. Master's level preparation is preferred. Physical therapists are licensed by the state.

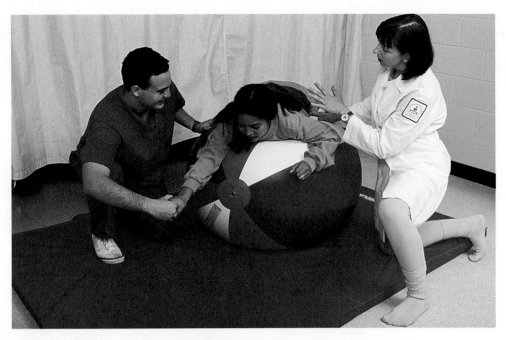

Figure 30-1 A physical therapist working with a patient.

Box 30-1 Rehabilitative Health Careers

Art therapist
Audiologist
Audiometrist
Corrective therapist
Dance therapist
Drug preparation inspector
Drug preparation utility worker
Educational therapist
Horticultural therapist
Industrial therapist
Manual arts therapist
Medication aide
Music therapist
Occupational therapist
Occupational therapy aide
Occupational therapy assistant
Orientation therapist for the blind
Orthoptist
Orthotic assistant
Orthotic technician

Pharmacist
Pharmacologist
Pharmacy assistant
Pharmacy helper
Physical-integration practitioner
Physical therapist
Physical therapy aide
Physical therapy assistant
Physiologist
Prosthetic assistant
Prosthetic technician
Recreational therapist
Speech pathologist
Teacher of the blind
Teacher of the deaf
Teacher of the handicapped
Teacher of home therapy
Teacher of vocational training
Voice pathologist

Physical therapy assistants provide routine treatments under the supervision of a physical therapist. This work includes application of hot and cold packs, ultraviolet and infrared light treatments, ultrasound and electrical stimulation, and **hydrotherapy.** Assistants observe patients during treatment and record performance. Accredited programs that prepare physical therapy assistants require 2 years of college-level training and award an associate degree.

Kinesiotherapists work under the direction of a physician. They help patients strengthen and coordinate body movements using exercise. Kinesiotherapists specialize in maintaining muscle endurance, mobility, strength, and coordination. Their patients include those who are geriatric, have psychiatric needs, have physical or developmental disabilities, are striving for cardiac recovery, have been injured in sports, and have had amputations. Education for the kinesiotherapist includes a bachelor's degree in exercise physiology or physical education that includes an internship of at least 1000 hours of training. Certification is desirable but not required for all employment opportunities. National registration is available through the American Kinesiotherapy Association.

Orientation and mobility instructors or specialists help visually impaired and blind individuals to move about independently. Methods used to improve mobility include use of a cane, sensors, guide dogs, and electronic travel aids to help interpret the environment. A bachelor's degree is minimal for entry-level positions, and a master's degree is preferred. Certification for the orientation and mobility instructor is voluntary. Rehabilitation counseling provides the patient with career guidance and help in locating services that are needed for successful employment.

Orthotist and Prosthetist

Orthotist and prosthetist practitioner programs usually require a baccalaureate degree. Certification is available through the American **Orthotic** and **Prosthetic** Association after successful completion of an approved program, 1 year of experience, and a certification examination. Technicians help to produce the appliances designed by the professional, but they are not responsible for patient assessment. Registration is possible but not required for technicians.

Certified orthotists (COs) provide services for patients with disabling conditions of the limbs or spine. They design, fabricate, and fit braces or strengthening apparatus. Additionally, the orthotist supervises support personnel and laboratory activities necessary to develop new devices for straightening a distorted part (orthosis).

Certified prosthetists (CPs) provide care to patients with partial or total absence of a limb and who use an artificial limb **(prosthesis).** Responsibilities of the prosthetist in-

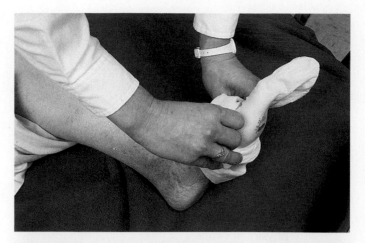
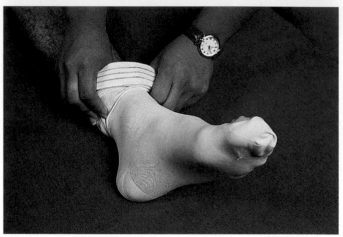

Figure 30-2 Elastic stockings help to prevent the development of emboli.

clude design, material selection, production, instruction on use, and evaluation of the appliance. *Myoelectronics* is the technical term for electromechanical prostheses. Myoelectronic technology amplifies and transfers nerve impulses from the body into electrical current to drive a motor. Parts of the body that have been lost can be replaced with artificial devices. Prostheses can also be specially designed for sports activities, including swimming, skiing, running, and climbing.

Corrective therapists conduct physical exercise programs to prevent muscle deterioration in inactive patients. The corrective therapist teaches the use of braces, crutches, and canes. Elastic stockings may be used for patients with limited mobility to decrease the chance of embolus development (Figure 30-2; Skill 30-1). Corrective therapists may complete bachelor's or master's degrees.

Pedorthists modify and provide footwear to patients with imperfectly formed feet. Some conditions that might require specially fitted shoes include arthritis, injury, and congenital defects. Pedorthists follow the prescription of a physician.

Skill 30-1

Applying Elastic Stockings

1. Maintain medical asepsis by using the guidelines provided in the Standard and Transmission-Based Precautions, including good handwashing technique and use of gloves as needed.

2. Verify physician's orders for usage of antiembolic or elastic stockings, which are used to prevent the development of blood clots in the legs.

3. Identify the patient and explain the procedure.

4. Raise the bed to a comfortable working height.

5. Position the patient in a supine position.

6. Expose the leg to be covered with the stocking while draping other parts of the body with linens.

7. Gather the stocking into one hand so that the toe of the foot can be inserted directly into the toe of the stocking.

8. Slip the stocking over the foot while supporting the foot in one hand and moving the stocking with the other. Adjust the stocking as needed so that the heel of the foot fits into the heel of the stocking.

9. Pull the stocking over the remainder of the leg, making sure it is not twisted or wrinkled. Twisting or wrinkling of the stockings may cause discomfort or cut off circulation to an area of the leg.

10. Repeat the procedure for the other leg.

11. Lower the bed. Position the patient for safety and comfort.

12. Record the time of stocking application. Antiembolic stockings are removed at intervals to allow free circulation of blood to the legs.

There are no educational requirements for this work, and it can be learned through seminars. Although not required, certification is recommended and is based on successful examination by the Board of Certification in Pedorthics.

Occupational Therapist

Occupational therapy helps patients reach the highest level of independent living by overcoming physical injury, birth defects, aging, or emotional and developmental problems. Occupational therapy uses activities to help a person develop, maintain, or regain skills that enable satisfying and independent living. Specific programs are developed to permit work, leisure, and play activities. Occupational therapists use adaptive equipment such as splints, wheelchairs, canes, walkers, and prosthetic devices. They evaluate patients, plan the programs, and supervise or provide treatment. Occupational therapists analyze an activity to determine the adaptive skills required for the patient to perform it. Occupational therapists may be registered after successful completion of an accredited 4-year baccalaureate program, a minimum of 6 months' clinical training, and a national examination. Master's and doctoral programs are available for specialized practice and top-level employment. Most states require licensure to practice as an occupational therapist.

Occupational therapy assistants may be trained in programs that include a minimum of 2 months of supervised field training. Occupational therapy assistants instruct and assist patients to perform activities of daily living (ADLs). Assistants help to design and adapt living and working environments to meet the needs of the disabled patient. Certification of occupational therapy assistants (COTA) is possible after completion of an approved 2-year program. Certification is obtained by passing a national examination. Occupational therapy aides are trained on the job. They assist with transportation, equipment assembly, and maintenance of work areas.

Athletic Trainer

Athletic trainers work under the supervision of the team physician in a variety of amateur and professional sports and other settings. High schools, colleges, professional sports teams, and other athletic agencies employ trainers. Many athletic trainers at the high school level also teach classes. The trainer's role includes prevention of injury and emergency treatment. Athletic trainers use methods that include corrective exercise, conditioning, rehabilitation, and nutrition counseling. Often the athletic trainer is also responsible for ordering and maintaining supplies and equipment for the training room.

The trainer works with the physician, athletes, and coaches and must be able to communicate well. The trainer must also possess manual dexterity and the ability to work in stressful situations. Athletic trainers work long and irregular hours.

There are about 90 undergraduate university programs for athletic trainers that include a minimum of an 1800-hour internship over at least 2 academic years. These programs may also lead to teaching certification in one of the sciences for physical education. Most athletic trainers who work for colleges or professional teams have a master's or doctoral degree. Certification of athletic trainers is available but not required.

Pharmacist

Pharmacists mix and **dispense** drugs according to prescriptions written by physicians, veterinarians, dentists, and other authorized professionals. They also provide information to the consumer about side effects of medications, food and drug interactions, dosing schedules, and health care supplies. **Pharmacology** prepares the professional as a specialist in the science of drugs. Six of every 10 pharmacists are employed in small community pharmacies. Hospital pharmacists may specialize in the areas of nuclear drugs, poison control, or intravenous therapy. The pharmacist must be good with detail and conscientious about checking and rechecking work. Accuracy, neatness, and cleanliness are very important to ensure safe medication. Accredited schooling in pharmacology lasts a minimum of 5 years after a minimum of 1 year of college-level preparation. Two degrees are awarded in pharmacology. The bachelor of science in pharmacology (BS Pharm) or the doctor of pharmacology (PharmD) qualifies an individual to take the licensing examination. The doctor of pharmacology degree is the highest level of entry to practice, requiring 6 years of education. Residency programs are available after graduation in general, clinical, and specialty areas.

Pharmacy technicians assist the pharmacist in processing prescriptions and distribution of medication. Skills of the pharmacy technician include maintaining inventory and packaging, labeling, ordering, and stocking supplies. Pharmacy technicians may attend a 1-year vocational or community college program.

Pharmacy helpers assist the pharmacist by waiting on patients and maintaining the inventory of supplies under the direction of the pharmacist and technician. There is no standard educational experience for a pharmacy helper and on-the-job training is possible.

The pharmaceutical industry also employs pharmacists for research and product development. These individuals are called *pharmacologists* or *toxicologists*. Pharmacologists differ from pharmacists because they work with the clinical science of how the drug works rather than preparing or dispensing medications. Pharmacologists generally earn a pharmacy or medical degree and then specialize in this area.

Another group who works with medications is pharmaceutical industry workers. They produce medicines, remedies, nutritional supplements, and health care products. Some examples of the duties of industry workers are filling and examining vials and ampules and running the machines that fill capsules. Many pharmaceutical companies offer on-the-job training, but employment is competitive. A bachelor's degree in one of the sciences may be required.

Speech and Language Pathologist

Speech and language pathology and **audiology** provide evaluation, treatment, and research in communication and related disorders. The certificate of clinical competence (CCC) is the only credential recognized by every state for speech and language pathologists and audiologists. Qualifications for the voluntary certification include successful completion of a master's degree, 9 months of supervised experience, and successful completion of a national examination. More than 35 states require licensure for speech and language pathologists and audiologists. Doctoral preparation is required for research and teaching on the university level.

Researchers in communications disorders have made great advances. These professionals also may be called *speech, language,* or *hearing scientists.* Research has led to the development of better hearing aids, electronic voice boxes, and other technological devices to assist communication.

Speech pathologists diagnose language problems. They also plan and direct treatment designed to overcome the problems. They treat disorders such as delayed language development, the inability to speak (aphasia), stuttering, and **articulation** problems. Speech pathologists complete a master's degree and an internship. For employment in a school, speech pathologists must also qualify for a teaching certificate.

Audiologists specialize in prevention, identification, assessment, and rehabilitation of hearing disorders. This work includes prescribing and dispensing hearing aids. Audiologists test hearing and determine the level of hearing function. They serve as consultants to the government in areas of noise pollution and environmental influences on hearing. Audiometrists screen hearing under the supervision of the audiologist. This work includes fitting earphones, providing instruction, and recording the results of testing. Audiometrists may be trained on the job.

Respiratory Therapist

Respiratory therapists evaluate the patient to administer respiratory care and operate life support equipment under the supervision of a physician (Figure 30-3). The therapist monitors the respiratory equipment and observes the patient's response to treatment. Some treatments performed by respiratory therapists include oxygen administration, incentive spirometry, tracheotomy care, and mechanical ventilation (Figure 30-4; Skill 30-2). Respiratory therapists are trained in vocational programs, community colleges, and universities. Certification and registration are possible after completion of a program approved by the American Medical Association in addition to 1 year of experience. Twenty-five states require licensure.

Respiratory therapy technicians administer routine respiratory care under the supervision of a therapist. Technician programs are usually found in community colleges and are 1 year in length. Respiratory therapy assistants do not give direct care to patients but help by cleaning and storing equipment.

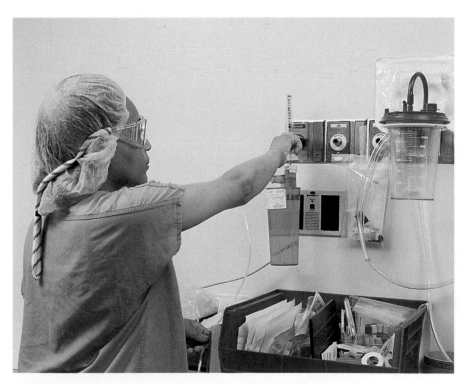

Figure 30-3   The rate of oxygen flow is ordered by the physician and is determined by the method of administration.

Skill 30-2

Assisting with Incentive Spirometry

1. Maintain medical asepsis by using the guidelines provided in the Standard and Transmission-Based Precautions, including good handwashing technique and use of gloves as needed.

2. Identify the patient and explain the procedure. Incentive spirometry is used to increase the breathing depth.

3. Instruct the patient to inhale deeply until the ball is raised to the top of the chamber and to hold the ball in that position for 6 seconds.

4. Instruct the patient to repeat this process 10 times.

5. The patient should repeat the procedure several times daily according to the physician's orders.

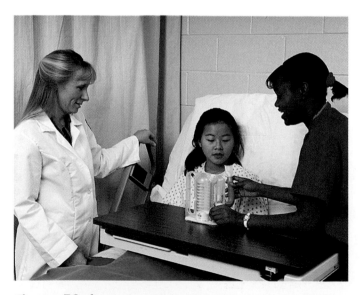

Figure 30-4   An incentive spirometer is used to help improve the depth of each inspiration.

Other Rehabilitative Personnel

Industrial rehabilitation specialists include vocational rehabilitation, manual arts, and horticultural therapists. Under the supervision of a physician, therapists in manual arts work to prevent physical deterioration of skills. Areas of training include woodworking, photography, metalworking, agriculture, electricity, and graphic arts. Employment as a manual arts therapist requires a bachelor's degree in the area of instruction plus experience.

Rehabilitation teachers work with blind and visually impaired adults. The visually impaired may need to learn Braille and how to organize the home for independent living. Use of community resources and management of activities may be taught by the rehabilitation teacher.

Art therapists use art activities as a method for nonverbal expression and communication to understand emotional conflicts and to promote personal growth. Entry-level education includes master's degree preparation in art and psychology with clinical training. Art therapists plan activities, provide instruction, and observe and record behavior. Most art therapists are employed in psychiatric clinics, but they also may work in extended care facilities or schools. National registration is possible for art therapists.

Dance and movement therapy uses movement to improve the emotional and physical rehabilitation of an individual. Dance therapy is a form of psychotherapy. It differs from educational and recreational dance by the focus on nonverbal behavior and use of movement as a method of intervention. Registered dance therapists (DTR) must complete graduate-level preparation and examination. Although licensure is not required, most dance therapists are licensed in a related field such as psychology.

Recreational therapists plan, organize, and direct medically approved recreation programs in hospitals and other institutions. The recreational therapist must design programs according to the abilities of the patient and record observations regarding the success of the activities. Educational programs for recreational therapists are available in community colleges and universities. Advanced degree preparation is necessary for top-level positions.

Music therapists plan, organize, and direct music activities and learning experiences for patients. The music therapist analyzes the patient's reaction to activities and records the findings. A bachelor's degree is the minimum for entry-level positions, and a master's degree is preferred for most employment opportunities.

Radiation therapy is the use of radiation to treat or relieve the pain of cancer and other diseases. The radiation technologist helps to plan and administer the treatment in addition to providing support for the patient. Education and training in this area may be completed in a 2-year community college or 4-year university. Some 1-year hospital based programs are available for graduates of a radiography program. The American Registry of Radiological Technicians certifies radiation therapists.

Dialysis technicians set up and run artificial kidneys for patients requiring assisted filtering of wastes from the blood. The dialysis technician must be familiar with sterile technique and follow instructions for the procedure exactly. Some of the job duties include monitoring vital signs and performing the venipuncture to start the dialysis. Dialysis technicians may be trained on the job.

The perfusionist, or extracorporeal circulation technician, manages the heart-lung machine during surgery and respiratory failure. The perfusionist works under the direction of the surgeon to regulate blood circulation and composition. During the extracorporeal circuit, the perfusionist may administer blood products, anesthetic agents, and drugs under the direction of the surgeon or anesthesiologist. The perfusionist monitors the oxygen and carbon dioxide content of the blood and may induce hypothermia by cooling the blood if so directed. Perfusionists are trained in programs, usually associated with a medical school, after a minimum of 1 year of college work in the basic sciences. Programs last from 1 to 2 years. Most perfusionists have been trained in a related health field such as medical technology, respiratory therapy, or nursing. Several states require licensure for the perfusionist. Certification through the American Board of Cardiovascular Perfusion is possible, after completion of acceptable education and training.

Content Instruction

Pharmacology

Pharmacology is the study of drugs, their actions, **dosages,** side effects, indications, and contraindications. Drugs are organic and inorganic materials that may be used for treatment or therapy in illness and injury. Prescription and administration of drugs are under the supervision of the Food and Drug Administration (FDA) of the federal government. Medications may be administered by licensed health care practitioners and by certain assistants under the supervision of a physician. Physicians, veterinarians, dentists, and their authorized agents such as physician assistants and nurse practitioners may prescribe medications. Enforcement of the drug laws is the responsibility of the Drug Enforcement Administration (DEA). The Controlled Substance Act of 1970 was enacted to regulate drugs capable of causing dependence. Medications that may be sold without a prescription are called *over-the-counter (OTC) drugs.*

Medications have generic, chemical, and trade names. The chemical name is based on the composition of the substance. The generic name is the common name of the drug, as consumers know it. The manufacturer owns the trade name. For example, the chemical name of a common drug that reduces fever (antipyretic) is acetylsalicylic acid. The generic name is aspirin. The drug may be bought over the counter under several brand- or trade-name labels. The trade name is registered and patented with the U.S. government. Drugs are classified according to the primary action that results in the body when used (Table 30-1).

Some common drug references used in pharmacology include the *United States Pharmacopoeia-Dispensing Information* (USP-DI) and the *Physician's Desk Reference* (PDR). The USP-DI is produced by a private group called the *United States Pharmacopeial Convention,* whereas the PDR is a collection of inserts from medications produced by pharmaceutical companies. The PDR is cross-referenced in sec-

Table 30-1   Common Drug Types and Actions

Drug Type	Action
Analgesic	Relieves pain
Anesthetic	Diminishes sensation
Antacid and acid reducer	Relieves excess stomach acid
Antibiotic	Combats infection
Anticholinergic	Blocks action of acetylcholine
Anticoagulant	Inhibits formation of clots
Anticonvulsive	Controls tremors and seizures
Antidepressant	Relieves mental depression
Antidiarrheal	Reduces diarrhea
Antiemetic	Reduces nausea
Antihistamine	Relieves allergic reactions
Antihypertensive	Reduces blood pressure
Antiinflammatory agent	Reduces inflammation
Antineoplastic agent	Destroys new growths
Antipyretic	Reduces fever
Antitussive	Reduces coughing
Bronchodilator	Opens respiratory tract
Central nervous system depressant	Reduces effects of central nervous system
Central nervous system stimulant	Relieves fatigue, elevates mood
Coagulant	Causes blood clotting
Decongestant	Constricts nasal membranes
Desensitization agent	Reduces allergic reactions
Diuretic	Reduces fluid in body
Emetic	Induces vomiting
Hormones and hypoglycemics	Balance hormonal components
Hypnotic	Produces sleep
Laxative	Induces fecal excretion
Sedative	Diminishes responses to stimuli
Sulfonamide	Cures bacterial infections
Vaccines and immunizations	Build immunity to infections
Vasodilator	Dilates blood vessels
Vitamins and minerals	Supplement inadequate diet

Table 30-2   Drug Administration Methods

Route	Description
Buccal	Inside the cheek; rapid administration
Inhalation	Breathed in the lungs; useful in dilating bronchial tubes
Internal	Inserted into a body opening (orifice); rapid absorption
Inunction	Applied topically; used mostly for dermatology conditions
Oral	Given by mouth; easy to administer; slow absorption
Parenteral	Injection; may be given into any layer of tissue—intradermal, intramuscular, intravenous, subcutaneous
Sublingual	Under the tongue; rapid absorption

tions that list the drugs by their manufacturer, brand name, generic name, and drug classification.

The dispensing of drugs must be correct to ensure the safety of their use. Prescriptions are valid when written on a printed form containing the name and address of the patient, date of the prescription, the superscription (Rx), list of ingredients (inscription), directions for preparation (subscription), directions for use (sig.), and physician's signature. The medication is labeled with the patient name, medication name, dosage, method of administration (route), and intervals for administration. Latin abbreviations and terms are used for prescriptions. Drugs may be administered by several routes (Table 30-2). Dosages are calculated using three systems of measurement (see Table 30-3).

Some medications are prepackaged or put into individual doses for convenience and accuracy before distribution. Techniques of medical asepsis are used during prepackaging to prevent contamination of medications. A laminar flow hood, which moves air in a parallel movement, may be used for some preparations to ensure cleanliness. All medications prepared for unit dosage are labeled with the drug name, amount, strength, dosage form, expiration date, and pharmacy control number.

Speech Pathology

Nearly 10 million people in the United States have speech and language disorders. Each year 60,000 people in the

United States lose the ability to speak (aphasia) because of stroke or head injury. The number of cases of laryngeal cancer increases by 8000 each year.

Speech disorders may result from congenital problems, illness, or injury. Some common speech disorders include difficulty with articulation (dysarthria), delayed speech, aphasia, cleft palate speech, stuttering, and voice problems. Speech problems may be detected with tests such as the *Wepman Auditory Discrimination Test,* which requires discrimination between similar sounding words. If the speech disorder is severe or permanent, manual or sign language can be learned for communication purposes (Figure 30-5).

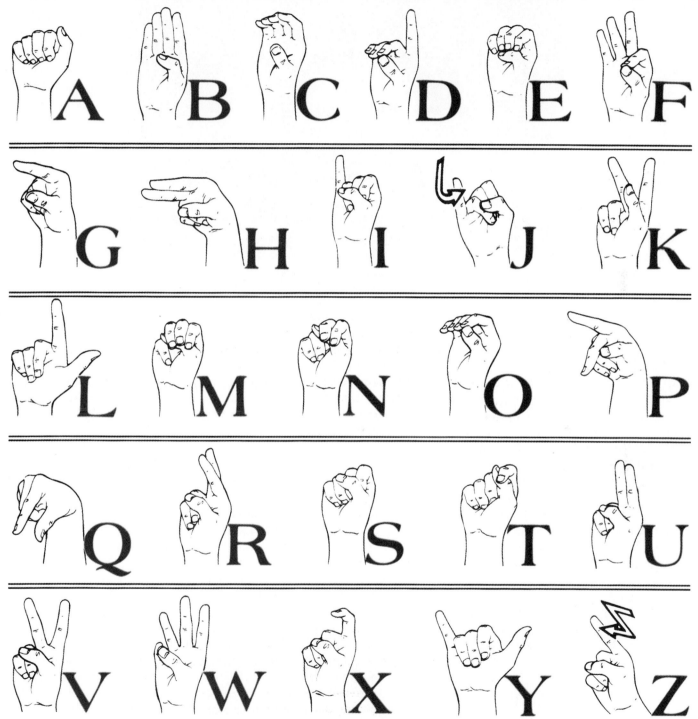

Figure 30-5   The manual alphabet is used as a form of communication by the majority of persons who do not hear. *(Courtesy The National Association for the Deaf, Silver Spring, Md.)*

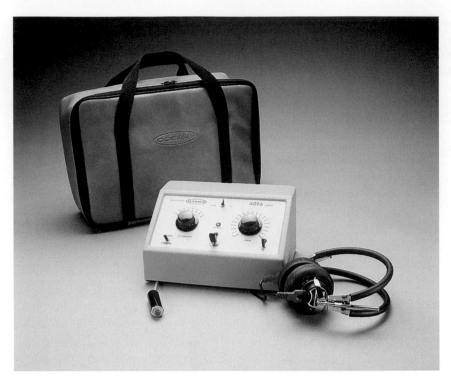

Figure 30-6 An audiometer is used to test hearing. *(Courtesy AMBCO Electronics, Tustin, Calif.)*

Hearing

More than 17 million people in the United States have hearing loss in one or both ears. Almost half of these people are older than 65 years of age. Hearing may be tested using an audiometer (Figure 30-6). Audiograms measure the ability to hear pure tones in each ear. A complete audiogram tests both bone conduction and air conduction. The bone conduction test measures the ability to hear a sound transmitted through bone, while the air conduction test determines the ability to hear sounds transmitted through the air. The results of the two tests may help determine whether hearing loss is due to an inability to conduct the sound (conductive hearing loss) or if it is due to the inner ear or nerve that sends sound signals to the brain (sensorineural hearing loss).

The flexibility of the eardrum may be measured using a tympanogram. This test measures the amount of sound reflected from the tympanic membrane at various levels of air pressure.

Respiratory Therapies

Breathing treatments include the intermittent positive pressure breathing (IPPB) procedure that increases the concentration of oxygen in the lungs. Pursed lip breathing is taught to prevent collapse of small air passages in the lungs. The procedure involves exhaling at a slow rate with lips shaped as for whistling to keep the pressure even. Chest physical therapy (CPT) includes postural drainage and percussion. Respiratory therapists may use percussion on the chest to loosen secretions or to determine the location of fluid or air in the respiratory system. Using a vibrator or striking the body with the fingers or hands to cause vibrations accomplishes percussion.

The amount of oxygen, carbon dioxide, and the pH value of the blood can be measured by using a blood gas analyzer. Respiratory personnel administer gases following the order of a physician. Gases that are used medicinally include oxygen, compressed air, and some air mixtures. The Department of Transportation (DOT) regulates the manufacture, testing, transportation, and marking of medical gas cylinders. The storage of cylinders is regulated to prevent fire and explosion of the gases. The cylinders containing medical gases are labeled by color to prevent confusion. Flow-regulating devices (flow meters) determine the amount of gas administered from the cylinders.

Oxygen may be delivered by several methods including nasal cannula or prongs, mask, and tent (Figure 30-7). Some masks are modified to allow insertion of medication. Humidifiers and **nebulizers** are used to administer water or medication into the lungs. Nebulizers are atomizers or devices that throw a spray of fluid. Humidifiers place moisture into the air that is breathed.

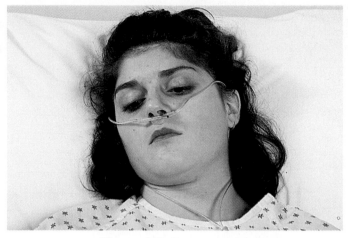 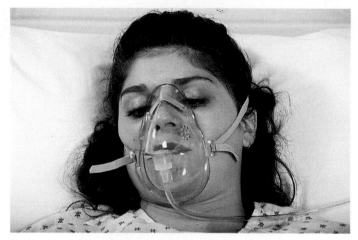

A   B

Figure 30-7   Methods of administration include **A**, nasal cannula or nasal prongs, and **B**, mask.

Performance Instruction

Application of Heat and Cold

Heat and cold applications are used in physical therapy to allow increased movement of joints. Heat and cold may be applied using aquamatic pads, ice bags, or water baths. Application must be done carefully as tissue may be damaged if the temperature is too extreme or maintained for too long. The skin on the area of application is checked frequently for redness, paleness, or blistering throughout the treatment (Figure 30-8).

Figure 30-8   Applications of heat and cold should never touch the skin directly.

Skill 30-3

Teaching Crutch Walking

1. Maintain medical asepsis by using the guidelines provided in the Standard and Transmission-Based Precautions, including good handwashing technique and use of gloves as needed.

2. Identify the patient and explain the procedure.

3. Measure the crutches for proper fit. The crutch length should be measured with the patient wearing walking shoes. The height is measured from 2 inches (5 cm) outside the tip of the toe and 6 inches (15 cm) ahead of this mark. The distance from this mark to 2 inches (5 cm) below the axilla is the proper crutch length.

Crutch Walking

Several gaits or methods of using crutches are possible. The type of injury and area that is not to bear weight during ambulation determine the method used. Crutches must be measured for proper fit while the patient is wearing walking shoes. Some examples of crutch gaits include the four-point, two-point, three-point, and tripod (Skill 30-3).

Medication Calculations

Medications may be given or administered only in a health care facility by licensed personnel. In some cases the medication dosage must be calculated using a conversion formula (Table 30-3). Accuracy of the conversion should be verified with another worker if possible.

Testing Hearing

To test hearing the patient is seated in a quiet room wearing the earphones of an audiometer. The machine is set to test each ear separately to detect sounds at 20 decibels (dB) and higher at a **frequency** of 1000 hertz (Hz). The procedure can be repeated at higher and lower frequencies. The patient indicates when the sound has been heard by raising a hand.

4. Teach the patient the four-point crutch gait sequence of right crutch, left foot, left crutch, right foot. There are several crutch gaits possible. The four-point gait is slow but stable. The patient must be able to move both legs separately and bear weight on each leg.

5. Teach the patient the two-point crutch gait sequence of right crutch and left foot followed by left crutch and right foot simultaneously. This method is faster but requires greater balance.

6. Teach the patient the three-point crutch gait sequence of simultaneously moving both crutches and the weaker extremity, followed by the stronger extremity. This is a rapid gait but requires that the arms be strong enough to support the entire body weight.

7. Teach the patient the tripod crutch gait sequence of both crutches forward followed by both legs swinging forward.

8. Instruct the patient to alternate methods to reduce fatigue and soreness.

Table 30-3 Conversion Units for Medications

Apothecary Units	Metric Units	Household Units
15-16 minims (min)	= 1 mL (cc)	
1 fluid dram	= 4 mL (cc)	= 1 teaspoon or 60 drops (gtts)
	16 mL	= 1 tablespoon
1 fluid ounce	= 30 mL	
1 quart (qt)	= 1000 mL (1 L)	
$\frac{1}{60}$ grain (gr)	1 mg	
1 gr	= 0.065 gram (g)	
15 gr	= 1 g	
2.2 lb	= 1 kg	
Examples	Because 1 kg = 2.2 lb, change pounds to kilograms by dividing the number of pounds by 2.2.	
	120 lb/2.2 kg = 54.05 kg	
	Because 1 ounce = 30 mL, change ounces to milliliters by multiplying the number of ounces by 30.	
	8 oz × 30 mL = 240 mL	

Review Questions

1. Use each of the following terms in one or more sentences that correctly relate their meaning.
   Dispense
   Dosage
   Frequency

2. Describe the function of the rehabilitative health care team.

3. Describe the role of each of the members of the rehabilitative health care team.

4. Describe the benefits of the wheelchair, crutches, Braille, sign language, and similar devices for the person with disabilities.

5. Describe two types of hearing loss and two methods used to assess hearing.

6. List 10 common categories of drugs and the action of each.

7. List the information needed to write a legal prescription.

8. Describe incentive spirometry, nebulizer, and percussion treatments.

Critical Thinking

1. Investigate and compare the cost of various types of treatments related to rehabilitative health care.

2. Contact the local city building inspector to obtain the specifications for construction of facilities for the disabled. Measure a public facility such as a restroom to determine if it meets the requirements of accessibility for the disabled.

3. Analyze a common activity of daily living such as eating a meal or changing clothes. Prepare a plan that would allow adaptation of the activity to meet the needs of an individual with varied disabilities.

4. Investigate a common speech disorder, including its cause and methods of improvement for the disorder.

5. Investigate the cost of educational preparation and job outlook for various rehabilitative health care personnel.

31

Emergency Health Careers

Learning Objectives

Define at least 10 terms related to emergency health care.

Specify the role of the emergency medical technician, and emergency room personnel, including personal qualities, levels of education, and credentialing requirements.

Identify three components of first aid.

Identify at least six types of external wounds and first aid treatment for each.

Identify at least three types of burns and first aid treatment for each.

Describe at least five ways in which poisoning may occur and first aid treatment for each.

Describe at least five causes of shock, the physical reaction to and first aid treatment for each.

Identify three types of fractures and first aid treatment for each.

Describe the effects of extreme cold and heat on the body and first aid treatment for each.

Describe the signs, symptoms, and treatment for a stroke and seizure activity.

Key Terms

Aspiration
(as-per-AY-shun) Act of inhaling foreign matter, usually emesis, into the respiratory tract

Aura
(ARE-uh) Subjective sensation or motor phenomenon that precedes and marks the onset of a seizure

Cardiopulmonary
(kar-dee-o-PUL-mun-ayr-ee) Pertaining to the heart and lungs

Consciousness
(KON-shus-ness) Responsiveness of the mind and to the impressions made by the senses

Critical
(KRIT-ih-kul) Pertaining to a crisis or danger of death

Endotracheal Intubation
(end-o-TRAKE-ee-ul in-too BAY-shun) Placing a tube within or through the trachea

Hemorrhage
(HEM-uh-ruj) Abnormal external or internal bleeding

Mottled
(MOT-uld) Spotted, with patches of color

Resuscitation
(ree-sus-ih-TAY-shun) Restoration of life or consciousness of a person who is apparently dead by using artificial respiration and cardiac massage

Seizure
(SEE-zhur) Sudden attack of a disease; uncontrolled muscle movements of epilepsy

Shock
(shok) Condition of acute failure of the peripheral circulation

Tourniquet
(TUR-nik-et) Instrument used to compress a blood vessel by application around an extremity

Toxin
(TOKS-in) Poison produced by animals, plants, or bacteria

Emergency Health Careers Terminology*

TERM	DEFINITION	PREFIX	ROOT	SUFFIX
Anaphylactic	Condition of not being protected against disease	an	aphylact	ic
Cardiopulmonary	Referring to the lungs and heart	cardio	pulmon	ary
Cyanoderm	Blue skin	cyan/o	derm	
Hematemesis	Vomiting of blood	hemat	eme	sis
Hemorrhage	Copious loss of blood		hemo	rrhage
Hypothermia	Condition of being below normal temperature	hypo	therm	ia
Midline	Median plane	mid	line	
Pneumothorax	Pertaining to the lungs and chest	pneumo	thorax	
Semiconscious	Partially aware of sensations	semi	consc	ious
Ventral	Abdomen; front side		ventr	al

*A transition phrase or vowel may be added to or deleted from the word parts to make the combining form.

Abbreviations for Emergency Health Careers

ABBREVIATION	MEANING
ACLS	Advanced cardiac life support
AED	Automated external defibrillator
AHA	American Heart Association
AKA	Above knee amputation
ARC	American Red Cross
EMT-A	Emergency medical technician—ambulance
EMT-I	Emergency medical technician—intermediate
EMT-P	Emergency medical technician—paramedic
ER	Emergency room
Fx	Fracture

Box 31-1 Emergency Health Careers

Ambulance attendant
Emergency medical technician
Emergency medical services coordinator
First-aid attendant
Flight nurse
Flight surgeon
Hospital entrance attendant
Paramedic

Careers

Accidents are one of the five leading causes of death in the United States. They account for 50% of the fatalities of those 15 to 24 years of age. Injuries can result from automobile and home accidents, falls, fires, explosions, natural disasters, and industrial mishaps. Snow, water, and other athletic sports also account for injuries that require emergency care. Common injuries caused by accidents include bone fractures, cuts, poisoning, reactions to heat and cold, problems associated with medical conditions, and loss of vital functions.

The goal of modern emergency care is immediate aid, or first aid, at the scene of injury rather than just the transportation of the victim to a medical facility. Levels of care have developed to provide this immediate care. These include the bystanders or first responders with knowledge of first aid and **cardiopulmonary resuscitation** (CPR), emergency medical technicians, and advanced emergency personnel (Box 31-1). Emergency medical services (EMS) are present in many communities. The EMS system is a coordinated response by all levels of practitioners to accidents and sudden illness. In most areas of the United States, emergency medical services are

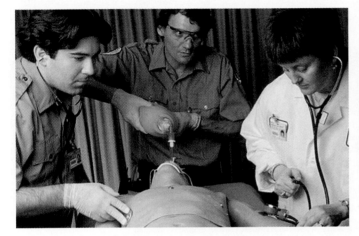

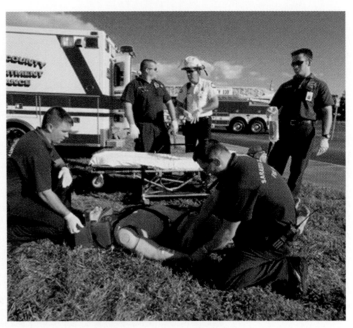

Figure 31-1   The Human Patient Simulator is used as a learning tool for EMTs. The lifelike mannequin physically represents the patient. Clinical features (such as palpable pulses and heart sounds, monitored parameters, electrocardiogram, and pulmonary artery catheter) bring the patient to life. Sophisticated physiological models of the body systems simulate normal and pathophysiological responses to drugs, mechanical ventilation, and other therapies. *(Courtesy Medical Education Technologies, Sarasota, Fla.)*

initiated by the use of the 9-1-1 telephone call. Personnel answering 9-1-1 calls are trained to determine the type of rescue personnel needed, location of the emergency, and other pertinent information. In some instances, they may even be able to direct the caller on methods for giving aid to the victim.

Emergency Medical Technician

Emergency medical technicians (EMTs) work under the supervision of a physician to provide care to the acutely ill or injured person in the prehospital setting. They respond to medical emergencies, give immediate care, and transport the victim to the hospital. Technicians also maintain the rescue vehicles and equipment. Some emergency medical technicians are employed by ambulance companies, emergency centers, and in industry. There are four classifications of emergency technicians recognized by the National Registry of Emergency Medical Technicians (NREMT): the First Responder, EMT-Basic, EMT-Intermediate, and EMT-Paramedic.

All emergency medical technicians must be alert to details and be able to manipulate small objects skillfully. The job is physically demanding and requires heavy lifting. The work is usually arranged in shifts and includes irregular hours.

The role of the EMT-First Responder is to provide care in cases of acute illness and injury until more qualified per-

sonnel are available. Skills such as CPR, first aid for fractures and bleeding, treatment of **shock**, and assistance with childbirth are included in the training (Figure 31-1).

EMT-Basic personnel perform all of the skills of the EMT-First Responder. In addition, the EMT-Basic may care for the person at an accident scene and provide transport in an ambulance.

In addition to the training of the EMT-Basic, the EMT-Intermediate (EMT-I) may establish intravenous lines, assess trauma victims, and apply inflatable antishock garments.

The EMT-P, or paramedic, provides advanced life support. The paramedic must be skilled in all the duties of the other EMT personnel, as well as in monitoring electrocardiograph readings and defibrillation. EMT-P may be employed by fire and police departments or may act as community volunteers. Paramedics may administer medications and perform **endotracheal intubation.**

Some states vary in their requirements for emergency medical technician training, which may limit EMT's opportunities to move to other areas. In some states, applicants must be at least 18 years of age and have a high school diploma. Standards for the educational requirements of EMTs are set by the U.S. Department of Transportation. Thirty-eight states require registration with the National Registry of Emergency Medical Technicians for certification. Training also includes a supervised internship. Certification of EMTs is required by all states. Proof of continuing education is required for recertification.

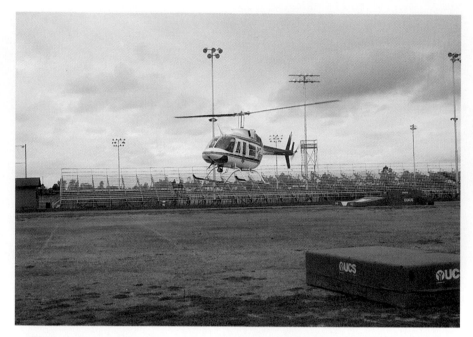

Figure 31-2 The helicopter is used in emergencies to transport victims.

EMT personnel may be categorized into four levels. When this type of naming system is used, the lowest level is the EMT-First Responder. These individuals have training in basic first aid and might be firefighters, policemen, or others who are the first to respond to an emergency. The first level of the emergency medical technician training system is the EMT-1, which is the same as the EMT-Basic. The EMT-Intermediate is divided into two levels (EMT-2 and EMT-3), depending on the training received. The EMT-4 level is the EMT-paramedic.

Other Emergency Personnel

Flight rescue professions have evolved as a career opportunity with the use of helicopters to transport victims to emergency facilities (Figure 31-2). The emergency rescue team usually includes a nurse and a paramedic. It may also include a respiratory therapist.

The minimum requirement for flight nursing includes being a registered nurse with several years of **critical** care experience. Advanced certified life support (ACLS) and critical care certification (CCRN) are often required of the registered nurse. Most emergency rescue facilities provide clinical and classroom instruction covering the specific training relating to flight and air rescue. Flight paramedics are also required to hold ACLS certification and have prior field experience. National Registry Paramedic Certification and previous flight experience are preferred in most employment opportunities. Flight respiratory therapists must be certified and have critical care experience. It is preferred

that candidates for flight rescue be registered respiratory therapists.

On arrival at the hospital the victim is admitted by the emergency personnel. Treatment is continued by emergency nurses and physicians who specialize in emergency and trauma care. Emergency medicine was recognized as a board-certified specialty for physicians in 1979.

Content Instruction

Emergency Procedures

First aid is the immediate care given to the victim of injury or sudden illness. The purpose of first aid is to sustain life and prevent death. It includes the prevention of permanent disability and the reduction of time needed for recovery. First aid provides basic life support and maintenance of vital functions.

Certification in first aid is awarded by several accredited agencies, including the American Red Cross and the American Heart Association. Content of the Red Cross course includes basic first aid for injuries, illness, and cardiopulmonary resuscitation (CPR) procedures.

Basic first aid training includes prevention, assessment, and treatment of illness and injury. *Triage* is the term used for setting priorities for care of the victim or victims. First aid training teaches treatment of wounds, poisoning, burns, shock, fractures, temperature alterations, illness caused by medical conditions, and other injuries.

Table 31-1   Emergency Assessment and Treatment

Emergency	What to Do	Why
Triage	1. Remove victim from immediate danger	It should be assumed that neck and back injuries have occurred in all accidents; move the victim only if in immediate danger
	2. Check level of consciousness	
	3. Establish an airway if needed	
	4. Check pulse and breathing	
	5. Treat severe bleeding	Severe loss of blood can lead to shock and death within minutes
	6. Treat poisoning	
	7 Treat burns	
	8. Treat for the signs and symptoms of shock; apply a blanket and do not give any beverages	Alcohol may cause greater injury or prevent medical personnel from providing treatments immediately
	9. Treat fractures	
	10. Treat other injuries as needed	

Emergency Assessment and Treatment

The first aid rescuer assesses the scene of injury or illness to determine the necessary action (Table 31-1). The first priority of the rescuer is to remove the victim from any immediate danger (Figure 31-3). The level of **consciousness** of the victim is the second consideration. An airway is established and pulse is assessed. The EMS system is activated at the earliest moment after breathing and circulation have been established or attempted. In most areas of the United States, the 9-1-1 emergency number may be used to summon help. When reporting an incident, the rescuer states the location, his or her name, the number of victims involved, and the nature of the incident. The rescuer waits for the EMS to disconnect the phone first. Because the rescuer may be visiting in the victim's home, all homeowners should place their name and address on each phone.

If there is more than one victim, the unconscious victim takes priority over the conscious one. If all victims are breathing and have a pulse, bleeding is the next consideration, then burns and other injuries.

Wounds

Wounds result when tissue is damaged externally or internally (Table 31-2). An example of an internal wound is a contusion, or bruise. Six types of external wounds result in different bleeding situations. These wound classifications are abrasion, incision, laceration, puncture, avulsion, and amputation.

Abrasions result from the scraping of skin or mucous membrane from the surface of the body. Bleeding from an abrasion is minimal, but infection may result. An incision is a cut made with a surgical instrument, knife, or glass. It results in a wound with straight edges. Bleeding is rapid and heavy. Lacerations are irregularly shaped cuts made with a sharp object and, of the various wounds, lacerations generally bleed the most. When bleeding has been controlled, bandages protect the wound from infection (Figure 31-4).

Puncture wounds are made when an object pierces the skin. The skin may close around the area and limit the bleeding. Punctures provide a high risk of infection. An avulsion is the traumatic tearing away of part of the body. Bleeding is rapid and heavy. The body part may be reattached or reinserted in some instances. An amputation is the surgical severing or cutting away of part of the body.

Bleeding occurs from all three types of blood vessels. Arterial bleeding is bright red and pulses as the heart beats and is the most serious type. Venous blood is darker in color and does not pulse. Capillary bleeding oozes at the surface of the skin. Shock and loss of consciousness can result from loss of blood in a short amount of time.

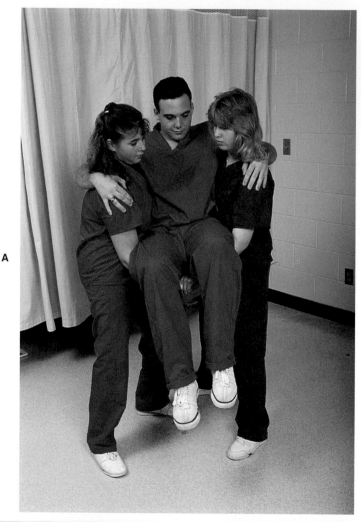

A

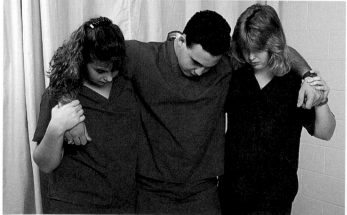

B

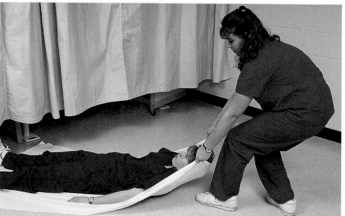

C

Figure 31-3   If the victim of an emergency must be moved, triage determines the correct method. **A,** The two-man carry. **B,** The two-man assistance. **C,** The one-man transfer.

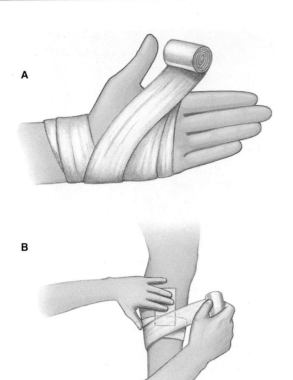

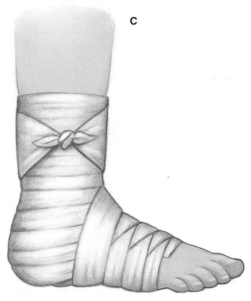

Figure 31-4   Methods of bandaging vary with the areas of injury. **A**, A simple figure eight. **B**, A dressing held in place with wrapping toward the heart. **C**, The tie is placed to locate the area of injury.

Table 31-2   Wounds

Emergency	What to Do	Why
Bleeding wound	1. Apply direct pressure to the wound using the cleanest dressing or hand available	Most bleeding can be stopped by direct pressure to the wound
	2. Do not remove the dressing	Dressing removal may interrupt clot formation
	3. Elevate the injured area	Elevation reduces the blood pressure and flow to the area
	4. Apply pressure to the pressure point closest to the wound	Direct pressure, elevation, and pressure on the artery control bleeding in 90% of all cases
	5. Apply a tourniquet above the level of the wound only as a last resort; use only if loss of life may occur from further blood loss. **Once applied, a tourniquet must never be removed**	A tourniquet may damage tissues beyond repair
	6. Cool any avulsed tissue or parts and transport them with the victim. **Do not place tissues directly on ice**	Many parts can be reattached if preserved from further tissue damage

Burns

Burns may result from exposure to heat, chemicals, or radiation (Table 31-3). The severity of a burn is determined by the location, depth, and size (Figure 31-5). Injury to the face, arms, legs, and genitals are the most critical. Burns that cover more than 10% of the body surface generally require hospitalization. Burns are classified into three degrees according to their depth.

First-degree burns affect only the outer layer of skin tissue. The skin becomes red and discolored, and some slight swelling may occur. Healing of first-degree burns is generally rapid. Examples of a first-degree burn are sunburn and the burn caused by immersing part of the body very briefly into hot water.

A second-degree burn is one that breaks the surface of the skin and injures the underlying tissue. Second-degree burns may result from a severe sunburn and exposure to hot liquids or heat. The appearance of blisters commonly indicates a second-degree burn. The skin is red or **mottled** in appearance. The skin may become wet when plasma is lost through the damaged skin. There is greater pain and swelling with this type of burn.

Third-degree burns are deep enough to damage the nerves and bones. Tissue burned to the third degree is charred and white in color. There may be less pain from a third-degree burn because the nerves are damaged. Third-degree burns may result from exposure to fire, very hot water, hot objects, or electricity.

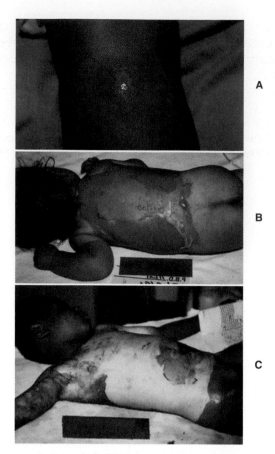

A

B

C

Figure 31-5   For legend see opposite page.

Table 31-3   Burns

Emergency	What to Do	Why
First-degree burn	1. Immerse affected area in cool water	
	2. Apply a dressing to the area	
Second-degree burn	1. Immerse affected area in cool water	
	2. Do not open blisters or apply ointments	Open wounds or ointments may increase the risk of infection
	3. Elevate the affected area	Elevation reduces swelling
	4. Seek medical attention if the affected area is large	
Third-degree burn	1. Do not remove any clothing adhering to the burn	Removing clothing can lead to tissue damage and fluid loss
	2. Cover the burn with a clean, dry dressing	Dressing the wound reduces pain and risk of infection
	3. Elevate if possible	
	4. Do not apply ointments, water, or butter	This application may increase the risk of infection
	5. Seek medical attention as soon as possible	Third-degree burns must be treated to prevent infection and permanent damage to tissues

Figure 31-5, cont'd   Thermal burns are those caused by contact with hot liquids, objects, electricity, or fire. They are classified according to the depth of damage to the skin. **A,** First-degree burns are minor, involving only the outer layers of the skin (epidermis). **B,** Second-degree burns affect the deeper layers of the epidermis and dermis and are very painful. **C,** Third-degree burns are those that affect not only the skin but also the muscle and bone. *(Courtesy St. John's Mercy Medical Center, St Louis, Mo.)*

Poisoning

Poisoning may occur in several ways and most poisoning occurs in the home (Table 31-4). Poison can be ingested, inhaled, absorbed, injected, or obtained by radiation. Ingestion is the taking in of a substance by eating or drinking. Signs and symptoms of poisoning include discoloration or burns on the lips, unusual odor, vomiting (emesis), or presence of a suspicious container.

Table 31-4	Poisoning	
Emergency	**What to Do**	**Why**
Ingestion	1. Save the suspected source of poison	EMS personnel can estimate type and amount of toxin ingested
	2. If at home, give the victim water or milk (if the victim is conscious without convulsions)	If unconscious, the victim may be in danger or aspiration (breathing of vomitus into the lungs)
	3. Contact poison control or the emergency room for a suggested treatment; if vomiting is suggested, give syrup of ipecac (vomit inducer) and then water. **Do not induce vomiting if poison is an acid, alkali, or petroleum product**	Tissue damage may occur as the substance passes through the esophagus again
	4. If the poison is a medicine, do not give anything by mouth without professional advice	A counteractive treatment may be administered
Inhalation	1. Move the victim to fresh air	
	2. Establish an airway; loosen clothing	Using the head-tilt chin-lift method to open an airway avoids injury to the spinal column
	3. Begin mouth-to-mouth artificial respiration if breathing is absent; give one breath every 5 seconds for adults and one breath every 3 seconds for children and infants	The rate of breathing, determined by the victim's age, provides adequate oxygen
Contact	1. Flood affected area with water for at least 10 minutes; cleanse with soap; do not attempt to neutralize the toxin with acids or alkalis	
	2. Remove contaminated clothing and jewelry	Clothing and jewelry will continue to poison the skin if left in place
	3. Flush a contaminated eye from the inner to the outer aspect for at least 20 minutes; do not force the eye open	Flushing from the inner to the outer aspect prevents contamination of the other eye

Table 31-5 Inadequate Circulation Due to Shock

Emergency	What to Do	Why
Shock	1. Eliminate cause if possible	
	2. Keep the victim lying down with feet slightly elevated (8 to 12 inches)	Elevating the legs allows blood to accumulate around the heart and brain
	3. Maintain the airway	
	4. Cover the victim with a blanket	Covering the victim helps maintain body temperature that has been lowered by reduced circulation
	5. Do not give any fluids to the victim	Victims of traumatic injury may require surgery; fluids can be a significant risk in such cases

Shock

Shock is the response of the cardiovascular system to the presence of adrenalin resulting in capillary constriction (Table 31-5). It may result in inadequate circulation to the body tissues, lowered blood pressure, and decreased kidney function. Shock can result from trauma, electrical injury, insulin shock, **hemorrhage,** or as a reaction to drugs. It may occur in conjunction with other injuries or illness such as respiratory distress, fever, heart attack, and poisoning. Anaphylactic shock is the response of the body to an allergen such as a medication.

Early signs and symptoms of shock include pale and clammy skin, weakness, and restlessness. The pulse and respiratory rate are rapid, and vomiting may occur. Late signs of shock include apathy, unresponsiveness, dilated pupils, mottled skin, and loss of consciousness. Shock may result in death if the condition is not reversed.

Fractures

Breakage of a bone is called a *fracture* (Table 31-6). Fractures can be classified as closed or open (Figure 31-6). Simple, or closed, fractures do not penetrate the skin. In open, or compound, fractures the bone breaks through the skin and is exposed. Open fractures present a greater chance of infection.

Other injuries to the bones and muscle tissue include muscle strains, sprains, and dislocation. Muscle strains result from injury to the muscle tissue, usually from overuse. Muscle strain causes pain and possibly cramping on movement. Sprains result from injury to the ligaments, or the attachments between the muscle and bones. Sprains result in a rapid swelling and pain when the joint is moved. Dislocation occurs when a bone moves out of a joint. Signs and symptoms of dislocation include swelling, pain, and discoloration.

Table 31-6   Fractures

Emergency	What to Do	Why
Closed fracture	1. Splint the fracture in the position found	Immobilization reduces pain and risk of injury
	2. Seek medical attention as soon as possible	Fractures must be set to prevent deformity
Open fracture	1. Stop the bleeding if necessary; do not replace a protruding bone in the tissues	Movement may damage tissues
	2. Immobilize the fracture	Immobilization reduces pain and further injury

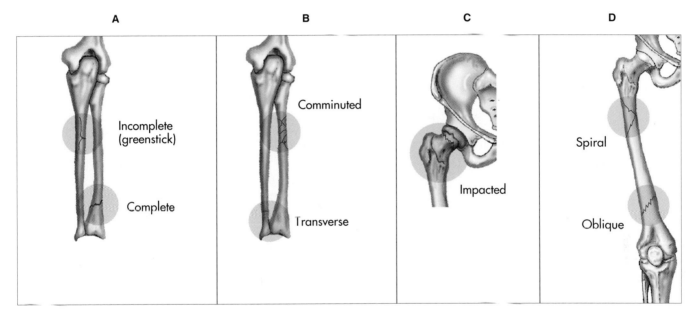

Figure 31-6   Types of fractures. **A,** Incomplete (greenstick) and complete. **B,** Comminuted and transverse. **C,** Impacted. **D,** Oblique and spiral. *(From Sanders MJ:* Mosby's paramedic textbook, *ed 2, St Louis, 2000, Mosby.)*

Temperature Alteration

The human body works well at a specified temperature (Table 31-7). If the temperature varies too much, the body cannot function. Exposure to heat can result in muscle cramping, heat exhaustion, or heat stroke. Muscle cramping results from an electrolyte imbalance caused by loss of salt from sweating. Muscle cramping causes pain and inability to use the muscle.

Signs and symptoms of heat exhaustion include perspiration (diaphoresis) and pale and clammy skin, even though the body temperature is normal. The victim may feel weak and nauseated.

In heat stroke, the skin is dry and flushed in appearance. The pulse is fast and strong. The internal temperature can rise to 106° F or more, resulting in death of brain tissue. Death may result from heat stroke if it is not treated quickly.

Table 31-7   Temperature Alteration

Emergency	What to Do	Why
Heat cramps	1. Massage the affected muscle area	Massage increases circulation and brings oxygen to the tissues
	2. Administer small amounts of salty water	Salt helps retain water; lack of water usually causes heat cramps
Heat exhaustion	1. Move victim to a cooler area	The reduction of temperature is the best treatment
	2. Sponge the skin with cool water	
	3. Seek medical attention	
Heat stroke	1. Move victim to a cooler area	
	2. Immerse in cool water or apply ice packs	
	3. Monitor vital signs; seek medical attention	Heat stroke results in life-threatening increase in body temperature and may cause death if not treated immediately
Hypothermia	1. If necessary, remove victim from cold water	
	2. Remove wet clothing	Wet clothing retains cold temperatures
	3. Cover the victim with a warm blanket or immerse in water	
	4. Give warm fluids if the victim is conscious	
	5. Monitor vital signs; seek medical attention	
Frostbite	1. Bring victim inside	Continued exposure to cold increases the tissue damage
	2. Cover the affected area with a blanket or cloth or immerse in slightly warm water; **do not rub**	Rubbing may damage the frozen tissue and increase the risk of gangrene infection
	3. Give warm fluids if the victim is conscious	
	4. Discontinue warming when skin becomes flushed	Swelling occurs as the tissues recover
	5. Elevate and cover the affected area loosely with a dry dressing	

Exposure to cold temperatures can result in frostbite or hypothermia. Frostbite occurs when the water in the body tissues freezes. When the tissue does not get oxygen because of the freezing, the tissue will die. The tissues of the nose, ears, fingers, and toes are the most susceptible. Early signs and symptoms of frostbite include redness and tingling. As damage progresses, the tissue becomes pale and numb.

Hypothermia is an abnormal lowering of body temperature, usually resulting from immersion in cold water or being stranded in subzero weather. Signs and symptoms include shivering, numbness, confusion, paleness, and eventual loss of consciousness.

Miscellaneous Injuries

Other injuries include those to the eyes, nose, jaw, neck, and chest and to those who are drowning (Table 31-8). These injuries may require special treatment techniques. Any object that penetrates the body should not be removed until professional medical help is available.

Bites can occur from animals or insects. Bites caused by animals and humans require medical attention to ensure prevention of infection and possibly to reattach a severed part. Snake or insect bites require medical attention if the venom is poisonous.

Table 31-8   Miscellaneous Injuries

Emergency	What to Do	Why
Nosebleed	1. Have victim sit up or lie down with head and shoulders raised	Raising the head decreases the blood flow to the area
	2. Lean the head forward slightly	
	3. Apply direct pressure against the bleeding nostril at the midline	Most bleeding can be stopped with direct pressure
	4. Apply a cold compress to the face and nose	The reduced temperature decreases blood flow to that area
Near drowning	1. Remove the victim from the water	
	2. Assess respirations; if heartbeat is absent, begin CPR	
	3. Keep the victim as cool as possible	Reduction in body temperature decreases the need for oxygen
Penetrating eye injury	1. Do not rub or rinse the injured eye	
	2. Do not remove foreign objects	
	3. Keep victim lying flat	
	4. Cover both eyes loosely with clean dressing, paper cups, or a similar device that does not place pressure on the eyes	Movement of the eye may cause further damage; both eyes are covered because the eyes move together when just one is covered
Insect and snake bites	1. Keep the victim lying flat with the affected part higher than the level of the heart	Raising the area of the bite slows circulation to and from that area
	2. Apply a band that constricts part of the circulation above the level of the bite	The constricting should not cut off circulation because tissue damage could occur
	3. Apply an ice pack to the area of the bite	Ice can reduce circulation of blood and toxins through the body
	4. Seek medical treatment of bites from poisonous snakes and insects	Toxin damage may not be evident

Marine Injuries

With the increase in numbers of people pursuing marine sports such as skin and scuba diving, safety and first aid measures for this particular area has become more important (Table 31-9). Most injuries by marine life and during diving are caused by the victim, because aquatic life is rarely aggressive. The Divers Alert Network (DAN) provides insurance and consultation for members regarding marine injuries throughout the world.

In scuba diving, air embolism and decompression illness resulting from rapid ascent is a major concern. A diver should never rise to the surface faster than the air bubbles and must breathe continuously during descent and ascent and take a precautionary decompression stop at 15 feet for 3 minutes at the end of all dives. Additionally, divers should always have a "buddy" who is within sight at all times. Treatment of decompression sickness and air embolism requires immediate, specialized advanced life support techniques of a recompression chamber to restore the normal composition of air in the blood.

Aquatic life differs from one ocean location to another, so consultation with local health care professionals and divers is important in determining treatment (Figure 31-7). The three main types of marine injuries are stings, punctures, and bites. Puncture wounds might be caused by sea urchins, stingrays, or spiny fish that are stepped on or touched. Stings from jellyfish or coral may occur when touched. Aquatic life may be venomous (designed to kill prey) or poisonous (causing harm if eaten because of **toxins** in the tissues). Some aquatic animals, including fish, bite when threatened or if food is held in the diver's hand.

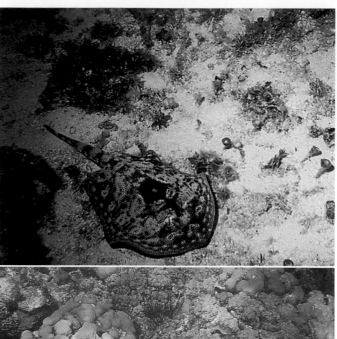

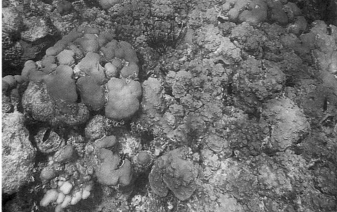

Figure 31-7   Aquatic life can contribute to marine injuries.

Table 31-9   Aquatic Injuries

Emergency	What to Do	Why
Marine injuries	1. Treat all victims of aquatic injury for the signs and symptoms of shock	
	2. If possible, remove any materials from puncture and stings from the wound	Projectiles with toxin continue to poison the wound
	3. Soak the wound in warm water for 20 minutes	Water will help remove toxins
	4. Pain may be relieved with vinegar or diluted ammonia and an application of baking soda paste	Other home remedies include a paste of meat tenderizer and water
	5. Bites are treated to control the bleeding	
	6. Seek medical attention if the wound is severe or if there is an allergic reaction	

Table 31-10   Medical Conditions

Emergency	What to Do	Why
Stroke	1. Assess and establish vital functions	Strokes often affect vital functions
	2. Activate EMS system	Medical attention is a priority
	3. Treat the victim for the signs and symptoms of shock	
	4. Position the victim on the affected side	Secretions may block the airway
Seizure	1. Prevent the victim from self-injury by cushioning the head and arms if possible; do not restrain the victim	The victim does not recognize the damage done by movement; restraining may lead to injury
	2. Observe and monitor vital functions; do not insert anything into the mouth	Respirations may stop during a grand mal seizure, but they could resume in the clonic phase; items placed in the mouth may cause further injury and obstruction of the airway
	3. Assist the victim to lie on the side or abdomen as seizure activity subsides	Saliva may accumulate in the mouth and may cause choking

Medical Conditions

First aid may be necessary in the case of illness caused by a sudden medical condition such as a stroke or a **seizure** activity (Table 31-10). Strokes, or cerebrovascular accidents, occur from spontaneous rupture of a blood vessel or clot formation in the brain. Signs and symptoms may include loss of consciousness, paralysis, difficulty breathing, slurred speech, loss of bladder control, and unequal pupil size. The condition may threaten the victim's life.

Seizure, or uncontrolled muscle activity, may be preceded by an **aura** and may occur in several patterns. Convulsions are the uncoordinated movement of groups of muscles usually resulting from poisoning (drug overdose) or elevated temperature. Coordinated seizure activity may occur in individuals with epilepsy. The International Classification of Epileptic Seizures divides seizures into two types based on the area of the brain from which they originate. Partial seizures start in a specific area of the brain and may cause motor or sensory symptoms such as automatic actions, hallucinations, or twitching of muscle groups. Tonic-clonic (grand mal), absence (petit-mal), and myoclonic seizures involve larger areas of the brain and are categorized as general. Uncontrolled movement of the body and loss of consciousness may occur with generalized seizures.

Performance Instruction

All emergency workers use substance isolation precautions to prevent the spread of microorganisms. This includes the use of gloves when body fluids are touched or breaks are present on the skin. Body fluids include blood, urine, vomitus, feces, and any materials contaminated by these substances. The hands are washed thoroughly after the gloves are removed. Masks, goggles, or face shields may be worn if splattering of body secretions is possible. Barrier devices such as resuscitation masks are used to administer mouth-to-mouth breathing.

Some of the methods of emergency care may be performed by bystanders or first responders trained in first aid. These include the assessment of the type and severity of injuries or triage. If breathing and heartbeat are absent from any victim, cardiopulmonary resuscitation or CPR is initiated (Table 31-11; Skills 31-1 and 31-2). After establishing the order of treatment of victims involved in the emergency, bleeding is treated first. Most bleeding from wounds may be stopped with a combination of direct pressure and elevation of the wounded area. Pressure may also be placed on the major arteries that supply the affected

Skill 31-1

Performing Cardiopulmonary Rescue*

1. Maintain medical asepsis by using the guidelines provided in the Standard and Transmission-Based Precautions, including good handwashing technique and use of gloves as needed.

2. Check to see if the person is responsive by gently shaking him or her and shouting.

3. Call 9-1-1 or have someone else do it.[†]

4. Get an AED[‡] if available.

5. Open the victim's airway by using a head tilt-chin lift movement. (Use a jaw thrust technique if the victim may have a neck injury.)

6. Look at the victim's chest to see if it is moving. Listen and feel for air from the victim's airway.

7. If the victim is not breathing, give two slow rescue breaths. (Use a barrier device if available.)

8. Check for circulation by feeling the carotid artery for no more than 10 seconds.

9. If no pulse is found, provide cycles of 15 chest compressions to 2 rescue breaths until the victim recovers or you are instructed to stop by advanced emergency personnel. (Check for a pulse after the first minute of compressions and ventilations.)

10. If the victim recovers and there are no other signs of injury to the back or neck, turn the victim to his or her side.

11. Continue monitoring breathing until instructed to stop by advanced emergency personnel.

---

*These are general guidelines for administering CPR. An authorized course given by the American Heart Association or American Red Cross should be successfully completed before using this skill.

[†]Two-rescuer CPR may be performed. One rescuer assesses the victim and performs breathing while the other performs chest compressions using the same ratio of chest compressions to breaths (15:2).

[‡]Automated External Defibrillators (AEDs) can be safely used by lay rescuers with a few hours of training. When the device is attached to the victim with two adhesive pads, it analyzes the heart activity and determines whether shock is necessary.

Table 31-11   Differences in CPR Between Adults, Children, and Infants*

Action	Adult (more than 8 years old)	Child (1 to 8 years old)	Infant (less than 1 year old)
Activate EMS	Activate EMS as soon as victim is found	Give 1 minute of CPR then activate EMS	Give 1 minute of CPR then activate EMS
Breaths	2 seconds each; 10 to 12 per minute	1 to 1 1/2 seconds each; 20 per minute	1 to 1 1/2 seconds each; 20 per minute
FBAO	Abdominal thrusts	Abdominal thrusts	Back blows or chest compressions
Pulse assessment	Carotid pulse	Carotid pulse	Brachial pulse
Compressions	Landmark is lower half of sternum; use heel of one hand with other hand on top; 1 1/2 to 2 inches depth; 100 per minute	Landmark is lower half of sternum; use heel of one hand; 1/3 to 1/2 depth of chest; 100 per minute	Landmark is one finger width below nipple line; use two fingers; 1/3 to 1/2 depth of chest; at least 100 per minute
Compression-ventilation ratio	15:2	15:2	5:1

*These are general guidelines for administering CPR. An authorized course given by the American Heart Association or American Red Cross should be successfully completed before using this skill.

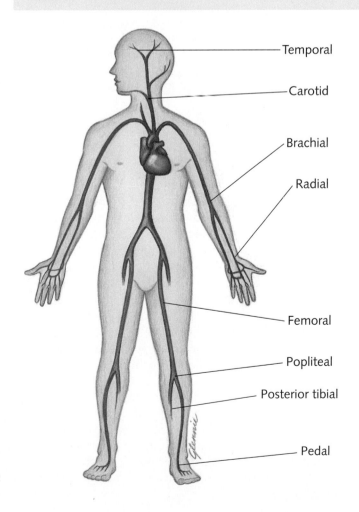

Temporal

Carotid

Brachial

Radial

Femoral

Popliteal

Posterior tibial

Pedal

Figure 31-8   Pressure on artery points may be used to stop bleeding in 90% of bleeding wounds.

Skill 31-2

Performing Foreign-Body Airway Obstruction Rescue

1. Maintain medical asepsis by using the guidelines provided in the Standard and Transmission-Based Precautions, including good handwashing technique and use of gloves as needed.

2. Assess whether assistance is needed.

3. If the victim cannot speak or cough forcefully, perform abdominal thrusts until the object is dislodged.

4. Lower the victim to the ground if unresponsiveness occurs.

5. Call 9-1-1 or have someone else do it.

6. Get an AED if available.

7. Attempt CPR.* Look for a foreign body each time rescue breaths are attempted. Remove the object if seen.

---

*These are general guidelines for administering CPR. An authorized course given by the American Heart Association or American Red Cross should be successfully completed before using this skill.

area (Figure 31-8). In only the most extreme cases when death resulting from bleeding is probable, a **tourniquet** may be used. The application of a tourniquet damages the tissues below the area where applied, so it is not recommended unless all other methods have failed to stop bleeding.

Treatment for burns varies with the type and amount of tissue damage. A first-degree burn causes the skin to redden and is treated by applying cool water to the area. Second-degree burns result in blisters and may also be treated with cool water and elevation of the area affected. Third-degree burns cause extensive damage to the skin and tissues beneath it. Clothing and material that adheres to a third-degree burn should not be removed. The burned area may be covered with a clean, dry cloth of dressing and elevated to reduce swelling. Advanced medical treatment is needed as soon as possible in the case of a third-degree burn. Ointments and other materials are not applied to any burn without medical direction.

Poisoning by ingestion may result from household materials, medications, and other items. The victim of poisoning should be given milk or water if fully conscious and without convulsions. No liquids are given to an unconscious person. Vomiting should not be encouraged unless medically directed to do so because the substance may further damage the body during vomiting if caustic. As treatment of poisoning depends on the type of poison ingested, advanced medical attention should be sought as soon as possible. Other types of poisoning that may need treatment include inhalation and contact poisoning.

All victims of trauma should be treated for shock. The victim is encouraged to lie down with the feet and legs slightly elevated. The victim may be lightly covered with a blanket. No fluids are given to a victim of trauma unless it is specifically indicated as in poisoning.

The main focus of the treatment of fractures is immobilization of the injured area (Figure 31-9). A closed fracture does not penetrate the skin. An open fracture may require the stopping of bleeding before immobilization. All fractures should be treated with advanced medical support as soon as possible.

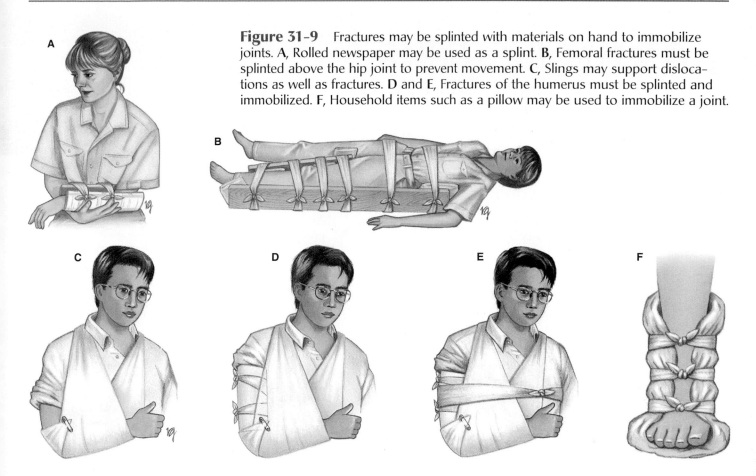

Figure 31-9 Fractures may be splinted with materials on hand to immobilize joints. **A,** Rolled newspaper may be used as a splint. **B,** Femoral fractures must be splinted above the hip joint to prevent movement. **C,** Slings may support dislocations as well as fractures. **D** and **E,** Fractures of the humerus must be splinted and immobilized. **F,** Household items such as a pillow may be used to immobilize a joint.

Heat cramps may appear in muscles. The affected area may be massaged to bring oxygen to the area and a small amount of slightly salty water may help to increase the fluid balance in the body. Heat exhaustion and heat stroke are more severe reactions to exposure to heat. The victim should be moved to a cooler area and sponged with cool water. Medical attention for heat exhaustion is needed as soon as possible. In heat stroke, the victim's body temperature should be lowered as soon as possible with cool water or ice packs. Heat stroke is life threatening, and advanced medical attention should be sought as soon as possible.

Hypothermia and frostbite result with exposure to cold temperatures. The victim of hypothermia should be treated by removal to a warm area if possible. Wet clothing is removed and a warm blanket applied. If the victim is fully conscious, warm fluids may help increase body temperature. Frostbite results in tissue damage because of freezing of body fluids. The area affected should not be rubbed to prevent further damage. A warm blanket may be applied to the affected area. If the victim is conscious, warm fluids may be given to raise body temperature. Advanced medical attention may be needed for both hypothermia and frostbite injuries.

Other miscellaneous emergencies that may occur include nosebleeds, drowning, eye injuries, and insect or snake bites. A nosebleed may be treated by having the victim sit or lie down with the head and shoulders raised. With the head slightly forward, the victim may apply direct pressure to the nostrils at the midline. A cold compress on the nose may also help stop bleeding. Victims of drowning are removed from the water as soon as possible and artificial respiration started. First responders should not remove objects that penetrate the eye. Additional damage to the eye may be prevented by loosely covering both eyes to prevent movement of the injured area. Eye injuries require advanced medical treatment as soon as possible. Insect and snake bites may be treated by the application of cold to and elevation of the affected area. A restricting band may be placed between the bite and the heart to slow the poison's spread, as long as it does not cut off all circulation to the area. Ice placed on the bite may also reduce the poison's circulation from the area. Advanced medical attention is necessary for many snake and insect bites.

Some medical conditions that may require emergency care include stroke and seizures. The stroke victim should be monitored for vital signs while emergency personnel are responding. The person may be placed on the affected side to promote easier breathing and prevent **aspiration.** Response to seizure activity involves protecting the victim from injury by removing articles that might be in the way of movement or providing a cushioned area when possible. Nothing should be inserted into the victim's mouth nor should any restraint be applied to stop movement. When the seizure activity has stopped, the person may be turned on one side to promote easier breathing.

Review Questions

1. Use each of the following terms in one or more sentences that correctly relate their meaning.
   Consciousness
   Critical
   Hemorrhage
   Shock
   Tourniquet

2. Describe the members of the emergency health care team including education, role, and credentialing requirements.

3. Describe the purpose of the emergency health care team.

4. Define first aid and list its three components.

5. Describe six types of external wounds.

6. Describe three ways used to determine the severity of burns and the three degrees of burns.

7. Describe five ways that poisoning may occur.

8. Describe the effect that shock has on the body and list five causes.

9. Describe three types of fractures and treatment for each.

10. Describe the effects of extreme cold and heat on the body.

Critical Thinking

1. Investigate and compare the cost of various types of emergency care treatments.

2. Research and describe five common medications used in emergency health care.

3. Investigate and compare the cost of education for five emergency health care professionals.

4. Describe the certification requirements for first aid and cardiopulmonary resuscitation.

5. Research and report the poisonous plants, reptiles, and insects local to the area.

32

Information and Administration Careers

Learning Objectives

Identify at least 10 terms related to health care information and administration.

Specify the role of selected information and administrative health care workers, including personal qualities, levels of education, and credentialing requirements.

Identify three personal characteristics needed in an efficient health occupations clerk.

Identify at least five forms used as part of the medical record.

Describe at least three methods of payment for health care.

Key Terms

Administration

(ad-min-ih-STRAY-shun) Management, performance of executive responsibilities and duties

Benefit

(BEN-uh-fit) Financial help in time of illness, retirement, or unemployment

Chart

Collection of written materials relating to the health care of a patient

Confidential

(kon-fuh-DEN-shul) Private and secret; may be protected by law

Customary

(KUS-tum-ay-ree) Fee charged by similar practitioners for a service in the same economic and geographical area

Deficient

(deh-FISH-unt) Lacking some important part

Dictation

(dik-TAY-shun) Speaking words to be written by another person; may be recorded

Insurance

(in-SHUR-ins) Payment by contract by one party to another in which the second party guarantees the first party against financial loss from a specific event

Reasonable

(REE-sun-uh-bul) Fee that considers both the usual fee charged by a practitioner for a particular service and the fee charged by other practitioners for the same service

Transcribe

(tran-SKRIBE) To make a written copy of dictated or recorded matter

Information and Administration Careers Terminology

TERM	DEFINITION	PREFIX	ROOT	SUFFIX
Abduction	Move away	ab	duc	tion
Adduction	Move toward	ad	duc	tion
Arthritis	Inflammation of the joint		arthr	itis
Arthrodesis	Fixation of the joint		arthr/o	desis
Cervical	Pertaining to the neck		cervic	al
Hypertrophy	Above normal amount of growth	hyper	troph	y
Myelogram	Picture of the bone marrow		myelo	gram
Neuralgia	Painful nerve		neur	algia
Osteopathy	Disease of the bone	osteo	path	y
Terminology	Study of words		termin	ology

*A transition phrase or vowel may be added to or deleted from the word parts to make the combining form.

Abbreviations for Information and Administration Careers

ABBREVIATION	MEANING
ART	Accredited records technician
CAAHEP	Commission on Accreditation of Allied Health Education Programs
CEO	Chief executive officer
CPT	Current procedure terminology
CTS	Carpel tunnel syndrome
HUC	Health unit coordinator
RHIT	Registered health information technician
RRA	Registered records administrator
RSI	Repetitive stress injury
URC	Usual, reasonable, customary

Careers

Even though health care administrators and information personnel often do not have direct contact with the patients, they are of critical importance to the quality of care delivered. Health care managers need to be organized to work quickly and accurately. Good communication skills are needed to provide information and leadership in the health care setting. Administrators must be able to form and maintain good working relationships with those in subordinate positions. With the exception of high-level managers, most health information and administrative service personnel work regular hours. Some examples of careers in **administration** include the health care facility managers, supervisors, medical secretaries, unit coordinators, and medical records personnel (Box 32-1).

Health Service Managers

Administrators and managers are needed in all health care facilities including clinics, health maintenance organizations, hospitals, home care agencies, private practices, rehabilitation agencies, hospice services, long-term medical day care, and ambulatory care settings. The top executive is often referred to as the *chief executive officer* (CEO). Administrators develop and expand services with authority given to them by the governing board or agency owner. Administrators manage the facility budget, programs, and personnel. They are responsible for relations with other agencies and organizations.

Administrators coordinate services, hiring, and training of personnel (Figure 32-1). Administrators may be responsible for establishing the policies and procedures of the facility. The CEO must demonstrate public relations skills as well as leadership ability. Long, irregular hours are often required for public speaking and travel.

Box 32-1   Information and Administration Careers*

Administrator, drug and alcohol facility
Administrator, hospital
Biological photographer
Biophysicist
Chemist, food
Chief of nuclear medicine
Clerk, medical records
Coordinator of rehabilitation services
Coroner
Dietary manager
Dietician, research
Director, counseling
Director, community health nursing
Director, diagnostics clinics
Director, nursing registry
Director, nursing service
Director, occupational health nursing
Director, outpatient services
Director, pharmacy service
Director, placement
Director, radiology
Director, school of nursing
Director, speech and hearing
Director, volunteer services
District advisor
Executive director, Nurses Association
Food and drug inspector
Health physicist
Health unit coordinator
Hospital registration staff
Information scientist

In-service coordinator, auxiliary personnel
Instructor, psychiatric aides
Laboratory manager
Librarian
Librarian, special
Library technical assistant
Manager, dental laboratory
Medical physicist
Medical records administrator
Medical records technician
Medical technologist teaching supervisor
Nurse, consultant
Nurse, evening supervisor
Nurse, head
Nurse, instructor
Nurse, supervisor
Nursing home administrator
Patient resource agent
Photographer, scientific
Public relations representative
Radiology administrator
Rehabilitation center manager
Secretary, medical
Supervisor, artificial breast fabrication
Supervisor, central supply
Supervisor, hearing aid assembly
Supervisor, laundry
Utilization review coordinator
Ward clerk
Ward service supervisor

*Health information and administrative occupations cover a broad spectrum of careers in which individuals have advanced to leadership positions.

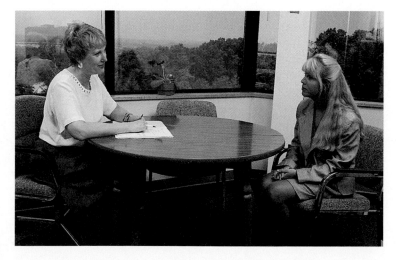

Figure 32-1   Administrators often participate in hiring decisions.

Preadmission Form

Patient Information	Last Name First Middle Address City State Zip County Telephone Social Security # Date of Birth Maiden Name Reason for Admission OB/GYN Patients: Date of last menstrual cycle OB/GYN's name OB Due Date Religion (optional) Notify clergy ____ yes ____ no Telephone Spouse's Name Social Security #
Employment Information	Occupation Employer Address City State Zip Telephone Spouse's Occupation Spouse's Employer Telephone Address City State Zip
Person Responsible for Payment	Name (if other than yourself) Address City State Zip County Telephone Relationship to Patient Occupation Employer Employer's Address City State Zip Telephone How long employed?
Emergency Contact	Name (relative or friend) Address City State Zip Telephone
Insurance Information	Subscriber's name Relationship to Policy Holder Subscriber's Identification/Member Number Effective Date Type of Policy ____ individual ____ group Group Number Employer (if group policy)
Other Insurance	Insurance company Policy Holder's Name Relationship to Policy Holder Policy Number Effective Date Type of Policy ____ individual ____ group Group Number Employer (if group policy)
Medicare	Name (exactly as shown on card) Claim Number Effective Date
Previous Admissions	Have you ever been admitted to this hospital before? ____ yes ____ no
Accident Information	Date of accident Time of accident Is accident job related? ____ yes ____ no How did accident happen?
Signature	_____ Date _____

Figure 32-2   The patient may complete the admissions form alone or with help from a health care worker.

Positions for health managers who have obtained 4-year bachelor's degrees are available in small institutions, but master- or doctoral-level preparation is preferred for employment in large facilities. Employment opportunities for managers will grow the fastest in residential care facilities and practitioner's offices and clinics. More than 190 colleges and universities offer advanced degree programs that specialize in health care administration. Master's level preparation is also available in long-term care administration, public health, public administration, or business administration. Other managers may study business, public administration, or human resources administration before becoming employed in the health care industry. An internship is required by many administrative programs, and postgraduate residents and fellows may occupy middle-management positions as part of the educational program. Although regulations vary from state to state, licensing is usually required for administrators of long-term care facilities. Duties of the health care manager may include hiring and coordination of personnel, budget preparation and implementation, and public relations.

Patient representatives, or advocates, help patients to understand the health care policies and procedures of the facility, obtain services, and make informed decisions about their care. The work of the patient representative is varied based on the needs of the current patients. Some duties might include assisting with the drafting of a living will, resolving a conflict between the facility staff and patient, or simply assisting the patient to complete forms (Skill 32-1). Hospitals and other facilities set their own requirements for the education and experience background of this individual. Many of the patient representatives have a master's degree in a health-related field.

Support Personnel

Health services clerks or office managers may have the duties of receptionist, accountant, and assistant. The clerk or manager is responsible for the smooth operation of the services. The clerk must be dependable and take initiative in making sure the office runs well. It is important that the office personnel arrive on time and give the impression of being ready to give eager and efficient care. The clerk

working in a private office locates and organizes the **charts** of patients who are expected to visit that day.

Hospital registration staff record and manage the admission of patients. Admission staffs convey the first impression of the facility. The admitting clerk should be calm, patient, pleasant, and efficient. Duties of the admissions clerk include pre-registration interviewing, verifying insurance, arranging transportation, and in some instances, assigning beds for the hospital stay (Figure 32-2). To complete **insurance** forms, the clerk must first verify the type of insurance and obtain the correct form (Figure 32-3). The clerk may complete some information, using information contained in the patient's record. Signatures of the patient and spouse, if any, are needed to authorize release of medical information during care. The forms must be completed accurately, because the code used for reimbursement for services is determined in part by use of the insurance forms. Clerks may also assist with completion of forms for death and birth records. Most clerks learn their responsibilities on the job, but managers usually have a college degree in a health-related field.

The medical secretary is employed by institutions and private facilities, such as a doctor's office, to assist in administration of services. Duties of the medical secretary include taking **dictation,** using transcription skills to compile reports and charts, assisting the physician with medical reports, articles, and conference proceedings, and preparing correspondence (Figure 32-4). For this occupation, knowledge of medical terminology supplements the associate degree or vocational training of a general secretary. Secretaries also may file records using a variety of systems that may be narrative or numerical. The charts may be cross-referenced and marked with a locator card when removed to ensure easy retrieval. If the secretary is also responsible for keeping the budget records, a fee schedule must be established. Although the American Medical Association provides the Current Procedure Terminology (CPT) code, which gives a schedule for fees for services, the practitioner may have one that differs. The federal government has a system of determining payment for services based on time, skill, expenses of maintaining a practice, and malpractice costs. This system is called the *resource-based relative value scale* (RBRVS) and is replacing the usual, **reasonable, and customary** (URC) practices of the past. All patients are given a receipt

Medical Benefits Request

Return To: Any Insurance Co.
Any Road
Any Town, USA 12345

Complete section 1-6.

Sign section 7 to have benefits paid to your doctor.

Complete Employee Information on reverse side.

If you have submitted a request for benefits to another plan, including Medicare, attach a copy of the bills you submitted to the other plan and the explanation of benefits you received from the other plan.

Attach itemized bills or ask your health care provider to complete the applicable section on the reverse side. The bills must include:
-patient's name   -relationship to employee
-date of service   -type of service rendered
-condition being treated
If this information is missing, write it on the bill and sign your name.

If prescription drugs are covered under your plan, submit receipts or a Prescription Drug Record form. Receipts must contain:
-drug name   -purchase date   -quantity
-dose per/day   -strength   -physician name
-charge   -prescription number -pharmacy name/address
-nature of illness or injury
This information can be copied from the prescription bottle or box.

Incomplete forms will delay payment.

1. Employer Information	Name (as shown on ID card)	Policy/Group Number

2. Employee Information	Social Security Number - - ___Active ___Retired Date if retirement:	Name Address (include zip code) ___Address is new	Birth Date Daytime Phone ( )

3. Patient Information	Social Security Number - - Relationship to Employee (circle) Self Spouse Child Other Sex (circle) Male Female Is patient employed? (Circle) No Yes Date of Retirement:	Name Address (if different from employee) Full Time Student (circle) Expected Graduation Date Yes No Name/Address of Employer	Birth Date School Name Marital Status

4. Other Coverage Information

Are any family members expenses covered by another group health plan, group pre-payment plan (Blue Cross-Blue Shield, etc.), no fault auto insurance, Medicare or any federal, state or local government plan? (circle)
                                               No   Yes

If yes, list policy or contract holder, policy or contract number(s) and name/address of insurance company or administrator:

Insured's Social Security Number	Insured's Name	Insured's Birth Date

5. Claim Information

If claim for a laboratory test or doctor's office visit, state diagnosis or nature of illness: Is claim related to employment? (circle)
                                                              No   Yes

Is claim related to an accident? (circle)
  No   Yes   If yes, date   Time   am   pm
Description of Accident:

6. Release

To all providers of health care:
You are authorized to provide Any Insurance Company, and any independent claim administrators and consulting health professionals and utilization review organizations with whom Any Insurance Company has contracted information concerning health care advice, treatment or supplies provided the patient (including that relating to mental illness and/or AIDS/ARC/HIV). This information will be used to evaluate claims for benefits. Any Insurance Company may provide the employer named above with any benefit calculation used in payment of this claim for the purpose of reviewing the experience and operation of the policy or contract. This Authorization is valid for the term of the policy or contract under which a claim has been submitted. I know that I have a right to receive a copy of this authorization upon request and agree that a photographic copy of this authorization is as valid as the original.
Patient's or Authorized Person's Signature_____ Date _____

7. Assignment

I authorize payment of medical benefits to the physician or supplier of service.
Patient's or Authorized Person's Signature_____ Date _____
Any person who knowingly and with intent to defraud or deceive any insurance company files a statement of claim containing any materially false, incomplete or misleading information is guilty of a crime.

Figure 32-3 Accurate completion of insurance forms determines whether or not claims will be paid promptly.

Skill 32-1

Assisting the Patient with Insurance Forms

1. Gather all equipment and supplies, including the correct form and a pen. A clipboard may be used to provide a writing surface if desired.

2. Obtain the correct form for the patient's insurance coverage. The format of forms may differ, although the information required is fairly consistent.

3. Copy available information from the patient's registration slip and insurance identification card neatly and accurately. Follow the order described on the form. The patient who is not required to complete the same information more than once will be impressed by your competence and courtesy.

4. Interview the patient for any corrections and missing information in the following categories:

   Insured: The patient's policy information or relationship to the insured is required.

   Other insurance: Some coverage may be excluded or added if the patient or patient's spouse has an additional policy.

   Signatures: The patient's (and spouse's) signature is required to authorize the release of medical information as needed during care.

   Medical information: The nature of the complaint (signs and symptoms), length of duration, first time of treatment, history of prior illnesses and injuries, and care provider identification number are noted.

   Coding of treatment: Correct codes for the diagnosis and treatment determine the billing and must be completed carefully.

   Financial agreement: The method of payment for services excluded in the insurance coverage must be designated in the record of patient care.

5. Verify all information before completing the interview.

6. The care provider's identification information may be completed by the assistant but requires the signature of the professional.

GAMMA   A DIVISION OF THE MERCY HOSPITAL SYSTEM

February 19, 1996

Ms. Miller
Nursing Coordinator
Horizon Medical Center
11204 Sunset Drive
St. Louis, MO 63179

Dear Ms. Miller:
Reference Line (if any)

Body of Letter

Closing,

Susan Williams
Director of Radiology

enclosure

Figure 32-4   Business correspondence reflects the relationship of the health care worker with the patient.

for payment if cash or a check is used for payment. Bills are then issued each month for patients with outstanding debt to the practitioner (Figure 32-5, Skill 32-2).

The health unit coordinator (HUC) performs nonclinical activities for the nursing unit. Nonclinical activities are those that do not involve direct contact with the patient. The coordinator's duties include assembling and maintaining patient charts, transcribing physician's orders, and acting as receptionist and secretary on the unit. Part of maintaining the chart includes determining if any part of the chart is missing. The person responsible for that part of the chart is then notified to correct the **deficiency.** Health unit coordinator and management certification is available on completion of a 2-year college program. The health unit manager coordinates the nonclinical activities for several

units. The duties of the manager include establishing policies and procedures for unit coordinators, managing personnel, and preparing the budget.

Medical Records Personnel

Medical records personnel organize, analyze, and generate data relating to patient records. The greatest use of medical records personnel is in hospitals, although other employment opportunities are available in medical offices and health maintenance organizations. Medical records and health information technicians are projected by the U.S. Department of Labor to be one of the fastest growing occupations through 2010.

Registered records administrators (RRAs) are responsible for management of the information system. They create

Skill 32-2

Preparing a Business Letter

1. Select the appropriate stationery for the letter required. The letter must be correct in content and uniformly displayed to look professional. Paper that is 8½ × 11 inches is standard for business letters.

2. Type the letter following the format preferred by the health care professional. Although there may be more than one acceptable letter format, a professional appearance includes the addressee information, date, salutation, body, closing, signature, and enclosures when needed.

3. Proofread the letter for accuracy and format.

4. Address an envelope to accompany the letter.

Daily Record of Charges and receipts
July 18, 1998

45-613 Eye-Ease®
46-713 20/20 Buff
Made in USA

	Patient	Charges / Adjustments	Cash	Check	Office visit	Lab	X-ray	Ecg	Medication	Non-Office visit	Receipt No.
			Receipts		Memo of Charges by type of Service rendered						
1	Brown, John	3500		3500	3500						1051
2	Black, James	12200		5000	4000	4200	4000				1052
3	Doe, Jane	7500			3500			4000			
4	Smith, Robert	3500		3500		2000			1500		1053
5	Goode, Alice	3500	3500		3500						1054
6	Jones, Mary	9800			3000		5000		1800		
7	Small, Joseph	4000	2000					4000			1055
8	Biggs, Barney (home)	4500								4500	
9											
10	Mail										
11	White, Willie			4500							
12	Green, Gordon			5500							
13	Blue Shield (Check totalling $ 115.38										
14	Sampson, Sam			4388							
15	Vinson, Vera	(1050)		6950		(1050)					
16	Medicare (Check totalling $ 100.05										
17	Grey, Gertrude	(1225)		4775							
18	Reddy, Ruth	(1770)		5430	(950)		(1225)				
19								(1220)			
20											
21	Totals for the day	44455	5500	43343	16950	5150	7775	6780	3300	4500	
22											
23											
24											
25											
26											
27											

Figure 32-5 Records for charges and payments are used to provide accurate billing. *(From Cooper MG, Cooper DE, Burrows NJ: The medical assistant, ed 6, St Louis, 1993, Mosby.)*

policies and procedures to ensure adequate departmental efficiency. Additionally, the records administrator may be responsible for employee evaluation and budget preparation. Education for the records administrator is a 2-year college certificate or 4-year college or university degree. There are 52 colleges and universities offering programs approved by the American Medical Records Association. Supervised clinical experience is required in an accredited program. The American Medical Records Association offers a registration examination to graduates of accredited programs.

The Commission on Accreditation of Allied Health Education Programs (CAAHEP) has accredited 177 programs for health information technicians. The Registered Health Information Technician (RHIT) may also specialize in coding by completing a voluntary certification program. The accredited record technician (ART) performs the technical functions of medical records maintenance. This includes organizing, analyzing, and evaluating records using established standards under the direction of a registered record administrator. In a small facility, the records technician may have the full responsibility of the medical records department. Medical records technicians may be educated in a 2-year program or through an independent study program offered by the American Medical Records Association. Completed over 3 years, the independent study program must include supervised clinical experience.

The medical transcriptionist, also called *medical stenographer,* listens to and types information to provide a permanent record from a variety of audio equipment. Most health care providers use digital or analog dictating equipment. However, the use of the Internet and speech-recognition software has provided quicker return of documents. Knowledge of medical terminology and computer skills such as keyboarding and word processing is required for accurate transcription of the records. Medical records clerks or transcriptionists may sometimes learn on the job because the duties performed are limited in number. Associate degree programs in transcription are offered through some community colleges and vocational programs. Certification is voluntary and provided through the American Association for Medical Transcription. Medical transcription employment opportunities are projected to grow faster than average through 2010. This field may provide flexibility in the hours worked or employment from home.

Health Information and Communication

One of the fastest growing fields in the health care industry is the management of information. Communication of health-related information is the function of several disciplines including health science librarians, educators, in-service personnel, public relations personnel, biomedical photographers, illustrators, and writers.

Health science librarians provide access to information by practicing professionals, researchers, and students. The librarian locates information in journals, books, computer resources, and audiovisual media. Librarians may also be responsible for planning, budgeting, and purchasing the resources. Librarians must have good organizational and communication skills to store the information logically and to teach others how to locate desired information. Specialties in health library science include reference, collection development, acquisitions (purchasing), serials (periodicals), and education. Other librarians may function as catalogers, audiovisual technicians, or medical historians. Clinical librarians may accompany the physician on hospital rounds to assess information needs of specific patients. The minimum level of education for health science librarians is a master's degree. Certification is available and must be maintained through a yearly examination.

Educators teach new and experienced health personnel at all employment levels. Health educators may specialize in fields of practice such as personal, community, consumer, environmental, or public health. Most public schools require standard teacher certification, which includes a bachelor's degree in education, for employment as a health educator. A master's degree is required for many positions.

Public health educators plan, organize, and direct health education programs for group and community needs. They determine and set goals for the health needs of the community. They prepare and distribute teaching materials in schools, industries, and community agencies. Public health educators may have a bachelor's or master's degree.

Public health educators may work with community health providers to design ways to increase the use of public health resources. The health educator may be responsible for orientation of new employees of the public health department as well as for educational programs to inform personnel of new developments in the health field. Public health educators may be responsible for development of brochures, pamphlets, and other teaching materials for educating the community.

Public relations representatives plan and conduct programs to create a favorable image of the agency. Public relations includes sending press releases to news media and planning new advertising strategies. Minimal educational requirements include a bachelor's degree in public relations. The education for public relations provides skills in journalism and public speaking. Public relations specialists often work long and irregular hours to be available when special events occur. Media relations and marketing may be part of public relations services.

Biological photographers document life-related health events with a variety of production equipment. This may include producing slides, photographs, prints, transparencies, videotapes, and computer graphics. Photomicrography is taking photographs through a microscope. Electron microscopy can record images without the use of light. Biophotographers often specialize in one area such as animal, plant, or surgical photography. The education is usually 2 to 4 years of college for training in photography and basic sciences, especially biology. Certification and registration are available through the Biological Photographers Association.

Medical illustrators are specialized artists who use a variety of visual materials to communicate vital information regarding biosciences. Illustrators provide sketches, paintings, drawings, computer images, and three-dimensional models. Advanced functions of medical illustrators include production of instructional models of artificial body parts. Medical illustrators must be talented artists with education in anatomy, art, and general medicine. The five accredited schools available for this area of specialization require applicants to have a bachelor's degree for admission.

Medical writers create and edit technical material for educational and marketing materials. Individuals with a master's degree are preferred for employment as medical writers. Doctoral-level education in health science and related writing areas is available. Many medical writers first enter the health professions as technicians, scientists, or engineers in an area of interest. Job opportunities for the medical writer are available in universities and private industries such as pharmaceutical companies.

Public health statisticians gather, analyze, and present public health data used to uncover trends in health and in the causes of disease. Statisticians may be employed by voluntary organizations, government, or health departments to plan health care services. A doctorate in public health (DPH), which includes biostatistics training, is necessary for this profession.

Content Instruction

Office Management

Orderliness of equipment and supplies used in the work area provides a secure environment for maintaining the **confidentiality** of patient records. Various systems may be used to record appointments and billing information. This information may be kept in written form or stored in computerized systems. Filing may be numerical, alphabetical, or both (Figure 32-6). Cross-referencing of records in several locations may be necessary for prompt retrieval. Any filing system must be up to date to be useful (Skill 32-3).

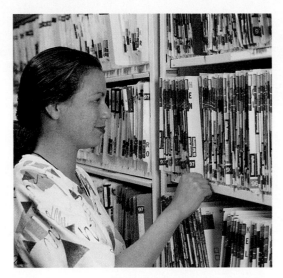

Figure 32-6   Many different filing systems work well if items are filed promptly and in the correct location. *(From Kinn ME, Woods M: The medical assistant, ed 8, Philadelphia, 1999, WB Saunders.)*

Jonesville Medical Center

John Jones, MD
1000 Center Street
Jonesville, ST 22222

❖ ❖ ❖

Your next appointment is:

_____ at _____ o'clock

Please notify the office at least 24 hours in advance if you are unable to keep the appointment.

Figure 32-7   After the necessary information is gathered, some offices provide the patient with a card as a reminder of the next visit.

Most agencies maintain an appointment procedure that includes a card given to the patient, a confirmation telephone call, and a daily log (Figure 32-7). Records of daily appointments usually cover at least 1 year to enable planning in advance. Appointment records are often written in pencil so that they can be erased in the case of a cancellation. Patients who are kept waiting because of overbooking or errors in scheduling appointments may become dissatisfied with the service. Some facilities charge patients a percentage of the fee if they miss appointments or fail to provide advance notice (no-show). The patient must be made aware of such a policy before the appointment date. When

Skill 32-3

Filing Forms

1. Establish a filing system by alphabetic or numeric order. Files should be maintained so that an item can be found immediately.

2. File items immediately after use. Filing trays may be needed if time does not permit immediate placement in files, but they should be emptied daily.

3. Place an "out" card (or placeholder) in the location of a file that is removed from the system. Another employee may seek the chart and waste time looking if it has been removed.

4. Establish rules for filing and cross-referencing files. All employees should use the same rules and system for locating and placing files.

making an appointment, the clerk records information such as the date, time, and purpose of the visit as well as the referring individual, if any. Many offices call the individual to confirm the appointment 1 or 2 days before the scheduled date (Skill 32-4).

In addition to scheduling appointments, the clerk or office manager is responsible for scheduling laboratory tests and other procedures. The patient must be consulted regarding convenient locations and times of additional appointments. The clerk should also inform the patient of the approximate time needed for the testing and when the results will be available. The clerk can help ensure the best possible care for patients who are sent to other agencies by properly planning the visit and by maintaining a positive relationship with the other agency personnel.

Records Management

Many forms are used to provide information about the health care patient. When placed in a folder or notebook, the information is considered to be the chart, or medical record (Figure 32-8).

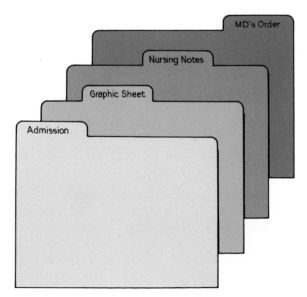

Figure 32-8 The medical record may be made up of several different forms, and the types of forms may vary according to the care needed.

Skill 32-4

Scheduling an Appointment

1. Obtain and write down all pertinent information when the appointment is made, including the full name, address, telephone number, purpose of the visit, and referring person, if any.

2. Assign the earliest time available that meets the patient's needs. Schedules should be realistic for needed services and should allow for emergency treatment.

3. Enter the required information, including the time and the patient's full name, telephone number, and reason for visit in the appointment book in pencil. Using pencil permits appointments to be changed neatly if conflicts occur.

4. Prepare an appointment card to be given or sent to the patient. A visual reminder may ensure that the patient does not make a conflicting appointment.

5. Call the patient to confirm the appointment 1 or 2 days before it is scheduled. Confirming appointments helps ensure that both the patient and health care practitioner keep to the schedule.

Skill 32-5

Completing Forms

1. Seat the patient in a comfortable chair away from distractions. Patient records should be kept confidential.

2. Ask the patient about each item on the form. Explain any items that are unclear. Terminology that is common to health care personnel may not be understood by the patient.

3. Allow the patient to answer completely. Information that is not immediately familiar may require time for recall.

4. Verify insurance coverage and expiration date by checking the insurer's card.

5. Obtain the patient's signature to guarantee payment by an insurance program or by the patient. Insurance providers will not supply information or payment without a release signature from the patient.

6. Code forms with the appropriate payment number for billing. The coding may determine the amount, promptness, and acceptability of the coverage.

7. Terminate the interview by informing the patient how, when, and by whom the service will be rendered.

If the patient is able to understand and complete the forms without assistance, he or she may do so. The clerk or health care worker may complete some forms during an interview or when the care is given. Minors may not give legal consent for treatment except in special situations determined by the laws of the state. The clerk must explain all forms regarding payment, release of information, and other nonmedical concerns to the patient in a way that can be easily understood (Skill 32-5).

Records management is the responsibility of every health care worker. The medical record for a patient is used in every aspect of health care. The chart contains the medical history and physical assessment, test results, surgery reports, and notes about the patient's condition and course of treatment (Box 32-2). Any form that is part of the chart is important because it contains information necessary to provide the best care possible. Not all charts contain all possible forms. Out-patient, obstetric, and other specialized charts may vary. The chart is considered the legal record, and information on the chart is considered to be confidential. Confidential information may not be given to anyone other than those authorized by the patient and health care practitioner managing the care. With authorization, information from the medical record may be used for billing, education, planning, and research.

Records must be accurate, legible, complete, and organized to provide efficient care (Box 32-3). Some medical information may be assembled in verbal form by using dictaphone machinery. The oral record must be **transcribed** or written in permanent form to become part of the legal record. The dictating practitioner should ensure accuracy by checking the record that is transcribed from verbal information. Information that a clerk transcribes or copies from one written record to another is checked by authorized personnel.

Box 32-2   Inpatient Chart Order

1. Fact sheet (information sheet)
2. Diagnosis-related group (DRG) worksheet
3. Emergency room record
   a. Paramedic transport record
   b. Nursing notes
4. Death
   a. Autopsy report
   b. Autopsy release
   c. Release of body
5. Discharge summary (typed)
6. History and physical (typed)
7. Consultation(s) (typed)
8. Physician orders
9. Progress notes
10. Dialysis progress notes
11. Operative procedures
    a. Consent for procedure
    b. Consent for transfusion
    c. Preoperative checklist
    d. Operative record
    e. Anesthesia record
    f. Operative report (typed)
    g. Postanesthesia record
    h. Pathology report(s)
12. Outside laboratory report(s)
13. Laboratory reports (computerized)
14. Radiograph
15. Electrocardiogram
16. Holter monitor echo report
17. Nutritional progress notes
18. Social service notes
19. Respiratory therapy
    a. Progress notes
    b. Continuous therapy notes
    c. Arterial blood gases
    d. Pulmonary function report
    e. Ventilator flow sheet
20. Physical therapy
    a. Continuous therapy notes
21. Speech therapy
22. Graphic record
23. Medication sheets
24. Intravenous flow
25. Intake and output sheet
26. Cardiac arrest sheet
27. Nursing Kardex care plan
28. Nursing Kardex treatments
29. Nursing assessment sheet
30. Nursing flow sheet
31. Diabetic flow sheet
32. Nurses notes
33. Miscellaneous
    a. Consents
    b. Releases
    c. Transfers
    d. Records from other facilities
34. Discharge instruction sheet

Methods of Payment

In the United States more than a billion dollars a day is spent on health care. Health care costs account for more than one tenth of the national economy. Methods of payment for health costs have changed with growth of the industry. Payment may be made on a fee-for-service basis or through a prepaid **benefit** package. Fee-for-service payment requires that money be received at the time of service. A prepaid benefit package may be obtained through insurance or a health maintenance organization. The fee for services in a prepaid system is not based on the type of treatment.

Insurance is payment in advance for services in the event that they are needed. Insurance may be obtained through groups, privately, or from government benefits (Table 32-1). Group insurance benefits may be obtained through benefit programs arranged by the employing agency. Private insurance packages are obtained from the insurance company directly. In the United States, the federal Medicare and Medicaid programs provide health insurance for many individuals. State laws vary but all provide worker's compensation and disability programs.

An insurance company may not pay a certain part of the cost of treatment as a condition of its terms. The amount that must be paid by the patient before the insurance company begins to pay is called the *deductible*. Some insurance packages require that a percentage of each transaction be paid by the insured (co-payment). Individuals may have

Box 32-3   Guidelines for Charting

1. Print in black ink.
2. All entries must be timed, dated, and signed.
3. Leave no blanks between notes or at the end of a line.
   Correct: 9:30 am c/o pain rt hand, rt leg. Able to sit up in bed unassisted. _____ J. Smith, SNA
4. Chart in accurate, clear, and brief manner. Avoid unnecessary words such as *and, the,* and *a.*
5. Use only standard abbreviations.
6. Use the patient as the subject of each statement. The word *patient* is assumed, not written.
7. Be objective, not subjective. Record information and treatments that can be seen, heard, felt, smelled, or measured.
8. Avoid words that interpret or make judgments such as "seems," "appears," and "normal."
   Incorrect: 9:50 am Appears to be in pain when moving.
   Correct: 9:50 am Facial grimace and wincing noted on movement.
9. Document each treatment and activity even if it is part of routine care.
   Correct: 9:55 am Side rails up.

10. Use a direct quote to express the patient's reaction to care.
11. Sign each note at the time it is written using first initial, last name, and professional designation.
    Correct: J. Smith, SNA
12. Correct errors by making one line through the mistake, writing "ERROR" above it. Initial the change.
    ERROR *JS*
    Correct: 10:00 am c/o pain rt ~~forearm~~ wrist.
13. Do not write above or below the line to insert a forgotten word.
    Incorrect: 10:10 am Urine clear, small amount. Stool . . .   └─►yellow
14. Record that unusual treatments or activities were reported to supervising personnel.
    Correct: 10:15 am c/o severe pain rt elbow. Team leader notified.
15. Do not chart activities and treatments performed by other health personnel.

The chart is the medical and legal record of health care. Legally, services not charted were not performed.

Table 32-1   Types of Health Insurance

Type	Description
Group or private	Open to company employees and their dependents; coverage usually includes medical and hospital care; may require deductible or co-payment
Blue Cross and Blue Shield	Open to employees of prepaid companies or to individuals at higher rate; may require deductible or co-payment; in some states, Blue Cross and Blue Shield are separate agencies
Medicare	Federal program through Social Security Act to provide health care to those over 65 years of age; provides specified fee for services; may require deductible
Medicaid	State program to supplement Social Security Act to provide health care to those who cannot afford it; eligibility varies state to state; usually no deductible, but varies with coverage
Worker's compensation	Required in all states to provide insurance for employees injured on the job; not all doctors accept worker's comp, but those who do must register each year; coverage includes all services necessary to treat industrial injury; no deductible or co-payment
CHAMPUS*	A cost-sharing program in which federal government pays part of charges; remainder paid by recipient of the care; provides benefits for those in the uniformed services and their dependents

*Civilian Health and Medical Program of the Uniformed Services.

coverage from more than one insurance program. Without insurance, the patient is responsible for full payment of the cost of care. Inability to pay may lead health care workers to refuse uninsured, nonemergency treatment and to offer less than optimal health care.

Not all procedures and treatments are covered by insurance companies. Billing codes are used to designate the type of treatment and to determine whether coverage is allowed. Diagnostic-related groupings (DRGs) have been established by the federal government to determine a usual, reasonable, and customary (URC) fee for services for Medicare recipients. Many insurance companies use this fee structure to determine the allowable payment. Health care providers in private practice and other agencies may establish a different fee schedule for services.

Performance Instruction

All patients that visit the health care facility are greeted by name and asked to log in their time of arrival (Figure 32-9). Some patients may need help with completion of the forms necessary for care. If it is the first visit, the clerk or receptionist may make the patient feel more comfortable by introducing the practitioner.

The clerk or receptionist uses the telephone to obtain and give information to patients and other health care professionals. Good communication skills are needed to perform these duties well (Figure 32-10). Some people may not welcome information regarding billing, records, and scheduling, so the health services clerk must be able to work well with various and difficult personalities. Courtesy and efficiency are necessary at all times regardless of the responses of others. The importance of the call must be determined by the clerk to decide if it is an emergency or routine call. Good communication skills include stating the name of the facility and personal title when answering the call as well as speaking slowly and clearly. All information gathered should be repeated to ensure accuracy. Information received and given during telephone calls is always confidential. A well-timed and caring sense of humor may be helpful in dealing with difficult telephone conversations.

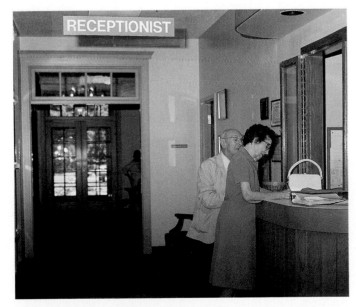

Figure 32-9   At the reception desk, the patient is greeted and asked to sign the log.

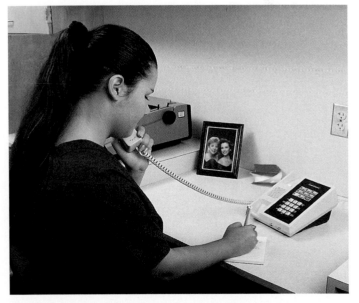

Figure 32-10   The foundation of good telephone etiquette is built on courtesy, accuracy, and thoroughness.

Review Questions

1. Use each of the following terms in one or more sentences that correctly relate their meaning.

   Benefit

   Customary

   Insurance

   Reasonable fee

2. Describe the role of health information and administrative health care workers.

3. List at least five occupations in health information and administrative health care and include the personal qualities, levels of education, and credentialing requirements for these workers.

4. List five forms that make up part of the medical record.

5. Describe three methods used to pay for health care services.

6. Define insurance and the possible consequences of lacking adequate insurance and the inability to pay for health care services.

7. Describe the funding structure relating to diagnostic-related groupings.

8. List five rules for maintaining an accurate medical record.

Critical Thinking

1. Investigate and compare the cost of education for at least three of the health care information and administrative health care workers.

2. Establish and maintain a filing system for classroom notes or club activities.

33

Environmental Careers

Learning Objectives

Define at least eight terms relating to environmental health care.

Describe the function of the environmental health care team.

Specify the role of the environmental health care team members, including personal qualities, educational requirements, responsibilities, and credentialing requirements.

Identify at least five areas of pollution control that are monitored and regulated by environmental health services.

List at least five health conditions that are affected by environmental pollution.

Describe the natural recycling process or chain of life in an ecosystem.

Key Terms

Biosphere
(BIE-us-fere) Part of the universe, including the air (atmosphere), earth (lithosphere), and water (hydrosphere), in which living organisms exist

Decibel
(DES-ih-bul) Unit used to express ratio of power between two sounds

Ecosystem
(EE-ko-sis-tum) Living organisms and nonliving elements interacting in a specific area

Hydrocarbon
(HIE-dro-kar-bun) Organic compound made of hydrogen and carbon only

Mutagen
(MYOO-tuh-jen) Physical or chemical agent that induces genetic mutation or change

Particulate
(par-TIK-yoo-lut) Composed of separate particles or pieces

Pesticide
(PES-tih-side) Poison used to destroy pests of any kind

Pollution
(puh-LOO-shun) Condition of being defiled or impure

Environmental Careers Terminology*

TERM	DEFINITION	PREFIX	ROOT	SUFFIX
Aquatic	Pertaining to the ocean		aquat	ic
Asepsis	Pertaining to absence of pathogens	a	sep/s	is
Atmosphere	Pertaining to the air	atmo	sphere	
Biomedical	Pertaining to medicine and life	bio	medic	al
Ecology	Study of environment		ec	ology
Hydrocarbon	Pertaining to hydrogen and carbon	hydro	carbon	
Hydrosphere	Pertaining to the earth and water	hydro	sphere	
Lithosphere	Pertaining to the earth and rock	lith/o	sphere	
Mutagen	Originating mutation	muta	gen	
Ultrasonic	Pertaining to sound beyond the range (of human hearing)	ultra	son	ic

*A transition phrase or vowel may be added to or deleted from the word parts to make the combining form.

Abbreviations for Environmental Careers

ABBREVIATION	MEANING
CBET	Certified biomedical equipment technician
CLES	Clinical laboratory equipment specialist
CO	Carbon monoxide
CRES	Certified radiological equipment specialist
CST	Certified surgical technologist
dB	Decibel
EMF	Electromagnetic field
EPA	Environmental Protection Agency
ORT	Operating room technologist
pH	Potential or partial concentration of hydrogen ions

Box 33-1 Environmental Health Careers*

Dietetic consultant
Dietetic intern
Dietetic technician
Dietician, chief
Dietician, clinical
Dietician, teaching
Ecologist
Food management aide
Food service worker
Health equipment servicer
Industrial hygienist
Industrial safety health teacher
Medical coordinator, pesticides
Microbiologist, public health
Pollution control engineer
Public health dentist
Public health educator
Public health service officer
Safety manager
Sanitarian
Sheltered works director

*The environmental health care team works to create a supportive environment for the patient.

Skill 33-1

Planning Menus

1. Maintain medical asepsis by using the guidelines provided in the Standard and Transmission-Based Precautions, including good handwashing technique and use of gloves as needed.

2. Distribute meal requisitions (menus) early in the day. The type of meal requisition is determined by the physician's diet order and special needs of the patient.

3. Collect meal requisitions when completed. Patients may need assistance with completion of meal forms.

4. Determine the number of meals needed according to the number of patients (census). Tally the number of food portions required for each of them. Establish a schedule for the food preparation. Salads and fresh fruits should be prepared as late as possible to ensure freshness.

Careers

Environmental careers create a supportive environment for the patient. Support services or ancillary health workers are needed in all aspects of health care. Most ancillary workers are not seen by the person receiving the service (Box 33-1). Many of the assistant level workers providing care in other career areas maintain the equipment and supplies needed for optimal care. In addition to the specific skills and knowledge needed in each specialty area, ancillary workers must know basic medical terminology and principles of asepsis.

Nutrition Services

Dietitians provide nutritional counseling and services in a variety of settings. They supervise food operations to meet the patients' needs and provide counseling on nutrition. Dietitians manage the nutritional services of the health care system. The goals of the dietitian include promotion and maintenance of health, prevention and treatment of illness, and assistance in rehabilitation through nutritional education and diet. Dietitians may specialize in clinical, commu-

nity, management, business, education, or consulting services. Dietitians must successfully complete a minimum of 4 years in a bachelor's degree program in dietetics, nutrition, or food systems management. Part of the dietitian program includes an internship in the health care industry. A master's or doctoral degree is preferred in many employment opportunities. Registration is available after successful completion of an accredited program and examination.

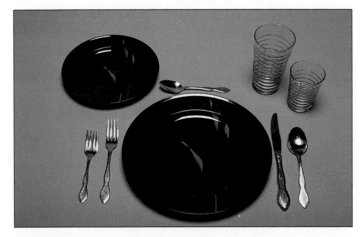

Figure 33-1 Using the proper place setting can make food more appealing to patients.

Skill 33-2

Preparing the Dining Area

1. Maintain medical asepsis by using the guidelines provided in the Standard and Transmission-Based Precautions, including good handwashing technique and use of gloves as needed. The hands should be washed after cleaning the surfaces of the table and chairs because the utensils for setting the table are cleaner than the furniture.

2. Arrange the chairs for easy access. Patients may require enough space for access by a wheelchair. Use separate cloths to clean the top of the table and chairs. Separate cleaning cloths are used for the table and chair seats because the tabletop is generally cleaner than the chairs.

3. If desired, spread a tablecloth.

4. Select the correct flatware, dinnerware, and glassware. Handle utensils by the stem. Utensils should be handled so that the area that touches the mouth is not touched by the hands.

5. Set the places correctly. A proper place setting provides all materials needed for the patient to eat the meal and helps to create a pleasant environment to encourage eating.

6. If needed, assist the patient with opening containers, cutting food, placing a napkin, and eating.

7. When the meal is finished, thoroughly clean the area and return used items to the designated location.

Dietary technicians complete a 2-year associate degree program. They plan menus and supervise the production of food (Skill 33-1). Food service workers or dietary assistants prepare and deliver the meal trays to patients or prepare the dining area (Figure 33-1; Skill 33-2). They may also help the patient select a menu and process the order. Food service workers may prepare food and beverages. Collecting the empty meal trays and washing the dishes are also duties of the food service worker. On-the-job training is available for some of the entry-level dietary positions.

Dietitians are assisted by others in the facility to distribute meal requisitions to patients early in the day (Figure 33-2). The type of meal plan is determined by the physician's order and special needs of the patient. When the diet menus are completed, they are collected and the amount of food portions needed to complete the meals may be determined and prepared.

Weight reduction specialists counsel patients to lose weight using dietary and activity guidelines. These individuals may be called *nutritionists*, *dietary consultants*, or *weight counselors*. The person giving weight loss counseling must be outgoing, sincere, and patient. Weight loss programs vary greatly, as do the qualifications of these specialists. Some weight loss centers hire individuals who have gone through a weight loss program and have had some training sponsored by the organization. Weight loss specialists in private practice may be registered dietitians. Licensing for diet counselors is either in place or under consideration in 25 states.

The food scientist-technologist evaluates the safety of food processing and ingredients in the industry setting. This worker also develops new foods and new methods for producing known foods. Food scientist-technologists complete a minimum of 2 years of college. Bachelor's degrees are available in the area of food technology.

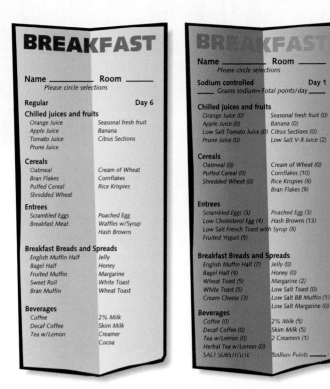

Figure 33-2   Well-planned meal requisitions allow a variety of food choices within the limits of the individual diet.

Environmental Control

The **pollution** control engineer analyzes contamination problems to establish methods and equipment to prevent pollution. Engineers review data from potential sources of contamination such as industrial plants. They calculate the pollutants being produced and may recommend denial of operating permits in plants that cause excessive amounts of pollution. A bachelor's degree is minimal for entry-level employment as a pollution control engineer.

The environmental engineer modifies facilities for environmental protection. The responsibilities include recommending methods for insect and rodent control and providing for safe disposal of radioactive waste materials. The environmental engineer researches factors concerning population growth, industrial planning, and natural environments. The duties of an environmental engineer include recommendation of equipment to meet the standards set by government agencies. A master's degree is recommended for entry-level employment as an environmental engineer.

Industrial hygienists conduct health programs in manufacturing plants and government agencies. Hygienists identify, control, and eliminate health hazards and diseases in the workplace. Responsibilities of an industrial hygienist include collection and analysis of dust, gases, and other possibly harmful substances. Consideration is given to ventilation, radiation, noise, exhaust, lighting, and other items that may affect the workers' health. Industrial hygienists prepare reports and recommend actions to eliminate potential hazards. Employment may be possible with a bachelor's degree, but master's level preparation is preferred.

Safety engineers are employed in all work environments. They identify existing and potential hazards in conditions and practices. Additionally, safety engineers develop, implement, and evaluate methods to control hazards. More than 100 universities offer degrees in safety engineering or safety management. Most safety engineers are employed by manufacturing, insurance, construction, or government agencies.

Health and regulatory inspectors enforce laws and regulations concerning employment hazards. Inspectors work for the local, state, or federal government. Health inspectors regulate consumer products such as food, drugs, and cosmetics. They also regulate quarantine for imported products and for people from other countries. Environmental health inspectors ensure that food, water, and air meet government standards. Health inspectors may specialize in such areas as dairy, food, waste, and air or in institutional or occupational health.

Radiation monitors, also called *health physics technicians,* test air, soil, water, floors, walls, and other areas of human contact for radiation. Most radiation monitors have at least 2 years of college education with a degree in nuclear technology. Most employers train radiation monitors on the job in the specific procedures used to detect radiation. Certification is available through the National Registry of Radiation Protection Technologists.

Ecologists analyze and regulate the quality of the environment as it is affected by living organisms. Some areas of specialization include air pollution analysis, water quality analysis, soil analysis, forest ecology, aquatic ecology, plant ecology, and animal ecology. Most ecologists work in the habitat to be studied such as the forest, large city, ocean, and so forth. Ecologists earn a baccalaureate degree in one of the major sciences with emphasis on courses in the area of specialization. Most ecologists are employed by the government or private industry such as petrochemical companies.

Sanitarians plan, develop, and execute environmental health programs. Their work includes organizing waste disposal procedures for schools and governments and for community, industrial, and private organizations. Sanitarians set and enforce standards concerning food, sewage, and waste disposal. Bachelor's preparation in environmental science is minimal for entry-level appointments. Advancement requires a master's degree in public health. Sanitation engineers may be educated in civil engineering.

Using the Epidemiological Approach

1. Identify the health problem, disease, or illness. The person, place, and time are needed to identify and solve the problem, just as the signs and symptoms of disease are needed to determine the condition.

2. Identify the source of the problem by interviewing the affected individuals, checking public records, and making observations.

3. Plan a method to prevent the problem from recurring. Methods of prevention may include changing the environment to eliminate the causative agent or educating the affected population about methods of prevention.

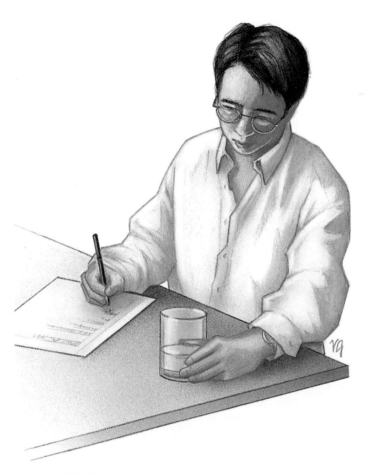

Figure 33-3 Water may be analyzed for its quality, bacterial content, or other pollutant content.

Environmental health technicians collect and analyze air and water samples under the supervision of the sanitarian (Figure 33-3). Training for the environmental health care technician is available in post-secondary vocational programs. Training may also be offered in the community college and result in an associate degree. Environmental health assistants perform routine tasks under the supervision of the sanitarian. Environmental health assistants learn on the job.

Public health microbiologists conduct tests and study the relationship of people to organisms that cause pollution, disease, or epidemics to prevent the same problems in the future (Skill 33-3). Microbiologists in public health usually work for some level of government. Some examples of the work done by microbiologists include testing foods, monitoring the sludge from sewage treatment, and identifying organisms that cause widespread disease. Microbiologists must have at least a bachelor's degree in biological or life science. However, most microbiology study is completed on the graduate level. Some states require public health microbiologists to be licensed. Certification as a Specialist in Public Health may be granted by the Academy of Microbiology.

Other Support Service Personnel

Other support service personnel are found in all areas of the health care facility. Some of the departments of support personnel include sterile supply, central service, biomedical engineering, laundry, security, and maintenance operations. Ancillary services also include groundskeeping, housekeeping, and other personnel needed to run a large institution (Skill 33-4). On-the-job training is available for many of the entry-level support services positions.

Some 2-year colleges work in cooperation with local hospitals to offer a degree in biomedical equipment technology. On-the-job training may be possible in some areas. These biomedical equipment technicians work with the biomedical engineering staff to service and maintain equipment in the facility. Duties of the equipment technician include installing, calibrating, and inspecting and maintaining electrical, mechanical, hydraulic, and pneumatic equipment. The equipment includes electrocardiogram, blood gas analysis, radiological, anesthetic, and other apparatus. Voluntary certification of technicians by the Society of Biomedical Equipment Technicians is available in three areas of specialization. Areas of certification are certified biomedical equipment technician (CBET), clinical laboratory equipment specialist (CLES), and certified radiological equipment specialist (CRES).

The surgical technician or operating room technologist (ORT) works under the direction of the surgeon. The duties of the surgical technician include maintaining the sterile field and passing instruments to the surgeon during an operation. The role may include cleaning and restocking the operating rooms. Knowledge of surgical procedures is necessary to anticipate the needs of the surgeon. Most surgical technicians complete a vocational or hospital-based training program lasting 9 to 12 months. In some states, the surgical technologist may serve as the circulator or primary nonsterile member of the surgical team. Certification is available through the Association of Surgical Technologists and may result in a higher salary for the certified surgical technologist (CST).

Central service or sterile supply technicians sterilize, assemble, clean, and store diagnostic and surgical equipment (Figure 33-4). Training of central service technicians includes isolation, aseptic, and decontamination techniques. Training is available through vocational and 2-year college programs or on the job.

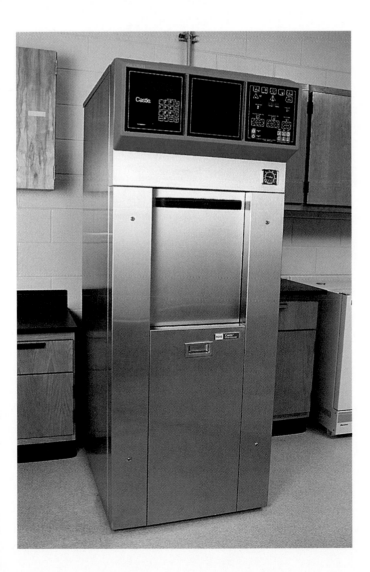

Figure 33-4   The autoclave sterilizes instruments by using steam under pressure to kill all microorganisms, including viruses and spores.

Skill 33-4

Housekeeping: General Rules

1. Maintain medical asepsis by using the guidelines provided in the Standard and Transmission-Based Precautions, including good handwashing technique and use of gloves as needed.

2. Establish and maintain a cleaning schedule. A clean and sanitary facility provides a safe and comfortable environment for the patient.

3. Place contaminated wasted in the designated container immediately. Clean all contaminated equipment and supplies and return them to the designated location. Use the appropriate container for disposal of biohazardous waste.

4. Disinfect all work surfaces.

5. Handle contaminated linens as little as possible.

6. Report any exposure to contaminated materials to the supervisor immediately.

7. Maintain the patient's privacy and confidentiality while providing care at all times.

Central supply assistants inventory, receive, store, and distribute the equipment and products needed in large health care institutions (Figure 33-5). The educational requirement for the central supply clerk is minimal as the work is repetitive. On-the-job training is possible for central supply assistants.

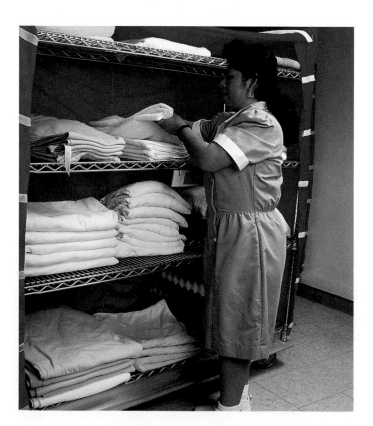

Figure 33-5 Central supply assistants help with the distribution of linens for the health care facility.

Content Instruction

Environmental Resources and Hazards

There is a limited supply of air, water, and land on the earth. These resources are constantly being used and reused (recycled). The **biosphere** is the air, crust of the earth, and water. It is made up of **ecosystems**, or the living and nonliving parts of the environment that support a chain of life in a selected area (Figure 33-6). Ecology is the study of living organisms and how they relate to their environment. Humans produce more waste than can be recycled through natural processes. Pollution of the water, air, and land now endangers life as it is known. The goal of the public health programs that control the environment is to protect life and preserve the resources necessary for it. The Environmental Protection Agency (EPA) is the federal agency that sets and regulates the standards for environmental factors.

There are many diseases and health conditions linked to environmental conditions. Emphysema and other lung disorders may be caused or worsened by air pollution. Lead poisoning has resulted from paint and gasoline additives. Because of government programs to reduce the blood level of lead in the population, it has decreased in adults since 1970. According to Centers for Disease Control estimates, 890,000 U.S. children between the ages of 1 and 5 have elevated lead levels in their blood. Carbon monoxide from car exhaust is linked to heart disease. As a waste product of manufacturing, mercury has been linked to nerve disorders. Lung cancer has been known to result from exposure to asbestos fibers, which, in the past, were used for insulation. Chemicals found in the environment act as **mutagens** and cause many cancers.

Air pollution is composed of dust and soot (**particulates**), carbon monoxide, **hydrocarbons,** and nitrogen oxides. It is estimated that three out of five Americans live in areas that do not meet the national standards set by the Clean Air Act of 1970. Thinning of the protective ozone layer of the atmosphere has resulted from the contaminants released from automobile exhaust, aerosol propel-

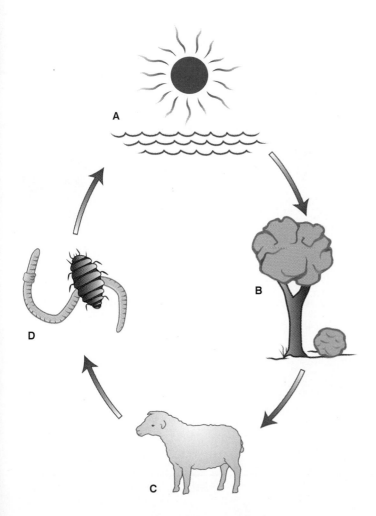

Figure 33-6   The chain of life—ecosystem. The chain of life is composed of the following elements. **A,** Sunlight, water, oxygen, carbon dioxide, organic compounds, and nutrients found in the ecosystem. **B,** Plants or "producers" on land and in water convert carbon dioxide and other nutrients from the ecosystem in carbohydrates through photosynthesis, releasing oxygen. **C,** Herbivores (cows, sheep), carnivores, and other consumers feed on the producers and on each other. **D,** "Decomposers," such as bacteria, fungi, and insects, break down dead producers and consumers thereby returning their compounds into the ecosystem for reuse.

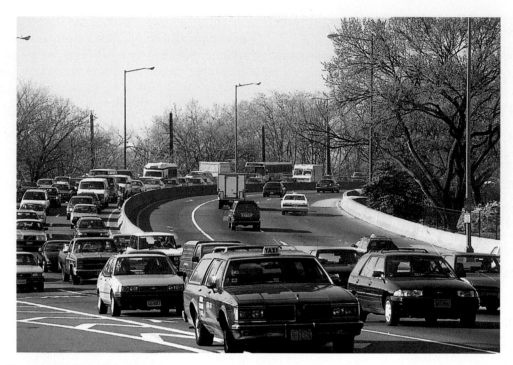

Figure 33-7 Pollution of the air, caused partly by automobile exhaust, has become a significant health factor.

Table 33-1 Air Pollution Facts

Body System	Effect of Air Pollution
Respiratory	Ozone reduces the body's ability to remove toxins and infectious agents
Sensory	Chemicals in air pollution irritate the eyes
Nervous	Carbon monoxide in air pollution disturbs coordination and concentration
Cardiovascular	Carbon monoxide in air pollution takes the place of red blood cells on the hemoglobin molecule, reducing the blood level of oxygen

Index Rating	Smog Index Meaning
0-50	Good
51-100	Moderate
101-199	Unhealthful—People with heart or respiratory problems are encouraged to limit activity
200-299	Very unhealthful—Elderly people and those with heart or respiratory problems are encouraged to stay inside
300+	Hazardous—Everyone should avoid outdoor activities

Table 33-2   Sources and Effects of Noise

Sound	Noise Level (dB)	Effect
Firecracker, balloon pop, shotgun blast	150	Pain, hearing loss from unprotected exposure
Jet engine (near)	140	Pain, hearing loss from unprotected exposure
Jet takeoff (100-200 feet), stock car races	130	Pain, hearing loss from unprotected exposure
Thunderclap (near), nightclub	120	Sensation felt
Power saw, rock music band, snowmobile, leaf blower, car horn, video arcade	110	More than 1 minute unprotected exposure risks permanent hearing loss
Garbage truck	100	More than 15 minute unprotected exposure risks hearing loss
Motorcycle, shop tools, lawnmower, subway	90	Very annoying
Electric razor	85	Hearing damage occurs
Traffic noise, garbage disposal, telephone ring	80	Annoying, interferes with conversation
Vacuum cleaner, hair dryer	70	Interferes with telephone conversation
Normal conversation, typewriter, sewing machine	60	Comfortable
Office, air conditioner, rainfall, refrigerator, air conditioner	50	Comfortable
Whisper, quiet library	30	Very quiet
Normal breathing	10	Just audible
	0	Threshold of normal hearing

lants, and painting materials (Figure 33-7). The decrease in the ozone layer has increased the intensity of ultraviolet rays reaching the surface of the earth and leading to a higher incidence of skin cancer. Much of the air pollution in cities results from the burning of fuels such as oil. Air pollution in rural areas is caused by agricultural, mining, and lumbering activities. The physical effects of air pollution have been documented (Table 33-1).

Sound is a form of energy measured by pitch and loudness. Pitch, or the quality of the sound that is heard, is determined by the speed of the vibrations against the eardrum. Loudness is the intensity of the sound waves or how hard the sound waves strike the eardrum. Loudness of sounds is measured in **decibels** (dB) (Table 33-2). The lowest sound level that can be heard by the healthy human ear under quiet conditions is 1 dB. More than 23 million Americans have some hearing loss, more than 1 million of those are less than 18 years of age. One third of these hearing losses are linked to environmental causes and could be prevented.

Inside the cochlea of the ear, microscopic hairs move back and forth, stimulating nerve fibers that transmit

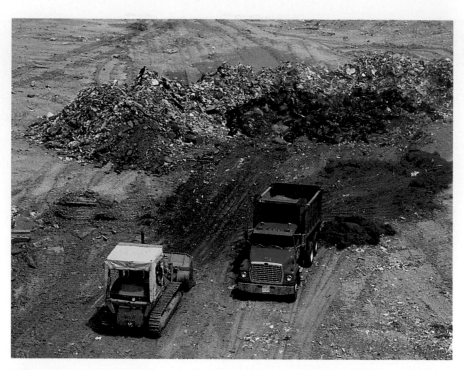

Figure 33-8 Disposal of waste in public landfills provides a reservoir for disease-causing organisms.

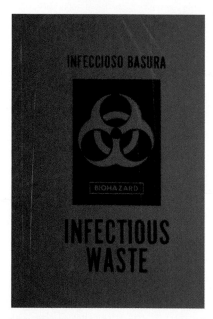

Figure 33-9 A biohazard symbol.

Box 33-2 **Ten Leading Work-Related Diseases and Injuries**

1. Occupational lung diseases
2. Musculoskeletal injuries
3. Occupational cancers other than lung cancer
4. Severe traumatic injury
5. Cardiovascular disease
6. Disorders of reproduction
7. Neurotoxic disorders
8. Noise-induced hearing loss
9. Dermatology conditions
10. Psychological disorders

From National Institute for Occupational Safety and Health.

sound to the brain. The hairs can be damaged when too great a force is created by loud sounds. The ear protects itself by changing the loudness of the sound with the ossicles, or small bones of the ear. If the sound is too loud, this cannot be done. Hearing loss, caused by exposure to noise in cities, has been reported. There is excessive noise in homes and offices as well as in traffic and outdoor environments. Environmental noise in homes results from ap-

pliances, tools, and music equipment. At sound levels about 40 dB, noise disturbs a sleeping person, and above 50 dB it disturbs conversation. At levels above 85 dB, stress reactions caused by noise may be expected. Damage to the ear that results in hearing loss occurs at 80 dB. At about 120 dB the ear feels pain, and small animals die when exposed to 165 dB. Other adverse effects of excessive noise include cardiovascular, endocrine, and neurological reac-

Skill 33-5

Preparing Meals

1. Maintain medical asepsis by using the guidelines provided in the Standard and Transmission-Based Precautions, including good handwashing technique and use of gloves as needed.

2. Assemble equipment and supplies needed for the recipe.

3. Measure the ingredients as required for the number of portions needed.

4. Prepare the food according to the recipe.

5. Store the food appropriately until the time of use.

6. Clean the countertops and equipment with disinfectant.

7. Return the equipment and supplies to the designated storage area.

---

tions that are similar to exposure to continuous stress. When a "temporary threshold shift" or muffling, bussing, or fullness is felt after exposure to noise, damage to the ear has been done.

Water is tested for its quality, bacteria, and pollutants. The quality is determined by the water temperature, turbidity, odor, animal and plant life, pH, and presence of debris. Water can be contaminated directly by industrial plants, oil discharges, **pesticides,** fertilizers, and heat from plants producing electricity. Water can also be polluted when chemicals and waste seep into the ground water, which supplies wells and springs. Standards for acceptable drinking water are set by the federal government.

Each year more than 4 billion tons of solid waste are produced in the United States. This represents 1300 pounds per person. Waste may be incinerated or stored in landfills. Approximately 6000 landfills are being used (Figure 33-8). Two thirds of those created were filled by the end of the 1980s. This waste includes many materials, such as plastic containers, cans, and paper products, that do not break down easily into recyclable compounds. When stored, the waste produces a reservoir for disease-causing organisms. Disposal of radioactive and other hazardous waste materials has become a concern of the environmental health services (Figure 33-9).

Controversy still exists regarding the possible harmful effect of electromagnetic fields (EMFs) generated by power lines, computers, hair dryers, and other electrical devices. Electromagnetic fields are low-frequency energy emissions. Some research has associated exposure to electromagnetic fields to cancers such as leukemia, miscarriages, and birth defects.

Work-related injuries and illnesses are the concern of public health personnel. The National Institute for Occupational Safety and Health has identified 10 leading causes of work-related disorders and injuries (Box 33-2). Some agents that lead to lung damage include silica dust and asbestos. Cancers induced by work-related exposure to agents include liver, larynx, blood, and bone. Cardiovascular disease is aggravated in the workplace by exposure to solvents, carbon monoxide, noise, and psychosocial stress.

Performance Instruction

Food Preparation

Food may be prepared by a food service worker under the supervision of the dietary department. Medical asepsis may be maintained by using good handwashing technique as well as wearing nets to contain the hair and gloves to protect the food. Recipes may be used to measure the ingredients to make food items. All prepared food is stored ap-

Skill 33-6

Analyzing Water

1. Maintain medical asepsis by using the guidelines provided in the Standard and Transmission-Based Precautions, including good handwashing technique and use of gloves as needed.

2. Collect a water sample in a sterile container to prevent contamination from other sources. Elements of the water that may indicate pollution include the presence of animal and plant life.

3. Observe and record the temperature of the water. Water temperature varies with the climate, oxygen content, and depth of the water sample.

4. Observe and record the turbidity of the water. The turbidity or clarity of the water can be determined by the amount of light that passes through it or by use of a Secchi disk. Water with high turbidity may be unacceptable for use by humans.

5. Observe and record the odor of the water. Odor may result from chemicals, organisms, or organic materials in the water. Odor does not necessarily indicate pollution of the water, but it is undesirable.

6. Using a microscope, observe the water and record the presence of life forms in the sample. The animals and plants that live in a body of water are indicators of its oxygen and other contents.

7. Observe and record the uses of the water sample area. Water may be used for recreational or industrial purposes. Litter in the water may indicate pollution from inappropriate use.

8. Measure and record the pH of the water sample. Litmus paper can be used to indicate the concentration of acid or alkaline materials in the water sample. The acidity of the water determines whether algae will grow and relative quantity of minerals or hardness of the water.

9. Prepare and incubate a streak culture plate to determine the presence of microscopic bacteria in the sample. Record the results.

10. Determine the acceptability of the water sample for its intended use. Drinking water should have a neutral pH, be free of microorganisms, have no odor, and be at an appropriate temperature.

propriately to prevent contamination until it is used. The counters and equipment in the kitchen area are cleaned and disinfected to prevent contamination of food items (Skill 33-5).

Water Analysis

Water analysis involves the collection of a water specimen to determine the presence of pollution in the form of animal or plant waste. Some of the tests performed in water analysis include determination of the turbidity, odor, presence of microorganisms, and pH. Water that is suitable for one purpose, such as swimming, might not be acceptable for another, such as drinking (Skill 33-6).

Instrument Maintenance

When the operative or medical procedure is completed, it is the task of the surgical technician, central supply worker, or other designated personnel to clean and prepare the instruments or equipment for further use. Medical asepsis is maintained throughout the cleaning procedure by using good handwashing techniques and wearing disposable gloves. Contaminated materials are removed from the instruments by rinsing them in cold water first because warm water may cause some materials to harden. Rinsing the instruments is followed by scrubbing them with a brush in warm, soapy water. Small instruments may be cleaned in an ultrasonic cleaner which uses vibration at high frequency to remove debris (Figure 33-10). Instruments are dried well with a clean cloth or in a hot air oven. Some instruments may require oiling according to the manufacturer's instructions. Surgical instruments are arranged in trays to make a set needed for a specific operation such as an eye, abdominal, or dental procedure. Other instruments may be wrapped and then sterilized using steam or chemicals (Figure 33-11). Soiled water and materials used in cleaning are disposed of in an appropriate manner to avoid contamination of the cleaning area. Chemicals that sterilize may be used to decontaminate some instruments and the cleaning area (Skills 33-7 and 33-8).

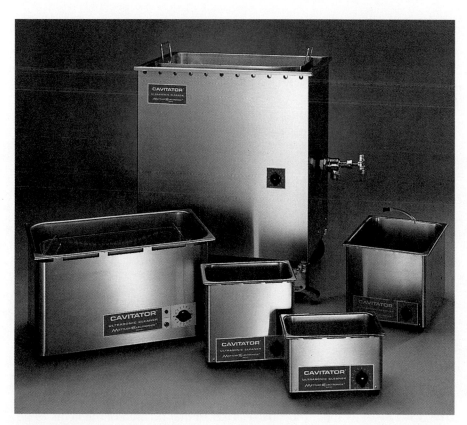

Figure 33-10 Ultrasonic cleaning removes debris by vibration. *(Courtesy Mettler Electronics, Anaheim, Calif.)*

Skill 33-7

Cleaning Instruments

1. Maintain medical asepsis by using the guidelines provided in the Standard and Transmission-Based Precautions, including good handwashing technique and use of gloves as needed. If the instruments are contaminated with body secretions, wear gloves to prevent the spread of microorganisms.

2. Remove all contaminating materials from the instruments by rinsing them in cold water. Contaminating materials may be more difficult to remove if warmed beforehand.

3. Scrub instruments with a brush in warm, soapy water. If necessary, place small instruments in a sonic cleaner for cleaning by vibration. Dry instruments well with a towel or in hot-air oven. Oil instruments according to the manufacturer's instructions. Arrange instruments on trays or return them to the designated area. Instruments may be stored on trays for convenient use, for example, in abdominal, eye, or dental procedures.

4. Dispose of soiled water and linens appropriately because pathogens can be carried on moist surfaces.

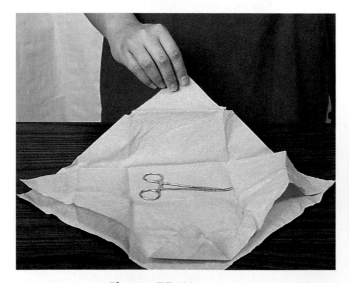 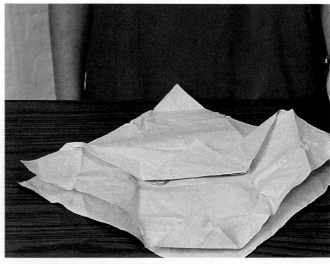

Figure 33-11 A wrapper must be selected so that no area of the items to be sterilized remains uncovered. Many items are wrapped twice to provide easier use after sterilization.

Skill 33-8

Wrapping Packages for Sterilization

1. Maintain medical asepsis by using the guidelines provided in the Standard and Transmission-Based Precautions, including good handwashing technique and use of gloves as needed. Wrapping packages for sterilization is a clean procedure requiring that the hands and instruments be as free from microorganisms as possible.

2. Select clean instruments for sterilization. Instruments may be arranged into sets for convenient use in particular procedures.

3. Select a wrapping towel or drape that is large enough to cover all contents completely. Drapes for autoclave sterilization may be made of cotton or specialized disposable material. Draping materials must allow penetration by the pressurized steam or gas.

4. Place instrumentation and sterilizing indicator diagonally in the center of the wrapping materials. The outside indicating tape does not ensure that the inner contents have been sterilized.

5. Fold the corners of the draping material into the center of the tray. The near edge is folded first, sides next, and the far edge last. The package should be neat and tight, with no exposed edges of the wrapping materials. Tuck the last edge into the pocket formed by the first three sides.

6. Seal the package with indicator tape. Secure tape so that the package will not be pulled open when the tape is removed.

7. Label the tape with the date and time of sterilizaiton, contents, and the initials of the preparer. Items are not considered sterile indefinitely.

8. Place the package in the appropriate location for articles requiring sterilization.

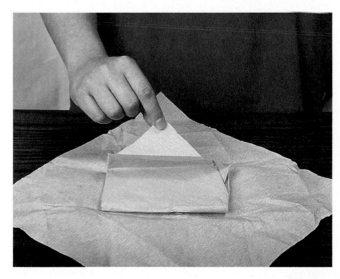
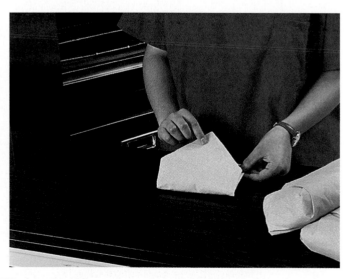

Figure 33-11, cont'd

Review Questions

1. Use each of the following terms in one or more sentences that correctly relate their meaning.
   Decibel
   Ecosystem
   Hydrocarbon
   Particulate
   Pesticide
   Pollution

2. Describe the role of at least three members of the environmental health care team.

3. Describe the function of the environmental health care team.

4. Describe the role of agencies that control the quality of the air, water, noise, food, and soil.

5. Describe the effects of atmospheric, water, noise, food, and soil pollution on the health of the community.

6. Identify the chain of life of an ecosystem in the local community.

7. List the departments and functions of the federal government's environmental health services.

Critical Thinking

1. Investigate and compare the cost of various types of environmental health care services.

2. Keep a log of particulate values from local weather reports for 1 week. Investigate the cause of the most prevalent types of particulates in the area.

3. Test the noise level production of various sites in the environment. Record observations about the feeling various noises produce.

4. Investigate the services provided by environmental health care agencies in the community.

34
Biotechnology Careers

Learning Objectives

Define at least 10 terms relating to biotechnology.

Identify the function of the biotechnological health care team.

Describe the role of at least five of the biotechnological health care team members, including personal qualities, levels of education, and credentialing requirements.

Describe the structure, function, and method of replication of DNA.

Describe three research techniques used by biotechnologists.

Describe at least three ethical concerns that have been raised since the beginning of DNA research.

Key Terms

Artificial Insemination
(art-uh-FISH-ul in-sem-ih-NAY-shun) Injection of semen into the uterine canal, unrelated to sexual intercourse

Deoxyribonucleic Acid (DNA)
(dee-ok-see-rie-bo-noo-KLAY-ik AS-id) Large nucleic acid molecule that makes up chromosomes

Electrophoresis
(ee-lek-tro-fore-EE-sis) Movement of charged suspended particles through a medium in responses to an electric field

Enzyme
(en-ZIME) Protein that acts as a catalyst in the cell

Eugenics
(yoo-JEN-iks) Study of the methods for controlling the characteristics of humans

Fermentation
(fer-men-TAY-shun) Chemical change that is brought about by the action of an enzyme or microorganism

Forensics
(fore-EN-ziks) Pertaining to the courts of law

Monoclonal Antibody
(mon-o-KLO-nal AN-tee-bod-ee) Identical cells or cells originating from the same cell

Selective Breeding
(seh-LEK-tiv bree-ding) Choosing the parents of offspring to enhance development of desired traits

Biotechnology Careers Terminology*

TERM	DEFINITION	PREFIX	ROOT	SUFFIX
Antibody	Against substances	anti	body	
Biodiversity	Variety of life	bio	divers/it	y
Biotechnology	Study of technology and life	bio	tech/n	ology
Congenital	Born with	con	gen/it	al
Dystrophy	Painful or difficult growth or nutrition	dys	troph	y
Endocrine	To secrete inside	endo	crine	
Eugenics	Pertaining to new origins	eu	gen	ics
Genetic	Pertaining to the origin		gen/et	ic
Neoplasm	New growth	neo	plasm	
Transgenic	Pertaining to cross origins	trans	gen	ic

*A transition phrase or vowel may be added to or deleted from the word parts to make the combining form.

Abbreviations for Biotechnology Careers

ABBREVIATION	MEANING
AIDS	Acquired immune deficiency syndrome
CBER	Center for Biologics Evaluation and Research
CF	Cystic fibrosis
DNA	Deoxyribonucleic acid
ELISA	Enzyme-linked immunosorbent assay
FDA	Food and Drug Administration
GM	Genetically modified
HIV	Human immunodeficiency virus
MD	Muscular dystrophy
NIH	National Institutes of Health

Careers

Biotechnology applies scientific and engineering techniques to the manipulation of the genes of living organisms. Various surveys indicate that 1 in 200 live births have a chromosomal abnormality. Biotechnology includes a broad range of improvements that may be applied to plants or animals and their products. Biotechnologists alter the cells of living things to discover and improve genetic traits (Box 34-1).

Biotechnologist

Scientists have been using natural techniques of biotechnology such as **fermentation, selective breeding,** and **artificial insemination** for many years. This emerging field began to take form as a separate discipline in the early 1980s with the development of cloning and recombinant DNA techniques of gene manipulation (Box 34-2). Other personnel are filling positions to design, manufacture, and operate the equipment needed to make these techniques possible. Personnel in biotechnology must show great creativity and logical thought and be able to work independently and as part of a team. The work takes great concentration and perseverance because the results may not be available immediately.

Because of the competitive nature of the field, most biotechnology labs use elaborate safety and security systems. Safety guidelines for the transfer and manipulation of DNA have been established by the National Institutes of Health (NIH). Some of these precautions include the use of laminar flow hoods to vent and filter air, strict sterilization, and careful planning to ensure all microorganisms are harmless. To date, no incident of a safety problem has been documented.

Biotechnologists also face criticism within their own profession. Many researchers believe that too much money is being spent duplicating work. For example, more than a dozen laboratories recently worked in competition rather than in cooperation to identify a gene that causes breast cancer.

Biotechnologists face a unique challenge as professionals in the health care field. Unlike any other area of health care practice throughout history, biotechnology has made many complex advances faster than they can be communicated to the public. There are more than 1000 biotechnology companies in the United States, most working in therapeutic and diagnostic areas of the field. More than 600 vaccines and therapeutic drugs are currently on the market as a result of biotechnology research. Lack of understanding has contributed to some rejection and fear of the progress being made in this area.

Biotechnologists also face ethical concerns about the control of human characteristics (**eugenics**) and the safety of organisms produced by gene manipulation. Some concerns include the counseling of couples to not have children if a faulty gene is present, insurance carriers refusing to cover offspring born after detection of a known genetic defect, and selection of offspring before implantation based on favorable traits such as gender. Some controversial

genes are being researched, such as those that may influence characteristics, such as obesity, violence, and hyperactivity.

Biotechnologists may work in many fields of practice including research, **forensics**, immunology, and teaching. Health professionals from other disciplines may specialize in the field of biotechnology. Biotechnologists may also work for regulating agencies such as the Food and Drug Administration (FDA) and National Institutes of Health (NIH).

Medical biotechnologists work with the production of antibodies for diagnosis or treatment of disease. Immunologists have used the skills of biotechnology to produce **monoclonal antibodies** for the treatment of many disorders such as cancer and acquired immune deficiency syndrome (AIDS). Other medical biotechnologists work to produce methods and products to treat diabetes, blood diseases, and heart disease.

Research biotechnologists supervise the work of associates and assistants in industry and health care to find better products and solutions to disorders. One product of genetic research is the development of transgenic animals.

Through the process of genetic transfer, animals that contain new genetic information can be bred. One example is the manipulation of the shriverer mouse. These mice are naturally born with a condition that prevents production of myelin sheath on nerves and is soon fatal. The species has been genetically altered to produce the myelin. Other mice have been genetically engineered to produce monoclonal antibodies and, yet others, to carry the gene for muscular dystrophy to allow research in that area.

Biotechnologists in forensics use biological samples from a crime scene such as hair, skin, and blood to identify suspects. The technique of DNA fingerprinting makes this possible, because each person has segments of DNA that carry a specific message unique to that person. These segments can be separated in a process called **electrophoresis**, which uses the natural electrical charge of molecules to separate them. The biotechnologist can then take photographic images of DNA fragments that are unique to each person.

Biotechnologists must complete a minimum of a master's degree but usually hold a doctoral degree in biotechnology or a related field such as biochemistry or genetics. Biotechnologists are not currently licensed.

Associates in biotechnology (biotechnicians) perform complex procedures of DNA extraction and cloning. They may be responsible for analyzing the data gathered using computer technology. Research associates usually hold a master's degree in biotechnology or a related field.

Assistants in biotechnology perform routine work of gene manipulation including combining bacteria with nutrients or **enzymes** in petri dishes, photographing projects, and performing simple tests. They also perform laboratory duties such as cleaning and sterilizing of glasswork. Assistants in biotechnology usually hold a bachelor's degree in biotechnology or a related field such as biochemistry or

molecular biology. At least 15 universities offer a 4-year degree in biotechnology.

Geneticists study patterns of inheritance and develop methods to influence genetic information. Geneticists may work as counselors for individuals with a family history of genetic abnormalities. Some of the techniques used by geneticists include isolation of genes and genetic manipulation. Some areas of specialization for geneticists include human, medical, molecular, cell, or population genetics. Geneticists may also specialize in genetic engineering. Geneticists are usually required to hold a doctoral degree for employment in research, teaching, or administration. Licensure and certification are not required for geneticists.

Support Personnel

Biomedical engineers or bioengineers design, develop, and help maintain instruments and machines that are used to monitor and treat disease in health care. Some examples of technological devices include lasers, pacemakers, and artificial hearts and kidneys.

Another development is the use of biosensors, or biological structures that recognize other structures such as enzymes, antibodies, and receptors. The biosensor converts the information to a voltage charge, sound, or light emission. The glucose meter that diabetics use to check their blood for sugar is a type of biosensor. The enzyme glucose oxidase binds with the blood that produces an electrochemical reaction in the meter to indicate the sugar level.

Recently technology has led to the development of robotic surgical instrumentation that can be used to visualize the surgery site from a distance. It is possible that this type of surgery may allow telecommunication of surgical skills in the future. Specialties for biomedical engineers include

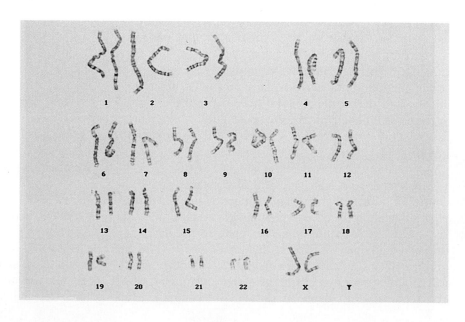

Figure 34-1 The karyotype may be used to show genetic abnormalities. *(Courtesy Wards Natural Science Establishment, Rochester, NY.)*

medical, clinical, and rehabilitation practice. They may also work in research to design new devices.

Most biomedical engineers work for hospitals. Education and training for this emerging field vary greatly. Most biomedical engineers hold at least a 4-year university degree. Some areas of study are engineering biophysics, bioinstrumentation, biothermodynamics, biotransport, biomechanics, and biomedical computers. Biomedical engineers working in health care must be registered. Licensing as a professional engineer is preferred. Voluntary certification is available.

Biomedical equipment technicians and repairers inspect and adjust the equipment used in health care. The equipment includes such items as the heart monitors and radiologic equipment. The education for biomedical equipment repairers is usually an associate degree in that area. An apprenticeship may be required. Voluntary certification is available on passing an examination and documentation of experience.

Bioprocess engineers design and operate the equipment used to ferment organisms used in biotechnology. They may also collect and purify the products for use. Some examples of products produced by fermentation include insulin and human growth hormone.

Content Instruction

Cell Genetics

Deoxyribonucleic acid (DNA) is a molecule that, by the sequencing of its components, determines all of the characteristics of living things. A nucleic acid is made of a nitrogen base that is attached to a sugar and phosphate. Each strand of DNA is formed in a double helix of chains of these nucleotides. The DNA conveys its message by unfolding and breaking into two strands. Special units of three nucleotides replicate or form a messenger to leave the strand. The new messenger makes a protein that directs a body function. The genetic information of humans is found in the nucleus of the cell in 23 pairs of chromosomes (Figure 34-1). Each chromosome is made up of a chain of DNA. The protein messages expressed by the sequencing of the DNA determines characteristics and directs the body processes. There are more than 100,000 genes on the human chromosome.

Each single chromosome contains 3 billion phosphate base pairs that make up the 100,000 genes (Figure 34-2).

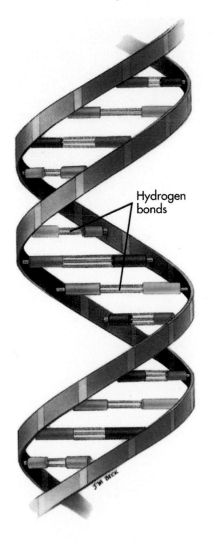

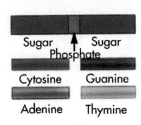

Hydrogen bonds

Figure 34-2 DNA holds the individual genetic code for each person. Each strand of DNA is made up of a series of neucleotides. The sequence of neucleotides determines which protein is synthesized. *(Courtesy Joan M. Beck.)*

Table 34-1 Mapped Genes

Chromosome Number	Genetic Information Influenced
1	Rh blood type—blood protein Thyroid-stimulating hormone—metabolism Amylase—starch digestion
2	Myosin—coats neurons Antibodies—fight infection Glucagon—sugar storage
3	Rhodopsin—light-sensitive pigment
4	Huntington's disease—neurotransmission defects Alcohol dehydrogenase—breaks down alcohol in body Red hair color
6	Major histocompatibility complex—antibodies Several reproductive hormones
7	Collage production Trypsin—digestive enzyme Cystic fibrosis
9	ABO blood grouping
10	Hexokinase enzyme—hemolytic anemia
11	Hemoglobin—sickle-cell anemia or thalassemia Insulin Parathyroid hormone Albinism
12	Phenylketonuria (PKU)
14	Antibody production
15	Tay-Sachs disease—neurological disorder
16	Chymotrypsinogen—protein digestion
17	Neurofibromatosis—nerve tissue tumors Growth hormone
18	Tourette syndrome—neurological disorder
19	Familial hypercholesterolemia Brown hair color Green-blue eye color
20	Adenosine deaminase—immunodeficiency disease
X	Duchenne muscular dystrophy Red-green color blindness Hemophilia

Table 34-2   Types of DNA Tests

Disease	Description
Adult polycystic disease	Multiple kidney growths
Alpha-1-antitrypsin deficiency	Can cause hepatitis, cirrhosis of the liver, emphysema
Charcot-Marie-Tooth disease	Progressive degeneration of muscles
Familial adenomatous polyposis	Colon polyp by age 35 years, often leading to cancer
Cystic fibrosis	Lungs clog with mucus; usually fatal by 40 years of age
Duchenne/Becker muscular dystrophy	Progressive degeneration of muscles
Hemophilia	Blood fails to clot properly
Fragile X syndrome	Most common cause of inherited mental retardation
Gaucher's disease	Mild to deadly enzyme deficiency
Huntington's disease	Lethal neurological deterioration
Amyotropic lateral sclerosis (ALS; "Lou Gehrig's" disease)	Fatal degeneration of the nervous system
Myotonic dystrophy	Progressive degeneration of muscles
Multiple endocrine neoplasia	Endocrine gland tumors
Neurofibromatosis	Café-au-lait spots to large tumors
Retinoblastoma	Blindness; potentially fatal eye tumors
Spinal muscular atrophy	Progressive degeneration of muscles
Tay-Sachs disease	Lethal childhood neurological disorder
Thalassemia	Mild to fatal anemia
Future Tests	
Alzheimer's disease	Most likely multiple genes involved
Breast cancer	5%-10% of cases are thought to be hereditary
Diabetes	Most likely multiple genes involved
Nonpolyposis colon cancer	Several genes cause up to 20% of all cases
Manic depression	Most likely multiple genes involved

A single gene, such as that for cystic fibrosis, is made up of 6100 base pairs. Some genes are expressed at one stage of development and no other. Ninety percent of the genome does not express itself at all.

The Human Genome Project, begun in 1988, is a multibillion dollar international effort to identify and sequence all of the human chromosomes. This process is called *gene mapping* (Table 34-1). Computerization of the sequencing techniques has allowed biotechnologists to identify gene sequences at a much more rapid rate than in the past. Researchers involved in this project report the identification of at least 18 genes involved in insulin-dependent diabetes. Scientists have also identified the location of a gene called *BRCA1* that causes 5% of all breast cancers. At least one gene that makes people susceptible to allergies and asthma also has been identified. In all, more than 50 genetic diseases can now be identified using DNA testing (Table 34-2).

Products that may serve as pharmaceuticals are being developed with biotechnology techniques in the emerging discipline called *pharmacogenomics*. Some genetically modified (GM) foods in development include edible vaccines, therapeutic proteins, and antibodies produced by plants. For example, the ProdiGene company (College Station, Tx) is developing vaccines and insulin to be produced by corn plants. CropTech is trying to grow plants that produce enzymes and anticancer proteins. Other researchers are developing bananas grown to contain the hepatitis B vaccine. However, a market for genetically modified plants has not been established. Although it may help prevent cancer, a GM tomato rich in the anti-oxidant nutrient (beta-carotene) has not been accepted by the American public.

Techinques of Biotechnology

Some of the techniques of biotechnology include gene cloning and gene splicing or recombinant DNA. Biotechnologists have been cloning plants for many years. This process involves removing a small number of meristem or growing plant cells and, by manipulation with hormones, creating a complete new plant. The similar process has been used to produce cattle by separating the cells of an *in vitro* embryo to create several embryos with exactly the same genetic information. Genetically identical tadpoles have also been cloned from the stomach lining cells of a single donor. Sea urchins have been reproduced by chemical manipulation of cells from one individual. In 1993 scientists split an early stage human embryo that was defective into single cells. Each was then coated in an artificial gel and continued to develop for several days before being discarded.

Gene splicing is moving genes from one location to another in the same or a different organism. An enzyme is used to "cut" a section of DNA open, allowing another to take its place. Free-floating rings of DNA called *plasmids* from an organism such as *Escherichia coli* can be used to introduce new genetic information. This process is called *transformation,* or recombinant DNA, as the genetic message in the organism is changed in the process. More than 80 specific enzymes, called *restriction enzymes,* have been identified to cut DNA at specific locations.

One example of the application of gene manipulation is the production of human growth hormone by *E. coli.* In the past, human growth hormone was harvested from pituitary glands donated at the time of death. It takes 80 to 100 pituitary glands to treat one child for 1 year. Most treatment plans last 8 to 10 years. The shortage of donated pituitaries and cost of the process made the treatment difficult. Through the process of recombinant DNA, the common bacteria *E. coli* has been given the genetic direction to make the human growth hormone. Fermentation processes allow large quantities to be produced. The quality of the hormone produced is consistent and economical.

Some other applications of biotechnology research include the use of early detection pregnancy tests and the enzyme-linked immunosorbent assay or (ELISA) technique, which can be used to detect the presence of HIV and other viruses.

More than 3000 people have been treated using one of several techniques called *gene therapy* (Box 34-3). Gene therapy is used to treat diseases such as heart disease, cystic fibrosis, infectious disease, and cancer. In cancer, genes may be inserted into a tumor using a virus to "infect" the cell with new information. Treatment with gene therapy is very expensive. The cost of one treatment may range from

---

Box 34-3 Disorders Approved for Treatment With Gene Therapy*

Cancer
Cystic fibrosis
Enzyme deficiency
Heart disease
Hemophilia
HIV
Transplant rejection

*Sample listing of 244 therapies approved by the NIH since 1989.

Box 34-4 Preclinical Gene Therapy Trials*

Rheumatoid arthritis
Diabetes
Other neurogenerative disorders
Hepatitis
Parkinson's disease
Hyperlipidemia/cholesteremia
Anemia
Non-specific bacterial infection
Musculoskeletal disorders
Tuberculosis
Herpes
Alzheimer's disease
Urinary incontinence
Chlamydiosis
Gastrointestinal ulcer
Osteoporosis

*Trials are listed in order of prevalence according to IMS Health, a pharmaceutical company.

Skill 34-1

Extracting DNA

1. Maintain medical asepsis by using the guidelines provided in the Standard and Transmission-Based Precautions, including good handwashing technique and use of gloves as needed. The National Institutes of Health has established safety guidelines for the handling and transfer of DNA.

2. Prepare a culture of nonpathogenic bacterial broth. Acceptable nonpathogenic bacteria, solution qualities, and percentages should be obtained by a qualified instructor or laboratory personnel.

3 Place a small amount of bacterial broth into a test tube and add a small amount of dishwashing solution to it. The dishwashing solution disrupts the cell membrane, opening the cells.

4. Place the test tube in a hot water bath for 15 minutes.

5. Use an eye dropper to pour a small amount of alcohol on top of the solution.

6 Carefully move a glass rod through the alcohol into the bacteria solution and turn it gently.

7. Continue to move the rod gently through the alcohol into the solution. The fiberlike DNA strands will "spool" around the glass rod for collection.

8. This DNA may be treated and stained to verify components of deoxyribose or phosphates.

9. Clean all materials and return them to the designated location for storage.

$150,000 to $300,000. The Center for Biologics Evaluation and Research (CBER) regulates human gene therapy products (Box 34-4). As of July 2002, no gene therapy product had been approved for sale.

Performance Instruction

Electrophoresis

To determine a genetic "fingerprint," the DNA must first be removed from the nucleus of the cell (Skill 34-1). This is accomplished by using a compound that has properties similar to a detergent that breaks the cell membranes open. An enzyme is then used to separate the DNA strands into segments. The DNA is then removed using a centrifuge to separate the heavier cell part away from it. Once removed the DNA may be placed in a solution for electrophoresis (Figure 34-3). A gel bed is prepared through which the DNA will move (Skill 34-2). Templates are used during the preparation to make "wells," or spaces in which the DNA samples are placed. The electrical current of the electrophoresis technique draws the DNA through the gel. Once completed, the gel bed may be dyed to compare the bands from each DNA sample (Skill 34-3).

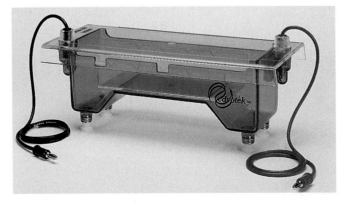

Figure 34-3 Electrophoresis uses a slight charge to separate DNA into a pattern that is unique to each individual. *(Courtesy of Edvotek, Bethesda, Md.)*

Skill 34-2

Preparing Agarose Gel for Electrophoresis

1. Maintain medical asepsis by using the guidelines provided in the Standard and Transmission–Based Precautions, including good handwashing technique and use of gloves as needed.

2. Prepare an electrophoresis gel bed for use by taping the ends of the box to form a square.

3. Dilute the concentrated buffer with distilled or deionized water according to the manufacturer's instructions.

4. Weigh the agarose powder to obtain the concentration required by the experiment being performed.

5. Add the weighed powder to the diluted buffer solution.

6. Heat the mixture, swirling gently, to dissolve the agarose completely.

7. Cool the hot agarose to 50° C.

8. Pour the cooled agarose into the gel bed. Use a pipette to line the edges of the gel bed. Allow 2 to 3 minutes for the gel to solidify.

9. Place templates *(combs)* into the designated location in the electrophoresis gel bed to form wells.

10. Allow the gel to set or harden before use.

Skill 34-3

Using a Micropipette

1. Maintain medical asepsis by using the guidelines provided in the Standard and Transmission-Based Precautions, including good handwashing technique and use of gloves as needed.

2. Unlock the pipette by pulling the control button out and turning it to adjust the volume setting. Micropipettes may range from small volumes such as 0.5 μL to 2500 μL (microliters).

3. Lock the volume setting in place by pushing the control button down.

4. If dispensing a liquid against the inside dry surface of a vessel, prerinse the pipette tip with water before using it. Do not prerinse the tip if a liquid is already present in the vessel.

5. Press the control button down to the first stop.

6. Hold the pipette in a vertical position and immerse the pipette 2 to 3 mm into the liquid to be dispensed.

7. Allow the control button to glide back slowly, pulling the liquid into the pipette.

8. Touch the tip of the pipette to the side of the vessel while pulling it out.

9. Wipe off any external droplets of fluid from the tip with a lint-free tissue.

10. Hold the tip of the pipette against the wall of the vessel or on the surface of the liquid in the vessel where it is to be dispensed.

11. Slowly press the control button to the first stop, releasing the fluid. Wait 1 to 3 seconds.

12. Continue to press the control button down to the second stop to remove any remaining fluid.

13. While continuing to hold the control button down, remove the pipette by sliding the tip along the side of the vessel.

14. Remove the pipette by pressing the control button down to the final stop.

15. Clean the pipette by wiping it with a soap solution or isopropanol.

16. Rinse the pipette with distilled water and lubricate the piston slightly with silicone grease.

17. Return the pipette to the designated storage area.

Review Questions

1. Use each of the following terms in one or more sentences that correctly relate their meaning.
   Electrophoresis
   Eugenics
   Forensics
   Selective breeding

2. Describe the duties, educational preparation, lines of authority, and credentialing of five biotechnology health care personnel.

3. Write a paragraph that describes the relationship of the following terms.
   Chromosome
   Deoxyribose
   DNA
   Gene
   Helix
   Nucleic acid
   Phosphate

4. Describe the method and use of the techniques of cloning, genetic engineering, and gene therapy.

5. Describe three ethical concerns regarding DNA research.

Critical Thinking

1. Investigate and compare the cost of various types of biotechnology tests and procedures.

2. Research and report the cost of education for two biotechnological health care professionals.

3. Identify a "scare story" from the media regarding biotechnology. For example, the media reported the impending extinction of monarch butterflies because of pollen of genetically engineered corn. It was also reported that genetically engineered corn that was accidentally introduced into grain used in tacos caused allergic reactions. Investigate and report the facts of the story chosen.

4. Investigate and report the incidence of researchers failing to report "adverse events" involving gene therapy trials to the NIH. For example, the FDA stopped research by scientists at Tufts University in 2000 because it was believed that they did not report the deaths of two volunteers being treated with gene therapy to grow new blood vessels.

Common Prefixes, Word Roots, and Suffixes

Word Root Examples

Root	Meaning	Example	Meaning
A			
aden	gland	adenoma	tumor of the gland
adren	adrenal gland	adrenalectomy	removal of the adrenal gland
angi	vessel	angiogram	picture (x-ray) of a vessel
appendic	appendix	appendectomy	removal of the appendix
arter	artery	arteriosclerosis	hardening of the artery
arthro	joint	arthritis	inflammation of the joint
aur	ear	auricle	pertaining to the ear
B			
bio	life	biology	study of life
blephar	eyelid	blepharospasm	uncontrolled muscle contraction of the eyelid
bronch	bronchus	bronchitis	inflammation of the bronchus
bucc	cheek	buccal	pertaining to the cheek
C			
calc	stone	renal calculus	kidney stone
carcin	cancer	carcinoma	tumor that is cancerous
cardio	heart	cardiology	study of the heart
cephal	head	encephalitis	inflammation on the inside of the brain
cerebr	brain	cerebrospinal	pertaining to the spine and brain
cervix	neck	cervical	pertaining to the neck
cheil	lip	cheilorrhaphy	suture of the lip
chole	bile	cholecystectomy	removal of the bile sac (gallbladder)
chondr	cartilage	chondrectomy	removal of cartilage
col	colon	colocentesis	surgical puncture of the colon
colpo	vagina	colporrhaphy	repair of the vagina
cost	rib	intercostal space	space between the ribs
cranio	skull	craniotomy	incision into the skull
cut	skin	cutaneous	pertaining to the skin
cysto	bladder	cystoscopy	examination of the bladder
cyt	cell	cytology	study of the cell

Word Root Examples—cont'd

Root	Meaning	Example	Meaning
D			
dactyl	finger	dactyledema	swelling of the finger
dent	tooth	dentiform	shape of a tooth
derm	skin	dermatitis	inflammation of the skin
dors	back	dorsolateral	pertaining to the side and back
dyn	pain	acrodynia	pain in the extremities
E			
emesis	vomiting	hematemesis	vomiting of blood
endarter	inside lining	endarterectomy	removal of the inside lining
enter	intestine	enteritis	inflammation of the intestines
erythro	red	erythrocyte	red blood cell
G			
gastr	stomach	gastritis	inflammation of the stomach
gen	originate, born	congenital	born with
gingiv	gums	gingivitis	inflammation of the gums
gloss	tongue	subglossal	below the tongue
glyc	sweet, sugar	glycogen	formed of sweet, sugar
gyne	woman	gynecology	study of woman
H			
helio	sun	heliotherapy	sun treatment
hemo	blood	hemogram	picture (x-ray) of the blood
hepato	liver	hepatomegaly	enlargement of the liver
histo	tissue	histoma	tumor of the tissue
hydro	water	hydrotherapy	water treatment
hypno	sleep	hypnotic	pertaining to sleep
hyster	uterus, womb	hysterectomy	removal of the uterus, womb
L			
laparo	abdomen	laparotomy	incision into the abdomen
later	side	lateral	pertaining to the side
lingua	tongue	sublingual	below the tongue
lip	fat	lipoid	resembling fat
lith	stone	lithotomy	incision into a stone
M			
mamm	breast	mammography	picture (x-ray) of the breast
manus	hand	manipulation	move about with the hands
mast	breast	mastitis	inflammation of the breast
meningo	membrane	meningitis	inflammation of the meninges
metra	uterus	myometrium	muscle of the uterus
myco	fungus	mycology	study of fungus
myelo	marrow	myelogram	picture of the bone marrow
myo	muscle	myoma	tumor of the muscle
myring	eardrum	myringotomy	incision into the eardrum

Continued

Word Root Examples—cont'd

Root	Meaning	Example	Meaning
N			
naso	nose	nasal	pertaining to the nose
nephr	kidney	nephrology	study of the kidney
neuro	nerve	neuralgia	painful nerves
noct	night	nocturia	urination at night
O			
ocul	eye	ocular	pertaining to the eye
odont	tooth	odontology	study of tooth
onco	mass, tumor	oncology	study of mass, tumor
oophor	ovary	oophorectomy	removal of the ovary
ophthalm	eye	ophthalmologist	specialist in the eye
orch	testicle	orchitis	inflammation of the testicle
orchido	testicle	orchidectomy	removal of a testicle
orth	straight, correct	orthopedics	dealing with straightening of bones
oss	bone	ossicle	small bone
osteo	bone	osteoarthritis	inflammation of the bone and joints
oto	ear	otoscope	instrument to view the ear
P			
pan	complete, all	panhysterectomy	complete removal of the uterus
Pap	papanicolaou smear		
path	disease	pathologist	one who studies disease
pedes	foot	pedicure	foot grooming
pepsi, pept	digest	peptic	pertaining to digestion
pharynx	throat	pharyngitis	inflammation of the throat
phlebo	vein	phlebitis	inflammation of the vein
phob	fear	phobia	fear of
phren	diaphragm, mind	phrenic	pertaining to the diaphragm
pleura	rib, side	pleuritis	inflammation of the rib, side
pnea	breathing	bradypnea	slow breathing
pneumo	air, lung	pneumonectomy	removal of the lung
pod	foot	podiatry	diagnosis and treatment of the foot
procto	rectum	proctoscopy	examination of the rectum
pseud	false	pseudocirrhosis	false condition of the liver
psora	itch	psoriasis	skin condition characterized by itching
psych	mind	psychology	study of the mind
pulmon	lung	pulmonary	pertaining to the lung
pyelo	kidney, pelvis	pyelonephrectomy	removal of the kidney
pyo	pus	pyuria	pus in the urine

Word Root Examples—cont'd

Root	Meaning	Example	Meaning
Q			
quadr	four	quadriceps	four heads (muscle)
R			
ren	kidney	renal	pertaining to the kidney
retr	back, behind	retrograde	situated behind
rhin	nose	rhinoplasty	plastic repair of the nose
S			
salping	fallopian tube	salpingectomy	removal of the fallopian tube
sarc	flesh	sarcoma	tumor of the flesh
sebum	oil	sebaceous	pertaining to oil
sedat	quiet, calm	sedation	calmed with medication
somni	sleep	insomnia	lack of sleep
splen	spleen	splenectomy	removal of the spleen
spondyl	vertebrae	spondylitis	inflammation of the vertebrae
stoma	mouth	stomatitis	inflammation of the mouth
T			
thorac	chest	thoracentesis	surgical puncture into the chest
thorax	chest	thoracotomy	incision into the chest
thromb	clot	thrombitis	inflammation of a clot
tox	poison	toxin	poisonous
trachea	windpipe	tracheotomy	incision into the windpipe
trophy	growth, nutrition	hypertrophy	above normal amount of growth
tympano	eardrum	tympanitis	inflammation of the eardrum
U			
utero	uterus	uteropexy	fixation of the uterus
V			
valv	valve	valvotomy	incision into a valve
vaso	vessel	vasectomy	removal of a vessel
vena	vein	venipuncture	puncture into a vein
ventr	front, abdomen	ventral	pertaining to the abdomen
vesic	bladder	vesicotomy	incision into the bladder
viscero	organ	visceral	pertaining to organs
vit	life	vital	pertaining to life

Prefix Examples

Prefix	Meaning	Example	Meaning
A			
a-	without	atrophy	without growth
ab-	away from	abduction	move away from
acro-	extremities	acromegaly	enlargement of the extremities
ad-	toward	adduction	move toward
ambi-	both	ambidextrous	able to use both hands
an-	without	anorexia	without appetite
ante-	before	antenatal	before birth
anti-	against, opposing	antiemetic	against emesis (vomiting)
astr-	star	astrocyte	star-shaped cell
auto-	self	autohemotherapy	transfusion using blood from self
B			
bi-	two, both	bilateral	both sides
brachy-	short	brachymorphic	pertaining to a short form
brady-	slow	bradycardia	slow heart rate
C			
capit-	head	biceps	two head (muscle)
con-	with	congenital	born with
contra-	against	contraception	against conception
cryo-	cold	cryotherapy	treatment with cold
cyan-	blue	cyanoderm	blue skin
D			
dys-	bad, out of order	dyspepsia	digestion that is bad (indigestion)
dys-	painful	dyspnea	painful respiration
E			
ecto-	on the outside	ectopic	on the outside of the normal location
en-	inside	encephalotomy	incision into the inside of the head (brain)
end-	inside	endocardium	inside of the heart
epi-	upon, in addition to	epigastric	upon the stomach
erythro-	red	erythrocyte	red cell
eu-	normal	eupnea	normal breathing
ex-	out, away from	exogenic	produced away from

Prefix Examples—cont'd

Prefix	Meaning	Example	Meaning
H			
hemi-	half	hemiplegia	paralysis of half the body
hyper-	above, more than	hyperglycemia	above the normal amount of sugar in the blood
hypo-	under, beneath	hypoglycemia	under the normal amount of sugar in the blood
I			
inter-	between	intercostal	between the ribs
intra-	within	intravenous	within the vein
L			
leuk-	white	leukopenia	decrease in number of white blood cells
M			
melan-	black	melanoma	black tumor
micro-	small	microencephaly	small brain
N			
neo-	new	neoplasm	new tissue
P			
para-	beside, by the side	paraplegia	paralysis beside
peri-	around, about	periodontal	around a tooth
poly-	many, much	polydactyly	many fingers
post-	after, behind	postnatal	after birth
pre-	before, in front of	prenatal	before birth
pro-	in front of	prolapse	an organ's slipping in front of its usual position
S			
semi-	half	semicomatose	half conscious
sub-	under	subglossal	under the tongue
supra-	above, over	supracostal	above the ribs
T			
tachy-	fast	tachycardia	fast heart rate

Suffix Examples

Suffix	Meaning	Example	Meaning
A			
-ac	pertaining to	cardiac	pertaining to the heart
-al	pertaining to	cervical	pertaining to the neck
-algia	pain	neuralgia	pain of the nerve
-ar	pertaining to	muscular	pertaining to the muscles
-asthenia	weakness, lack of	myasthenia	muscle weakness
C			
-cele	tumor or swelling	cystocele	tumor or swelling of the bladder
-centesis	surgical puncture	arthrocentesis	surgical puncture into a joint
-cle	small, little	ossicle	small bone
-crine	to secrete	endocrine	to secrete inside
D			
-desis	surgical union or fixation	arthrodesis	fixation of a joint
E			
-eal	pertaining to	esophageal	pertaining to the esophagus
-ectasis	expansion,	nephrectasis	enlargement of the kidney
-ectomy	removal of	chondrectomy	removal of a rib
-emia	blood condition	anemia	blood condition of too few cells
-esthesia	sensation	anesthesia	lack of sensation
G			
-genic	originating from	carcinogenic	originating from cancer
-gram	record	angiogram	record of a vessel
-graphy	recording	mammography	recording of a breast
I			
-iasis	condition resulting	lithiasis	condition resulting in a stone
-ic	pertaining to	enteric	pertaining to the intestines
-ist	one who practices	neurologist	one who practices study of nerves
-itis	inflammation of	myositis	inflammation of the muscle
L			
-lysis	loosening, destruction of	hemolysis	destruction of red blood cells
M			
-malacia	softening	adenomalacia	softening of the gland
-megaly	enlargement	cardiomegaly	enlargement of the heart

Suffix Examples—cont'd

Suffix	Meaning	Example	Meaning
O			
-oid	like, resembling	lipoid	resembling fat
-ologist	specialist in the study of	radiologist	specialist in the study of radiographs
-ology	study of	pathology	study of disease
-oma	tumor	adenoma	glandular tumor
-orrhea	discharge	rhinorrhea	discharge from the nose
-osis	condition of	nephrosis	condition of the kidney
-ostomy	opening into	colostomy	opening into the colon
-otomy	incision into	arthrotomy	incision into a joint
-ous	pertaining to, containing	sebaceous	pertaining to oil
P			
-pathy	disease of	osteopathy	disease of the bone
-penia	decrease, deficiency	leukopenia	deficiency of white blood cells
-pexy	surgical fixation	nephropexy	surgical fixation of the kidney
-phobia	fear	photophobia	fear of light
-plasty	surgical repair	rhinoplasty	surgical repair of the nose
-plegia	paralysis	hemiplegia	paralysis of half the body
-ptosis	drooping	blepharoptosis	drooping eyelid
R			
-rrhexis	breaking, bursting	cardiorrhexis	breaking of heart
-rrhaphy	suture	herniorrhaphy	suture of a swelling
S			
-sclerosis	hardening	atherosclerosis	hardening of the vessels
-scopy	look, observe	cystoscopy	look into the bladder
-spasm	involuntary contraction	cardiospasm	involuntary contraction of the heart
-stasis	halting	hemostasis	halting the flow of blood
-stenosis	narrowing	arteriostenosis	narrowing of the artery
U			
-ular	pertaining to	valvular	pertaining to a valve
-uria	presence of (a substance) in urine	hematuria	blood in the urine

Abbreviations and Symbols

Treatments and Tests

Abbreviation	Meaning	Abbreviation	Meaning
A			
ab	abortion	ASA	aspirin
abd	abdominal	asap, (ASAP)	as soon as possible
ABG	arterial blood gas	AST	asparate aminotranferase (formerly SGOT)
ABC	aspiration biopsy cytology	as tol	as tolerated
ABO	blood group classification system	ATD	admission, transfer, discharge
ac (a.c.)	before meals	ATP	adenosine triphosphate
ac & cl	acetest and clinitest	Av (AV)	atrioventricular, arteriovenous
ACTH	adrenocorticotrophic hormone	ax	axillary
ADH	antidiuretic hormone		
ADL	activities of daily living	**B**	
ad lib	as desired	Bact	bacteriology
adm	admission	BE	barium enema
ADP	adenosine diphosphate	b.i.d.	twice a day
AED	automated external defibrillator	bil	bilateral
AFB	acid-fast bacillus	BK	below knee
AKA	above the knee amputation	bl	blood
alb	albumin	bl wk	blood work
ALT	alanine aminotransferase (formerly SGPT)	BM	bowel movement
alt dieb	alternate days (every other day)	BMR	basal metabolic rate
am	morning	BP	blood pressure
amal	amalgam	Bpm	beats per minute
amb	ambulate	BR	bed rest
amt	amount	BRP	bathroom privileges
ANS	autonomic nervous system	BS	blood sugar, bowel sounds, breath sounds
ant	anterior	BSA	body surface area
Ap	apical	BSI	body substance isolation
AP	anteroposterior	BSO	bilateral salpingo-oophorectomy
A & P	anterior and posterior, anatomy and physiology	BSP	body substance precautions
		BUN	blood, urea, nitrogen
Aq (AQ)	aqueous, water	Bx (BX)	biopsy

Treatments and Tests—cont'd

Abbreviation	Meaning	Abbreviation	Meaning
C		**E**	
C & S	culture and sensitivity	EBL	estimated blood loss
CAB	coronary artery bypass	ECF	extracellular fluid
cal	calorie	ECG	echocardiogram
caps	capsules	ECT	electroconvulsive therapy
CAT	computerized axial tomography	EEG	electroencephalogram
cath	catheter	EKG	electrocardiogram
CBC	complete blood count	ELISA	enzyme linked immunosolvent assay
CC (C.C.)	chief complaint	EMF	electromagnetic field
CHO	carbohydrate	EMG	electromyogram
chol	cholesterol	ERV	expiratory reserve volume
circ	circumcision	ESR	erythrocyte sedimentation rate
cl liq	clear liquid	etiol	etiology
CNS	central nervous system	exam	examination
c/o	complaint of	exc	excision
CO	carbon monoxide, cardiac output	exp	exploratory
COMP	compound	ext	external, extract, extraction
CPK	creatine phosphokinase		
CPR	cardiopulmonary resuscitation	**F**	
CPT	chest physical therapy, current procedure terminology	FBAO	foreign body airway obstruction
		FBS	fasting blood sugar
CSF	cerebrospinal fluid	FBW	fasting blood work
CT	computer tomography	FF (F.Fl.)	force fluids
CVS	chorionic villus sampling	FHT	fetal heart tone
cx	cervix	FIFO	first in, first out
CXR	chest x-ray	FSH	follicle-stimulating hormone
cysto	cystoscopy		
		G	
D		GB	gallbladder
D & C	dilatation and curettage	GFR	glomerular filtration rate
DAT	diet as tolerated	GH	growth hormone
D/C	discontinue	GHB	gamma hydroxybutyric acid
del	delivery	GI	gastrointestinal
diff (DIFF)	differential	GM	genetically modified
DNA	deoxyribonucleic acid	GTT	glucose tolerance test
DNR	do not resuscitate	gtt(s)	drop(s)
DP	dorsalis pedis	GU	genitourinary
DPT	diphtheria, pertussis, tetanus		
DRG	diagnosis-related grouping	**H**	
D/S	dextrose in saline	H & H	hemoglobin and hematocrit
DSA	digital subtraction angiography	Hb	hemoglobin
D/W	dextrose in water	HCG	human chorionic gonadotrophin
dx	diagnosis	Hct (HCT)	hematocrit
		HDL	high-density lipoprotein

Continued

Treatments and Tests—cont'd

Abbreviation	Meaning	Abbreviation	Meaning
H—cont'd		**L**	
Hgb	hemoglobin	lap	laparotomy
HGH	human growth hormone	lat	lateral
HOB	head of bed	LDH	lactic dehydrogenase
hr	hour	LDL	low-density lipoprotein
HR	heart rate	LH	luteinizing hormone
hs (h.s.)	hour of sleep, at bedtime	liq	liquid
ht	height	LLL	left lower lobe
hx	history	LLQ	left lower quadrant
hypo	hypodermic injection	LMP	last menstrual period
hyst	hysterectomy	LOC	level of consciousness
		LP	lumbar puncture
I		lt, L	left
IABP	intra-aortic balloon pump	LUL	left upper lobe
ICF	intracellular fluid	LUQ	left upper quadrant
ICS	intercostal space	LV	left ventricle
I & D	incision and drainage		
I & O	intake and output	**M**	
ICSH	interstitial cell-stimulating hormone	MC (MCH)	mean corpuscular hemoglobin
IgG	immunoglobulin	MCHC	mean corpuscular hemoglobin concentration
IM	intramuscular		
inf	inferior	MCV	mean corpuscular volume
ing	inguinal	MN	midnight
inj	injection	MOM	milk of magnesia
IPPB	intermittent positive pressure breathing	MRI	magnetic resonance imagery
irrig	irrigation	MSH	melanocyte-stimulating hormone
IRV	inspiratory reserve volume		
IS	intercostal space	**N**	
isol	isolation	neg	negative
IT	inhalation therapy	neuro	neurology
IU	international unit	NG	nasogastric
IUD	intrauterine device	NGT	nasogastric tube
IV	intravenous	noc(t)	night
IVP	intravenous pyelogram	NPO	nothing by mouth
		NS	normal saline
K		nsg	nursing
kcal	kilocalorie	NVS	neurological vital signs
KO	keep open		
KUB	kidneys, ureters, bladder	**O**	
		o.d.	right eye
		oint	ointment
		OOB	out of bed
		o.s.	left eye
		os	bone
		OTC	over the counter
		o.u.	both eyes

Treatments and Tests—cont'd

Abbreviation	Meaning
P	
P	pulse, phosphorus, pressure
PABA	para-aminobenzoic acid
$Paco_2$	(Pco_2) partial pressure of carbon dioxide
Pao_2 (PO_2)	partial pressure of oxygen
PBI	protein-bound iodine
pc (p.c.)	after meals
PCV	packed cell volume
PDR	physician desk reference
PERLA	pupils equally reactive to light
Perrla	pupils equal, round, react to light and accommodation
PET	positron emission tomography
PKU	phenylketonuria
pm	between noon and midnight
PNS	peripheral nervous system
po	by mouth
post (pos)	posterior
pp (p.p.)	postprandial (after eating)
ppm	parts per million
PRBC	packed red blood cells
PRN (p.r.n.)	as needed
pro time (PT)	prothrombin time
pt	patient
PTH	parathyroid hormone
PTT	partial thromboplastin time
Q	
q	every
q.d.	every day
q.h.	every hour
q._____h.	every _____ hours
q.i.d.	four times a day
q._____m.	every _____ minutes
qns	quantity not sufficient
q.o.d.	every other day
qs	quantity sufficient
R	
r (R)	rectal
R (resp)	respiration
RAIU	radioactive iodine uptake
RBC	red blood cell, red blood count
RBRVS	resource based relative value scale
reg	regular
REM	rapid eye movement
Rh	rhesus

Abbreviation	Meaning
RK	radial keratotomy
RLL	right lower lobe
RLQ	right lower quadrant
RNA	ribonucleic acid
RO	reality orientation
R/O	rule out
ROM	range of motion
rt, Ⓡ	right
RUL	right upper lobe
RUQ	right upper quadrant
RV	residual volume
Rx	prescription
S	
SA	sinoatrial
sc	subcutaneous
sec	second
sed rate	sedimentation rate
SGOT	(see AST)
SGPT	(see ALT)
SI	système international (metric system)
sig.	directions for use of prescription
SMAC	sequential multiple analysis computer
spec	specimen
spG (sp gr)	specific gravity
sq	subcutaneous
S & S	signs and symptoms
SSE	soap suds enema
stat	immediately
STH	somatotropic hormone
sup	suppository
SVD	spontaneous vaginal delivery
SVN	small volume nebulizer
sx	symptoms
T	
T	temperature, thoracic
T & A	tonsillectomy and adenoidectomy
Tabs	tablets
T & C	type and crossmatch
TCDB	turn, cough, deep breath
temp (T)	temperature
TH	thyroid hormone
THC	tetrahydrocannabinol
t.i.d.	three times a day
TLC	tender loving care
TAH	total abdominal hysterectomy

Continued

Treatments and Tests—cont'd

Abbreviation	Meaning	Abbreviation	Meaning
T—cont'd		**V**	
T.O.	telephone order	vag	vaginal
tol	tolerated	VC	vital capacity
TPN	total parenteral nutrition	VDRL	Venereal Disease Research Laboratory (test for syphilis)
TPR	temperature, pulse, respiration		
trach	tracheotomy, tracheostomy	vit	vitamin
TSH	thyroid-stimulating hormone	VO	verbal order
tsp	teaspoon	vol	volume
TURP	transurethral resection prostate	VS	vital signs
TV	tidal volume	**W**	
TVH	total vaginal hysterectomy		
TWE	tap water enema	WA	while awake
tx	traction	WBC	white blood cell, white blood count
U		wt	weight
UA (U.A.)	urinalysis		
ung	ointment		
ur	urine, urinary		
URC	usual, reasonable, customary		

Conditions and Diagnoses

Abbreviation	Meaning	Abbreviation	Meaning
A		**E**	
ABE	acute bacterial endocarditis	EE	equine encephalomyelitis
AFIB (Afib)	atrial fibrillation	EP	ectopic pregnancy
AFL	atrial flutter	**F**	
AHD	arteriosclerotic heart disease		
AI	aortic insufficiency	FAE	fetal alcohol effect
AIDS	acquired immunodeficiency syndrome	FAS	fetal alcohol syndrome
ALL	acute lymphocytic leukemia	FIP	feline infectious peritonitis
AMI	acute myocardial infarction	FL	feline leukemia
AML	acute myelocytic leukemia	FP	feline panleukopenia
AP	angina pectoris	FTT	failure to thrive
ARC	AIDS-related complex	FUO	fever of unknown origin
ARDS	acute respiratory distress syndrome	FUS	feline urologic syndrome
ARM	artificial rupture of membranes	FVR	feline viral rhinotracheitis
ASCVD	arteriosclerotic cardiovascular disease	fx, (Fr)	fracture
ASD	atrial septal defect	**G**	
ASHD	arteriosclerotic heart disease	GC	gonorrhea
AUL	acute undifferentiated leukemia		
		H	
B		H/A	headache
BA	bronchial asthma	HB	heart block
BOM	bilateral otitis media	HCVD	hypertensive cardiovascular disease
BPH	benign prostatic hypertrophy	HDN	hemolytic disease of the newborn
		HIV	human immunodeficiency virus (virus causing AIDS)
C			
CA (Ca, ca)	cancer, carcinoma		
CAD	coronary artery disease	**I**	
CBS	chronic brain syndrome	IBD	irritable bowel disease
CF	cystic fibrosis	IHD	ischemic heart disease
CHB	complete heart block	IRDS	infant respiratory distress syndrome
CHD	coronary heart disease	**J**	
CHF	congestive heart failure		
CI	coronary insufficiency	JRA	juvenile rheumatoid arthritis
CLL	chronic lymphocytic leukemia	**L**	
COLD	chronic obstructive lung disease		
COPD	chronic obstructive pulmonary disease	lac	laceration
CPD	cephalopelvic disproportion	LE	lupus erythematosus
CPV	canine parvovirus	**M**	
CTS	carpel tunnel syndrome		
CVA	cerebrovascular accident	MD	muscular dystrophy
		MI	myocardial infarction
D		MS	multiple sclerosis
DIC	diffuse intravascular coagulation	**N**	
DM	diabetes mellitus		
DOA	dead on arrival	NF	neurofibromatosis
DT	delirium tremens		

Continued

Conditions and Diagnoses—cont'd

Abbreviation	Meaning	Abbreviation	Meaning
O		**T**	
OD	overdose	TB	tuberculosis
P		TIA	transient ischemic attack
PD	Parkinson's disease	TMJ	temporomandibular joint
PID	pelvic inflammatory disease	**U**	
PMS	premenstrual syndrome	URI	upper respiratory infection
PP	postpartum	UTI	urinary tract infection
PVC	premature ventricular contraction	**V**	
PVD	peripheral vascular disease	VD	venereal disease
R		Vfib	ventricular fibrillation
RA	rheumatoid arthritis	VSD	ventricular septal defect
RDS	respiratory distress syndrome	VT	ventricular tachycardia
RF	rheumatic fever		
RHD	rheumatic heart disease		
S			
SBE	subacute bacterial endocarditis		
SIADH	syndrome of inappropriate antidiuretic hormone		
SIDS	sudden infant death syndrome		
SLE	systemic lupus erythematosus		
SOB	shortness of breath		
S/S	signs and symptoms		
STD	sexually transmitted disease		

Titles of Associations and Personnel

Abbreviation	Meaning	Abbreviation	Meaning
A		CPU	central processing unit
AA	Alcoholics Anonymous	CRES	certified radiological equipment specialist
AART	American Association for Respiratory Therapy	CRNA	certified registered nurse anesthetist
		CRTT	certified respiratory therapy technician
AATA	American Art Therapy Association	CS (R)	central supply (room)
ACLS	advanced cardiac life support	CST	certified surgical technologist
ACSM	American College of Sports Medicine	CT	certified technologist
ACSW	Academy of Certified Social Workers	CVT	certified veterinary technician
ADA	American Dental Association, American Dietetic Association	**D**	
AHA	American Heart Association, American Hospital Association	DA	dental assistant
		DC	doctor of chiropractic
AHT	animal health technician	DDS	doctor of dental surgery
AMA	American Medical Association	DEA	Drug Enforcement Agency
AMRA	American Medical Records Association	DH	dental hygienist
AN	associate nurse	DHHS	Department of Health and Human Services
ANA	American Nurses Association	DMD	doctor of medical dentistry
APA	American Psychiatric Association, American Psychological Association	DO	doctor of osteopathy
		DOT	Dictionary of Occupational Titles, United States Department of Transportation
ARC	American Red Cross	DPH	doctorate of public health
ART	accredited record technician	DPM	doctor of podiatric medicine
ASCP	American Society of Certified Pathologists	DSW	doctor of social work
ASHBEAMS	American Society of Hospital Based Emergency Air Medical Services	DTR	dance therapist registered
		DVM	doctor of veterinary medicine
B		**E**	
BCLS	basic certified life support	ED	emergency department
BPA	Biological Photographers Association	EdD	doctor of education
BS Pharm	bachelor of science in pharmacology	EENT	ears, eyes, nose, throat
BSW	bachelor of social work	EMS	emergency medical services
C		EMT—First Responder (EMT-1)	emergency medical technician-first responder
CAHEA	Committee on Allied Health Education Accreditation	EMT-1	emergency medical technician-basic
		EMT-2 (EMT-3)	emergency medical technician-intermediate
CBET	certified biomedical equipment technician	EMT-P (EMT-4)	emergency medical technician-paramedic
CCC	certificate of clinical competence	ENT	ears, nose, throat
CCRN	certified critical registered nurse	EPA	Environmental Protection Agency
CCU	coronary care unit, critical care unit	**F**	
CDC	Centers for Disease Control and Prevention	FDA	Food and Drug Administration
CENSHARE	Center for the Study of Human-Animal Relationships	**G**	
CEO	chief executive officer	GP	general practitioner
CLES	clinical laboratory equipment specialist	Gyn (GYN)	gynecologist, gynecology
CMA	certified medical assistant	**H**	
CNP	certified nurse practitioner	HHA	home health assistant
CO	certified orthotist	HHS	health and human services
COTA	certified occupational therapy assistant		
CP	certified prosthetist		
CPT	chest physical therapy		

Continued

Titles of Associations and Personnel—cont'd

Abbreviation	Meaning	Abbreviation	Meaning
H—cont'd		ORT	operating room technician
HIPPA	Health Insurance Portability and Accountability Act	OSHA	Occupational Safety and Health Administration
HMO	health maintenance organization	OT	occupational therapy (therapist)
HOSA	Health Occupations Students of America	OTR	occupational therapist registered
HT	histology technician	**P**	
HUC	health unit coordinator (clerk)	PA	physician assistant
I		PAR	postanesthesia room
ICU	intensive care unit	PCA	personal care assistant
J		PCT	patient care technician
JCAHO	Joint Commission on Accreditation of Healthcare Organizations	PEDS (peds)	pediatrics
		PharmD	doctor of pharmacy
L		PhD	doctor of philosophy
lab	laboratory	PPO	preferred provider organization
L & D	labor and delivery	PsyD	doctor of psychology
LPN	licensed practical nurse	PT	physical therapy, physical therapist
LVN	licensed vocational nurse	PWA	person with AIDS
M		**R**	
MA	medical assistant	RCT	registered care technician
Mat	maternity	RDA	recommended daily allowance
MD	medical doctor	RHIT	registered health information technician
MLT	medical laboratory technician	RN	registered nurse
MSW	master of social work	RR	recovery room
N		RRA	registered records administrator
NA	nurse assistant	RRT	registered respiratory therapist
NATA	National Athletic Trainers Association	RSI	repetitive stress injury
NB	newborn	RT	respiratory therapy (therapist)
NCHSW	National Commission for Human Service Workers	RVT	registered veterinary technician
NCRP	National Council on Radiation Protection	**S**	
NFNA	National Flight Nurses Association	SBB	specialist in blood banking
NICU	neurological intensive care unit, neonatal intensive care unit	SICU	surgical intensive care unit
		SkillsUSA-VICA	SkillsUSA-Vocational Industrial Clubs of America
NIH	National Institutes of Health		
NIMH	National Institute of Mental Health	**U**	
NIOSH	National Institute of Occupational Safety and Health	USDA	United States Department of Agriculture
		USPHS	United States Public Health Service
NMT	nuclear medicine technologist	**V**	
NREMT	National Registry of Emergency Medical Technicians	VDM	Veterinarian Medical Degree
		VDRL	venereal disease research laboratory
O		VICA	Vocational Industrial Clubs of America
OB	obstetrician, obstetrics	**W**	
OBRA	Omnibus Budget Reconciliation Act	WHO	World Health Organization
OD	doctor of optometry		
opth	opthalmology		

Symbols

Abbreviation	Meaning	Abbreviation	Meaning
↑	higher	Hz	hertz
↓	lower	K^+	potassium ion
<	decrease, less than	kg	kilogram
>	increase, greater than	L	liter
@	at	lb	pound
C	Centigrade or Celsius	m	meter, minim
c̄	with	mEq	milliequivalent
Ca^{++}	calcium ion	μg	microgram
cc	cubic centimeter	mg	milligram
cg	centigram	Mg^{++}	magnesium ion
Cl^-	chloride ion	mL	milliliter
cm	centimeter	mm	millimeter
CO	carbon monoxide	μm	millimicron (nanometer)
CO_2	carbon dioxide	N	nitrogen
cu	cubic	Na^+	sodium ion
dB	decibel	NaCl	sodium chloride, salt
dL	deciliter	O_2	oxygen
F	Fahrenheit	oz (℥)	ounce
Fe^+	iron ion	p̄	after
ft	foot	P	phosphorus
g (gm)	gram	P_{CO_2}	partial pressure carbon dioxide
gr	grain	pH	potential of hydrogen; indicates hydrogen ion concentration
gt (gtt)	drop(s)		
H^+	hydrogen ion	P_{O_2}	partial pressure oxygen
HCl	hydrochloric acid	$PO_4^=$	phosphate ion
H_2O	water	pt	pint
H_2O_2	hydrogen peroxide	RAM	random access memory
HCO_3^-	bicarbonate ion	ROM	read only memory
Hg	mercury	s̄	without
Hr (hr)	hour	$SO_4^=$	sulfate ion
		s̄s̄	one half

Vitamins and Minerals

Vitamins

Nutrition	Function	Food Sources	Deficiency
Vitamin A (retinol)	Form and repair skin, membranes, eye tissue; resist infection; form visual purple (dim vision); produce corticosterone	Liver, carrots, sweet potaotes, greens, butter, margarine	Night blindness; retarded growth; infection; respiratory problems; rough, dry skin
Vitamin D (calciferol)	Help absorb calcium; build bones, teeth	Enriched milk, fish, liver oils, sunshine on skin	Rickets; weak bones, teeth
Vitamin E (tocopherol)	Protect structure of Vitamin A and unsaturated fatty acids; antioxidant	Vegetable oils, green leafy vegetables, whole grain cereals, wheat germ, egg yolk, butter	Anemia
Vitamin K	Blood clotting; liver function	Liver, milk, eggs, soybean oil, green leafy vegetables, fruits	Slow clotting, hemorrhages
Vitamin B (niacin)	Use nutrients; make fat; healthy skin, tongue, nerves; digestion	Liver, meat, poultry, fish, peanuts, enriched cereals	Pellagra; emotional, nervous disorders
Vitamin B_1 (thiamin)	Use energy; normal appetite; function of the nervous system	Lean pork, milk, yogurt, enriched cereals	Retarded growth; loss of appetite; nerve disorders; fatigue; beriberi; poor memory
Vitamin B_2 (riboflavin)	Produce energy; healthy skin, eyes; clear vision	Liver, milk, yogurt, cottage cheese	Reddened eyes; crackled skin; inflamed tongue; dry, scaly skin
Vitamin B_3 (pantothenic acid)	Regulate use of nutrients; production of cholesterol, adrenal steroids, hemoglobin	Meat, egg yolk, whole-grain cereal	Fatigue; cramps; respiratory infection; burning feet
Vitamin B_4	Form red blood cells; regulate nutrient use	Meat, soybeans, lima beans, whole-grain cereals	Muscle weakness
Vitamin B_6 (pyridoxine)	Use of nutrients; production of antibodies, form red blood cells	Liver, yeast, wheat germ, milk, potatoes, legumes	Skin disorders; anemia; weakness
Vitamin B_{12} (cyanocobalamin)	Blood formation; maintain nerve tissue; metabolism of iron	Meat, fish, milk products	Pernicious anemia; sores on mouth; loss of coordination
Biotin	Carbohydrate use; form and use fatty acids	Kidney, liver, milk, eggs, vegetables	Skin disorders; anemia; depression; sleeplessness; muscle pain
Folic acid (folacin)	Blood formation	Green leafy vegetables, dry legumes, nuts, whole-grain cereals, oranges	Anemia
Vitamin C (ascorbic acid)	Form collagen, blood vessels; promote healing; resist infection; help use iron	Broccoli, oranges, grapefruit, papayas, mangoes, strawberries	Rickets, bruising, scurvy; slow healing

Minerals

Nutrition	Function	Food Sources	Deficiency
Calcium	Form bones, teeth; stop bleeding; muscle contraction; nerve transmission; absorbs vitamin B_{12}	Milk products, cheese, sardines, dark green vegetables, fish	Rickets, poorly formed bones, teeth; slow clotting; osteoporosis
Chlorine	Water balance; electrolyte balance; part of acid in stomach; formation of enzymes	Table salt	Unknown in humans
Chromium	Metabolism of glucose	Meat, cheese, whole grain bread, peanuts, yeast	Type 2 diabetes
*Cobalt	Part of Vitamin B_{12}; erythrocyte production	Animal flesh and products, milk	Anemia
Copper	Storage and release of iron; development of bones, nervous tissue	Seafood, oysters, meat, eggs, whole grain cereals, nuts, raisins	Anemia; abnormal structure; abnormal hair color
Fluorine	Bone strength; healthy teeth	Fish, tea, meat, fluoridated water	Dental caries; brittle bones
Iodine	Form thyoxine	Seafood, iodized salt	Goiter; cretinism
Iron	Use energy; form hemoglobin (carry oxygen); resist infection; ability to concentrate	Liver, lean beef, oysters, dried beans, peas, lentils, dark green vegetables, whole grain cereals, egg yolk	Anemia; fatigue; shortness of breath; poor skin color
Magnesium	Regulate use of nutrients; function of nerves, muscles; assist enzymes; preserve tooth enamel; bone formation	Whole grain cereals, seafood, nuts, legumes, green vegetables, milk, tea, bananas	Tremors; foot cramps; convulsions; irregular heartbeat
Molybdenum	Enzyme component	Organ meats, greens, green leafy vegetables	Unknown
Phosphorus	Form bones, teeth; absorption of nutrients; metabolism of nutrients	Milk products, cereals, legumes, eggs, fish, meat, nuts	Rickets; poorly formed bones; loss of appetite; bone pain
Potassium	Muscle, nerve function	Fruits, vegetables, cereals, coffee, meat	Muscle weakness; irregular heart
*Selenium	Part of enzymes		Unknown
Sodium	Electrolyte balance, water balance; absorption of glucose; nerve function	Table salt, processed foods, canned foods, brown sugar	Dehydration; shock; weakness; cramps; nervous disorders
Sulfur	Form blood clots; healthy skin, hair, nails	Beef, wheat germ, beans, peas	Unknown in humans
Zinc	Part of enzymes, insulin	Meat, eggs, milk, seafood, whole-grain cereal	Loss of appetite; decrease taste; poor wound healing

A

abduct to draw away from median plane

abrasion wound characterized by the scraping of skin or mucous membrane from the surface of the body

abscess localized collection of pus in a cavity, formed by destruction of tissue

absorption uptake of substances into or across tissues

academic associated with a school of higher learning such as a university

accessory supplementary, complementary

accommodation focusing of the eye for varied distances

accreditation official authorization or approval

acetylcholine neurotransmitter between muscles and nerves

acquired not innate; not born with, but received from an outside source

active transport movement of materials across cell membrane and epithelial layers requiring energy

acuity sharpness or clearness

acute having a short and relatively severe course

addiction dependency on some habit; may be physical, psychological, or both

adduct draw toward the middle, or median plane

adenohypophysis anterior pituitary

adhere to stick to something

adipose of a fatty nature; fat

administration management performance of executive responsibilities and duties

adolescence period of growth from appearance of secondary gender characteristics to cessation of body (somatic) growth; roughly 12 to 18 years of age

adrenalin epinephrine; hormone that relaxes airways and constricts blood vessels

advocacy pleading the case of another; support

aerobic presence of oxygen

aerosol continuous dispersion of gas; atomization

afferent moving toward a center

agar dried product of algae capable of supporting bacterial growth

agoraphobia fear of being in a place where escape may not be possible

airborne present in the air, may be carried in respiratory droplets

alactasia malabsorption of lactose caused by a deficiency of the enzyme lactase

albuminuria excess protein in the urine

alignment arrangement of a group of points or objects along a line

allergen substance capable of inducing hypersensitive or allergic reaction

alloy solid mixture of two or more metals

alternative something different, substitute for something else

alveoli bony cavities in maxilla and mandible in which the roots of the teeth are attached; site of gas exchange in lungs

ambulatory walking or able to walk

amenorrhea complete loss of menstrual cycle

amino acids chemical compounds needed to build muscle, bone, blood, and antibodies

amputation the severing or cutting away of part of the body

amylase enzyme that is secreted by the salivary glands to begin the chemical portion of the digestive process

anabolism any constructive process by which simple substances are converted by living cells into more complex compounds

anaerobic absence of oxygen

analgesic pain reliever

analytical able or inclined to separate things into parts to study or examine them

analyze to examine a complex whole and compare the components

anaphylactic shock the response of the body to an allergen such as a medication

ancillary providing support for something

androgen any substance that possesses masculinizing activities

anemia below normal number of red blood cells

anesthesia loss of feeling or sensation

angina chest pain characterized by the feeling of choking and suffocation

anorexia eating disorder characterized by loss of appetite

antagonist muscle that acts in opposition to the action of another muscle, its agonist

antecubital area in front of the elbow

anterior in front or in the forward part of an organ; toward the head of the body

antibody substance produced in the body as a reaction to a specific antigen

anticoagulant substance preventing the coagulation or clotting of blood

antidiuretic substance suppressing the rate of urine formation

antigen substance that causes the formation of antibodies

antiinflammatory counteracting or suppressing inflammation

anuria complete suppression of excretion by kidneys; absence of urine

anus opening to the rectum between the buttocks

anxiety a feeling of fear or apprehension

apathy lack of feeling or emotion; indifference

apex narrowed and pointed end; tip

aphasia inability to speak

apical pertaining to, or located at, the apex of the heart

apiculture study of bees

apnea cessation of breathing

apocrine sweat gland that is attached to hair follicles

apparatus set of materials or instrument for a specific operation

apprehensive anxious or fearful about the future; uneasy

aptitude general suitability; ability to learn

arrhythmia variation in the normal pattern of the heartbeat

arteries blood vessels that carry blood away from the heart

articulation place of junction between two bones, joint; enunciation of words and syllables, how sounds are spoken

asbestos a chemical-resistant mineral form made of magnesium silicate that separates into long flexible fibers

asepsis freedom from infection; the methods used by health care workers to prevent the spread of microorganisms

aspirate remove by suction

aspiration act of inhaling foreign matter, usually emesis, into the respiratory tract

assertiveness technique to reduce the inner stress caused by inaccurate communication or lack of communication

astringent causing contraction, usually locally after topical application

asymmetry lack of sameness on both sides of the body in size, shape, and relative position

asymptomatic showing or causing no subjective evidence (symptom) of a condition or disease

atrium chamber of the heart

atrophy wasting away; decrease in size

attitude mental position or feeling with regard to a fact or situation

audiology science of hearing

auditory pertaining to the sense of hearing

aura subjective sensation or motor phenomenon that precedes and marks the onset of a seizure

auscultation listening to sounds produced in the body cavities using a stethoscope

autoclave machine that uses steam under pressure to sterilize materials

autoimmune directed against the body's own tissue

autonomic involuntary

autonomic nervous system portion of nervous system that regulates the activity of the cardiac muscle, smooth muscle, and glands

autopsy examination of parts of dead body to determine cause of death and pathological conditions

autosome any one of 22 paired chromosomes that are not sexual

autotransfusion the collection and transfusion of a person's own blood

aversion desire to avoid something that is disliked

avulsion the traumatic tearing away of part of the body

axilla the space under the arms; armpit

B

baccalaureate a bachelor's degree

bacteria single-celled organism that is neither plant nor animal; the most common cause of human disease and infection; classified by shape (bacilli, cocci, spirilla)

balance ability to maintain a steady position that does not tip

basal metabolic rate minimal energy expended for respiration, circulation, peristalsis, muscle tone, body temperature, and glandular activity of the body at rest

behavior conduct, actions that can be observed

benefit financial help in time of illness, retirement, or unemployment

benign not malignant or cancerous, not recurring

bevel slant or incline

bile fluid that helps digest fat in the small intestine; produced in the liver and stored in the gallbladder

binocular using both eyes

biochemical relating to the chemical substances present in living organisms

biological death death caused by the absence of breathing and heartbeat due to the loss of cell function

biopsy removal and examination of living tissue

biosphere part of the universe, including the air (atmosphere), earth (lithosphere), and water (hydrosphere), in which living organisms exist

birth canal the passageway for delivery of the fetus

blood pressure pressure of the blood on the walls of the artery, depending on energy of the heart action, elasticity of the walls of the arteries, and volume and viscosity of the blood

bolus the portion of food mixed with saliva that is swallowed

botany study of plant life

bovine pertaining to cattle

Braille system of writing that uses raised characters as letters

bronchodilator medication to dilate the bronchi and bronchioles for easier breathing

bulimia excessive, binge eating that may be followed by self-induced vomiting or purging

bursa saclike cavity filled with fluid to prevent friction

bylaws rules adopted by an organization to regulate its business

C

calculus calcium phosphate and carbonate with organic matter, deposited on the surfaces of teeth; tartar

calibrate to mark or determine gradations or units of measurement

calorie unit of heat

cancellous having a spongy or latticelike structure

canine pertaining to dogs

capacity holding power

capillaries blood vessels that receive blood from the arteries and carry it to the veins

carbohydrates starches, sugars, cellulose, and gums

carcass dead body of an animal, other than human

cardiac arrest period when the heart has stopped functioning entirely

cardiopulmonary pertaining to heart and lungs

cardiopulmonary resuscitation (CPR) a combination of mouth-to-mouth breathing and chest compressions that supplies oxygenated blood to the brain

cardioversion restoration of normal rhythm of the heart by electrical shock

career an occupation or profession

caries decalcification of the surface of the tooth followed by disintegration of the inner part of the tooth

carnivore animal that eats animals

carrier an animal that harbors or hosts a microorganism or gene without self-injury

cartilage specialized fibrous connective tissue

catabolism a breaking-down process by which complex substances are converted by living cells into more simple compounds

catalyst substance, usually used in small amounts relative to the reactants, that modifies and increases the rate of a reaction without being consumed in the process

catheter tube for injecting fluid into or removing fluid from a cavity (e.g., bladder or heart)

caustic capable of destroying or burning

cautery the application of heat that burns tissue

cavity hollow space

cellulose complex carbohydrate derived from plant walls

Celsius one measurement for temperature; 0 degrees is the freezing point of water and 100 degrees is the boiling point of water

centrifuge machine that separates lighter portions of a solution, mixture, or suspension by centrifugal force

cerebrospinal fluid fluid contained in the brain's ventricles, intracranial spaces, and central canal of the spinal cord

certification documentation of having met certain standards

ceruminous pertaining to earwax

character distinctive qualities that make up an individual

chart collection of written materials relating to the health care of a patient

chemotherapy treatment of disease by a chemical agent

cholecystectomy surgical removal of the gallbladder

cholesterol pearly, fatlike steroid alcohol found in animal fats and oils; precursor of bile acids and hormones

chronic persisting over a long period of time

chyme thick, semiliquid contents of stomach during digestion

cilium hairlike projection from the surface of a cell

circumcision the removal of the prepuce of the penis

clarity quality of being clear; lucid

client person who engages the professional services of another

climacteric menopause

clinical death death from the loss of brain activity (for a specified amount of time)

clone genetically identical cells descended from a single cell

clonic pertaining to alternate muscular contraction and relaxation in rapid succession

coagulation process of clot formation

coarctation narrowing of a vessel

coccygeal pertaining to the tail bone

cognitive relating to the process of acquiring knowledge by reasoning

collagen white protein fibers of the skin, tendons, bone, and cartilage (connective tissue)

combustion burning

communicable capable of being transmitted from one person or animal to another

communication exchange of information

compact having a dense structure

compassion sympathy with another's distress and a desire to remove it

compensate to make satisfactory payment or reparation to; recompense or reimburse

complementary accessory; health care used along with conventional practices

composition arrangement into proper proportion or relation; qualitative and quantitative makeup of a chemical compound

compound (open) fracture fracture in which the bone breaks through the skin and is exposed

comprehensive covering all areas; inclusive

conception onset of pregnancy; union of sperm and egg (ovum)

condition change from normal function that cannot be cured

confidential private and secret; may be protected by law

confinement restriction or limitation within the boundaries or scope of something

conformation particular shape

confusion loss of orientation

conscientious meticulous or careful; guided by conscience

consciousness responsiveness of the mind to the impressions made by the senses

consistency constitution or character; description of something's composition

constipation difficult or inadequate passage of fecal material

consumer one who uses goods or services produced by another

contagious capable of being transmitted from one person to another

contaminate to soil, make unclean, or infect with pathogens

continuum uninterrupted ordered sequence

contraceptive agent that prevents conception or pregnancy

contract shorten; reduce in size

contracture permanent shortening of tendons and ligaments of a joint resulting from atrophy of muscle

contusion an internal wound; a bruise

convergence coordinated movement of two eyes toward fixation on the same near point

convex evenly curved, resembling part of a sphere

convulsion the uncoordinated movement of groups of muscles usually resulting from poisoning or elevated temperature

coordinate put into order or rank to provide for smooth operation

coronary pertaining to the heart

coroner public officer whose primary function is to inquire about any death that may have occurred from unnatural cause

corpuscle any small mass or body

corrosive able to cause burning damage

creatinine end product of metabolism, found in muscle and blood and excreted in urine

credential document showing that a person is entitled to credit or to exercise official power

criterion an accepted standard used in making decisions or judgments about something

critical pertaining to a crisis or to danger of death

cryotherapy therapeutic use of cold

customary fee charged by similar practitioners for a service in the same economic and geographic area

cutaneous pertaining to the skin

cystocentesis process in which urine is obtained by a surgical puncture of the urinary bladder with a sterile needle

D

debris the scattered remains of something broken or destroyed; rubble or wreckage

decibel unit used to express relative power intensity of sounds

defecation evacuation of waste or fecal material from rectum

defibrillation termination of atrial or ventricular fibrillation usually by electroshock; cardioversion

deficient lacking some important part

deficit difference in amount

deformity distortion of any part or disfigurement of the body

degeneration deterioration; change from higher to lower (less functional) form

deglutition act of swallowing

delinquency antisocial or illegal behavior or acts

dementia organic loss of intellectual function

demographic pertaining to the study of people as a group, especially of statistical groupings according to age, gender, and environmental factors

dentition used to designate natural teeth in the mouth

deoxygenate act of depriving of oxygen

depilatory substance with the ability to remove hair

dermabrasion treatment of severe acne by removing the top layers of scarred skin

dermatitis inflammation of the skin

dermis corium, layer of skin beneath the epidermis

detoxify to treat (an individual) for alcohol or drug dependence, usually in a medically supervised program designed to rid the body of intoxicating or addictive substances

dexterity skill and ease in using body parts; mental skill or quickness

diagnosis methods used to discover cause and nature of an illness

diagnosis-related grouping predetermined payment structure for health care services established by the federal government

dialysis separating particles from a fluid by filtration through a semipermeable membrane

diaphoresis perspiration

diastole dilation of the heart; resting phase of the ventricles; alternates with systole

dictation words spoken or recorded to be written by another person

differentiate see or show the differences between two or more things

diffusion process of being widely spread; spontaneous movement of molecules or other particles in solution to reach uniform concentration

dilate stretch beyond normal dimension

dipping act of placing chewing tobacco or smokeless tobacco between the lower lip and teeth

disability lack of ability to function in the manner that most people function physically or mentally

discretionary offering the freedom to make a decision according to individual circumstances

discriminate to make distinctions based on differences

discrimination unfair treatment of one person or group, usually because of prejudice

disease interruption of normal function of the body usually caused by a factor that can be treated such as microorganisms

dislocation injury in which a bone moves out of a joint

dispense prepare, package, compound, or label for delivery according to a lawful order of a qualified practitioner

distend stretch out; inflate

diuresis increased excretion of urine

divergence simultaneous abduction of both eyes

diverticulum pouch that results from the weakening of the colon wall

dogmatism unwarranted or arrogant positiveness of opinion

domestic relating to the household or the family

domesticated animal that has been trained to live with people

dominant gene trait that appears when carried by only one in the pair of chromosomes

donor a person who supplies living tissue or who furnishes blood for transfusion to another

dopamine neurotransmitter in central nervous system

dosage regulation of size, frequency, and amount of medication

duct tube for passage of excretions or secretions

dysarthria difficulty with articulation

dysfunction disturbance, impairment, or abnormality in functioning of an organ

dysphagia difficulty swallowing

dyspnea difficult or labored breathing

dystocia abnormal labor

dystrophy disorder resulting from defective or faulty nutrition

dysuria painful or difficult urination

E

eccrine sweat gland that secretes onto the skin

echocardiography recording the position and motion of the heart walls or its internal structure using ultrasonic waves

ecosystem living organisms and nonliving elements interacting in a certain specific area

ectoparasite parasite that lives on the outside of the body, such as a tick

ectopic located away from normal position

edema swelling

efferent moving away from the center

effusion oozing fluids from blood or lymph vessels into body cavities

elasticity quality or condition of being able to stretch and resume original shape

electrocardiogram graphic tracing of the electrical activity of the heart

electrocardiography field of diagnostic health care in which the heart is monitored

electroencephalography field of diagnostic health care in which the brain is monitored

electrolysis destruction of hair by passage of an electrical current through the follicle

electrolyte substance that separates into ions in solution and is capable of conducting electricity

elongate to become or be made longer

embolism blockage of an artery, usually by a blood clot

embryo the young of any organism at an early stage of development

emesis act of vomiting; vomit

emmetropia normal vision; 20/20 vision

empathy ability to understand another person's feelings

endocrine secreting internally into blood or lymph

endometrium the lining of the uterus

endorphin one of the neuropeptides released by the brain that reduces pain

endoscopy visual inspection of a body cavity

endospore form assumed by some bacteria that is resistant to heat, drying, and chemicals; spore

endosseus referring to the inside of the bone

endotracheal intubation placing a tube within or through the trachea

enema liquid instilled into the rectum

engorge fill to capacity

enkephalin pain-relieving pentapeptide released by the brain

entomology study of insects

enzyme protein that accelerates specific chemical reaction

epidemic an outbreak of disease that affects a large number of people in one area

epidemiology the study of relationships of factors that determine the frequency and distribution of disease in a human community

epidermis outermost and nonvascular layer of skin

epilepsy transient disturbances of brain function

equilibrium state of balance

equine pertaining to horses

equivalent equal in value

erectile capable of becoming rigid and elevated when filled with blood

erratic characterized by a lack of consistency

erythrocyte red blood cell or corpuscle

Escherichia coli a microorganism that is non-pathogenic if found in the intestines, but pathogenic if found in the urinary tract

essential basic and necessary

esthetic pertaining to sensation, beauty, or improvement of appearance

ethics dealing with what is good or bad; determining moral duty and obligation

eupnea easy or normal breathing

euthanasia the induction of death in a sick, severely injured, or unwanted animal

exocrine secrete outwardly via a duct

exophthalmos abnormal protrusion of the eyeball

expenditure amount of money spent, as a whole or on a particular thing

expiration act of breathing out; exhalation

extract to obtain from a substance by chemical or mechanical action

extremity distal or terminal portion; arm or leg

extrinsic coming from or originating outside

F

fabrication created, invented, made from parts

farrier one who shoes horses

fat adipose tissue; reserve supply of energy

fatigue increased discomfort and decreased efficiency caused by prolonged or excessive exertion; exhaustion

feces excrement discharged from intestines

federal referring to the central unit of government of the United States

feedback a method to determine if a message was received accurately; a response by the receiver to indicate how the information was understood

feline pertaining to cats

fertility capacity to conceive or induce conception

fetal pertaining to an unborn baby from 2 months of gestation to birth

fever an elevation of body temperature

fibrillation quivering or spontaneous contraction of individual muscle fibers

fibroid tissue composed of threadlike, fibrous structure

filtration passage of liquid through a filter by gravity, pressure, or suction

first aid the immediate care given to the victim of injury or sudden illness

first-degree burn burn that affects only the outer layer of skin tissue

fissure cleft or groove; linear ulcer

flaccid weak; soft

flatulence excessive air or gas in stomach or intestines leading to distention of organs

fluoride chemical compound consisting of fluorine and another element

fluoroscope device used to examine deep structures by means of radioactive waves

follicle sac or pouchlike depression or cavity

fomite inanimate or nonliving object that transfers infectious microorganisms

forensic relating to, used in, or appropriate for courts of law or for public discussion or argumentation

formed element solid part of blood; red and white blood cells and platelets

fracture breakage of bone

fray to wear away the edge or surface of cloth or rope by friction

frequency the number of times an event occurs in a given period; in hearing, measure of cycles per second (hertz)

friction act of rubbing

frostbite exposure to cold that causes the water in the body tissues to freeze

functional having practical application or serving a useful purpose

fungus microorganism that grows in groups or colonies on other organisms; includes yeasts and molds

fusion merging of different elements into a union

G

gastric pertaining to the stomach

gender sex of an individual; male or female

genital reproductive organ

genome complete set of chromosomes with the associated genes

genotype genetic pattern of an individual

geriatric referring to all aspects of aging

gestation development of young from conception to birth, pregnancy

gingiva gum of the mouth; mucous membrane with supporting fibrous tissue

glucose simple sugar

glycosuria presence of sugar in urine

gonad sex glands that produces gametes

gonadotropin any hormone that stimulates the reproductive organs

gout swelling of the joints resulting from a buildup of uric acid caused by some metabolic disorder

grand mal seizure seizure that is preceded by an aura and results in semiconsciousness

grief the process that gradually resolves a sense of loss

grievance complaint; injustice

groin depression between thigh and trunk, inguinal region

growth hormone somatotropic hormone; secreted by the anterior pituitary gland

gustatory pertaining to the sense of taste

H

halitosis offensive or bad breath

hallucination imaginary visions

hay fever seasonal rhinitis usually caused by pollen in the air

hearing the auditory sense; the primary function of the ear

heat exhaustion condition characterized by perspiration, pale and clammy skin, and weakness

heat stroke condition characterized by dry skin, strong pulse, and a high internal temperature

hematology the study of the components of solid, or formed, elements of blood and blood-forming tissues

hematuria presence of blood in urine

hemodialysis filtration of the blood using an artificial membrane

hemolysis rupture of red blood cells

hemopoiesis process in which blood forms and develops

hemorrhage abnormal external or internal bleeding

herbal consisting of or made with aromatic plants

herbivore animal that eats plants

hereditary passed genetically, from one generation to another

heredity genetic transmission of trait or particular quality from parent to offspring

herniation abnormal protrusion of an organ or other body structure through a defect or natural opening in a covering membrane, muscle, or bone

heterosexual person who is attracted to the opposite sex

hierarchy arrangement into a graded series or levels of differing worth

hirsutism abnormal or excessive hair placement or growth

homeostasis tendency of an organism to maintain the "status quo" or the same internal environment

homosexual person who is attracted to the same sex

hormone chemical substance produced in the body that has specific regulatory effect on the activity of a certain organ

horticultural pertaining to the growing of plants

hospice long-term care facility providing care for the terminally ill

hydrate to supply water to in order to restore or maintain fluid balance

hydraulic operated or moved using liquid as the source of transmitting power

hydrocarbon organic compound made of hydrogen and carbon only

hydrotherapy application of water for therapeutic purposes

hygiene proper care of the mouth, teeth, and other parts of the body for maintenance of health and the prevention of disease

hyperactivity behavior characterized by constant overactivity

hyperglycemia abnormally high sugar content in the blood

hyperplasia tissue overgrowth

hypertrophy enlargement or overgrowth of an organ or part caused by an increase in its cells

hypochondria the belief in imaginary illness

hypoglycemia abnormally low sugar content in the blood

hypophysis pituitary gland

hypothermia an abnormal lowering of body temperature

I

imaging storing of an image or visual representation of someone or something

immerse to place or plunge something into a liquid

immunity high level of resistance to certain microorganisms or diseases; security against a particular disease

immunization process of becoming secure against a particular disease or pathogen

immunoassay quantitative determination of antigenic substance by examination of blood

immunohematology specialized branch of immunology that studies and identifies blood groups

immunology the study of how the blood cells prevent disease caused by microorganisms

immunosuppression prevention or diminution of immune response

impair damage

impulse sudden pushing force; activity along nerve fibers

inanimate pertaining to a nonliving article

incentive something that stimulates an action

incinerate act of burning, cremation

incision wound characterized by a cut made with a surgical instrument, knife, or glass

incubation period of time when an infection shows its effects

incus one of the three auditory bones of the inner ear; called the "anvil"

industry employment or business involving a skill

infarction an area of tissue death (necrosis) caused by loss of oxygen (ischemia) as a result of obstruction of circulation to the area

infection invasion and multiplication of microorganisms in the body tissues

inferior lower than another; bottom part

inflammation localized protective response to injury or destruction of tissue resulting in pain, heat, redness, swelling, and loss of function

ingest to take food or medicine into the body by mouth; eat or drink

inhale take into lungs by breathing

initiate cause something, especially an event or process, to begin

initiative enterprise; displaying energy or aptitude

inlay solid filling of gold or porcelain, used in dentistry to fill a defective area

innate (inborn) born with; not acquired; having from birth

inorganic having no organs; not derived from hydrocarbons

inscription the list of ingredients

insemination deposit of seminal fluid within the vagina or cervix

inspiration act of drawing air into the lung; inhalation

inspire to stimulate to action; motivate

insurance payment for health care expenses, which may or may not occur, in return for a specified payment in advance

integrative combining parts or objects that work together

intercourse sexual union

internship period of initial training under the supervision of a qualified practitioner

interpret to explain the meaning of

interstitial placed between, usually referring to between tissues

intervention any act performed to prevent harm or to improve the mental, emotional, or physical function of a patient

intracranial situated within the cranium

intraocular within the eye

intravenous within a vein or veins

intrinsic situated entirely within or pertaining exclusively to a part

inventory to make a list or catalog of contents

ischemia insufficient blood to a body part caused by functional constriction or actual obstruction of a blood vessel

isolation separation from others of someone with an infection to prevent the spread of microorganisms

J

Jacksonian seizure seizure that causes muscle movements on one side of the body

jaundice yellow appearance resulting from bile pigment stored in the skin and sclera of the eyes

jurisprudence science or philosophy of law

K

keloid sharply elevated, irregularly shaped scar that progressively enlarges

keratinize to make into insoluble protein that composes hair, nails, epidermis, and enamel of the teeth

ketones the presence of sugar and waste products of fat metabolism in urine; may indicate uncontrolled diabetes mellitus

kidneys urinary organs that form and eliminate urine

kinesthetic pertaining to muscular sense of balance or movement

L

labyrinth system of communicating canals in the inner ear

laceration type of wound characterized by irregularly shaped cut made with a sharp object

lactation production and secretion of milk by the mammary glands (breasts)

laminar air flow filtered air moving in parallel flow to prevent bacterial contamination and collection of harmful fumes

laparoscopy examination of the internal organs of the abdomen using a scope

laser device that converts electromagnetic radiation of highly amplified ultraviolet, visible, or infrared radiation frequencies

laxative agent that acts to promote evacuation of the bowel; cathartic

legal deriving authority from or founded on law

legume fruit or seed from a leguminous plant; e.g., beans or peas

lethargy condition of drowsiness or indifference

leukocyte white blood cell or corpuscle

liable legally responsible

license legal authority to perform a function, usually based on experience and education and an examination

ligament band of fibrous tissue that connects bones and supports joints

lingua the tongue

lipoprotein protein that contains lipids

lithotripsy crushing of a stone in, for example, the kidney, followed by washing out of fragments

litigation legal dispute; lawsuit

logical based on otherwise known statements, events, or conditions

lunula general term for a small crescent or moon-shaped area of fingernail

M

malignant tending to become progressively worse and result in death

malleus one of the three auditory bones of the ear that is like a hammer

malpractice failure of professional skill or learning that results in injury, loss, or damage

mammography radiological view of breasts

mandible bone of the lower jaw

manipulative characterized by controlling or handling

marine pertaining to the sea

marrow soft organic material filling the cavities of bones

mastication process of chewing food

maxilla irregularly shaped bone that forms the upper jaw

mediastinum mass of tissues and organs separating the two lungs

Medicare federal program that provides financial assistance to those 65 years of age and older and certain specified others as part of the benefits of the Social Security Act

medium substance that transmits impulses or that serves as growth location for microorganisms

megadose overdose; 10 times the recommended dose

melanin dark, shapeless pigment of the skin

melatonin hormone derived from serotonin and secreted by the pineal gland

meninges three membranes that surround and protect the brain and spinal cord

menopause time of life during which menstruation stops permanently

menses normal flow of blood and uterine lining that occurs in cycles in women

menstrual cycle the recurring cycle of change of the reproductive organs induced by hormones in women

menstruation cyclic, physiological discharge through the vagina of blood and mucosal tissues from the nonpregnant uterus

mental health a state of mind in which a person can cope with problems and maintain emotional balance and satisfaction in living

mental hygiene methods used to preserve and promote mental health

metabolism sum of all the physical and chemical processes by which living organized substance is produced and maintained (anabolism) and the transformation by which energy is made available for the uses of the organism (catabolism)

metastasis transfer of disease from one organ or part to another not directly connected with it

metazoan multicellular worm that causes disease

microbes microorganisms

microorganism microscopic living organism; microbe

micturition passage of urine; urination

milestone a significant point in development

mineral nonorganic solid substance

mobility the ability to move

morals standards based on the experience, religion, and philosophy of the individual and the society

morbidity the rate of a sickness in relation to the rest of the population

mortality number of deaths in a given time or place

mortuary funeral home, place where bodies are stored until burial

mottling spotting, with patches of color

muscle cramping pain and inability to use the muscle when loss of salt from sweating causes an electrolyte imbalance

mutagen physical or chemical agent that induces genetic mutation or change

mutation permanent change in a gene or chromosome

myalgia muscle pain

mycostatic agent that inhibits the growth of fungus

myelography x-rays of the spinal cord after injection of a contrast medium

myoelectronics electromechanical prostheses

N

nebulizer device used to deliver a spray or mist of medication into the lungs

necrosis area of tissue death

negligence failure to execute the care that a reasonable (prudent) person exercises

neonate newborn; neonatal period is the first 28 days after birth

neurobiology the study of the brain's relationship to psychosocial behavior

neurohormone hormone that stimulates a neural reaction or mechanism

neurohypophysis the posterior pituitary

neurotransmitter chemical messages, released from the axon of one neuron, that travel to another nearby neuron

neutering surgical sterilization of male animals to prevent unwanted births

nonpathogen microorganism that does not produce disease

nonverbal not involving language to communicate

nucleic acid group of complex compounds found in all living cells and viruses, composed of purines, pyrimidines, carbohydrates, and phosphoric acid

nutrients proteins, carbohydrates, fats, vitamins, and minerals necessary for growth, normal functioning, and maintaining life

nutrition process of taking in nutrients and using them for body function

O

oath solemn pledge

obstetrician medical doctor specializing in delivery of babies

occupation vocation; activity in which one participates

ocular referring to the eyes

olfactory pertaining to the sense of smell

oliguria excretion of diminished amount of urine in relation to fluid intake

opaque substance that cannot be penetrated by visible light

optimal best possible

oral pertaining to the mouth

orchiectomy the removal of the testes

organic pertaining to an organ; having organized structure; chemical substances containing carbon

organism an individual living thing, plant, or animal

oropharynx section of the pharynx that contains the palatine tonsils and the lingual tonsils

orthopedic pertaining to the correction or prevention of deformities

orthosis device designed for straightening a distorted part

orthotics art or science of custom designing, fabrication, and fitting of braces

ossicle auditory bone of the ear

ova eggs

oviducts the fallopian tubes

ovulation release of the egg (ovum) from the ovary

oxidase enzyme that acts as a catalyst

oxygenate to add oxygen to

P

pallor lack of color; paleness

palpation act of feeling with the hand

panic disorder a condition of feeling an unreasonable fear with no known cause

papilla small, nipple-shaped projection or elevation

paralysis loss or impairment of motor function

paranoia the feeling of being persecuted or plotted against by others

paraprofessional worker who assists a professional in the performance of duties

parasite plant or animal that lives on or within another living organism at the expense of the host organism

particulate composed of separate particles or pieces

pasteurized process of heating milk or other liquids to a moderate temperature for a definite time to kill pathogenic bacteria

patent unobstructed opening such as a patent ductus arteriosus in the heart

pathogen microorganism that produces disease

patient person under medical care and treatment

pegboard paper forms, backed with carbon, that are aligned on a set of pegs to allow written information to appear on all sheets

perception process of using the senses to acquire information about the environment

percussion tapping or striking a body part to learn the condition of inner parts by analyzing the sound or to loosen secretions

perfusion the flow of blood through a specific area of the body

perinatal pertaining to the period shortly before and after birth

periodic occurring at regular intervals

periodontal situated or occurring around a tooth

periosteum specialized connective tissue covering all the bones of the body

peripheral pertaining to the extremities or edges; away from the center

peristalsis wave of contraction or wormlike movement of digestive system that propels the contents

peritoneal pertaining to the layer of membrane lining the abdominopelvic walls

peritoneum a flat serous membrane that surrounds the abdominal cavity

permanent dentition the teeth that erupt and take the place of primary dentition; secondary teeth

perseverance steady persistence in adhering to a course of action, a belief, or a purpose; steadfastness

personality set of traits, characteristics, and behaviors that make one person an individual

personnel people working in a unit or in a facility

pesticide poison used to destroy pests of any kind

petit mal seizure seizure that results in the momentary loss of consciousness marked by staring with rapid blinking

petroleum oily liquid similar to gasoline

pH symbol relating to the concentration of hydrogen ions or acidity of a solution

phagocyte cell that surrounds and destroys microorganisms and foreign particles

pharmacology the study of the actions and uses of drugs

phenotype an individual's physical, biochemical, and physiological configuration; determined by genes

phlebotomy incision into a vein to withdraw blood

phlegm thick mucus secreted by the tissues in the respiratory passages and usually discharged through the mouth

phobia persistent, abnormal dread or fear

photosynthesis process by which plants turn energy from the sun and elements from the soil into food

pigment organic material that gives color in the body

pilus hair

pipette narrow, usually calibrated glass tube into which small amounts of liquid are suctioned for transfer or measurement

placenta an organ, characteristic of mammals during pregnancy, joining mother and offspring

plague disease causing a high rate of death, or mortality

plaque mass adhering to surface of tooth, composed of bacteria, saliva, and organic waste

plasma fluid portion of blood

pneumatic operated or moved using air as the source of transmitting power

podiatry branch of medicine concerned with care and treatment of the feet

poison substance that impairs health or destroys life when ingested

polarity specialization of a nerve cell determining the flow of impulses; having opposite effects at two ends such as a magnet

pollution condition of being defiled or impure

polydipsia excessive thirst persisting for long periods of time

polyneuritis inflammation of many nerves at once

polyphagia excessive eating

polyuria passage of large amount of urine in a given time

population all the inhabitants of a certain region or country

porcine pertaining to pigs, swine

postmortem after death

post-secondary pertaining to after high school; college or vocational training

posture position or arrangement of the body parts

poultry domesticated birds kept for eggs or meat sources

practitioner one who has met educational and training requirements to practice health care

precursor one that comes before; substance used to make another structure

prejudice preconceived judgment or opinion

prepuce foreskin that forms a retractable casing

prerequisite something that must be accomplished before attempting another task or course of study

prescription written order for dispensing drugs

primary dentition the teeth that erupt first and are replaced by permanent dentition; deciduous teeth

prime mover muscle that acts directly to bring about a desired movement

profession occupation that requires specialized knowledge and often long and intensive academic training

projectile an item that is hurled or impelled forward

prolactin latogenic hormone; produced and secreted by the anterior pituitary

prominence protrusion, bump

proprioceptor receptor that responds to stimulus originating in the body itself, especially to pressure, position, and stretching

prospective expected in the future

prosthesis an artificial device applied to replace a partially or totally missing body part for functional or cosmetic purposes

prosthetics art or science of custom design, fabrication, and fitting of artificial limbs

protein group of complex organic compounds that are the main part of cell protoplasm

protoplasm cytoplasm; protein and other materials contained in cells

protozoan animallike, unicellular organism

protrusion something that sticks out from its surroundings

prudent reasonable; wise

psyche the mind

psychic pertaining to the mind; mental

psychology the study of human and animal behavior, both normal and abnormal

psychoneurosis functional disturbance of the mind in which the individual is aware that reactions are not normal

psychosis major mental disorder in which the individual loses contact with reality

psychosocial related to factors of both psychological and social nature

psychosomatic physical symptoms caused by the mind

psychotherapy treatment of discomfort, dysfunction, or diseases by methods designed to understand and cope with problems

puberty the period during which the secondary sexual characteristics begin to develop and the capacity of sexual reproduction is attained

pulmonary pertaining to the lungs

pulmonary circulation carrying venous blood from the right ventricle to the lungs and returning oxygenated blood to the left atrium of the heart

pulse heartbeat that can be felt, or palpated, on surface arteries as the artery walls expand with blood

puncture wound made when an object pierces the skin

purine colorless crystalline solid made from uric acid

putrid foul, unpleasant

pyloric pertaining to the distal opening of the stomach through which stomach contents are emptied into the intestine

pyramid a structure built on a broad supporting base and narrowing gradually to a point

pyuria pus in the urine

Q

quackery treatment that pretends to cure disease

quadrant one of four regions used to describe location in the abdomen

quantitative expressible by a measurement

quarantine period of detention or isolation as a result of disease suspected to be communicable

R

radiation emission of energy, rays, or waves

radiography making film records of internal structures by passing x-rays or gamma rays through the body to make images on specially sensitized film; roentgenography

radioisotope a type of chemical element that is radioactive

radiopharmaceutical chemical agent used for treatment or diagnosis

range of motion active or passive movement of muscle groups to full extent possible; used to prevent contracture

rate expression of speed or frequency of an event in relation to a specified amount of time

reagent substance used in a chemical reaction to detect, measure, examine, or produce other substances

reality orientation awareness of position in relation to time, space, and person

reasonable fee fee that considers both the usual fee charged by a practitioner for a particular service and the fee charged by other practitioners for the same service

receptacle container for disposal of used materials

receptor specific type of cell that responds to a specific stimulus

recessive gene trait that does not appear unless carried by both members of a pair of chromosomes

recipient one who receives from another, such as in a blood transfusion

recombinant genetically engineered DNA prepared by transplanting or splicing genes from one species into the cells of a host organism of a different species, becoming part of the host organism

reflex an involuntary action in response to a stimulus

refraction deviation of light when passing through a medium to another medium of a different density

regeneration natural renewal of a structure, as of lost tissue or part

registration official record of individuals qualified to perform certain services

rehabilitation restoration of normal form and function after injury or illness

remedy medication or treatment that cures disease or relieves pain

remission decrease in symptoms of a disease

renal pertaining to the kidney

repetitive involving things that are done over and over again

reservoir place or cavity for storage; alternative host or passive carrier of pathogenic organism

residency period of training in a specific area under the supervision of a qualified health care practitioner

resident microorganism that is always present

resonance an echo or other sound produced by percussion of an organ or cavity of the body; process of energy absorption by an object

resorption loss of bone tissue caused by the action of specialized cells

respiration exchange of oxygen and carbon dioxide between the atmosphere and the cells of the body; ventilation

restoration replacement of part of a tooth, usually with silver alloy, gold, or esthetic composite material

restrain to limit, restrict, or keep under control

resuscitation restoration to life or consciousness of one apparently dead by using artificial respiration and cardiac massage

retardation intellectual slowing

retrieve to bring back or recover

retrovirus large group of viruses containing RNA

rhythm measured movement; recurrence of an action or function at regular intervals

rickettsiae very small, bacterialike organisms that cannot live outside living tissue

rigor mortis temporary stiffness or rigidity of skeletal muscles occurring after death

ritual established ceremony

roughage indigestible material such as fiber in diet

rural relating to the country life or agriculture

S

salinity relative content of salt

sanitation promotion of hygiene and maintaining cleanliness

sarcoma cancer arising from connective tissues such as bone and muscle

sarcomere repeating units of muscle fibers with the ability to contract

schizophrenia psychotic disorder characterized by withdrawal from reality

sclerosis the hardening of tissue

sebaceous pertaining to sebum or a greasy lubricating substance

sebum oil secreted by the sebaceous glands

second-degree burn burn that breaks the surface of the skin and injures the underlying tissue

secretion process by which glands produce and add chemical substances into the blood

sedentary sitting habitually; inactive habits

sediment substance that settles at the bottom of a fluid

seizure sudden attack of a disease; uncontrolled muscle movements of epilepsy

self-actualization becoming the best possible person

semipermeable permitting the passage of certain molecules and not others

senile pertaining to or characteristic of old age; especially referring to memory loss or mental impairment

sensation the ability to feel

sensitize to make film react to light by coating it with an emulsion

septal pertaining to a wall separating two cavities such as in the nose or in the heart

sequence order of succession or arrangement

serology the study of antibody reactions in serum, whole blood, or urine

serum fluid portion of blood with clotting proteins removed

shock condition of acute failure of the peripheral circulation

shroud burial garment or dress

simple (closed) fracture fracture that does not penetrate the skin

simultaneous occurring at the same time

sitz bath apparatus to bathe the perineal area with continuous flow of fluid

skeletal pertaining to the framework of the body

sociobiology the study of the relationship of genes to psychosocial behavior

socioeconomic pertaining to the society and the effects on it of production, distribution, consumption of goods, and services

somatic voluntary; pertaining to the body

spasm sudden involuntary contraction of a muscle or group of muscles

spaying the process of surgical sterilization in females to prevent unwanted births

specific gravity weight of a substance compared to an equal volume of another substance (usually water) used as a standard

spectrophotometry measurement of quantity of matter in solution by passing light through spectrum

sperm the male gamete produced by the testes

sphincter ringlike band of muscle that closes a passage or opening

spinal pertaining to the spine

spirochete spiral bacterium; microorganism

sprain injury to the ligaments, or the attachments between the muscle and bones

sputum matter ejected from the respiratory tract through the mouth

stapes one of the three auditory bones in the inner ear; called the "stirrup"

statistics numerical data

stenosis narrowing or stricture of a duct or canal

sterile unable to produce offspring; free from living microorganisms

steroid group name for lipids that contain a specific compound

stethoscope an instrument of various forms and materials used to listen to body sounds (auscultation)

stillborn born dead

stimulus any agent, act, or influence that produces a change in the development or function of tissues

strain injury to the muscle tissue usually resulting from overuse

strenuous energetic, very active

subcutaneous beneath the skin

subluxations incomplete or partial dislocations of the spine

subordinate of a lower rank, under the authority of another

subscription directions for preparation

sudoriferous conveying sweat

superior higher than another; above

susceptible likely to be affected with; especially sensitive

swine hogs

synchronous occurring at the same time

syndrome group of signs and symptoms that characterize a condition or disease

synovial pertaining to transparent alkaline fluid contained in joints

systemic pertaining to a group of interdependent parts or organs

systemic circulation general circulation, carrying oxygenated blood from the left ventricle to tissues of the body and returning the venous blood to the right atrium of the heart

systole period of contraction of the ventricles of the heart; alternates with diastole

T

tachypnea excessively fast respiration

tactile pertaining to the touch

technological resulting from improvements in productivity of machines

temperature measurement of the heat production and loss in the body

tendon fibrous cord by which a muscle is attached to a bone

terminal illness or injury for which there is no reasonable expectation of recovery

testosterone an androgenic hormone that causes the appearance of secondary sexual characteristics

tetany prolonged muscle spasm or contraction

thanatology the study of death

therapeutic relating to treatment of disease or disorder by remedial methods

therapy treatment of disease; science and art of healing

theriogenology branch of veterinarian medicine dealing with reproduction

thermal pertaining to or characterized by heat

third-degree burn burn that is deep enough to damage the nerves and bones

thoracic pertaining to the chest

thrill a vibration caused by an abnormal flow of blood; felt over an artery

thrombocyte blood platelet

tolerance the decreasing effect of a drug due to constant use

tomography specialized use of x-rays to show structures in one plane of the body by blurring the image of other planes

tonic having muscle tone

tonometer instrument that measures tension or pressure

tonus slight, continuous contraction of muscle

tourniquet instrument used to compress a blood vessel by application around an extremity

toxicology study of poisons

toxin poison produced by animals, plants, or bacteria

tracheotomy an alternative opening made into the trachea for the exchange of gases

transaction business deal; communication or activity between two or more people

transcribe to make a written copy of dictated or recorded matter

transfusion introduction of whole blood or blood component into bloodstream

transgenic animal or plant that contains genes from different species

transient a microorganism that is found temporarily

translucent permitting passage of light but not transparent

transsexual person who changed their biologic sex

transverse situated at right angles, placed crosswise

trauma wound or injury, physical or psychic

triage the term used for setting priorities for care of the victim or victims

U

ulcer open sore or lesion

ultrasonography visualization of deep structures of the body by recording reflections of sound waves directed into the tissues

ultrasound mechanical radiant energy, sound waves beyond the range of the human ear

ultraviolet wavelengths from 5 to about 400 nanometers of the visible light spectrum

unit part of a facility, including equipment and supplies, organized to provide specific care

universal occurring everywhere and in all things

universe all matter and energy that exists in the vastness of space

urea white substance found in urine, blood, and lymph; end product of protein digestion

urinal container into which a person may urinate or void urine

urinalysis physical, chemical, or microscopic examination of urine

urination discharge or passage of urine

urologist a physician that specializes in urinary conditions

urticaria vascular reaction of the skin marked by smooth elevated patches which are redder or paler than surrounding skin and itching

utility usefulness, effectiveness; a service provided by a public company, such as supplying gas, electricity, or water

V

vaccination introduction of a microorganism that has been made harmless in order to cause immunity to develop

value rate of usefulness, importance, or general worth

vapor solid or liquid in gaseous state such as steam

vascularity containing blood vessels or indicative of a large blood supply

vector carrier that transfers an infective agent from one host to another

veins blood vessels that carry blood back to the heart

venereal pertaining to or resulting from sexual intercourse

venomous toxic fluid secreted by animal life

ventilator machine that produces or assists with breathing

ventral front side, anterior

ventricle small cavity of the brain, lower chamber of the heart

verbal relating to or consisting of words or sounds

vesicle small bladderlike cell or cavity

veterinary pertaining to animals and their diseases

vicious mean or uncontrolled

villus one of many tiny vascular projections on the surface of small intestine

virus microorganism that isn't really a cell, but contains genetic information that can reproduce and cause illness inside a cell of the body

visceral pertaining to any large interior organ in any one of the cavities of the body

viscosity property of a fluid showing density or thickness

vision act or faculty of seeing, sight

vital necessary to life

vitamins organic compounds needed by the body for metabolism, growth, and development

vocational education designed to provide the skills for a particular job or career

void to empty, urinate, or defecate

volume the amplitude of sound waves

voluntary under control of the conscious will

W

wheeze whistling sound made during respiration

whelping delivery of puppies by female dog

withdrawal extreme nervousness, uncontrollable trembling, excessive sweating, and painful cramps that result when a drug (substance) is not taken anymore

X

xiphoid bone at the end of the sternum; shaped like a sword

Z

zoology study of animal life

zoonosis disease carried by animals to humans